Peroxisome Proliferator-Activated Receptors: Recent Advances

Editor: Olivia Pitts

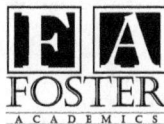

FA FOSTER ACADEMICS

www.fosteracademics.com

www.fosteracademics.com

FA
FOSTER
ACADEMICS

Cataloging-in-Publication Data

Peroxisome proliferator-activated receptors : recent advances / edited by Olivia Pitts.
  p. cm.
Includes bibliographical references and index.
ISBN 978-1-63242-910-0
1. Peroxisomes--Receptors. 2. Peroxisomes. 3. Hormone receptors. 4. Microbodies. I. Pitts, Olivia.
QH603.P47 P47 2020
571.655--dc23

Foster Academics,
118-35 Queens Blvd., Suite 400,
Forest Hills, NY 11375, USA

ISBN 978-1-63242-910-0 (Hardback)

Contents

Preface

The world is advancing at a fast pace like never before. Therefore, the need is to keep up with the latest developments. This book was an idea that came to fruition when the specialists in the area realized the need to coordinate together and document essential themes in the subject. That's when I was requested to be the editor. Editing this book has been an honour as it brings together diverse authors researching on different streams of the field. The book collates essential materials contributed by veterans in the area which can be utilized by students and researchers alike.

Gene expression can be regulated by the action of nuclear receptor proteins called peroxisome proliferator-activated receptors (PPARs). These function as transcription factors. They regulate cellular differentiation, nutrient metabolism and tumorigenesis. Three kinds of PPARs have been identified- PPARα, PPARβ/δ and PPARγ. PPARα is a nuclear receptor protein, which is important for the regulation of lipid metabolism in the liver. It is necessary for ketogenesis and is activated during a state of energy deprivation. By altering gene expression of a large number of target genes it influences biological processes. PPARδ is a nuclear hormone receptor, which may be involved in the pathogenesis of several chronic disease conditions, such as obesity, diabetes, atherosclerosis and cancer. PPARγ may be expressed in three distinct forms- PPARγ1, PPARγ2 and PPARγ3. It is responsible for the storage of fatty acid and glucose metabolism. This book is a valuable compilation of topics, ranging from the basic to the most complex advancements in the understanding of peroxisome proliferator-activated receptors. It presents this complex subject in the most comprehensible and easy to understand language. Coherent flow of topics, student-friendly language and extensive use of examples make this book an invaluable source of knowledge.

Each chapter is a sole-standing publication that reflects each author's interpretation. Thus, the book displays a multi-facetted picture of our current understanding of application, resources and aspects of the field. I would like to thank the contributors of this book and my family for their endless support.

Editor

Expression of GPR43 in Brown Adipogenesis is Enhanced by Rosiglitazone and Controlled by PPARγ/RXR Heterodimerization

Jiamiao Hu,[1,2] Arong Zhou,[1] Peter C. K. Cheung,[3] Baodong Zheng(iD),[1] Shaoxiao Zeng,[1] and Shaoling Lin(iD)[1]

[1]College of Food Science, Fujian Agriculture and Forestry University, Fuzhou, Fujian 350002, China
[2]Warwick Medical School, University of Warwick, Coventry, West Midlands, UK
[3]School of Life Sciences, The Chinese University of Hong Kong, Shatin, New Territories, Hong Kong

Correspondence should be addressed to Shaoling Lin; shaoling.lin@fafu.edu.cn

Academic Editor: Pascal Froment

GPR43, a G-protein coupled receptor recognizing short-chain fatty acids, has been reported to participate in many biological functions of white adipocytes, such as adipogenesis and lipolysis. However, the functional role of GPR43 in brown adipocytes is still not clear. In this study, we investigated the effects of the PPARγ agonist rosiglitazone on GPR43 expression in brown adipogenesis. The results demonstrated that GPR43 was expressed during the late phase of brown adipocyte differentiation, which could be further augmented by adipogenic agent rosiglitazone treatment. The PPARγ/RXR heterodimerization was found to be the key transcription factor for this enhancing effect of rosiglitazone on GPR43 expression. Taken together, these results suggested GPR43 levels might be regulated by PPARγ-activated events during brown adipocytes differentiation and reflect the adipogenesis status of brown adipocytes.

1. Introduction

In the last decades, several G-protein coupled receptors (GPCRs), i.e., GPR40, GPR41, GPR43, GPR84, and GPR120, were deorphaned as free fatty acids (FFAs) receptors [1–5]. Of these receptors, GPR43 is activated by short-chain fatty acids such as acetate, propionate, and butyrate [2–4]. RT-PCR analyses have demonstrated that GPR43 is expressed abundantly in spleen, bone marrow, liver, intestine, and adipose tissue [4, 6, 7].

So far, several independent studies have indicated a potential link between GPR43 expression and white adipogenesis. For example, GPR43 levels were significantly increased during the differentiation of 3T3-L1 adipocytes, which can be further upregulated by treatment with adipogenic agent such as troglitazone [8]. In mice fed with a high-fat diet (HFD), the augmented adiposity and adipocyte enlargement were observed with an overexpression of GPR43 in the subcutaneous white adipose tissue [6, 9]. In contrast, administration of inulin-type fructans could counteract this HFD-induced GPR43 overexpression and peroxisome proliferator activated receptor γ- (PPARγ-) related adipogenesis in the white adipose tissue of mice [9], suggesting GPR43 expression levels in white adipose tissue might reflect the obesity status in the animal's body. Furthermore, functional analyses have also suggested the promotive effects of short-chain fatty acids on adipogenesis via GPR43 in white adipocytes [8, 10]. However, up to date, most studies mainly focus on the potential functions of GPR43 in white adipocytes and the importance of GPR43 expression in brown adipocytes has not yet been thoroughly studied.

Recently, the promoter regions of GPR43 were determined in human monocytes, showing transcription factors including XBP1 were key transcription factors for the regulation of GPR43 expression [11]. Notably, transcription factor XBP1 was also found to play crucial roles in the adipogenesis [12–15]. In addition, the proadipogenic effects of short-chain fatty acids in brown adipogenesis were also reported by independent studies both *in vitro* and *in vivo* [16, 17]. These evidences together suggest the possible link between GPR43 expression with brown adipogenesis and its expression levels might also reflect the status of adipogenesis.

To test this hypothesis, in the present study we investigated the expression pattern of GPR43 during the differentiation of brown adipocyte precursor cells. We also examined the effect of adipogenic agent rosiglitazone on the regulation of GPR43 transcription in brown adipocytes to understand more about the possible underlying mechanism.

2. Methods and Materials

2.1. Materials. Rosiglitazone was purchased from Sigma-Aldrich; PPARγ antagonist GW9662 and RXR antagonist HX531 were purchased from Tocris Bioscience.

2.2. Cell Culture. The immortalized brown adipocyte cell line (IM-BAT) was constructed and a gift by Dr. Mark Christian (University of Warwick). Briefly, the primary brown preadipocytes were isolated from mice interscapular brown adipose tissue and cultured in DMEM/F12 medium containing 10% fetal bovine serum (FBS) and 1% antibiotic-antimycotic for 2 days before being immortalized by retroviral-mediated expression of temperature-sensitive SV40 large T antigen H-2kb-tsA58. Cells were continually cultured at 33°C and selected with G418 (100 mg/ml) for 2 weeks and maintained in 50 μg/ml of G418. IM-BAT cells were differentiated according to previous report [16] by treating with 500 μM 3-isobutyl-1-methylxanthine (IBMX), 250 nM dexamethasone, 170 nM insulin, and 1 nM 3,3′,5-triiodo-l-thyronine (T3) in DMEM/F12 medium containing 10% FBS for 2 days, followed by incubation with DMEM/F12 medium containing 170 nM insulin, 1 nM T3, and 10% FBS till clear lipid droplets could be seen under microscopy. Rosiglitazone, GW9662, or HX531 was dissolved in DMSO and then directly diluted in DMEM/F12 and treated during the course of differentiation. The final concentration of the DMSO did not exceed 0.1% for either the control or the treated cells for all experiments. All experiments were performed below passages 22.

The white adipocytes 3T3-L1 cells were purchased from ATCC and cultured in DMEM medium containing 10% newborn calf serum (NBCS). Cells were differentiated by treating with DMEM medium containing 500 μM IBMX, 1 μM dexamethasone, 1 μg/ml insulin, and 10% FBS for 2 days, followed by incubation with DMEM medium containing 1 μg/ml insulin and 10% FBS till lipid droplets were formed.

2.3. siRNA Transfection. To introduce siRNA into undifferentiated IM-BAT cells, siRNA was transfected with lipofectamine RNAiMAX according to manufacturer's manual. Briefly, IM-BAT cells were seeded to be 60–80% confluent at the time of transfection in DMEM:F12 medium containing 10% FBS without antibiotics. siRNA-lipid complexes were prepared and incubated at room temperature for 10 min before being added to cells. The cell culture medium was changed back into DMEM:F12 containing 10% FBS and 1%

penicillin/streptomycin after 6 h. 24 h after transfection, the cells were differentiated as described above. The efficiency of gene knockdown was measured by quantitative real-time PCR.

2.4. Oil Red O Staining. Lipid accumulation of differentiated adipocytes was visualized and determined by Oil Red O staining kit (ECM950, Millipore). Briefly, differentiated adipocytes were washed with PBS and fixed in 3.7% formaldehyde for 15 minutes, followed by staining with Oil Red O solution (3 g/L) for 15 minutes. After staining, cells were washed twice with water and photographed using a microscope (Axiovert 40CFL, Olympus).

2.5. Quantitative Real-Time PCR. Total RNA was extracted by using GenElute Mammalian Total RNA Miniprep Kit (Sigma). Complementary DNAs were synthesized by reverse transcription of 1 μg total RNA as templates using nanoScript 2 Reverse Transcription kits (Primerdesign). qRT-PCR was performed with Abi 7500 Fast Real-Time PCR System using SensiFAST SYBR (BIOLINE). Specific primers were designed in an intron-spanning manner for all possible cases. To avoid gDNA contamination during RNA extraction process, all RNA samples were treated with Precision DNase kits (Primerdesign). All primer pairs were confirmed not to self-dimerize by qRT-PCR using a nontemplate control. Expression levels were calculated according to the $2^{-\Delta\Delta Ct}$ method. The identity and purity of the amplified product were checked by analysing the melting curves carried out at the end of amplification.

2.6. Statistical Analysis. Results are presented as the mean ± SEM of at least triplicate samples in each experimental group; experiments were replicated to ensure consistency. Statistical significance of difference was determined using Student's t-test when comparing 2 groups or one-way ANOVA followed by post hoc Tukey's multiple comparison test when comparing more than 3 groups. Values were considered to be statistically significant if their P value was less than 0.05. All statistical calculations were analysed in GraphPad Prism 5.

3. Results

3.1. Rosiglitazone Treatment Significantly Increases GPR43 Expression in Brown Adipogenesis. We first measured the expression of GPR43 during the course of brown adipocytes differentiation by quantitative real-time PCR. Consistent with previous reports [16, 18], GPR43 mRNA expression was scarcely detected in the undifferentiated cells at day 0 but increased continuously throughout the differentiation period and was maintained at a high level after day 5 after differentiation (Figure 1(a)). Besides, our results also indicated that GPR43 expression in the differentiated brown adipocytes was much less (around 10-fold lower) than that in mature 3T3-L1 cells (white adipocytes cell line) while the levels of UCP1 were significantly higher in immortalized brown adipocytes (Figures 1(b) and 1(c)), showing that the brown adipocyte precursor cells are successfully differentiated.

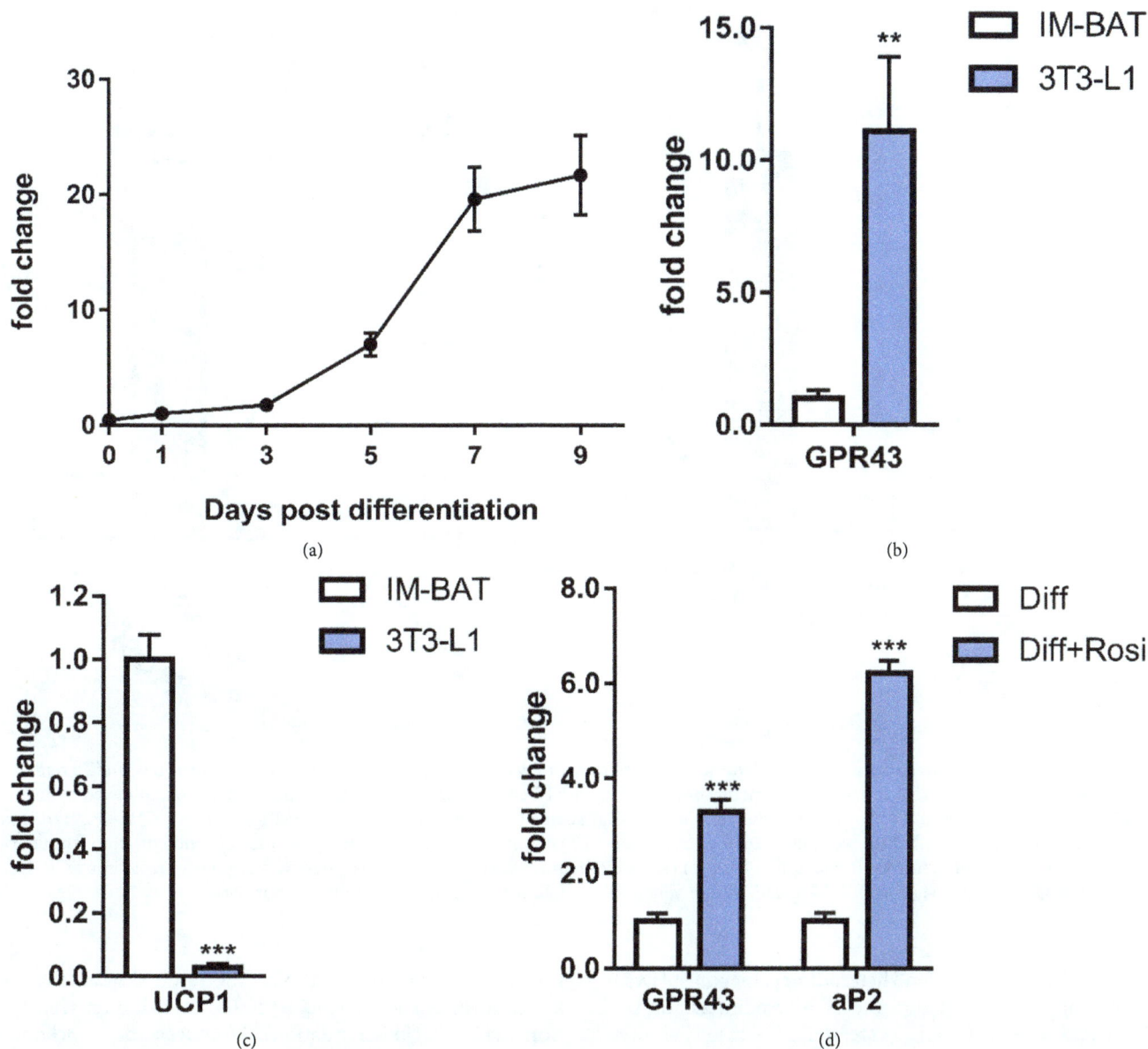

FIGURE 1: *Rosiglitazone treatment induces the increase of GPR43 transcription during the adipogenesis of brown adipocytes.* (a) mRNA transcription levels of GPR43 during the differentiation of IM-BAT adipocytes measured by quantitative real-time PCR. (b and c) Comparison of GPR43 (b) and UCP-1 (c) mRNA levels in mature IM-BAT adipocytes and 3T3-L1 adipocytes after 7 days of differentiation. (d) IM-BAT cells were differentiated with or without rosiglitazone (1 μM) from day 3 to day 7 before GPR43 and aP2 mRNA levels were measured on day 7 after differentiation. Data are expressed as mean ± SEM (n = 3). $^{**}P < 0.01$ and $^{***}P < 0.001$ by Student's t-test.

To further investigate the relationship between brown adipogenesis and GPR43 expression, the effects of the adipogenic agent rosiglitazone on GPR43 expression in brown adipocytes were evaluated. The results demonstrated that rosiglitazone treatment during differentiation induced a significant increase (~3.3-fold) in GPR43 expression compared to the normal differentiation condition in mature brown adipocyte (Figure 1(d)). Adipocyte Protein 2 (aP2), a PPARγ target gene known as a marker of adipocyte differentiation, also had ~6.2-fold increase in mature brown adipocytes treated with rosiglitazone, confirming the expected strong PPARγ activation induced by rosiglitazone (Figure 1(d)).

3.2. Rosiglitazone Upregulating GPR43 Expression Requires PPARγ and RXR Dimerization.

Studies have identified that the effects of rosiglitazone in adipocytes could be divided into PPARγ-dependent and PPARγ-independent ones. To elucidate the involvement of PPARγ in rosiglitazone-induced increase in GPR43 expression, PPARγ selective antagonist GW9662 was cotreated with rosiglitazone during the differentiation of brown adipocytes. The results indicated significant upregulation of GPR43 expression was only observed in cells treated with rosiglitazone but not in cells cotreated with GW9662, suggesting the upregulated GPR43 expression by rosiglitazone is PPARγ dependent (Figure 2(a)).

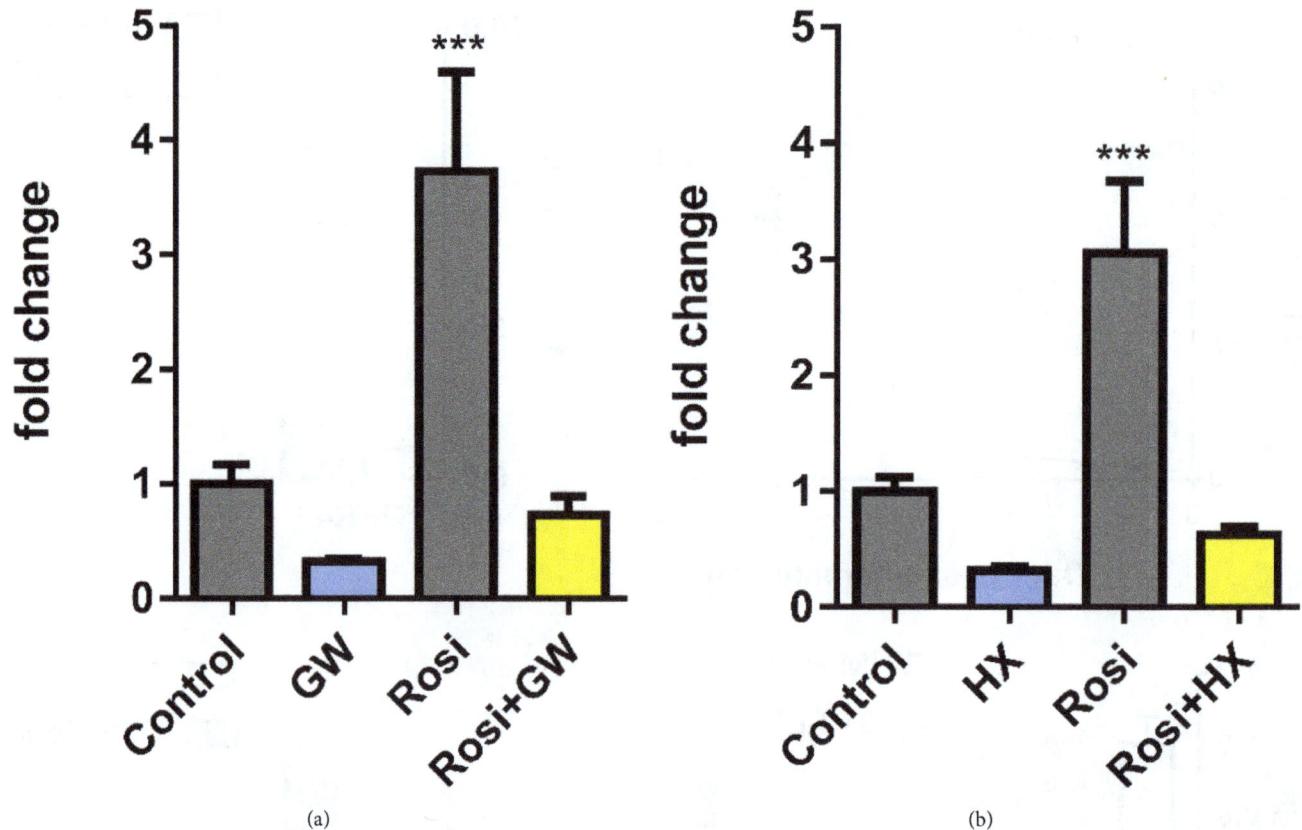

(a)

(b)

FIGURE 2: *Rosiglitazone-induced increase of GPR43 transcription requires dimerization of PPAR and RXR in brown adipocytes.* Undifferentiated IM-BAT cells were differentiated in IBMX, dexamethasone, insulin, and T3 containing DMEM:F12 medium for 2 days, followed by insulin and T3 containing medium in the absence or in the presence of rosiglitazone (1 μM) as indicated. The PPARγ antagonist GW9662 (1 μM) (a) or RXR antagonist HX531 (1 μM) (b) were also added to insulin and T3 containing medium during the course of differentiation from day 3 to day 7 after differentiation. mRNA transcription levels of GPR43 in mature adipocytes were measured by quantitative real-time PCR. Data are expressed as mean ± SEM ($n = 3$). $^{***}P < 0.01$ by one-way ANOVA followed by Tukey's multiple comparison.

Similarly, RXR homo- and heterodimer antagonist HX531 was also applied to test the role of heterodimerization of PPARγ and RXR in GPR43 expression. The results showed that cotreatment of HX531 with rosiglitazone also effectively inhibited rosiglitazone-induced GPR43 expression in brown adipocytes (Figure 2(b)). These evidences together suggested that the increase of GPR43 expression induced by rosiglitazone may require the formation of heterodimerization between PPARγ and RXR.

3.3. Rosiglitazone Overcomes the Effects of XBP1 Knockdown on GPR43 mRNA Expression in Brown Adipocyte. XBP1 has been recently identified as the key transcription factor for the expression of GPR43 in human monocytes [11]. Therefore, we next identified the role of XBP1 in rosiglitazone-induced increase of GPR43 expression in brown adipocytes. We firstly knocked down the expression of XBP1 in brown preadipocytes and then differentiated the knocked-down cells with or without rosiglitazone till day 5 as described above. To make sure of the duration of silencing after siRNA transfection, the expression of XBP1 was checked from day 1 to day 5 after differentiation. The XBP1 mRNA transcription levels were checked by real-time PCR and compared to cells

transfected with control siRNA. The result showed that the knockdown efficiency reached >60% at 48 h after transfection (24 h after differentiation). Moreover, the knockdown efficiency kept at >70% until day 5 after differentiation (Supplementary Figure 1), indicating the XBP1 gene silencing effect can last through the differentiation process of IM-BAT cells.

In accordance with previous findings, knockdown of XBP1 (Figure 3(b)) significantly impairs the differentiation of preadipocytes as demonstrated by oil accumulation (Figure 3(a)) as well as adipocyte differentiation marker aP2 transcription (Figure 3(d)). Accordingly, the expression level of GPR43 also significantly decreased in XBP1-knockdown cells (Figure 3(c)). Interestingly, in brown adipocytes transfected siRNA targeting XBP1, the rosiglitazone still led to a significant increase in GPR43 expression, indicating rosiglitazone can overcome the effects of the loss of XBP1 on GPR43 transcription (Figure 3(c)). Besides, we also tested the effect of rosiglitazone treatment on XBP1 splicing. The results also showed that there was no obvious XBP1 mRNA splicing detected (Figure 3(e)), suggesting rosiglitazone treatment has little effects on XBP1 activation. Taken together, these results suggest that rosiglitazone-induced GPR43 expression in

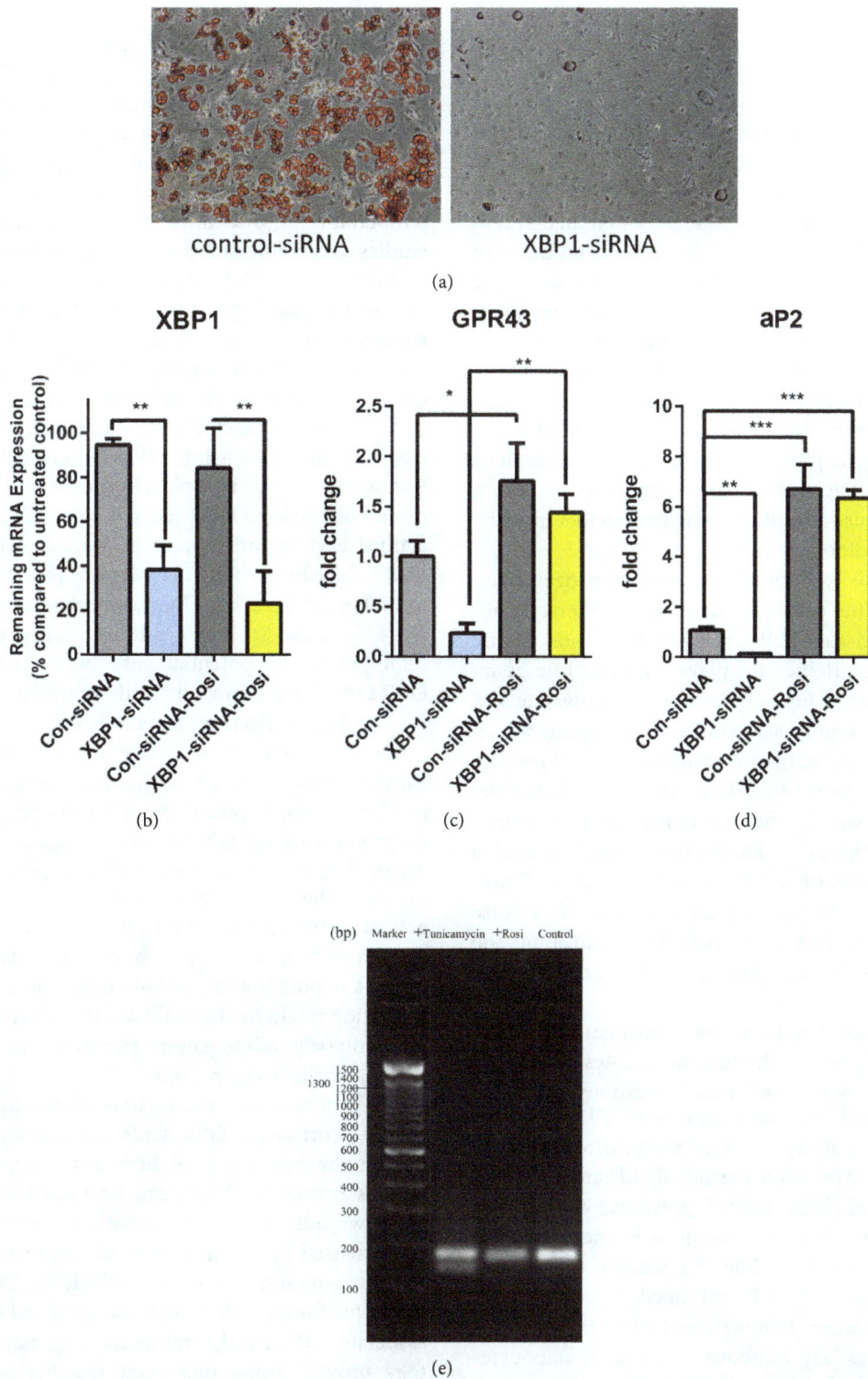

FIGURE 3: *Rosiglitazone-mediated increase of GPR43 transcription in adipocytes is XBP1 independent.* (a–d) IM-BAT adipocytes transfected with control siRNA or XBP1 siRNA were differentiated in the absence or in the presence of rosiglitazone (1 μM) during differentiation from day 3 to day 5 after differentiation. Accumulated lipids in the siRNA transfected IM-BAT adipocytes were measured by Oil Red O staining (a), while mRNA levels of XBP1 (b), GPR43 (c), and aP2 (d) in the transfected IM-BAT adipocytes were measured by quantitative real-time PCR. Data are expressed as mean ± SEM ($n = 3$). $^*P < 0.05$; $^{**}P < 0.01$; $^{***}P < 0.001$ by one-way ANOVA followed by Student's t-test. (e) Agarose gel of undifferentiated IM-BAT adipocytes treated with rosiglitazone (1 μM) for 6 h. Splicing of XBP1 mRNA was detected by RT-PCR. cDNA from preadipocytes treated with tunicamycin was used as positive control.

brown adipocytes might be mediated by XBP1-independent mechanism.

4. Discussion

It has been demonstrated that the activation of GPR43 in white adipose tissue promotes adipocyte differentiation and drives the inhibition of lipolysis [19]. However, little information has been known about the importance of this receptor in brown adipose tissue. Here, our results indicated that GPR43 expression was initiated in brown adipocytes from day 3 of postinduction period, while in white adipocytes abundant GPR43 expression was also observed in the late phase of differentiation [8]. Moreover, our results also demonstrated that the GPR43 expression was rapidly and consistently increased by rosiglitazone treatment in brown adipocytes, which is also similar to the effects of troglitazone in white adipocytes reported in previous studies [8]; these findings support the hypothesis that GPR43 expression in brown adipocytes might share a similar mechanism to that in white adipocytes during adipogenesis.

Rosiglitazone, a well-known antidiabetic drug, can upregulate the activities of PPAR-γ in many peripheral tissues (including adipose tissue) [20]. Since PPARγ is most highly expressed in adipose tissue and plays a crucial role as an adipogenic regulator during adipogenesis, rosiglitazone was also found to be a highly active adipogenic agent, which promotes adipocyte differentiation and activates adipocyte-specific genes expression [20]. Here, we observed that the GPR43 expression was significantly upregulated by rosiglitazone in brown adipocytes. Furthermore, our results also showed that the disruption of PPARγ and RXR heterodimerization almost abolished the rosiglitazone-induced increase in GPR43 expression in brown adipocytes, indicating the positive role of PPARγ activation in GPR43 expression in brown adipocytes.

XBP1 has been elucidated as a core *cis* element controlling the GPR43 transcription in human monocytes [11]. Here, our results also demonstrated that knockdown of XBP1 significantly impaired the expression of GPR43 in brown adipocytes. However, it seemed that rosiglitazone-induced augment of GPR43 expression was not significantly affected by the knockdown of XBP1. Indeed, previous evidence also suggested that XBP1 does not seem to be necessary for the proadipogenic effect of thiazolidinedione. For example, although deletion of XBP1 inhibited adipogenesis in adipocytes *in vitro*, such inhibitory effect could be overcome by thiazolidinediones [21]. Moreover, deletion of adipocyte-XBP1 *in vivo* did not affect body weight, adipose tissue mass, serum insulin, or glucose homeostasis, indicating XBP1 is not a contributing factor to the formation or expansion of adipose tissue *in vivo* [21]. Here, our findings are consistent with these previous results in that the increase of GPR43 expression by rosiglitazone seemed to be mediated at least partially by XBP1-independent mechanism.

In addition, the fact that short-chain fatty acids mediate a wide range of metabolic functions in white adipocytes and white adipose tissues *via* the GPR43 receptors [8, 19, 22] strongly supports the hypothesis that GPR43 acts as sensor that regulates energy metabolism in white adipose tissue. Brown adipose tissue also can regulate the metabolism and energy homeostasis by heat production when the body is exposed to cold temperature [23, 24]. Indeed, brown adipose tissue plays an important role in maintaining body temperature in rodentine mammals and infants. Recent studies also confirmed the presence of brown adipose tissue in human adults [25]. This discovery has drawn great interest in investigating its potential therapeutic application. Indeed, studies already suggested the regulation of GPR43 in brown adipocytes. It has been found that butyrate, an agonist of GPR43, increased *in vivo* adaptive thermogenesis, mitochondrial biogenesis, and UCP-1 expression in brown adipose tissue in mice [26], while HFD-fed GPR43 knock-out mice had significant lipid droplets in intrascapular brown adipose tissue compared to HFD-fed WT mice [27]. Recently, GPR43 agonist acetate and propionate were also found to prevent diet-induced metabolic disorders by induction of Cidea and mitochondrial marker Tfam expression as well as increasing Nrg4 secretion in brown adipose tissue, respectively [28], highlighting the potential links between the activation of GPR43 by short-chain fatty acids in brown adipose tissue and the regulatory effects on metabolism.

Notably, a previous study has reported that chronic PPARγ stimulation led to thermogenic gene expression in a subset of white precursor cells (Hoxc9 positive but Myf5 negative) from epididymal white adipose tissue depot [29]. Meanwhile, GPR43 activation has also been demonstrated to promote the beige adipogenesis *in vivo* [30]. Since PPARγ activation also contributes to the increase in GPR43 expression during brown adipogenesis, these evidences together imply a hypothesis that GPR43 expression driven by PPARγ activation might further enhance the effects of PPARγ stimulation on beige adipogenesis. However, this hypothesis needs further studies to be proven.

In summary, our results have shown that the expression of the short-chain fatty acids sensing GPR43 is initiated during the late phase of brown adipocyte differentiation and its expression levels can be used to reflect the status of brown adipocytes differentiation. GPR43 expression can be increased by the treatment of adipogenic agent such as rosiglitazone and controlled by PPARγ/RXR heterodimerization. Our findings that the levels of GPR43 expression were associated with the differentiation stages of brown adipocyte may provide some important insights into the complex roles of GPR43 in the brown adipogenesis. These results also suggest the functional roles of GPR43 in regulating metabolism in mature adipocytes.

Conflicts of Interest

The authors declare no conflicts of interest.

Acknowledgments

The authors are grateful to Dr. Mark Christian, who provided the immortalized brown adipocytes for the experiments. This research was supported by the National Natural Science Foundation of China (81703065), Natural Science Foundation of Fujian Province (2016J05067), High-Level University Construction Project (612014042), Fujian Provincial Key Laboratory of the Activity and Functional Component's Preparation from Marine Algae (2017FZSK06), and the Special Research Funds for Local Science and Technology Development Guided by Central Government (2017L3015).

Supplementary Materials

Supplementary Figure 1: duration of XBP1 silencing after XBP1 siRNA transfection. IM-BAT cells were transfected with XBP1 siRNAs (Santa Cruz, no. sc38628) or control siRNA (sc-37007) at 200 nM. On the next day, cells were differentiated as indicated. Cells were lysed on day 0 through day 5 after differentiation and XBP1 transcription levels were measured using the real-time PCR. Knockdown efficiency is expressed relative to expression from cells transfected with control siRNA. (*Supplementary Material*)

References

[1] C. P. Briscoe, M. Tadayyon, J. L. Andrews et al., "The orphan G protein-coupled receptor GPR40 is activated by medium and long chain fatty acids," *The Journal of Biological Chemistry*, vol. 278, no. 13, pp. 11303–11311, 2003.

[2] A. J. Brown, S. M. Goldsworthy, A. A. Barnes et al., "The orphan G protein-coupled receptors GPR41 and GPR43 are activated by propionate and other short chain carboxylic acids," *The Journal of Biological Chemistry*, vol. 278, no. 13, pp. 11312–11319, 2003.

[3] E. le Poul, C. Loison, S. Struyf et al., "Functional characterization of human receptors for short chain fatty acids and their role in polymorphonuclear cell activation," *The Journal of Biological Chemistry*, vol. 278, no. 28, pp. 25481–25489, 2003.

[4] N. E. Nilsson, K. Kotarsky, C. Owman, and B. Olde, "Identification of a free fatty acid receptor, FFA2R, expressed on leukocytes and activated by short-chain fatty acids," *Biochemical and Biophysical Research Communications*, vol. 303, no. 4, pp. 1047–1052, 2003.

[5] J. Wang, X. Wu, N. Simonavicius, H. Tian, and L. Ling, "Medium-chain fatty acids as ligands for orphan G protein-coupled receptor GPR84," *The Journal of Biological Chemistry*, vol. 281, no. 45, pp. 34457–34464, 2006.

[6] L. M. Cornall, M. L. Mathai, D. H. Hryciw, and A. J. McAinch, "Diet-induced obesity up-regulates the abundance of GPR43 and GPR120 in a tissue specific manner," *Cellular Physiology and Biochemistry*, vol. 28, no. 5, pp. 949–958, 2011.

[7] S. Karaki, R. Mitsui, H. Hayashi et al., "Short-chain fatty acid receptor, GPR43, is expressed by enteroendocrine cells and mucosal mast cells in rat intestine," *Cell and Tissue Research*, vol. 324, no. 3, pp. 353–360, 2006.

[8] Y.-H. Hong, Y. Nishimura, D. Hishikawa et al., "Acetate and propionate short chain fatty acids stimulate adipogenesis via GPCR43," *Endocrinology*, vol. 146, no. 12, pp. 5092–5099, 2005.

[9] E. M. Dewulf, P. D. Cani, A. M. Neyrinck et al., "Inulin-type fructans with prebiotic properties counteract GPR43 overexpression and PPARγ-related adipogenesis in the white adipose tissue of high-fat diet-fed mice," *The Journal of Nutritional Biochemistry*, vol. 22, no. 8, pp. 712–722, 2011.

[10] G. Li, W. Yao, and H. Jiang, "Short-chain fatty acids enhance adipocyte differentiation in the stromal vascular fraction of porcine adipose tissue," *Journal of Nutrition*, vol. 144, no. 12, pp. 1887–1895, 2014.

[11] Z. Ang, J. Z. Er, and J. L. Ding, "The short-chain fatty acid receptor GPR43 is transcriptionally regulated by XBP1 in human monocytes," *Scientific Reports*, vol. 5, no. 1, 2015.

[12] H. Sha, Y. He, H. Chen et al., "The IRE1α-XBP1 Pathway of the Unfolded Protein Response Is Required for Adipogenesis," *Cell Metabolism*, vol. 9, no. 6, pp. 556–564, 2009.

[13] J. E. Reusch, L. A. Colton, and D. J. Klemm, "CREB activation induces adipogenesis in 3T3-L1 cells," *Molecular & Cellular Biology*, vol. 20, no. 3, pp. 1008–1020, 2000.

[14] M. Kawai, N. Namba, S. Mushiake et al., "Growth hormone stimulates adipogenesis of 3T3-L1 cells through activation of the Stat5A/5B-PPAR pathway," *Molecular Endocrinology*, vol. 38, no. 1, pp. 19–34, 2007.

[15] W. C. Stewart, L. A. Pearcy, Z. E. Floyd, and J. M. Stephens, "STAT5A Expression in Swiss 3T3 Cells Promotes Adipogenesis In Vivo in an Athymic Mice Model System," *Obesity*, vol. 19, no. 9, pp. 1731–1734, 2011.

[16] J. Hu, I. Kyrou, B. K. Tan et al., "Short-chain fatty acid acetate stimulates adipogenesis and mitochondrial biogenesis via GPR43 in brown adipocytes," *Endocrinology*, vol. 157, no. 5, pp. 1881–1894, 2016.

[17] M. Sahuri-Arisoylu, L. P. Brody, J. R. Parkinson et al., "Reprogramming of hepatic fat accumulation and 'browning' of adipose tissue by the short-chain fatty acid acetate," *International Journal of Obesity*, vol. 40, no. 6, pp. 955–963, 2016.

[18] J. Hu, *The effects of short-chain fatty acid acetate on brown adipocytes differentiation and metabolism*, University of Warwick, 2016.

[19] H. Ge, X. Li, J. Weiszmann et al., "Activation of G protein-coupled receptor 43 in adipocytes leads to inhibition of lipolysis and suppression of plasma free fatty acids," *Endocrinology*, vol. 149, no. 9, pp. 4519–4526, 2008.

[20] H. Ohno, K. Shinoda, B. M. Spiegelman, and S. Kajimura, "PPARγ agonists induce a white-to-brown fat conversion through stabilization of PRDM16 protein," *Cell Metabolism*, vol. 15, no. 3, pp. 395–404, 2012.

[21] M. Gregor, E. Misch, L. Yang et al., "The Role of Adipocyte XBP1 in Metabolic Regulation during Lactation," *Cell Reports*, vol. 3, no. 5, pp. 1430–1439, 2013.

[22] N. Aberdein, M. Schweizer, and D. Ball, "Sodium acetate decreases phosphorylation of hormone sensitive lipase in isoproterenol-stimulated 3T3-L1 mature adipocytes," *Adipocyte*, vol. 3, no. 2, pp. 121–125, 2014.

[23] A. Bartelt, O. T. Bruns, R. Reimer et al., "Brown adipose tissue activity controls triglyceride clearance," *Nature Medicine*, vol. 17, no. 2, pp. 200–205, 2011.

[24] S. Enerbäck, "Brown Adipose Tissue In Humans: A New Target for Anti-Obesity Therapy," in *Novel Insights into Adipose Cell Functions*, Research and Perspectives in Endocrine Interactions, pp. 61–66, Springer Berlin Heidelberg, Berlin, Heidelberg, 2010.

[25] D. Chakraborty, A. Bhattacharya, and B. Mittal, "Patterns of brown fat uptake of 18F-fluorodeoxyglucose in positron emission tomography/computed tomography scan," *Indian Journal of Nuclear Medicine*, vol. 30, no. 4, p. 320, 2015.

[26] Z. Gao, J. Yin, J. Zhang et al., "Butyrate improves insulin sensitivity and increases energy expenditure in mice," *Diabetes*, vol. 58, no. 7, pp. 1509–1517, 2009.

[27] M. Bjursell, T. Admyre, and M. Göransson, "Improved glucose control and reduced body fat mass in free fatty acid receptor 2-deficient mice fed a high-fat diet," *American Journal of Physiology-Endocrinology and Metabolism*, vol. 300, no. 1, pp. E211–E220, 2011.

[28] K. Weitkunat, C. Stuhlmann, A. Postel et al., "Short-chain fatty acids and inulin, but not guar gum, prevent diet-induced obesity and insulin resistance through differential mechanisms in mice," *Scientific Reports*, vol. 7, no. 1, 2017.

[29] N. Petrovic, T. B. Walden, I. G. Shabalina, J. A. Timmons, B. Cannon, and J. Nedergaard, "Chronic peroxisome proliferator-activated receptor γ (PPARγ) activation of epididymally derived white adipocyte cultures reveals a population of thermogenically competent, UCP1-containing adipocytes molecularly distinct from classic brown adipocytes," *The Journal of Biological Chemistry*, vol. 285, no. 10, pp. 7153–7164, 2010.

[30] Y. Lu, C. Fan, P. Li, Y. Lu, X. Chang, and K. Qi, "Short Chain Fatty Acids Prevent High-fat-diet-induced Obesity in Mice by Regulating G Protein-coupled Receptors and Gut Microbiota," *Scientific Reports*, vol. 6, no. 1, 2016.

PPARs and Mitochondrial Metabolism: From NAFLD to HCC

Tommaso Mello,[1] **Maria Materozzi,**[1] **and Andrea Galli**[1,2]

[1]Clinical Gastroenterology Unit, Department of Biomedical Clinical and Experimental Sciences "Mario Serio", University of Florence, Viale Pieraccini 6, 50129 Florence, Italy
[2]Careggi University Hospital, Florence, Italy

Correspondence should be addressed to Tommaso Mello; tommaso.mello@unifi.it

Academic Editor: Daniele Fanale

Metabolic related diseases, such as type 2 diabetes, metabolic syndrome, and nonalcoholic fatty liver disease (NAFLD), are widespread threats which bring about a significant burden of deaths worldwide, mainly due to cardiovascular events and cancer. The pathogenesis of these diseases is extremely complex, multifactorial, and only partially understood. As the main metabolic organ, the liver is central to maintain whole body energetic homeostasis. At the cellular level, mitochondria are the metabolic hub connecting and integrating all the main biochemical, hormonal, and inflammatory signaling pathways to fulfill the energetic and biosynthetic demand of the cell. In the liver, mitochondria metabolism needs to cope with the energetic regulation of the whole body. The nuclear receptors PPARs orchestrate lipid and glucose metabolism and are involved in a variety of diseases, from metabolic disorders to cancer. In this review, focus is placed on the roles of PPARs in the regulation of liver mitochondrial metabolism in physiology and pathology, from NAFLD to HCC.

1. Introduction

Liver cancer is a major challenge in contemporary medicine. It represents the fifth most common cancer in men, the ninth in women, and the second most frequent cause of mortality among oncological patients. It was responsible for nearly 746,000 deaths in 2012, with an estimated incidence of over 780,000 new cases yearly worldwide [1]. The prognosis for liver cancer is extremely poor (overall ratio of mortality to incidence of 0.95), reflecting the absence of effective treatments. The most frequent type of primary liver cancer is hepatocellular carcinoma (HCC), accounting for up to 85% of total cancers [2].

Major risk factors include HBV or HCV infection, alcoholic liver disease, and most likely nonalcoholic liver disease (NAFLD) [2]. These and other chronic liver diseases lead to cirrhosis, which is found in 80–90% of HCC patients [2]. NAFLD is now the most common liver disease worldwide [3], with a global prevalence of about 25%. NAFLD is closely associated with other metabolic disorders such as obesity, metabolic syndrome, and type 2 diabetes [3]. Indeed, obesity and diabetes are now definitively recognized as independent risk factors for the development of HCC [4, 5]. NAFLD is histologically classified into nonalcoholic fatty liver (NALF), defined as the presence of steatosis in the absence of causes for secondary hepatic fat accumulation (i.e., alcohol consumption, steatogenic drugs, or genetic disorders), and nonalcoholic steatohepatitis (NASH), in which steatosis is complicated by inflammation and hepatocellular damage (ballooning hepatocytes), with or without fibrosis [6]. A relatively small portion of NAFL patients evolve into NASH, a progressive type of liver disease with the potential of evolving into cirrhosis and HCC. The cumulative incidence of HCC in NASH cirrhosis ranges from 2.4% to 12.8%, and although it is lower than in HCV cirrhotic patients, the absolute burden of NASH related HCC is higher due to the epidemic spread of NAFLD [7]. Moreover, NAFLD greatly increases the risk of HCC from other aetiologies, especially HCV and HBV. While the vast majority of HCC arise in cirrhotic livers, it can also occur in noncirrhotic patients [2]. Of notice, a significant amount of new HCC cases is diagnosed in patients with noncirrhotic NASH [4, 8]. The global incidence of HCC among NAFLD patients was recently estimated to be 0.44 per 1,000 person-year [3], which combined with the epidemic spread of metabolic disorders results in an enormous burden. The recent meta-analysis by Younossi et al. raised the question whether NAFLD could even precede the onset of metabolic syndrome rather than just being the hepatic manifestation of it [3].

The mechanisms that promote HCC development in NASH/NAFLD patients are complex and still poorly understood. A number of molecular mechanisms have been linked to obesity and related metabolic disorders that may accelerate the development of HCC, such as adipose-derived inflammation, lipotoxicity, and insulin resistance. These and other pathological events in obesity have complex interactions while their relative contribution to hepatocarcinogenesis in various stages of NAFLD progression remains to be determined.

Mitochondria can be seen as the energetic hub of the cell. As such, beyond their role in energy production, they play a central role in coordinating the cell anabolic and catabolic processes, in balancing the cell energetic demands in response to internal and external stimuli, and in the regulation of several cell signaling pathways. Deregulation of mitochondrial activity is a common trait to several human diseases, including cancer. Since Warburg, it has long been known that cancer cells undergo a radical metabolic shift toward glycolysis, irrespective of the oxygen availability (aerobic glycolysis) [9]. However, the actual significance of this metabolic remodeling, its consequences on cancer cell biology, and its plasticity have begun to be grasped only in recent years. The initial perception of the Warburg effects was that cancer cells rely primarily on glycolysis for energy production due to a defective mitochondrial respiration [10]. On the contrary, it is now clear that cancer cells hijack their mitochondria metabolism toward massive anabolic processes, in order to cope with the cell fast-growing rates [11]. In this line of view, exacerbate biosynthesis, in particular lipid biosynthesis, rather than glycolysis dependence, emerges as cancer metabolic hallmark.

Peroxisome proliferator activated receptors (PPARs) are master regulators of whole body and liver metabolism. Despite a similar structure, the three PPAR isotypes α, β/δ, and γ vary greatly in tissue distribution, pharmacological and endogenous ligands, and biological effects. In the past decades PPARs have been the focus of massive research effort that helped uncovering their contribution to cancer, metabolic, and cardiovascular diseases. The different PPAR isotypes regulate lipid metabolism by a number of mechanisms: (i) controlling the rate of FA disposal through mitochondrial and peroxysomal β-oxidation (FAO), (ii) regulating lipid biosynthesis via de novo lipogenesis, (iii) regulating FA uptake in peripheral tissue and in the liver, (iv) regulating whole body lipid trafficking through apolipoproteins, (v) interacting in complex regulatory network with other nuclear receptors (LXR, FXR), coactivators (PGC-1α and β, SREBP), or corepressors (NCOR) involved in the metabolic homeostasis. As liver is primarily a metabolic organ, PPARs-regulated processes are involved virtually in any liver disease.

This review summarizes current notions on the roles of PPARs in the regulation of liver mitochondrial metabolism in physiology and pathology, from NAFLD to HCC.

2. PPARs and Mitochondrial Metabolism in the Liver

2.1. PPARα. Peroxisome proliferator activated receptor α (PPARα) is the main PPAR isotype expressed in the liver and plays a major role in energy homeostasis, by regulating lipid metabolism and ketone body formation [12]. In mice but not in humans, PPARα also controls the glycolysis-gluconeogenesis pathway [13]. PPARα natural ligands are endogenous lipids such as fatty acids (FA) and their derivatives (eicosanoids, oxidized phospholipids) [14], while synthetic ligands include the class of hypolipidemic drugs fibrates, xenobiotic agents, and plasticizers.

Despite the fact that FA and derivatives can bind and activate PPARα in the liver, not all FA are created equal. Indeed, it has been now recognized that FA released in the bloodstream by the adipose tissue (i.e., during fasting or intense physical exercise) have little role as PPARα agonist [15], while preferentially activating PPARβ/δ, whereas fatty acids derived from dietary intake or de novo lipogenesis are efficient PPARα activators [15–18]. However, PPARα is absolutely required for the metabolic adaptation to fasting, since PPAR$\alpha^{-/-}$ mice, either full body [19] or liver-specific [20], develop steatosis with prolonged fasting. Moreover, the time course activation of PPARα in the liver mimics the kinetics of circulating FFA during fasting, and liver transcriptomic profiling revealed that the fasted state (versus fed or refed) triggered the broader PPARα-dependent response, strengthening the functional link between hepatic PPARα and adipose tissue-FA disposal [20]. Since activation of hepatic PPARα requires de novo lipogenesis [15, 21], the mechanisms that fine-tune PPARα activation in different metabolic conditions are still unclear and possibly involve separate pools of PPARα that can be activated in a context-dependent manner.

Moreover, the adipose tissue cross-talk with the hepatic PPARs can occur via adiponectin-induced FAO, which is dependent upon AdipoR2 subtype and requires PPARα induction [22], and via FGF21, produced mainly in the liver in a PPARα-dependent manner [20], which promotes both glucose uptake and lipolysis in the adipocytes [23], as well as hepatic lipid disposal [24].

In hepatocytes, PPARα promotes the expression of several genes involved in FA uptake, activation to acyl-CoA, and transport to the mitochondria or peroxisomes and subsequent β- or ω-oxidation, ketogenesis, and lipoprotein trafficking [25, 26] (Figure 1).

Many of the PPARα regulated genes directly modulate mitochondrial metabolism. Interestingly, among the many PPARα-regulated genes in hepatocytes, those involved in mitochondrial metabolic functions, especially in fatty acid oxidation, are consistently dependent upon PPARα regardless of the nutritional condition [20]. PPARα target genes are also carnitine palmitoyl transferase 1 (CPT-1) and carnitine palmitoyltransferase 2 (CPT-2) [19, 25], which mediate transport of long-chain fatty acids through the outer and inner mitochondrial membrane, respectively, to initiate their degradation in the β-oxidative pathway (Figure 1). The

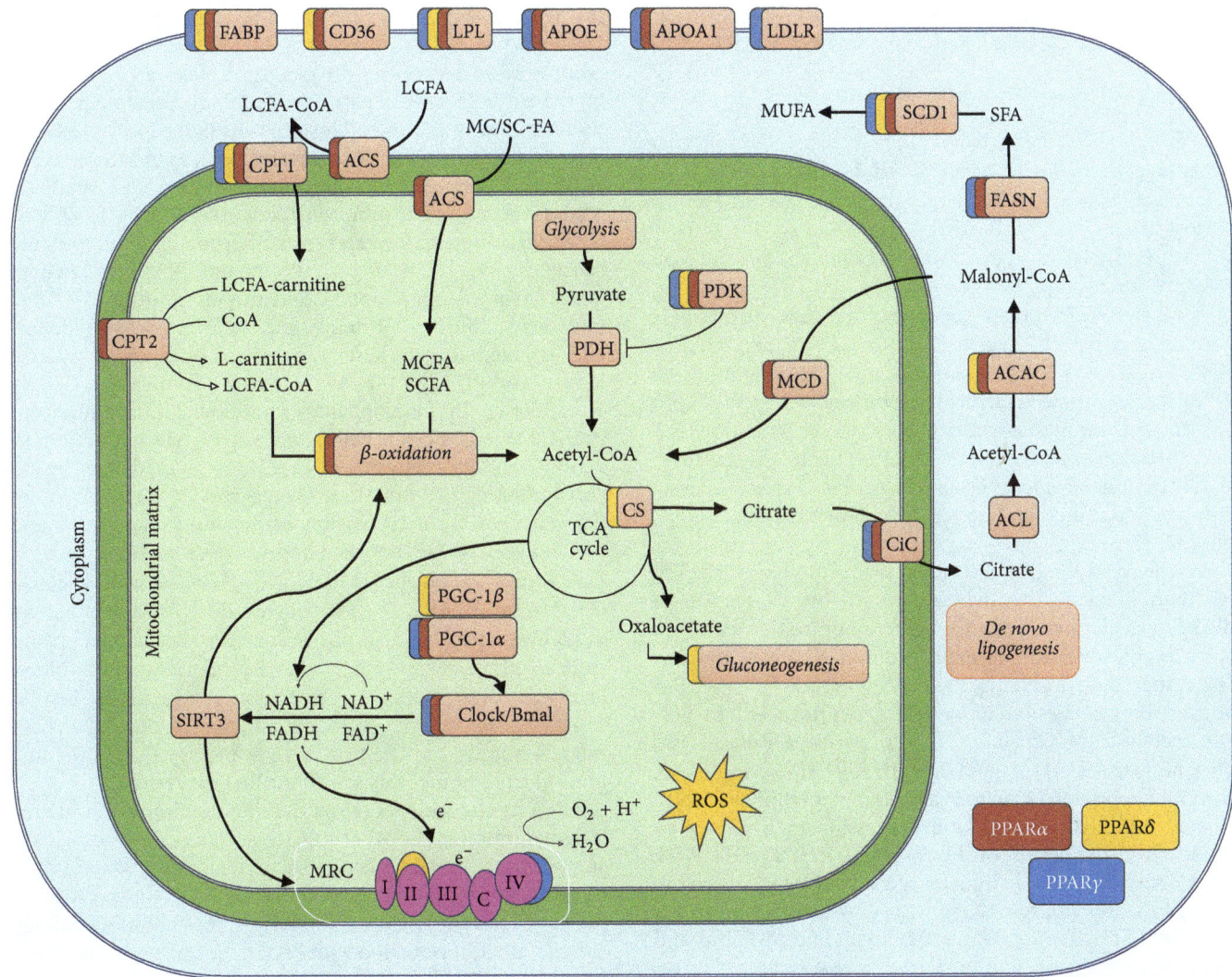

FIGURE 1: Role of hepatic PPARs in mitochondrial metabolism: fatty acid oxidation, circadian control of NAD+ dependent SIRT activity, de novo lipogenesis, and gluconeogenesis. Color-coding depicts PPAR isotypes-dependency of target genes.

β-oxidation cycle consists of four reactions, catalyzed by acyl-CoA dehydrogenases (ACADs), enoyl-CoA hydratases, L-3-hydroxyacyl-CoA dehydrogenase, and 3-ketoacyl-CoA thiolase, that sequentially remove two carbons—one acetyl-CoA molecule, until the acyl-CoA is completely converted to acetyl-CoA. The initial step of the β-oxidation cycle is catalyzed by length specific acyl-CoA dehydrogenases (such as ACADM, ACADS, and ACADVL), all of which are PPARα target genes [26]. The last three steps are carried on by the mitochondrial trifunctional protein (MTP), a large complex of four α and four β subunits. The expression of both subunits (encoded by genes HADHA, HADHB) as well as the MTP protein 3-ketoacyl-CoA thiolase (encoded by ACAA2) is regulated by PPARα [26].

The acetyl-CoA produced during FAO is then used to produce ketone bodies (acetoacetate and β-hydroxybutyrate) via mitochondrial HMG-CoA synthase, another PPARα regulated gene [27]. Ketone bodies are released in the blood

stream and, after conversion to citrate, fuel the TCA cycle in peripheral tissues (mostly heart, muscle, and brain).

FAO is functionally and physically linked to OXPHOS: the reducing equivalents produced by FAO are directly used by the electron transport chain (ETC); moreover, the two pathways are likely happening in large mitochondrial supercomplexes containing both FAO and ETC complexes [28]. Therefore, an unbalance in FAO or ETC directly affects the other pathway.

PPARα, as well as β/δ and γ, also induces the expression of all uncoupling protein (UCP-1, UCP-2, and UCP-3), of which UCP-2 is the main type expressed in liver [29, 30]. Uncoupling proteins allow protons to reenter the mitochondrial matrix without production of adenosine triphosphate, thus promoting energy expenditure and FA oxidation.

Paralleling its role in promoting energy expenditure through FA disposal, PPARα also inhibits the lipogenic pathway by induction of the malonyl-CoA decarboxylase which degrades malonyl-CoA, a precursor of FA biosynthesis and inhibitor of the mitochondrial transporter CPT-1 [31] (Figure 1).

2.2. PPARβ/δ. PPARβ/δ is ubiquitously expressed, often at higher level than PPARα or γ. Overall, PPARβ/δ role in lipid metabolism appears to be largely overlapping with PPARα in most tissues. Indeed, PPARβ/δ stimulates FAO in muscle and heart, the latter organ being extremely dependent on PPARβ/δ function [32].

Several PPARα target genes are thus not surprisingly induced also by PPPARβ/δ (UCP-1, UCP-2, and UCP-3, FABP, FAT/CD36, LPL, ACS, and CPT-1) [33, 34] and loss of PPARα in muscle is efficiently compensated by PPARβ/δ [33]. Indeed, numerous studies have shown that PPARβ/δ overexpression or activation in muscle dramatically improves FA utilization as energy source, reduces hyperlipidemia, improves endurance, and decreases insulin secretion from β-cells [32, 35–37].

However, in the liver PPARβ/δ seems to play a different role than PPARα. Adenoviral-mediated overexpression of PPARβ/δ in the liver enhanced glucose utilization either to increase glycogen storage or to promote de novo lipogenesis, rather than inducing FAO [38] (Figure 1). PPARβ/δ induced the expression of several genes involved in glucose metabolism (GLUT2, GK, and pyruvate kinase) and lipogenesis (FAS, ACC1, ACC2, SCD1, SREBP-1c, and PGC-1β) [38]. Conversely, gluconeogenesis genes (PEPCK, HNF-4) were inhibited by PPARβ/δ expression in hepatocytes. Importantly, the levels of PPARα and its target (CPT-1, acyl-CoA oxidase, and MCAD) were unaffected; therefore PPARβ/δ seems not to overlap with PPARα function in the liver [38]. Consistently, whole transcriptome profiling and liver metabolites analysis of PPARα$^{-/-}$ and PPARβ/δ$^{-/-}$ mice revealed clearly divergent roles [39]. Very interestingly, liver PPARβ/δ signals to PPARα and activates FAO in muscle via the lipid molecule PC (18:0/18:1), whose production in the liver is PPARβ/δ-dependent [40].

Different roles for PPARα and PPARβ/δ in mitochondriogenesis are also beginning to emerge. A transitory upregulation of PPARα, and consequent induction of PGC-1α, is necessary to promote mitochondriogenesis in the early steps of differentiating embryonic stem cells. A robust upregulation of PPARβ/δ is instead needed to promote mitochondriogenesis at later stages of cells differentiation and correlates with the expression of mature hepatocytic markers [41].

Functional peroxisome proliferator response elements have been identified in the distal promoter of PGC-1α, providing the mechanistic basis for PPAR-induced mitochondrial biogenesis. However, the contribution of the diverse PPAR isotypes to PGC-1α induction appears to be cell context-dependent. PGC-1α is activated by PPARα in brown adipose tissue [42] and by PPARγ in both white and brown adipose tissue [42]. In skeletal muscle, PPARβ/δ but not PPARα induce PGC-1α expression [43, 44].

In liver, PCG-1α is induced by fasting, paralleling PPARα activation, and promotes gluconeogenesis, a process mediated by PPARβ/δ [45].

2.3. PPARγ. PPARγ is the main PPAR isotype expressed in white and brown adipose tissue. It is the master inducer of adipogenesis and promotes glucose uptake and utilization in the novo lipogenic pathway, therefore regulating whole body lipid metabolism and insulin sensitivity. Natural PPARγ ligands are lipid molecules derivates, such as unsaturated FA, PGJ$_2$, and oxidized LDL [14, 46, 47] while potent synthetic ligands include the insulin sensitizer class of drug TZD [48].

PPARγ induces the expression of genes regulating glucose sensitivity (GLUT-4, IRS-1, IRS-2, and PI3K), as well as genes involved in FA uptake and mobilization (FAT/CD36, fatty acids binding proteins aP2, and lipoprotein lipase) and triglyceride synthesis (acyl-CoA synthetase, glycerol kinase, and PEPCK) [46, 49] (Figure 1). In the liver, PPARγ is expressed in macrophages, endothelial cells, quiescent (nonactivated) stellate cells, and hepatocytes. Its complex actions on liver physiology are mostly mediated by its anti-inflammatory functions on macrophages and endothelial cells, antifibrotic function in hepatic stellate cells, and metabolic cross-talk between hepatocytes and adipocytes via FGF family members (FGF21, FGF-1). Mice with selective deletion of PPARγ in hepatocytes developed relative fat intolerance, increased adiposity, hyperlipidemia, and insulin resistance. Loss of hepatic PPARγ increased TG blood level and redistribution to other tissues, aggravating insulin resistance in muscle and adipose tissue [50, 51]. These models highlighted the role of liver PPARγ in maintaining lipid/glucose homeostasis and insulin sensitivity.

PPARγ also induces the expression of mitochondrial proteins, common to the other PPARs, such as CPT-1 and UCPs, suggesting a possible degree of overlap in mitochondrial metabolism regulation with other PPAR members. Probably the most relevant function of PPARγ in mitochondria biology comes with its interaction with PGC-1 family members. PGC-1α was initially identified as a nuclear PPARγ coactivator in mitochondrial rich brown adipose tissue-tissue [52]. Since then, it has become clear that PGC-1α and β control virtually any aspect of mitochondria function and biogenesis [53], by thoroughly coordinating a plethora of nuclear receptors (including all three PPARs, EERα) and nonnuclear receptor protein [54]. Indeed, PPARγ can promote the expression of PGC-1α, which in turn potentiates PPARγ activity [55]. Recently, steatogenic FA were shown to induce PPARγ via PGC-1α, suggesting a link between mitochondria biogenesis and triglyceride accumulation [56].

3. Mechanisms of Mitochondrial Oxidative Stress Damage

Reactive oxygen species (ROS) are small reactive molecules generated by the normal cell metabolism, involved in homeostasis and signaling. ROS such as superoxide anion (O_2^-), hydrogen peroxide (H_2O_2), and hydroxyl radical ($HO^•$) consist of radical and nonradical oxygen species formed by the partial reduction of oxygen. Cellular ROS levels are controlled by antioxidant systems such as reduced/oxidized glutathione (GSH/GSSG), reduced/oxidized cysteine

(Cys/CySS), tioredoxin (Trx), peroxiredoxin (Prx), superoxide dismutase (SOD), and catalase.

An imbalance of the generation/neutralization of ROS, driven by an overproduction of ROS or a depletion of the antioxidant defenses, leads to a prooxidant state defined as "oxidative stress." Oxidative stress can directly damage proteins, lipids, and DNA, leading to damaged macromolecules and organelles, but also deranges the redox circuits that regulate many signaling pathways [57]. In fact, while excessively high levels of oxidative stress lead the cell to apoptosis, a controlled increase of ROS serves as critical signaling molecules in cell proliferation and survival [58]. ROS can be generated by growth factor signaling through activation of the NADPH oxidase NOX1 or through the mitochondria. In turn, they can induce cellular signaling cascades by oxidation of phosphatases such as PTEN or PTP or kinases such as Src. This leads to the activation of several pathways such as a Src/PKD1-dependent NF-κB activation mechanism, MAPK (Erk1/2, p38, and JNK), and the PI3K/Akt signaling. Aberrant levels of ROS induce a deregulation of these pathways, which are involved in several pathological conditions, such as NAFLD [59], diabetes [60], and cancer [58, 61].

Several different sources of ROS exist in mitochondria. ETC complex I and complex II, as well as other mitochondrial enzymes such as α-ketoglutarate dehydrogenase, pyruvate phosphate dehydrogenase, fatty acyl-CoA dehydrogenase, and glycerol 3-phosphate dehydrogenase, can produce $O_2^{\cdot-}$ as byproduct, releasing it within the mitochondrial matrix. Moreover, H_2O_2 is produced by the monoamine oxidases (MAOs) located in the outer mitochondrial membrane [62, 63]. Therefore, mitochondria can produce a significant amount of ROS during OXPHOS and FAO, especially in the context of reduced antioxidant defense such as depletion of the mitochondrial glutathione pool [64].

Four main alterations are the direct result of ROS formation: lipid, protein and DNA oxidation, and depletion of antioxidant molecules.

Mitochondrial DNA (mtDNA) is particularly susceptible to oxidative damage due to the absence of protective histones, incomplete DNA repair mechanisms, and the close proximity to ROS production site, which increase the risk of double-strand breaks and somatic mutations with increased ROS production [65]. Since the ETC proteins are encoded exclusively in mtDNA, oxidative damage leads to defective mitochondrial respiration and to a second burst of ROS production that damages mitochondrial membrane and eventually results in loss of mitochondrial membrane potential and activation of proapoptotic pathways due to the ROS induced-ROS-release avalanche [64, 65]. Indeed, depletion and mutation of mtDNA have been described in several type of liver injury, including NASH [66].

Lipid peroxidation is the process under which lipids, mainly polyunsaturated fatty acids, are attacked by oxidants such as ROS. These reactions can form a variety of primary and secondary products, among which malondialdehyde (MDA) appears to be the most mutagenic and 4-hydroxynonenal (4-HNE) the most toxic. MDA induced mutations are involved in cancer and other genetic diseases. 4-HNE can also act as a signaling molecule modulating many

pathways and inducing the expression of proteins, such as NF-κB, Akt, MAPK, JNK, and PPARs. Lipid peroxidation occurs through a radical reaction; it is therefore extremely harmful to biological membranes where the damage can rapidly spread.

The depletion of mitochondrial ROS scavenger is a key step in the pathogenesis of ROS-related liver disease.

In NASH animal model, depletion of mGSH occurs due to cholesterol accumulation in the mitochondrial membrane [67] that disrupts the functionality of GSH transport from cytosol to mitochondria. Depletion of mGSH and other antioxidant systems are documented in NASH patients [68].

ROS can also act as second messengers in cellular signaling oxidizing proteins on cysteine residues, resulting in protein activation or inhibition. High levels of ROS can therefore activate pathways in a signal-independent manner and self-sustain many proproliferative pathways highly involved in cancer and liver diseases such as NASH/NAFLD.

For example, it has been demonstrated that ROS can directly oxidize and activate complexes such as inflammasomes: protein platforms that assemble in the presence of exogenous or endogenous danger signals such as pathogen associated molecular patterns (PAMPs) and damage-associated molecular patterns (DAMPs) to activate and amplify inflammatory pathways [69]. Typically, inflammasomes consist of a sensor (NLRs, ALRs, and TLRs), an adaptor (ASC), and the effector molecule caspase-1 [70]. Once caspase-1 is recruited and activated through autocatalytic cleavage by the inflammasome, it can proteolytically process the inflammatory cytokines IL-1β and IL-18 that lead to a specialized form of cell death called pyroptosis. Pyroptosis causes the release of IL-1β and amplify the inflammatory response downstream of inflammasome activation [70]. In the liver, inflammasomes are expressed in hepatocytes as well as in immune cells and can also be activated by fatty acids through a mechanism involving mitochondrial ROS, decreased autophagy, and IL-1β secretion. Inflammasomes are found overexpressed in NAFLD and NASH and their silencing reduced hepatic injury, steatosis, and fibrosis [69]. Interestingly, agonists of PPARβ/δ were shown to reduce fatty acid induced inflammation and steatosis by inhibiting inflammasomes [69, 71].

Lipid overload in NAFLD and NASH leads to mitochondrial dysfunction and increased oxidative stress, which results from both increased electron flux through the ETC and depletion of the mitochondrial antioxidant defense systems [64].

Reduced levels of GSH, SOD, and catalase as well as increased protein oxidation, a hallmark of increased oxidative stress, are found in NASH patients [68]. Consistently, the mitochondria of NASH patients have altered morphology [72, 73], reduced or mutated mDNA content [66], and reduced oxidative phosphorylation capacity [74]. Oxidative stress constitutes one of the key factors driving NAFLD progression to NASH [75]. Indeed, histological markers of oxidative stress, such as oxidized phosphatidylcholine, localize into steatotic/apoptotic hepatocytes and macrophages and correlate with the degree of steatosis [76].

Depletion of mtGSH and mitochondria oxidative damage are recapitulated also in several animal models of NASH. Interestingly, Llacuna and colleagues highlighted that mitochondrial damage in diverse animal models of NASH seemed to be dependent more on mitochondria cholesterol accumulation (ob/ob mice or HFD administration), rather than only fatty acid/triglyceride overload (choline deficiency model) [67]. Consistently, statins reduced mitochondrial damage in ob/ob mice and HFD models.

This line of view is confirmed by a recent report highlighting the crucial role of dietary cholesterol in delivering the "second hit" for NASH onset, in context of moderate dietary fat administration (45% of total calories from fat) [77]. In this study, addition of a moderate level of cholesterol in HF elicits the onset of hepatocellular damage and inflammation through activation of the inflammasomes response, while neither dietary cholesterol nor HF alone produced the NASH phenotype. Importantly, addition of cholesterol to HF resulted in blunted adaptation of mitochondrial metabolism to HF and markedly reduced mitochondrial biogenesis, effects paralleled by a decrease in PGC-1α and TFAM expression levels [77]. Moreover, while hepatic inflammation recovered after removal of excess dietary cholesterol, mitochondrial functions remained hampered alongside elevated NRLP3 inflammasome protein levels, indicating slow recovery dynamics from mitochondrial damage.

Excess accumulation of free cholesterol in mitochondrial membranes emerges as a hallmark of cellular transformation, potentially fueling the metabolic derangement required for cancer cell growth and resistance to apoptosis [78].

4. PPARs and Mitochondrial Dysfunction, from NAFLD to HCC

4.1. PPARα. A role for PPARα in NASH pathogenesis in animal models has long been established.

PPARα$^{-/-}$ mice fed a MCD diet developed more severe NASH than WT mice, and Wy-14,643 administration completely prevented the development of NASH in WT mice, but not in PPARα$^{-/-}$ mice [79]. The protective effect of the PPARα agonist Wy-14,643 was unexpected, since the authors had foreseen a detrimental effect of the oxidative stress produced by peroxysomal ω-oxidation after PPARα activation. However, PPARα activation also resulted in increased hepatic lipid turnover through the β-oxidative pathway, preventing accumulation of lipoperoxides despite peroxysomal induction [79]. The beneficial effects of PPARα activation by Wy-14,643 were also confirmed in a severe NASH model with established fibrosis [80].

PPARα deletion in mice results in mild, age and sex-dependent, lipid accumulation in the liver [81]. Moreover, overnight fasting results in severe hypoglycemia, hypoketonemia, and increased plasma free FA levels, impaired β-oxidation, and ketogenesis in PPARα$^{-/-}$ mice [19]. As a result, HFD feeding worsens NAFLD in PPARα$^{-/-}$ mice [19, 82]. More recently, the use of a hepatocytic specific PPARα$^{-/-}$ mice model confirmed the protective role of PPARα in NAFLD induced by MCD and short-term HFD. Interestingly, PPARα$^{hep-/-}$ mice developed steatosis and hypercholesterolemia with aging similarly to whole body PPARα$^{-/-}$ mice but did not become obese nor hyperglycaemic [20], confirming that hepatocytic PPARα deletion by itself is a primary cause of liver steatosis.

On the other hand, in leptin deficient (ob/ob) and leptin resistant (db/db) mouse models, PPARα expression was found reduced, unchanged, or increased [83]. Rate of FAO also varies greatly depending on the study. While these discrepancies could be generated by different study protocols, they may be interpreted also in the light of different PPARα pools that can be differentially activated in the metabolism of dietary, versus adipose tissue-derived fatty acids.

Since FA can bind and activate PPARα, thus promoting mitochondrial and peroxysomal FAO, downregulation of PPARα in NASH mice models and patients may be counterintuitive. Moreover, high FAO can increase oxidative stress; therefore stimulating PPARα activity and FAO is somewhat expected to worsen the oxidative damage in hepatocytes. However, it should be recalled that although mitochondria are potentially a major source of ROS, they are also very well equipped with antioxidant defense systems. In fact, whether significant ROS production occurs in mitochondria in vivo is highly debated, and the endoplasmic reticulum is currently emerging as the major source or toxic ROS within the cell [64]. The current view is that liver triglycerides accumulation per se does not result in inflammation [84, 85]. Rather, accumulation of free fatty acids, in particular saturated fatty acids (SFA), results in marked lipotoxicity, hepatocellular damage, and inflammation [86, 87]. The onset of inflammation drives the progression from NAFLD to NASH and causes PPARα downregulation by TNFα [88]. Moreover, TNFα also reduces adiponectin levels. Adiponectin promotes FAO and blunts liver gluconeogenesis signaling through AdipoR2 receptor, which promotes PPARα activity [89] and depends upon PPARα induction. Thus, inflammation-mediated disruption of the metabolic cross-talk between the adipose tissue and the liver may account for reduced PPARα activity, mitochondrial dysfunction, and NASH development (Figure 2). A recent report by Ande and coworkers highlights the importance of the inflammatory cross-talk between adipose tissue and liver, in a sex-dependent manner, in the induction of hepatocytes mitochondrial dysfunction, NASH, and HCC development [90].

This line of view is consistent with the emerging role of PPARα in the control of inflammation [12] and provides additional rationale for pharmacological induction of PPARα in NASH treatment.

Reports on PPARα in human NAFLD are scarce. Very recently a thorough investigation of PPARs expression in NAFLD patients was assessed by Staels' group. The expression of PPARα, PPARβ/δ, and PPARγ was evaluated on mRNA extracted from paired liver biopsies collected 1 year apart in 85 patients. They found a significant association between decreased PPARα expression and histological severity of NASH. No correlation was found with PPARβ/δ or PPARγ expression [91].

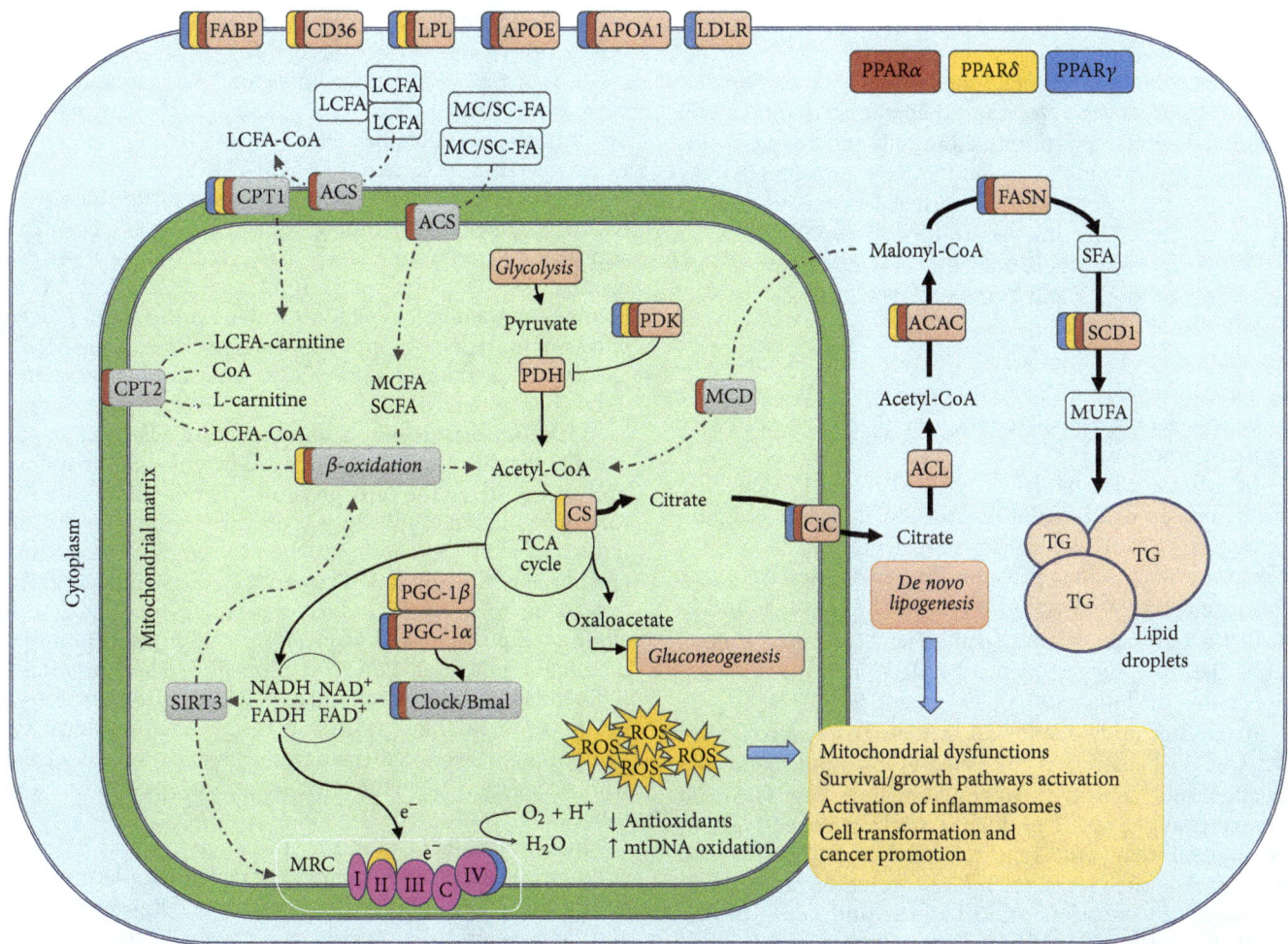

FIGURE 2: Altered mitochondrial metabolism in NASH and HCC: role of PPARs. Altered PPARs expression drives metabolic dysfunctions in the mitochondria leading to suppression of FAO, disruption of circadian rhythms, increased ROS levels, and upregulation of de novo lipogenesis. Color-coding depicts PPAR isotypes-dependency of target genes.

The PPARα agonists peroxisome proliferators exhibit liver cancerogenic activity when chronically administered in mice. The tumor promoting activity has been related to massive proliferation of peroxisomes, with consequent oxidative stress, and to inhibition of let-7c, a microRNA that represses c-myc expression [92]. Long-term HCC development was also found to be dependent with sustained PPARα activation in a transgenic model overexpressing the HCV core protein [93]. However, humans are resistant to peroxisome proliferation and indeed no association between fibrates and increased risk of any cancer has ever been found [94, 95].

Recently, PPARα$^{-/-}$ mice were found to be more susceptible to DEN-induced HCC, and PPARα anticancer activity was shown to be mediated by NF-kB inhibition [96].

Interestingly, PPARα regulation of mitochondrial metabolism may be exploited for cancer treatment. Many cancer types exhibit highly glycolytic metabolism, and cancer cell's mitochondria have a strong commitment toward anabolism and cataplerosis. Since TCA intermediates are used mainly in biosynthetic reactions, mitochondria of cancer cells often have scarce OXPHOS and rely mainly on glycolysis for ATP production. Activation of PPARα induces pyruvate dehydrogenase kinase 4 (PDK4) [97], which inhibits the pyruvate dehydrogenase complex, thus preventing pyruvate from glycolysis to enter mitochondria for acetyl-CoA synthesis and anaplerosis. The net result is the blockage of TCA and fatty acid synthesis, which requires acetyl-CoA, and the slowing-down of glycolytic rate [98].

Activation of PPARα suppresses anaplerosis from glutamine, by repressing the expression of glutaminase and glutamate dehydrogenase, thus potentially counteracting c-myc-dependent activation of glutaminolysis in tumor [97].

Therefore, the transrepression activity of PPARα on lipid biosynthesis and anaplerosis is just as relevant as its transactivation activity on FAO genes. The transrepression activity of PPARα indeed impacts on mitochondria metabolism through SIRT1, by competing with ERR transcriptional pathway [99]. Interestingly, Pawlak and colleagues recently showed that the transrepression activity of PPARα also regulates the inflammatory response in liver, preventing transition from NAFLD to NASH and fibrosis, and occurs independently on PPARα DNA binding activity and its lipid handling properties [100].

A very recent report established a direct connection between PPARα-driven FAO and hepatocyte proliferation. CyclinD1, expressed in proliferating cells and a typical protooncogene, was found to inhibit PPARα expression, thereby reducing β-oxidation, both in normal hepatocytes and in HCC cells lines. This link was confirmed also in liver after partial hepatectomy, where induction of CyclinD1 timed with a reduction of PPARα and its target genes [101].

4.2. PPARβ/δ. As summarized above, PPARβ/δ functions significantly overlap with PPARα in peripheral tissues, while in the liver its functions are more closely related to PPARγ regulated processes.

In genetic mice model of NAFLD (ob/ob), adenoviral overexpression of PPARβ/δ reduced the lipogenic program activated by SREBP-1c, via downregulation of the SREBP-1c activator insig-1, thus ameliorating hepatic steatosis [102]. Conversely, increased activation of SREBP-1c was found in PPARβ/δ$^{-/-}$ versus WT mice, fed either a control or ethanol liquid diet [103], suggesting that PPARβ/δ may play a role in suppressing the lipogenic pathway trough SREBP-1c.

In another study, adenoviral-mediated overexpression of PPARβ/δ in hepatocytes improved glucose utilization and hepatic insulin sensitivity. After overnight fasting, PPARβ/δ overexpressing livers had higher triglyceride and glycogen content than wild-type mice, while fatty acids and cholesterol level were similar [38]. Moreover, adenoviral-mediated overexpression in C57/BL6 mice induced SREBP-1c and PGC-1β expression. PPARβ/δ overexpression protected mice liver from fatty acid overload by promoting (i) FA conversion into nontoxic MUFA and (ii) FA storage into lipid droplets as triglycerides (Figure 2). As a result, activation of inflammatory pathways by FA overload was reduced in PPARβ/δ overexpressing mice fed HFD although steatosis was increased [38]. Treatment of db/db mice with the high affinity PPARβ/δ ligand GW501516 resulted in marked increase of genes involved in fatty acids synthesis and pentose phosphate pathways, promoting FA synthesis in the liver (in parallel with FA oxidation in muscle) [104].

These discrepancies are difficult to reconcile and might be related to the different mice model used, although in both genetic and dietary models PPARβ/δ has been shown to either promote or inhibit liver lipogenesis. Moreover, PPARβ/δ inhibits hepatic FGF21 expression [105], while PPARα is a potent activator of FGF21 [20]. Since FGF21 is known to inhibit SREBP-1c and several other lipogenic genes in the liver [106, 107], the potential cross-talk of different PPAR isotypes on FGF21 may contribute to eliciting context-dependent effects.

Despite these striking differences, activation of PPARβ/δ consistently resulted in a beneficial effect on liver damage.

Pharmacological activation of PPARβ/δ has been explored in several rodents and human studies. Administration of PPARβ/δ agonists improved hepatic steatosis and reduced insulin resistance and hepatic inflammation [71, 108–111].

Consistently, PPARβ/δ$^{-/-}$ mice were prone to inflammation derived liver damage.

In humans, PPARβ/δ agonists for NASH treatment are currently under investigation in clinical trials. The first evidence in men was obtained with GW501516, which proved to be equal to the PPARα agonist GW590735 in reducing plasma triglycerides levels and superior to the PPARα agonist in reducing cholesterol LDL, apolipoprotein B, liver fat content, and urinary isoprostane [112]. More recently, the PPARβ/δ agonist MBX-8025 was tested in 181 dyslipidemic patients in combination with atorvastatin or alone. MBX-8025 proved effective in reducing apolipoprotein B levels, non-HDL-cholesterol, triglycerides, free fatty acids, and high-sensitive C-reactive protein [113].

PPARβ/δ-driven mitochondriogenesis has been implicated in the differentiation of hepatic-like tissue from mouse of ES cells [41]. At the early phase of differentiation, a transitory upregulation of PPARα was observed, which resulted in induction of PGC-1α and mitochondriogenesis. Instead, the late phase of differentiation required a robust and sustained expression of PPARβ/δ, which was timely associated with albumin expression and acquisition of high mitochondrial membrane potential. PPARβ/δ agonists L165041 promoted differentiation into hepatic-like tissue that was abolished by PPARβ/δ inhibitor GSK0660 [41]. Therefore, PPARβ/δ may promote terminal hepatocyte differentiation associated with acquisition of mature mitochondria metabolism and function.

Indeed, PPARβ/δ$^{-/-}$ mice show a delay in liver regeneration after partial hepatectomy, associated with lack of Akt activation, lack of induction of glycolytic and lipogenic genes, and suppression of E2F transcription factors activation [114].

Interestingly, PPARβ/δ was associated with nonproliferating hepatocytes in a gene signature analysis of nuclear receptor in proliferating livers and HCC [115]. The authors analyzed the expression of all 49 members of the nuclear receptor superfamily in regenerating mouse liver and PPARβ/δ (together with TRα and FXRβ) was found consistently downregulated throughout the process. PPARβ/δ was found significantly reduced in a small series of HCC with respect to the surrounding nontumoral tissue and the PPARβ/δ agonist GW501516 suppressed CyclinD1 expression and cell proliferation in Hepa1-6 cells [115]. However, whether PPARβ/δ agonists suppress HCC cells growth is still controversial [116, 117]. Both PPARβ/δ and PPARγ have been implicated in mediating beta-catenin-Tcf/lef signaling [118].

Recently, PPARβ/δ was identified as a target gene of FHL2, a tumor suppressor gene also involved in hepatocellular carcinoma [119, 120].

4.3. PPARγ. The effectiveness of the insulin sensitizers TZD in ameliorating the lipidemic profile, inflammation, and steatosis in T2DM patients is well established. Several clinical trials have explored the potential of TZDs in the treatment of NASH and have recently been reviewed [121, 122].

A recent meta-analysis of RCT on TZD and NASH (3 with pioglitazone, 1 with rosiglitazone) confirmed the effectiveness of TZD in improving steatosis, necroinflammation, and hepatocyte ballooning [123]. A significant improvement in fibrosis was obtained only when the analysis was restricted to the pioglitazone studies only. Rosiglitazone failed to improve necroinflammation, ballooning, and fibrosis in the 1-year FLIRT trial [124] and even when treatment was extended for additionally 2 years [125]. Combinatory treatment of rosiglitazone with metformin or losartan did not improve the histological endpoint versus rosiglitazone alone [126]. A very recent report suggests that rosiglitazone administration may exert opposite outcome on liver steatosis depending on liver PPARγ expression levels: RGZ worsen steatosis in PPARγ overexpressing mice fed a HFD and protected mice with low PPARγ expression level [121, 127].

PPARγ is indeed markedly overexpressed in the liver of obese patients with NAFLD and NASH, and its expression positively correlates with plasma insulin, HOMA-IR, and SREBP1-c mRNA levels and inversely correlates with adiponectin [128]. High PPARγ levels, in particular of PPARγ2, promotes de novo lipogenesis and liver steatosis and is associated with HFD feeding in mice [129–131]. However as recalled above, induction of PPARγ by TZD, in particular pioglitazone, ameliorates steatosis and NASH. This discrepancy may be interpreted in the light of the double nature of PPARγ target genes, which comprises both genes of de novo lipid synthesis and mitochondrial genes promoting FAO [132]. Moreover, pioglitazone also binds and activates PPARα with low potency [133], which could explain its better performance than rosiglitazone in ameliorating steatosis. Mechanistically, induction of PPARγ in steatotic hepatocytes may serve as a protective mechanism to reduce liver FFA levels by storing them as less toxic triglycerides [134, 135]. Therefore, the prosteatotic action of PPARγ [136] may not be entirely detrimental. However, excess triglyceride accumulation eventually results in hepatocyte ballooning and necroinflammation, promoting transition to NASH.

The role of PPARγ in hepatocellular carcinoma is still debated. A large body of literature on PPARγ and cancer was produced using TZD, which eventually were proved to have several anticancer pleiotropic effects also independently of PPARγ [137–140].

We and others have investigated the role of PPARγ on hepatocarcinogenesis in mice harboring a hepatocyte specific deletion of PPARγ gene (PPARγ$^{hep-/-}$ mice). Yu and colleagues found increased DEN-induced HCC in mice lacking one PPARγ allele, thus suggesting a tumor-suppression function for PPARγ [141]. Moreover, RGZ reduced HCC development in DEN-treated WT mice but not in PPARγ$^{+/-}$ mice [141]. Using a transgenic model of HBV-related HCC, we found that RGZ or PGZ effectively reduced HCC onset [142]. Strikingly, TZD treatment resulted more effective in PPARγ$^{hep-/-}$ mice than in WT mice [142], highlighting that (i) TZD antitumor activity is independent of PPARγ; (ii) PPARγ expression reduced TZD activity; therefore in this model PPARγ may support, rather than inhibiting, tumor growth.

As the master regulator of adipogenic differentiation, PPARγ has been described to promote differentiation programs in a variety of tumor cell types [143, 144],

inducing cell-cycle arrest [145], apoptosis/anoikis [146–148], and inhibiting EMT [149, 150], angiogenesis [151], and metastasis [152].

However, several lines of evidence also support the notion that this nuclear receptor may support the growth in several cancer types. Conflicting results have been reported in breast cancer model. Recently, Avena et al. showed that breast cancer growth was inhibited by PPARγ overexpression epithelial cancer cells but promoted by PPARγ overexpression in cancer associated stroma [153]. The authors identify the tumor promoting role of PPARγ in the metabolic symbiosis between stoma and epithelial cancer cells, where cancer associated fibroblasts provided intermediates for mitochondrial metabolism to cancer cells [153]. Moreover, increased de novo lipogenesis, that is promoted by PPARγ, is now recognized as a metabolic hallmark of cancer cell [154], including HCC [155–159] (Figure 2). Indeed, de novo lipogenesis is activated downstream of the Akt/mTOR pathway, one of the most common signaling pathways altered in cancer. Forced activation of Akt/mTOR induces liver cancer [160, 161], a process mediated at least in part by activation of FASN [155, 156]. Consistently, inactivation of FASN was recently shown to completely inhibit Akt-driven HCC in mice [158]. Importantly, FASN is not oncogenic per se. However, when the PI3K/Akt/mTOR pathway becomes hyperactive, the induction of the de novo lipogenesis is a requisite for supporting cancer cell growth. Importantly, PPARγ is a direct transcriptional target of mTORC1 [162]. Moreover, in PTEN null mice PPARγ was found to directly induce the expression of key glycolytic gene HK and oncogenic PKM2, inducing hepatocyte steatosis, hypertrophy, and hyperplasia [163].

Therefore, PPARγ may inhibit or promote HCC development depending on the metabolic context, the cell type expressing it, the oncogenic signaling pathways involved, and dietary or pharmacological treatment. It is however conceptually very attractive to explore the therapeutic potential interference with the cancer cell lipid handling capacity, through modulation of mitochondrial FA, ketogenesis, and lipogenesis, as an integrated anticancer approach.

5. PPARs and Circadian Regulation of Mitochondria Metabolism

Many processes of our metabolism and physiology are regulated by circadian clocks, endogenous time-tracking systems that coordinate daily rhythms of rest, activity, feeding behavior, energy utilization, and storage. Although circadian rhythms are endogenous they respond to external stimuli, which include light, temperature, and redox cycles [164]. Circadian regulation is coordinated by the suprachiasmatic nucleus in the brain, but most peripheral organs contain their own independent pacemakers [165]. At a cellular level these oscillations are driven by transcriptional feedback loops associated with changes in chromatin remodeling, mRNA processing, protein turnover, and activity [166–169]. Main factors that control circadian rhythmicity in the cells include BMAL1 and CLOCK ("activators") and CRYs and PERs ("inhibitors"). Their effects are tissue-specific and in the liver they control approximately 10% of the transcriptome [170], influencing metabolic pathways by modifying the expression or activity of key enzymes and transporters involved in lipid, glucose, and mitochondrial oxidative metabolism. Reciprocally, intracellular metabolites and transcriptional factors modulate CLOCK activity in response to the energy status.

Circadian dysregulation of lipid metabolism, ROS production, and cell-cycle control is linked to various pathological conditions including metabolic syndrome, diabetes, chronic liver diseases, and cancer [171–173].

5.1. Clock and Lipid Metabolism: Regulation of PPARs and Mitochondrial Functions.

The redox state of the cell also seems to play an important part in the rhythmicity of metabolism, especially in the mitochondria. NAD+ levels oscillate and are under direct control of clock transcription factors that upregulate the rate-limiting enzyme in NAD^+ biosynthesis, NAMPT (nicotinamide phosphoribosyl transferase). In mitochondria NAD+ activates SIRT3, an important regulator of intrinsic mitochondrial function including FAO. In the cytoplasm NAD+ activates SIRT1 that operates a small feedback regulating Clock and Bmal. Disruption of circadian rhythms in mice leads to defects in mtFAO and decreased OCR mainly through deregulation of NAD+ dependent SIRT3 activity [174, 175] (Figure 2).

Several genes involved in lipid metabolism (such as SREBP, HMGCoAR, and FAS) are modulated by PPARα and display circadian fluctuations that are lost in PPARα-KO mice [176, 177].

PPARα is a direct transcriptional target of BMAL1 and CLOCK [178–180] and in the rodent liver operates a feedback loop binding BMAL1 and REV-ERBα gene promoters. BMAL1-KO and CLOCK-mutant mice display abolished PPARα oscillation and decreased expression in the liver, whereas PPARα-KO mice display altered oscillation of PER3 and BMAL1 [181]. Moreover, administration of PPARα agonists fenofibrates upregulates the expression of *Bmal1* in mouse liver [180].

Fatty acids are known to be PPARα activators, binding directly to the transcriptional factor. Interestingly, hepatic fatty acids are also produced in a circadian manner by acyl-CoA thioesterases (ACOTs) and lipoprotein lipases (LPLs).

The expression of both enzyme families displays circadian rhythmicity; it is regulated by PPARα and can in fact be induced by WY14643. Moreover, silencing members of ACOTs lead to a downregulation of Cyp4a10 and Cyp4a14, PPARa targets [182–186].

Another clock controlled gene, Nocturnin, binds to PPARγ modulating its transcriptional activity [187], and PPARγ systemic inactivation in mice leads to impaired rhythmicity of the canonical clock genes in liver and adipose tissues [188]. PGC-1α is also rhythmically expressed in mouse liver and muscle, upregulates circadian factors BMAL1, CLOCK, and REV-ERBα [189], and modulates the length of circadian oscillations by controlling Bmal1 transcription in a REV-ERB-dependent manner. Mice lacking PGC-1α show abnormal circadian rhythms and altered expression of metabolic genes [189]. Interestingly, circadian regulation was lost also in

mice lacking PGC-1β, but this resulted in markedly decreased activity during the dark cycle, as opposed to the hyperactive PGC-1α KO mice [190] (Figure 2).

The liver-specific deletion of PPARδ in mice showed that it is involved in the temporal regulation of several lipogenic genes, such as fatty acid synthase (FAS) and acetyl-CoA carboxylase 1 and acetyl-CoA carboxylase 2 [40]. BMAL1 also induces the expression of REV-ERBα, a nuclear receptor that downregulates BMAL1 itself, operating a negative feedback, and upregulates the expression of a liver-specific microRNA: miR-122 [191]. miR-122 is also involved in lipid metabolism in mouse liver [192] and PPARδ was proven to be one of its targets, suggesting that PPARδ plays a role in hepatic circadian regulation [193].

The circadian regulation of mitochondrial metabolism is still in its early days. Using a MS-based proteomic approach, the expression of rate-limiting enzymes and metabolites in mitochondria was quantitatively evaluated throughout the day [194]. Many key mitochondrial enzymes involved in carbohydrates and lipid metabolism were found to peak in the early morning period and to be regulated by PER2/3 proteins. Mitochondrial respiration displayed an oscillatory behavior, peaking several times of the day. In mice KO for Per2/3, as well as in those fed a HFD, period protein oscillation was lost, together with OXPHOS oscillation [194].

5.2. Circadian Disturbances in Liver Disease.

It is now clear that circadian rhythms are fundamental in liver physiology and their disruption is observed in many hepatic pathologic conditions, such as NASH, NAFLD, ALD, and HCC [110, 172, 195–198].

In a mouse model of NASH it was found that HFD induces the susceptibility to develop NASH through desynchronized Clock gene expression and altered cellular redox status, accompanied by reduced sirtuin abundance [197]. HFD in mice is sufficient to induce the loss of circadian fluctuations of insulin secretion [199]. Conversely, BMAL1 whole body-KO mice and Clock-mutant mice display hepatic steatosis, obesity, hypoinsulinemia, and increased glucose intolerance [200].

The molecular alterations found in the liver of HFD-fed mice include loss of oscillation or phase advance of rhythmicity of many genes involved in lipid and mitochondrial metabolism (such as NAMPT, acetyl-coenzyme A synthetase, and ornithine decarboxylase 1) and gain of oscillation of other genes such as PPARγ and its targets [201]. This transcriptional reprogramming relies on changes in the oscillation and chromatin recruitment of PPARγ that also induces the oscillation of *Cidec* (cell death activator CIDE-3) [201], a protein that is substantially elevated in the livers of the obese ob/ob mice [202]. Administration of GW9662, a specific PPARγ antagonist, into HFD-fed animals produced a decrease in PPARγ-induced Cidec expression [201]. The expression of another known PPARγ target, pyruvate carboxylase (Pcx), an important regulator of hepatic gluconeogenesis, was significantly elevated and rhythmic in livers of HFD-fed mice [201]. In Nocturnin-KO mice fed with HFD, liver PPARγ oscillation was abolished, accompanied by a reduced expression of many genes related to lipid metabolism and resistance to hepatic steatosis [203].

Accumulating evidence supports the importance of the disruption of circadian rhythms in various types in cancer. Specifically, in HCC patients, low expression of clock genes was observed in the cancerous tissue, but not in the non-cancerous liver tissue, and correlated with tumor size and tumor grade [204]. A number of mechanisms may explain the circadian control on HCC. For example, it was found that DEN exposure in mice is associated with circadian disturbance, suggesting that liver clocks are involved in the carcinogenesis [196]. Mutations and polymorphisms of the clock proteins are being screened to assess their association with HCC. Interestingly, a functional polymorphism of PER3 was recently associated with a lower risk of death in HCC patients treated with TACE [205].

6. Perspectives and Conclusions

It is now clear that expression or activation of nuclear receptors, including PPARs, is not sufficient to predict their biological output. The net effect of a nuclear receptor activation in a given cell actually depends on the context of coactivators, corepressors, dimerization events, availability of endogenous/synthetic ligands, posttranslational modifications, competition, and interactions with other NRs. This led to the development of partial agonist selective PPAR modulators (SPPARMs), a second generation of PPAR agonists able to selectively activate a subset of target genes downstream a specific PPAR isotype.

K-877 is a SPPARαM currently being tested in dyslipidemic patients that exhibits higher lipid lowering activity than fibrates and has a favorable risk profile [206, 207]. INT-131, SPPARγM, has potent glucose lowering effects not associated with TZD side-effects [208].

A different approach to PPAR modulation is to simultaneously activate, with different potency, more than one isotype: dual PPAR agonist or pan-agonists are currently under investigation. The dual PPARα/δ agonist GFT-505 is proving effective in reducing plasma triglyceride levels, improving insulin sensitivity, and increasing HDL-cholesterol in obese patients [209, 210] and showed promising results in mice model of NASH [211]. Very recently a phase 2 multicenter randomized controlled trial, enrolling 274 subjects with histologically proven NASH, showed that GFT505 produces a dose-dependent improvement in histology of patients with NASH [212].

As we gain knowledge of the metabolic circadian regulation and of its disruption in disease, an entire new area of intervention begins to emerge. Modulation of amplitude and phase of PPARs circadian regulation could be exploited to drive complex metabolic remodeling of mitochondrial metabolism in NASH and cancer models. Finally, the integration of the above-mentioned approaches with the metabolic and genetic profiling of cancers holds the promise for new therapeutic approaches that can selectively target the fuel requirements of HCC.

Abbreviations

ACAA2:	Acetyl-CoA acyltransferase 2
ACADM:	Medium-chain specific acyl-CoA dehydrogenase
ACADs:	Acyl-CoA dehydrogenases
ACADVL:	Very long-chain specific acyl-CoA dehydrogenase
ACC1 and ACC2:	Acetyl-CoA carboxylase 1 and acetyl-CoA carboxylase 2
ACS:	Acetyl-coenzyme A synthetase
AdipoR2:	Adiponectin receptor 2
MAL1:	Aryl hydrocarbon receptor nuclear translocator-like protein 1
CPT-1 and CPT-2:	Carnitine palmitoyl transferase 1 and carnitine palmitoyl transferase 2
DAMPs:	Damage-associated molecular pattern
ERRalpha:	Estrogen related receptor alpha
ETC:	Electron transport chain
FAO:	Fatty acid oxidation
FAS:	Fatty acid synthase
FAT/CD36:	Fatty acid translocase
FHL2:	Four and a half LIM domains protein 2
FXR:	Farnesoid X receptor
GK:	Glycerol kinase
GLUT2:	Glucose transporter 2
GLUT-4:	Glut transporter 4
HADHA and HADHB:	Trifunctional enzyme subunit alpha and beta
H-FABP:	Heart-type fatty acid-binding protein
HMGCoAR:	3-hydroxy-3-methylglutaryl-CoA reductase
HNF-4:	Hepatocyte nuclear factor 4-alpha
IRS-1, IRS-2:	Insulin receptor substrate 1 and insulin receptor substrate 2
JNK:	Jun N-terminal kinase
LC-FA:	Long-chain fatty acids
LPL:	Lipoprotein lipase
LXR:	Liver X receptor
M/S-FA:	Medium/short chain fatty acids
MAPK:	Mitogen-activated protein kinase 1
MCD:	Methionine and choline deficient diet
MDA:	Malondialdehyde

MTP:	Mitochondrial trifunctional protein
MUFA:	Monounsaturated fatty acids
NAD+:	Nicotinamide adenine dinucleotide
NAMPT:	Nicotinamide phosphoribosyltransferase
NCOR:	Nuclear receptor corepressor 1
NF-κB:	Nuclear factor NF-kappa-B
PAMPs:	Pathogen associated molecular patterns
PDK4:	Pyruvate dehydrogenase kinase 4
PEPCK:	Phosphoenolpyruvate carboxykinase
PGC-1α/β:	Peroxisome proliferator activated receptor gamma coactivator 1 α/β
PI3K:	Phosphatidylinositol 3-kinase
PKM2:	Pyruvate kinase M2
PTEN:	Phosphatidylinositol 3,4,5-trisphosphate 3-phosphatase and dual-specificity protein phosphatase
REV-ERBa:	Nuclear receptor subfamily 1 group D member 1
SCD1:	Acyl-CoA desaturase 1
SFA:	Saturated fatty acids
SIRT-1 andSIRT-3:	NAD-dependent protein deacetylase sirtuin-1 andNAD-dependent protein deacetylase sirtuin-3
SOD:	Superoxide dismutase
TRα:	Thyroid hormone receptor alpha (TR-alpha)
UCP-1, UCP-2, and UCP-3:	Mitochondrial uncoupling protein 3
4-HNE:	4-hydroxynonenal.

Competing Interests

The authors declare that they have no competing interests.

References

[1] J. Ferlay, I. Soerjomataram, M. Ervik et al., *GLOBOCAN 2012 v1.0, Cancer Incidence and Mortality Worldwide*, IARC Cancer-Base no. 11, International Agency for Research on Cancer, 2013, http://globocan.iarc.fr.

[2] H. B. El-Serag, "Hepatocellular carcinoma," *New England Journal of Medicine*, vol. 365, no. 12, pp. 1118–1127, 2011.

[3] Z. M. Younossi, A. B. Koenig, D. Abdelatif, Y. Fazel, L. Henry, and M. Wymer, "Global epidemiology of nonalcoholic fatty liver disease-meta-analytic assessment of prevalence, incidence, and outcomes," *Hepatology*, vol. 64, no. 1, pp. 73–84, 2016.

[4] B. Q. Starley, C. J. Calcagno, and S. A. Harrison, "Nonalcoholic fatty liver disease and hepatocellular carcinoma: a weighty connection," *Hepatology*, vol. 51, no. 5, pp. 1820–1832, 2010.

[5] H. B. El-Serag, T. Tran, and J. E. Everhart, "Diabetes increases the risk of chronic liver disease and hepatocellular carcinoma," *Gastroenterology*, vol. 126, no. 2, pp. 460–468, 2004.

[6] N. Chalasani, Z. Younossi, J. E. Lavine et al., "The diagnosis and management of non-alcoholic fatty liver disease: practice Guideline by the American Association for the Study of Liver Diseases, American College of Gastroenterology, and the American Gastroenterological Association," *Hepatology*, vol. 55, no. 6, pp. 2005–2023, 2012.

[7] M. Masarone, A. Federico, L. Abenavoli, C. Loguercio, and M. Persico, "Non alcoholic fatty liver: epidemiology and natural history," *Reviews on Recent Clinical Trials*, vol. 9, no. 3, pp. 126–133, 2014.

[8] N. Kawada, K. Imanaka, T. Kawaguchi et al., "Hepatocellular carcinoma arising from non-cirrhotic nonalcoholic steatohepatitis," *Journal of Gastroenterology*, vol. 44, no. 12, pp. 1190–1194, 2009.

[9] O. Warburg, "On the origin of cancer cells," *Science*, vol. 123, no. 3191, pp. 309–314, 1956.

[10] O. warburg, "On respiratory impairment in cancer cells," *Science*, vol. 124, no. 3215, pp. 269–270, 1956.

[11] C. S. Ahn and C. M. Metallo, "Mitochondria as biosynthetic factories for cancer proliferation," *Cancer & Metabolism*, vol. 3, no. 1, article 1, 2015.

[12] A. W. F. Janssen, B. Betzel, G. Stoopen et al., "The impact of PPARα activation on whole genome gene expression in human precision cut liver slices," *BMC Genomics*, vol. 16, no. 1, article 760, 2015.

[13] M. Rakhshandehroo, G. Hooiveld, M. Müller, and S. Kersten, "Comparative analysis of gene regulation by the transcription factor PPARα between mouse and human," *PLoS ONE*, vol. 4, no. 8, Article ID e6796, 2009.

[14] W. Wahli and L. Michalik, "PPARs at the crossroads of lipid signaling and inflammation," *Trends in Endocrinology and Metabolism*, vol. 23, no. 7, pp. 351–363, 2012.

[15] M. V. Chakravarthy, Z. Pan, Y. Zhu et al., "'New' hepatic fat activates PPARα to maintain glucose, lipid, and cholesterol homeostasis," *Cell Metabolism*, vol. 1, no. 5, pp. 309–322, 2005.

[16] D. Patsouris, J. K. Reddy, M. Müller, and S. Kersten, "Peroxisome proliferator-activated receptor α mediates the effects of high-fat diet on hepatic gene expression," *Endocrinology*, vol. 147, no. 3, pp. 1508–1516, 2006.

[17] P. G. P. Martin, H. Guillou, F. Lasserre et al., "Novel aspects of PPARα-mediated regulation of lipid and xenobiotic metabolism revealed through a nutrigenomic study," *Hepatology*, vol. 45, no. 3, pp. 767–777, 2007.

[18] L. M. Sanderson, P. J. de Groot, G. J. E. J. Hooiveld et al., "Effect of synthetic dietary triglycerides: a novel research paradigm for nutrigenomics," *PLoS ONE*, vol. 3, no. 2, Article ID e1681, 2008.

[19] S. Kersten, J. Seydoux, J. M. Peters, F. J. Gonzalez, B. Desvergne, and W. Wahli, "Peroxisome proliferator-activated receptor α mediates the adaptive response to fasting," *Journal of Clinical Investigation*, vol. 103, no. 11, pp. 1489–1498, 1999.

[20] A. Montagner, A. Polizzi, E. Fouche et al., "Liver PPARalpha is crucial for whole-body fatty acid homeostasis and is protective against NAFLD," *Gut*, vol. 65, no. 7, pp. 1202–1214, 2016.

[21] M. V. Chakravarthy, I. J. Lodhi, L. Yin et al., "Identification of a Physiologically Relevant Endogenous Ligand for PPARα in Liver," *Cell*, vol. 138, no. 3, pp. 476–488, 2009.

[22] T. Yamauchi, J. Kamon, Y. Ito et al., "Cloning of adiponectin receptors that mediate antidiabetic metabolic effects," *Nature*, vol. 423, no. 6941, pp. 762–769, 2003.

[23] P. Iglesias, R. Selgas, S. Romero, and J. J. Díez, "Biological role, clinical significance, and therapeutic possibilities of the recently discovered metabolic hormone fibroblastic growth factor 21," *European Journal of Endocrinology*, vol. 167, no. 3, pp. 301–309, 2012.

[24] F. M. Fisher, P. C. Chui, I. A. Nasser et al., "Fibroblast growth factor 21 limits lipotoxicity by promoting hepatic fatty acid activation in mice on methionine and choline-deficient diets," *Gastroenterology*, vol. 147, no. 5, pp. 1073.e6–1083.e6, 2014.

[25] E. Szalowska, H. A. Tesfay, S. A. van Hijum, and S. Kersten, "Transcriptomic signatures of peroxisome proliferator-activated receptor α (PPARα) in different mouse liver models identify novel aspects of its biology," *BMC Genomics*, vol. 15, no. 1, article 1106, 2014.

[26] S. Kersten, M. Rakhshandehroo, B. Knoch, and M. Müller, "Peroxisome proliferator-activated receptor alpha target genes," *PPAR Research*, Article ID 612089, 2010.

[27] D. G. Cotter, B. Ercal, X. Huang et al., "Ketogenesis prevents diet-induced fatty liver injury and hyperglycemia," *The Journal of Clinical Investigation*, vol. 124, no. 12, pp. 5175–5190, 2014.

[28] Y. Wang, A.-W. Mohsen, S. J. Mihalik, E. S. Goetzman, and J. Vockley, "Evidence for physical association of mitochondrial fatty acid oxidation and oxidative phosphorylation complexes," *Journal of Biological Chemistry*, vol. 285, no. 39, pp. 29834–29841, 2010.

[29] F. Villarroya, R. Iglesias, and M. Giralt, "PPARs in the control of uncoupling proteins gene expression," *PPAR Research*, vol. 2007, Article ID 74364, 12 pages, 2007.

[30] L. J. Kelly, P. P. Vicario, G. M. Thompson et al., "Peroxisome proliferator-activated receptors γ and α mediate in vivo regulation of uncoupling protein (UCP-1, UCP-2, UCP-3) gene expression," *Endocrinology*, vol. 139, no. 12, pp. 4920–4927, 1998.

[31] G. Y. Lee, N. H. Kim, Z.-S. Zhao, B. S. Cha, and Y. S. Kim, "Peroxisomal-proliferator-activated receptor α activates transcription of the rat hepatic malonyl-CoA decarboxylase gene: a key regulation of malonyl-CoA level," *Biochemical Journal*, vol. 378, no. 3, pp. 983–990, 2004.

[32] L. Cheng, G. Ding, Q. Qin et al., "Cardiomyocyte-restricted peroxisome proliferator-activated receptor-δ deletion perturbs myocardial fatty acid oxidation and leads to cardiomyopathy," *Nature Medicine*, vol. 10, no. 11, pp. 1245–1250, 2004.

[33] D. M. Muoio, P. S. MacLean, D. B. Lang et al., "Fatty acid homeostasis and induction of lipid regulatory genes in skeletal muscles of peroxisome proliferator-activated receptor (PPAR) α knock-out mice. Evidence for compensatory regulation by PPARδ," *Journal of Biological Chemistry*, vol. 277, no. 29, pp. 26089–26097, 2002.

[34] U. Dressel, T. L. Allen, J. B. Pippal, P. R. Rohde, P. Lau, and G. E. O. Muscat, "The peroxisome proliferator-activated receptor β/δ agonist, GW501516, regulates the expression of genes involved in lipid catabolism and energy uncoupling in skeletal muscle cells," *Molecular Endocrinology*, vol. 17, no. 12, pp. 2477–2493, 2003.

[35] B. Brunmair, K. Staniek, J. Dörig et al., "Activation of PPAR-delta in isolated rat skeletal muscle switches fuel preference from glucose to fatty acids," *Diabetologia*, vol. 49, no. 11, pp. 2713–2722, 2006.

[36] L. Jiang, J. Wan, L.-Q. Ke, Q.-G. Lü, and N.-W. Tong, "Activation of PPARδ promotes mitochondrial energy metabolism and decreases basal insulin secretion in palmitate-treated β-cells," *Molecular and Cellular Biochemistry*, vol. 343, no. 1-2, pp. 249–256, 2010.

[37] M. C. Manio, K. Inoue, M. Fujitani, S. Matsumura, and T. Fushiki, "Combined pharmacological activation of AMPK and PPARδ potentiates the effects of exercise in trained mice," *Physiological Reports*, vol. 4, no. 5, Article ID e12625, 2016.

[38] S. Liu, B. Hatano, M. Zhao et al., "Role of peroxisome proliferator-activated receptor δ/β in hepatic metabolic regulation," *Journal of Biological Chemistry*, vol. 286, no. 2, pp. 1237–1247, 2011.

[39] L. M. Sanderson, M. V. Boekschoten, B. Desvergne, M. Müller, and S. Kersten, "Transcriptional profiling reveals divergent roles of PPARα and PPARβ/δ in regulation of gene expression in mouse liver," *Physiological Genomics*, vol. 41, no. 1, pp. 42–52, 2010.

[40] S. Liu, J. D. Brown, K. J. Stanya et al., "A diurnal serum lipid integrates hepatic lipogenesis and peripheral fatty acid use," *Nature*, vol. 502, no. 7472, pp. 550–554, 2013.

[41] D.-Y. Zhu, J.-Y. Wu, H. Li et al., "PPAR-β facilitating maturation of hepatic-like tissue derived from mouse embryonic stem cells accompanied by mitochondriogenesis and membrane potential retention," *Journal of Cellular Biochemistry*, vol. 109, no. 3, pp. 498–508, 2010.

[42] E. Hondares, M. Rosell, J. Díaz-Delfín et al., "Peroxisome proliferator-activated receptor α (PPARα) induces PPARγ coactivator 1α (PGC-1α) gene expression and contributes to thermogenic activation of brown fat: involvement of PRDM16," *Journal of Biological Chemistry*, vol. 286, no. 50, pp. 43112–43122, 2011.

[43] M. Schuler, F. Ali, C. Chambon et al., "PGC1α expression is controlled in skeletal muscles by PPARβ, whose ablation results in fiber-type switching, obesity, and type 2 diabetes," *Cell Metabolism*, vol. 4, no. 5, pp. 407–414, 2006.

[44] E. Hondares, I. Pineda-Torra, R. Iglesias, B. Staels, F. Villarroya, and M. Giralt, "PPARδ, but not PPARα, activates PGC-1α gene transcription in muscle," *Biochemical and Biophysical Research Communications*, vol. 354, no. 4, pp. 1021–1027, 2007.

[45] S. Herzig, F. Long, U. S. Jhala et al., "CREB regulates hepatic gluconeogenesis through the coactivator PGC-1," *Nature*, vol. 413, no. 6852, pp. 179–183, 2001.

[46] M. T. Nakamura, B. E. Yudell, and J. J. Loor, "Regulation of energy metabolism by long-chain fatty acids," *Progress in Lipid Research*, vol. 53, no. 1, pp. 124–144, 2014.

[47] M. Ricote, A. C. Li, T. M. Willson, C. J. Kelly, and C. K. Glass, "The peroxisome proliferator-activated receptor-γ is a negative regulator of macrophage activation," *Nature*, vol. 391, no. 6662, pp. 79–82, 1998.

[48] R. E. Soccio, E. R. Chen, and M. A. Lazar, "Thiazolidinediones and the promise of insulin sensitization in type 2 diabetes," *Cell Metabolism*, vol. 20, no. 4, pp. 573–591, 2014.

[49] M. Ahmadian, J. M. Suh, N. Hah et al., "PPARγ signaling and metabolism: the good, the bad and the future," *Nature Medicine*, vol. 19, no. 5, pp. 557–566, 2013.

[50] O. Gavrilova, M. Haluzik, K. Matsusue et al., "Liver peroxisome proliferator-activated receptor γ contributes to hepatic steatosis, triglyceride clearance, and regulation of body fat mass," *Journal of Biological Chemistry*, vol. 278, no. 36, pp. 34268–34276, 2003.

[51] K. Matsusue, M. Haluzik, G. Lambert et al., "Liver-specific disruption of PPARγ in leptin-deficient mice improves fatty liver but aggravates diabetic phenotypes," *The Journal of Clinical Investigation*, vol. 111, no. 5, pp. 737–747, 2003.

[52] P. Puigserver, Z. Wu, C. W. Park, R. Graves, M. Wright, and B. M. Spiegelman, "A cold-inducible coactivator of nuclear receptors linked to adaptive thermogenesis," *Cell*, vol. 92, no. 6, pp. 829–839, 1998.

[53] J. St-Pierre, J. Lin, S. Krauss et al., "Bioenergetic analysis of peroxisome proliferator-activated receptor γ coactivators 1α

and 1β (PGC-1α and PGC-1β) in muscle cells," *The Journal of Biological Chemistry*, vol. 278, no. 29, pp. 26597–26603, 2003.

[54] W. Fan and R. Evans, "PPARs and ERRs: molecular mediators of mitochondrial metabolism," *Current Opinion in Cell Biology*, vol. 33, pp. 49–54, 2015.

[55] E. Hondares, O. Mora, P. Yubero et al., "Thiazolidinediones and rexinoids induce peroxisome proliferator-activated receptor-coactivator (PGC)-1α gene transcription: an autoregulatory loop controls PGC-1α expression in adipocytes via peroxisome proliferator-activated receptor-γ coactivation," *Endocrinology*, vol. 147, no. 6, pp. 2829–2838, 2006.

[56] H. Maruyama, S. Kiyono, T. Kondo, T. Sekimoto, and O. Yokosuka, "Palmitate-induced regulation of PPARγ via PGC1α: a mechanism for lipid accumulation in the liver in nonalcoholic fatty liver disease," *International Journal of Medical Sciences*, vol. 13, no. 3, pp. 169–178, 2016.

[57] P. D. Ray, B.-W. Huang, and Y. Tsuji, "Reactive oxygen species (ROS) homeostasis and redox regulation in cellular signaling," *Cellular Signalling*, vol. 24, no. 5, pp. 981–990, 2012.

[58] M. Schieber and N. S. Chandel, "ROS function in redox signaling and oxidative stress," *Current Biology*, vol. 24, no. 10, pp. R453–R462, 2014.

[59] L. Zeng, W. J. Tang, J. J. Yin, and B. J. Zhou, "Signal transductions and nonalcoholic fatty liver: a mini-review," *International Journal of Clinical and Experimental Medicine*, vol. 7, no. 7, pp. 1624–1631, 2014.

[60] I. Afanas'ev, "Signaling of reactive oxygen and nitrogen species in diabetes mellitus," *Oxidative Medicine and Cellular Longevity*, vol. 3, no. 6, pp. 361–373, 2010.

[61] I. Afanas'ev, "Reactive oxygen species signaling in cancer: comparison with aging," *Aging and Disease*, vol. 2, no. 3, pp. 219–230, 2011.

[62] J. St-Pierre, J. A. Buckingham, S. J. Roebuck, and M. D. Brand, "Topology of superoxide production from different sites in the mitochondrial electron transport chain," *The Journal of Biological Chemistry*, vol. 277, no. 47, pp. 44784–44790, 2002.

[63] E. B. Tahara, F. D. T. Navarete, and A. J. Kowaltowski, "Tissue-, substrate-, and site-specific characteristics of mitochondrial reactive oxygen species generation," *Free Radical Biology and Medicine*, vol. 46, no. 9, pp. 1283–1297, 2009.

[64] T. Mello, F. Zanieri, E. Ceni, and A. Galli, "Oxidative stress in the healthy and wounded hepatocyte: a cellular organelles perspective," *Oxidative Medicine and Cellular Longevity*, vol. 2016, Article ID 8327410, 15 pages, 2016.

[65] C. Ricci, V. Pastukh, J. Leonard et al., "Mitochondrial DNA damage triggers mitochondrial-superoxide generation and apoptosis," *American Journal of Physiology—Cell Physiology*, vol. 294, no. 2, pp. C413–C422, 2008.

[66] H. Kawahara, M. Fukura, M. Tsuchishima, and S. Takase, "Mutation of mitochondrial DNA in livers from patients with alcoholic hepatitis and nonalcoholic steatohepatitis," *Alcoholism: Clinical and Experimental Research*, vol. 31, supplement 1, pp. S54–S60, 2007.

[67] L. Llacuna, A. Fernández, C. V. Montfort et al., "Targeting cholesterol at different levels in the mevalonate pathway protects fatty liver against ischemia-reperfusion injury," *Journal of Hepatology*, vol. 54, no. 5, pp. 1002–1010, 2011.

[68] L. A. Videla, R. Rodrigo, M. Orellana et al., "Oxidative stress-related parameters in the liver of non-alcoholic fatty liver disease patients," *Clinical Science*, vol. 106, no. 3, pp. 261–268, 2004.

[69] J. Xiao and G. L. Tipoe, "Inflammasomes in non-alcoholic fatty liver disease," *Frontiers in Bioscience*, vol. 21, pp. 683–695, 2016.

[70] D. Sharma and T. Kanneganti, "The cell biology of inflammasomes: mechanisms of inflammasome activation and regulation," *The Journal of Cell Biology*, vol. 213, no. 6, pp. 617–629, 2016.

[71] M. Y. Lee, R. Choi, H. M. Kim et al., "Peroxisome proliferator-activated receptor delta agonist attenuates hepatic steatosis by anti-inflammatory mechanism," *Experimental & Molecular Medicine*, vol. 44, no. 10, pp. 578–585, 2012.

[72] S. Seki, T. Kitada, T. Yamada, H. Sakaguchi, K. Nakatani, and K. Wakasa, "In situ detection of lipid peroxidation and oxidative DNA damage in non-alcoholic fatty liver diseases," *Journal of Hepatology*, vol. 37, no. 1, pp. 56–62, 2002.

[73] S. H. Caldwell, R. H. Swerdlow, E. M. Khan et al., "Mitochondrial abnormalities in non-alcoholic steatohepatitis," *Journal of Hepatology*, vol. 31, no. 3, pp. 430–434, 1999.

[74] M. Pérez-Carreras, P. Del Hoyo, M. A. Martín et al., "Defective hepatic mitochondrial respiratory chain in patients with nonalcoholic steatohepatitis," *Hepatology*, vol. 38, no. 4, pp. 999–1007, 2003.

[75] R. Gambino, G. Musso, and M. Cassader, "Redox balance in the pathogenesis of nonalcoholic fatty liver disease: mechanisms and therapeutic opportunities," *Antioxidants and Redox Signaling*, vol. 15, no. 5, pp. 1325–1365, 2011.

[76] Y. Ikura, M. Ohsawa, T. Suekane et al., "Localization of oxidized phosphatidylcholine in nonalcoholic fatty liver disease: impact on disease progression," *Hepatology*, vol. 43, no. 3, pp. 506–514, 2006.

[77] S. Li, X.-Y. Zeng, X. Zhou et al., "Dietary cholesterol induces hepatic inflammation and blunts mitochondrial function in the liver of high-fat-fed mice," *Journal of Nutritional Biochemistry*, vol. 27, pp. 96–103, 2016.

[78] V. Ribas, C. García-Ruiz, and J. C. Fernández-Checa, "Mitochondria, cholesterol and cancer cell metabolism," *Clinical and Translational Medicine*, vol. 5, article 22, 2016.

[79] E. Ip, G. C. Farrell, G. Robertson, P. Hall, R. Kirsch, and I. Leclercq, "Central role of PPARα-dependent hepatic lipid turnover in dietary steatohepatitis in mice," *Hepatology*, vol. 38, no. 1, pp. 123–132, 2003.

[80] E. Ip, G. Farrell, P. Hall, G. Robertson, and I. Leclercq, "Administration of the potent PPARα agonist, Wy-14,643, reverses nutritional fibrosis and steatohepatitis in mice," *Hepatology*, vol. 39, no. 5, pp. 1286–1296, 2004.

[81] P. Costet, C. Legendre, J. Moré, A. Edgar, P. Galtier, and T. Pineau, "Peroxisome proliferator-activated receptor α-isoform deficiency leads to progressive dyslipidemia with sexually dimorphic obesity and steatosis," *The Journal of Biological Chemistry*, vol. 273, no. 45, pp. 29577–29585, 1998.

[82] M. A. Abdelmegeed, S.-H. Yoo, L. E. Henderson, F. J. Gonzalez, K. J. Woodcroft, and B.-J. Song, "PPARα expression protects male mice from high fat-induced nonalcoholic fatty liver," *The Journal of Nutrition*, vol. 141, no. 4, pp. 603–610, 2011.

[83] K. Begriche, J. Massart, M.-A. Robin, F. Bonnet, and B. Fromenty, "Mitochondrial adaptations and dysfunctions in nonalcoholic fatty liver disease," *Hepatology*, vol. 58, no. 4, pp. 1497–1507, 2013.

[84] M. Monetti, M. C. Levin, M. J. Watt et al., "Dissociation of hepatic steatosis and insulin resistance in mice overexpressing DGAT in the liver," *Cell Metabolism*, vol. 6, no. 1, pp. 69–78, 2007.

[85] W. Liao, T. Y. Hui, S. G. Young, and R. A. Davis, "Blocking microsomal triglyceride transfer protein interferes with apoB secretion without causing retention or stress in the ER," *Journal of Lipid Research*, vol. 44, no. 5, pp. 978–985, 2003.

[86] Z. Z. Li, M. Berk, T. M. McIntyre, and A. E. Feldstein, "Hepatic lipid partitioning and liver damage in nonalcoholic fatty liver disease: role of stearoyl-Coa desaturase," *Journal of Biological Chemistry*, vol. 284, no. 9, pp. 5637–5644, 2009.

[87] M. Sharma, S. Mitnala, R. K. Vishnubhotla, R. Mukherjee, D. N. Reddy, and P. N. Rao, "The riddle of nonalcoholic fatty liver disease: progression from nonalcoholic fatty liver to non-alcoholic steatohepatitis," *Journal of Clinical and Experimental Hepatology*, vol. 5, no. 2, pp. 147–158, 2015.

[88] K. Beier, A. Völkl, and D. Fahimi, "TNF-α downregulates the peroxisome proliferator activated receptor-α and the mRNAs encoding peroxisomal proteins in rat liver," *FEBS Letters*, vol. 412, no. 2, pp. 385–387, 1997.

[89] V. G. Giby and T. A. Ajith, "Role of adipokines and peroxisome proliferator-activated receptors in nonalcoholic fatty liver disease," *World Journal of Hepatology*, vol. 6, no. 8, pp. 570–579, 2014.

[90] S. R. Ande, K. H. Nguyen, B. L. Grégoire Nyomba, and S. Mishra, "Prohibitin-induced, obesity-associated insulin resistance and accompanying low-grade inflammation causes NASH and HCC," *Scientific Reports*, vol. 6, Article ID 23608, 2016.

[91] S. Francque, A. Verrijken, S. Caron et al., "PPARα gene expression correlates with severity and histological treatment response in patients with non-alcoholic steatohepatitis," *Journal of Hepatology*, vol. 63, no. 1, pp. 164–173, 2015.

[92] Y. M. Shah, K. Morimura, Q. Yang, T. Tanabe, M. Takagi, and F. J. Gonzalez, "Peroxisome proliferator-activated receptor α regulates a microRNA-mediated signaling cascade responsible for hepatocellular proliferation," *Molecular and Cellular Biology*, vol. 27, no. 12, pp. 4238–4247, 2007.

[93] N. Tanaka, K. Moriya, K. Kiyosawa, K. Koike, F. J. Gonzalez, and T. Aoyama, "PPARα activation is essential for HCV core protein-induced hepatic steatosis and hepatocellular carcinoma in mice," *The Journal of Clinical Investigation*, vol. 118, no. 2, pp. 683–694, 2008.

[94] F. J. Gonzalez and Y. M. Shah, "PPARα: mechanism of species differences and hepatocarcinogenesis of peroxisome proliferators," *Toxicology*, vol. 246, no. 1, pp. 2–8, 2008.

[95] S. Bonovas, G. K. Nikolopoulos, and P. G. Bagos, "Use of fibrates and cancer risk: a systematic review and meta-analysis of 17 long-term randomized placebo-controlled trials," *PLoS ONE*, vol. 7, no. 9, Article ID 0045259, 2012.

[96] N. Zhang, E. S. H. Chu, J. Zhang et al., "Peroxisome proliferator activated receptor alpha inhibits hepatocarcinogenesis through mediating NF-κB signaling pathway," *Oncotarget*, vol. 5, no. 18, pp. 8330–8340, 2014.

[97] M. C. Sugden and M. J. Holness, "Mechanisms underlying regulation of the expression and activities of the mammalian pyruvate dehydrogenase kinases," *Archives of Physiology and Biochemistry*, vol. 112, no. 3, pp. 139–149, 2006.

[98] M. Grabacka, M. Pierzchalska, and K. Reiss, "Peroxisome proliferator activated receptor α ligands as anticancer drugs targeting mitochondrial metabolism," *Current Pharmaceutical Biotechnology*, vol. 14, no. 3, pp. 342–356, 2013.

[99] S. Oka, R. Alcendor, P. Zhai et al., "PPARα-Sirt1 complex mediates cardiac hypertrophy and failure through suppression of the ERR transcriptional pathway," *Cell Metabolism*, vol. 14, no. 5, pp. 598–611, 2011.

[100] M. Pawlak, E. Baugé, W. Bourguet et al., "The transrepressive activity of peroxisome proliferator-activated receptor alpha is necessary and sufficient to prevent liver fibrosis in mice," *Hepatology*, vol. 60, no. 5, pp. 1593–1606, 2014.

[101] S. Kamarajugadda, J. R. Becker, E. A. Hanse et al., "Cyclin D1 represses peroxisome proliferator-activated receptor alpha and inhibits fatty acid oxidation," *Oncotarget*, vol. 7, no. 30, pp. 47674–47686, 2016.

[102] X. Qin, X. Xie, Y. Fan et al., "Peroxisome proliferator-activated receptor-δ induces insulin-induced gene-1 and suppresses hepatic lipogenesis in obese diabetic mice," *Hepatology*, vol. 48, no. 2, pp. 432–441, 2008.

[103] M. Goudarzi, T. Koga, C. Khozoie et al., "PPARβ/δ modulates ethanol-induced hepatic effects by decreasing pyridoxal kinase activity," *Toxicology*, vol. 311, no. 3, pp. 87–98, 2013.

[104] C.-H. Lee, P. Olson, A. Hevener et al., "PPARδ regulates glucose metabolism and insulin sensitivity," *Proceedings of the National Academy of Sciences of the United States of America*, vol. 103, no. 9, pp. 3444–3449, 2006.

[105] M. Zarei, E. Barroso, R. Leiva et al., "Heme-regulated eIF2α kinase modulates hepatic FGF21 and is activated by PPARβ/δ deficiency," *Diabetes*, vol. 65, no. 10, pp. 3185–3199, 2016.

[106] Y. Zhang, T. Lei, J. F. Huang et al., "The link between fibroblast growth factor 21 and sterol regulatory element binding protein 1c during lipogenesis in hepatocytes," *Molecular and Cellular Endocrinology*, vol. 342, no. 1-2, pp. 41–47, 2011.

[107] J. Xu, D. J. Lloyd, C. Hale et al., "Fibroblast growth factor 21 reverses hepatic steatosis, increases energy expenditure, and improves insulin sensitivity in diet-induced obese mice," *Diabetes*, vol. 58, no. 1, pp. 250–259, 2009.

[108] L. Serrano-Marco, R. Rodríguez-Calvo, I. El Kochairi et al., "Activation of peroxisome proliferator—activated receptor-β/-δ (PPAR-β/-δ) ameliorates insulin signaling and reduces SOCS3 levels by inhibiting STAT3 in interleukin-6-stimulated adipocytes," *Diabetes*, vol. 60, no. 7, pp. 1990–1999, 2011.

[109] X. Li, J. Li, X. Lu et al., "Treatment with PPARδ agonist alleviates non-alcoholic fatty liver disease by modulating glucose and fatty acid metabolic enzymes in a rat model," *International Journal of Molecular Medicine*, vol. 36, no. 3, pp. 767–775, 2015.

[110] H. J. Lee, J. E. Yeon, E. J. Ko et al., "Peroxisome proliferator-activated receptor-delta agonist ameliorated inflammasome activation in nonalcoholic fatty liver disease," *World Journal of Gastroenterology*, vol. 21, no. 45, pp. 12787–12799, 2015.

[111] L. A. Bojic, D. E. Telford, M. D. Fullerton et al., "PPARδ activation attenuates hepatic steatosis in $Ldlr^{-/-}$ mice by enhanced fat oxidation, reduced lipogenesis, and improved insulin sensitivity," *Journal of Lipid Research*, vol. 55, no. 7, pp. 1254–1266, 2014.

[112] U. Risérus, D. Sprecher, T. Johnson et al., "Activation of peroxisome proliferator-activated receptor (PPAR)δ promotes reversal of multiple metabolic abnormalities, reduces oxidative stress, and increases fatty acid oxidation in moderately obese men," *Diabetes*, vol. 57, no. 2, pp. 332–339, 2008.

[113] H. E. Bays, S. Schwartz, T. Littlejohn III et al., "MBX-8025, a novel peroxisome proliferator receptor-δ agonist: lipid and other metabolic effects in dyslipidemic overweight patients treated with and without atorvastatin," *Journal of Clinical Endocrinology and Metabolism*, vol. 96, no. 9, pp. 2889–2897, 2011.

[114] H.-X. Liu, Y. Fang, Y. Hu, F. J. Gonzalez, J. Fang, and Y.-J. Y. Wan, "PPARβ regulates liver regeneration by modulating Akt and E2f signaling," *PLoS ONE*, vol. 8, no. 6, Article ID e65644, 2013.

[115] M. Vacca, S. D'Amore, G. Graziano et al., "Clustering nuclear receptors in liver regeneration identifies candidate modulators of hepatocyte proliferation and hepatocarcinoma," *PLoS ONE*, vol. 9, no. 8, Article ID e104449, 2014.

[116] H. E. Hollingshead, R. L. Killins, M. G. Borland et al., "Peroxisome proliferator-activated receptor-β/δ (PPARβ/δ) ligands do not potentiate growth of human cancer cell lines," *Carcinogenesis*, vol. 28, no. 12, pp. 2641–2649, 2007.

[117] L. Xu, C. Han, K. Lim, and T. Wu, "Cross-talk between peroxisome proliferator-activated receptor δ and cytosolic phospholipase $A_2\alpha$/cyclooxygenase-2/prostaglandin E_2 signaling pathways in human hepatocellular carcinoma cells," *Cancer Research*, vol. 66, no. 24, pp. 11859–11868, 2006.

[118] S. Handeli and J. A. Simon, "A small-molecule inhibitor of Tcf/β-catenin signaling down-regulates PPARγ and PPARδ activities," *Molecular Cancer Therapeutics*, vol. 7, no. 3, pp. 521–529, 2008.

[119] C. Y. Cao, S. W.-F. Mok, V. W.-S. Cheng, and S. K.-W. Tsui, "The FHL2 regulation in the transcriptional circuitry of human cancers," *Gene*, vol. 572, no. 1, pp. 1–7, 2015.

[120] C.-F. Ng, P. K.-S. Ng, V. W.-Y. Lui et al., "FHL2 exhibits antiproliferative and anti-apoptotic activities in liver cancer cells," *Cancer Letters*, vol. 304, no. 2, pp. 97–106, 2011.

[121] H. Yau, K. Rivera, R. Lomonaco, and K. Cusi, "The future of thiazolidinedione therapy in the management of type 2 diabetes mellitus," *Current Diabetes Reports*, vol. 13, no. 3, pp. 329–341, 2013.

[122] D. M. Torres, C. D. Williams, and S. A. Harrison, "Features, diagnosis, and treatment of nonalcoholic fatty liver disease," *Clinical Gastroenterology and Hepatology*, vol. 10, no. 8, pp. 837–858, 2012.

[123] E. Boettcher, G. Csako, F. Pucino, R. Wesley, and R. Loomba, "Meta-analysis: pioglitazone improves liver histology and fibrosis in patients with non-alcoholic steatohepatitis," *Alimentary Pharmacology and Therapeutics*, vol. 35, no. 1, pp. 66–75, 2012.

[124] V. Ratziu, P. Giral, S. Jacqueminet et al., "Rosiglitazone for nonalcoholic steatohepatitis: one-year results of the randomized placebo-controlled Fatty Liver Improvement With Rosiglitazone Therapy (FLIRT) trial," *Gastroenterology*, vol. 135, no. 1, pp. 100–110, 2008.

[125] V. Ratziu, F. Charlotte, C. Bernhardt et al., "Long-term efficacy of rosiglitazone in nonalcoholic steatohepatitis: results of the Fatty Liver Improvement by Rosiglitazone Therapy (FLIRT 2) extension trial," *Hepatology*, vol. 51, no. 2, pp. 445–453, 2010.

[126] D. M. Torres, F. J. Jones, J. C. Shaw, C. D. Williams, J. A. Ward, and S. A. Harrison, "Rosiglitazone versus rosiglitazone and metformin versus rosiglitazone and losartan in the treatment of nonalcoholic steatohepatitis in humans: a 12-month randomized, prospective, open- label trial," *Hepatology*, vol. 54, no. 5, pp. 1631–1639, 2011.

[127] M. Gao, Y. Ma, M. Alsaggar, and D. Liu, "Dual outcomes of rosiglitazone treatment on fatty liver," *The AAPS Journal*, vol. 18, no. 4, pp. 1023–1031, 2016.

[128] P. Pettinelli and L. A. Videla, "Up-regulation of PPAR-γ mRNA expression in the liver of obese patients: an additional reinforcing lipogenic mechanism to SREBP-1c induction," *Journal of Clinical Endocrinology and Metabolism*, vol. 96, no. 5, pp. 1424–1430, 2011.

[129] M. Inoue, T. Ohtake, W. Motomura et al., "Increased expression of PPARγ in high fat diet-induced liver steatosis in mice," *Biochemical and Biophysical Research Communications*, vol. 336, no. 1, pp. 215–222, 2005.

[130] Y.-L. Zhang, A. Hernandez-Ono, P. Siri et al., "Aberrant hepatic expression of PPARγ2 stimulates hepatic lipogenesis in a mouse model of obesity, insulin resistance, dyslipidemia, and hepatic steatosis," *Journal of Biological Chemistry*, vol. 281, no. 49, pp. 37603–37615, 2006.

[131] A. Vidal-Puig, M. Jimenez-Liñan, B. B. Lowell et al., "Regulation of PPAR γ gene expression by nutrition and obesity in rodents," *The Journal of Clinical Investigation*, vol. 97, no. 11, pp. 2553–2561, 1996.

[132] G. P. Ables, "Update on Pparγ and nonalcoholic fatty liver disease," *PPAR Research*, vol. 2012, Article ID 912351, 5 pages, 2012.

[133] J. Sakamoto, H. Kimura, S. Moriyama et al., "Activation of human peroxisome proliferator-activated receptor (PPAR) subtypes by pioglitazone," *Biochemical and Biophysical Research Communications*, vol. 278, no. 3, pp. 704–711, 2000.

[134] E. Xu, M.-P. Forest, M. Schwab et al., "Hepatocyte-specific Ptpn6 deletion promotes hepatic lipid accretion, but reduces NAFLD in diet-induced obesity: potential role of PPARγ," *Hepatology*, vol. 59, no. 5, pp. 1803–1815, 2014.

[135] C. W. Wu, E. S. H. Chu, C. N. Y. Lam et al., "PPARγ is essential for protection against nonalcoholic steatohepatitis," *Gene Therapy*, vol. 17, no. 6, pp. 790–798, 2010.

[136] E. Morán-Salvador, M. López-Parra, V. García-Alonso et al., "Role for PPARγ in obesity-induced hepatic steatosis as determined by hepatocyte- and macrophage-specific conditional knockouts," *FASEB Journal*, vol. 25, no. 8, pp. 2538–2550, 2011.

[137] S. Kuntz, S. Mazerbourg, M. Boisbrun et al., "Energy restriction mimetic agents to target cancer cells: comparison between 2-deoxyglucose and thiazolidinediones," *Biochemical Pharmacology*, vol. 92, no. 1, pp. 102–111, 2014.

[138] A. Galli, T. Mello, E. Ceni, E. Surrenti, and C. Surrenti, "The potential of antidiabetic thiazolidinediones for anticancer therapy," *Expert Opinion on Investigational Drugs*, vol. 15, no. 9, pp. 1039–1049, 2006.

[139] C.-W. Wu, G. C. Farrell, and J. Yu, "Functional role of peroxisome-proliferator-activated receptor γ in hepatocellular carcinoma," *Journal of Gastroenterology and Hepatology*, vol. 27, no. 11, pp. 1665–1669, 2012.

[140] A. Laganà, S. Vitale, A. Nigro et al., "Pleiotropic Actions of Peroxisome Proliferator-Activated Receptors (PPARs) in dysregulated metabolic homeostasis, inflammation and cancer: current evidence and future perspectives," *International Journal of Molecular Sciences*, vol. 17, no. 7, p. 999, 2016.

[141] J. Yu, B. Shen, E. S. H. Chu et al., "Inhibitory role of peroxisome proliferator-activated receptor gamma in hepatocarcinogenesis in mice and *in vitro*," *Hepatology*, vol. 51, no. 6, pp. 2008–2019, 2010.

[142] A. Galli, E. Ceni, T. Mello et al., "Thiazolidinediones inhibit hepatocarcinogenesis in hepatitis B virus-transgenic mice by peroxisome proliferator-activated receptor γ-independent regulation of nucleophosmin," *Hepatology*, vol. 52, no. 2, pp. 493–505, 2010.

[143] E. Ceni, T. Mello, M. Tarocchi et al., "Antidiabetic thiazolidinediones induce ductal differentiation but not apoptosis in pancreatic cancer cells," *World Journal of Gastroenterology*, vol. 11, no. 8, pp. 1122–1130, 2005.

[144] X. Ren, D. Zheng, F. Guo et al., "PPARγ suppressed Wnt/β-catenin signaling pathway and its downstream effector SOX9 expression in gastric cancer cells," *Medical Oncology*, vol. 32, no. 4, 2015.

[145] K. Wu, Y. Yang, D. Liu et al., "Activation of PPARγ suppresses proliferation and induces apoptosis of esophageal cancer cells by inhibiting TLR4-dependent MAPK pathway," *Oncotarget*, 2016.

[146] S. Dionne, E. Levy, D. Levesque, and E. G. Seidman, "PPARγ ligand 15-deoxy-delta 12,14-prostaglandin J2 sensitizes human colon carcinoma cells to TWEAK-induced apoptosis," *Anticancer Research*, vol. 30, no. 1, pp. 157–166, 2010.

[147] O. Pellerito, A. Notaro, S. Sabella et al., "WIN induces apoptotic cell death in human colon cancer cells through a block of autophagic flux dependent on PPARγ down-regulation," *Apoptosis*, vol. 19, no. 6, pp. 1029–1042, 2014.

[148] D. M. Ray, S. H. Bernstein, and R. P. Phipps, "Human multiple myeloma cells express peroxisome proliferator-activated receptor γ and undergo apoptosis upon exposure to PPARγ ligands," *Clinical Immunology*, vol. 113, no. 2, pp. 203–213, 2004.

[149] A. Galli, E. Ceni, D. W. Crabb et al., "Antidiabetic thiazolidinediones inhibit invasiveness of pancreatic cancer cells via PPARγ independent mechanisms," *Gut*, vol. 53, no. 11, pp. 1688–1697, 2004.

[150] L.-Q. Cao, Z.-L. Shao, H.-H. Liang et al., "Activation of peroxisome proliferator-activated receptor-γ (PPARγ) inhibits hepatoma cell growth via downregulation of SEPT2 expression," *Cancer Letters*, vol. 359, no. 1, pp. 127–135, 2015.

[151] I. Cellai, G. Petrangolini, M. Tortoreto et al., "*In vivo* effects of rosiglitazone in a human neuroblastoma xenograft," *British Journal of Cancer*, vol. 102, no. 4, pp. 685–692, 2010.

[152] B. Shen, E. S. H. Chu, G. Zhao et al., "PPARgamma inhibits hepatocellular carcinoma metastases in vitro and in mice," *British Journal of Cancer*, vol. 106, no. 9, pp. 1486–1494, 2012.

[153] P. Avena, W. Anselmo, D. Whitaker-Menezes et al., "Compartment-specific activation of PPARγ governs breast cancer tumor growth, via metabolic reprogramming and symbiosis," *Cell Cycle*, vol. 12, no. 9, pp. 1360–1370, 2013.

[154] J. A. Menendez, "Fine-tuning the lipogenic/lipolytic balance to optimize the metabolic requirements of cancer cell growth: molecular mechanisms and therapeutic perspectives," *Biochimica et Biophysica Acta—Molecular and Cell Biology of Lipids*, vol. 1801, no. 3, pp. 381–391, 2010.

[155] D. F. Calvisi, C. Wang, C. Ho et al., "Increased lipogenesis, induced by AKT-mTORC1-RPS6 signaling, promotes development of human hepatocellular carcinoma," *Gastroenterology*, vol. 140, no. 3, pp. 1071–1083, 2011.

[156] J. Hu, L. Che, L. Li et al., "Co-activation of AKT and c-Met triggers rapid hepatocellular carcinoma development via the mTORC1/FASN pathway in mice," *Scientific Reports*, vol. 6, Article ID 20484, 2016.

[157] L. Li, L. Che, K. M. Tharp et al., "Differential requirement for *de novo* lipogenesis in cholangiocarcinoma and hepatocellular carcinoma of mice and humans," *Hepatology*, vol. 63, no. 6, pp. 1900–1913, 2016.

[158] L. Li, G. M. Pilo, X. Li et al., "Inactivation of fatty acid synthase impairs hepatocarcinogenesis driven by AKT in mice and humans," *Journal of Hepatology*, vol. 64, no. 2, pp. 333–341, 2016.

[159] D. Cao, X. Song, L. Che et al., "Both *de novo* synthetized and exogenous fatty acids support the growth of hepatocellular carcinoma cells," *Liver International*, 2016.

[160] J. Samarin, V. Laketa, M. Malz et al., "PI3K/AKT/mTOR-dependent stabilization of oncogenic far-upstream element binding proteins in hepatocellular carcinoma cells," *Hepatology*, vol. 63, no. 3, pp. 813–826, 2016.

[161] C. Wang, L. Che, J. Hu et al., "Activated mutant forms of PIK3CA cooperate with RasV12 or c-Met to induce liver tumour formation in mice via AKT2/mTORC1 cascade," *Liver International*, vol. 36, no. 8, pp. 1176–1186, 2016.

[162] M. Laplante and D. M. Sabatini, "Regulation of mTORC1 and its impact on gene expression at a glance," *Journal of Cell Science*, vol. 126, pp. 1713–1719, 2013.

[163] G. Panasyuk, C. Espeillac, C. Chauvin et al., "PPARγ contributes to PKM2 and HK2 expression in fatty liver," *Nature Communications*, vol. 3, article 672, 2012.

[164] D. P. King and J. S. Takahashi, "Molecular genetics of circadian rhythms in mammals," *Annual Review of Neuroscience*, vol. 23, pp. 713–742, 2000.

[165] U. Schibler and P. Sassone-Corsi, "A web of circadian pacemakers," *Cell*, vol. 111, no. 7, pp. 919–922, 2002.

[166] D. Feng and M. A. Lazar, "Clocks, metabolism, and the epigenome," *Molecular Cell*, vol. 47, no. 2, pp. 158–167, 2012.

[167] N. Koike, S.-H. Yoo, H.-C. Huang et al., "Transcriptional architecture and chromatin landscape of the core circadian clock in mammals," *Science*, vol. 338, no. 6105, pp. 349–354, 2012.

[168] J. Morf, G. Rey, K. Schneider et al., "Cold-inducible RNA-binding protein modulates circadian gene expression posttranscriptionally," *Science*, vol. 338, no. 6105, pp. 379–383, 2012.

[169] G. Rey, F. Cesbron, J. Rougemont, H. Reinke, M. Brunner, and F. Naef, "Genome-wide and phase-specific DNA-binding rhythms of BMAL1 control circadian output functions in mouse liver," *PLoS Biology*, vol. 9, no. 2, Article ID e1000595, 2011.

[170] H. Yoshitane, H. Ozaki, H. Terajima et al., "CLOCK-controlled polyphonic regulation of circadian rhythms through canonical and noncanonical E-boxes," *Molecular and Cellular Biology*, vol. 34, no. 10, pp. 1776–1787, 2014.

[171] Y. Tahara and S. Shibata, "Circadian rhythms of liver physiology and disease: experimental and clinical evidence," *Nature Reviews Gastroenterology and Hepatology*, vol. 13, no. 4, pp. 217–226, 2016.

[172] X. Tong and L. Yin, "Circadian rhythms in liver physiology and liver diseases," *Comprehensive Physiology*, vol. 3, no. 2, pp. 917–940, 2013.

[173] S. Sahar and P. Sassone-Corsi, "Metabolism and cancer: the circadian clock connection," *Nature Reviews Cancer*, vol. 9, no. 12, pp. 886–896, 2009.

[174] C. B. Peek, A. H. Affinati, K. M. Ramsey et al., "Circadian clock NAD$^+$ cycle drives mitochondrial oxidative metabolism in mice," *Science*, vol. 342, no. 6158, Article ID 1243417, 2013.

[175] M. D. Hirschey, T. Shimazu, J.-Y. Huang, B. Schwer, and E. Verdin, "SIRT3 regulates mitochondrial protein acetylation and intermediary metabolism," *Cold Spring Harbor Symposia on Quantitative Biology*, vol. 76, pp. 267–277, 2011.

[176] G. F. Gibbons, D. Patel, D. Wiggins, and B. L. Knight, "The functional efficiency of lipogenic and cholesterogenic gene expression in normal mice and in mice lacking the peroxisomal proliferator-activated receptor-alpha (PPAR-α)," *Advances in Enzyme Regulation*, vol. 42, pp. 227–247, 2002.

[177] D. D. Patel, B. L. Knight, D. Wiggins, S. M. Humphreys, and G. F. Gibbons, "Disturbances in the normal regulation of SREBP-sensitive genes in PPARα-deficient mice," *Journal of Lipid Research*, vol. 42, no. 3, pp. 328–337, 2001.

[178] K. Oishi, H. Shirai, and N. Ishida, "CLOCK is involved in the circadian transactivation of peroxisome-proliferator-activated receptor α (PPARα) in mice," *Biochemical Journal*, vol. 386, no. 3, pp. 575–581, 2005.

[179] P. Gervois, S. Chopin-Delannoy, A. Fadel et al., "Fibrates increase human REV-ERBα expression in liver via a novel peroxisome proliferator-activated receptor response element," *Molecular Endocrinology*, vol. 13, no. 3, pp. 400–409, 1999.

[180] L. Canaple, J. Rambaud, O. Dkhissi-Benyahya et al., "Reciprocal regulation of brain and muscle Arnt-like protein 1 and peroxisome proliferator-activated receptor α defines a novel positive feedback loop in the rodent liver circadian clock," *Molecular Endocrinology*, vol. 20, no. 8, pp. 1715–1727, 2006.

[181] L. Chen and G. Yang, "PPARs integrate the mammalian clock and energy metabolism," *PPAR Research*, vol. 2014, Article ID 653017, 6 pages, 2014.

[182] F. Gachon, N. Leuenberger, T. Claudel et al., "Proline- and acidic amino acid-rich basic leucine zipper proteins modulate peroxisome proliferator-activated receptor α (PPARα) activity," *Proceedings of the National Academy of Sciences of the United States of America*, vol. 108, no. 12, pp. 4794–4799, 2011.

[183] A. Benavides, M. Siches, and M. Llobera, "Circadian rhythms of lipoprotein lipase and hepatic lipase activities in intermediate metabolism of adult rat," *American Journal of Physiology—Regulatory Integrative and Comparative Physiology*, vol. 275, no. 3, part 2, pp. R811–R817, 1998.

[184] M. C. Hunt, P. J. G. Lindquist, J. M. Peters, F. J. Gonzalez, U. Diczfalusy, and S. E. H. Alexson, "Involvement of the peroxisome proliferator-activated receptor α in regulating long-chain acyl-CoA thioesterases," *Journal of Lipid Research*, vol. 41, no. 5, pp. 814–823, 2000.

[185] M. C. Hunt, K. Solaas, B. Frode Kase, and S. E. H. Alexson, "Characterization of an acyl-CoA thioesterase that functions as a major regulator of peroxisomal lipid metabolism," *Journal of Biological Chemistry*, vol. 277, no. 2, pp. 1128–1138, 2002.

[186] K. Schoonjans, J. Peinado-Onsurbe, A.-M. Lefebvre et al., "PPARα and PPARγ activators direct a distinct tissue-specific transcriptional response via a PPRE in the lipoprotein lipase gene," *The EMBO Journal*, vol. 15, no. 19, pp. 5336–5348, 1996.

[187] M. Kawai, C. B. Green, B. Lecka-Czernik et al., "A circadian-regulated gene, *Nocturnin*, promotes adipogenesis by stimulating PPAR-γ nuclear translocation," *Proceedings of the National Academy of Sciences of the United States of America*, vol. 107, no. 23, pp. 10508–10513, 2010.

[188] G. Yang, Z. Jia, T. Aoyagi, D. McClain, R. M. Mortensen, and T. Yang, "Systemic pparγ deletion impairs circadian rhythms of behavior and metabolism," *PLoS ONE*, vol. 7, no. 8, Article ID e38117, 2012.

[189] C. Liu, S. Li, T. Liu, J. Borjigin, and J. D. Lin, "Transcriptional coactivator PGC-1α integrates the mammalian clock and energy metabolism," *Nature*, vol. 447, no. 7143, pp. 477–481, 2007.

[190] J. Sonoda, I. R. Mehl, L.-W. Chong, R. R. Nofsinger, and R. M. Evans, "PGC-1β controls mitochondrial metabolism to modulate circadian activity, adaptive thermogenesis, and hepatic steatosis," *Proceedings of the National Academy of Sciences of the United States of America*, vol. 104, no. 12, pp. 5223–5228, 2007.

[191] H. R. Ueda, W. Chen, A. Adachi et al., "A transcription factor response element for gene expression during circadian night," *Nature*, vol. 418, no. 6897, pp. 534–539, 2002.

[192] C. Esau, S. Davis, S. F. Murray et al., "miR-122 regulation of lipid metabolism revealed by in vivo antisense targeting," *Cell Metabolism*, vol. 3, no. 2, pp. 87–98, 2006.

[193] D. Gatfield, G. Le Martelot, C. E. Vejnar et al., "Integration of microRNA miR-122 in hepatic circadian gene expression," *Genes and Development*, vol. 23, no. 11, pp. 1313–1326, 2009.

[194] A. Neufeld-Cohen, M. S. Robles, R. Aviram et al., "Circadian control of oscillations in mitochondrial rate-limiting enzymes and nutrient utilization by PERIOD proteins," *Proceedings of the National Academy of Sciences of the United States of America*, vol. 113, no. 12, pp. E1673–E1682, 2016.

[195] E. Filipski, P. F. Innominato, M. W. Wu et al., "Effects of light and food schedules on liver and tumor molecular clocks in mice," *Journal of the National Cancer Institute*, vol. 97, no. 7, pp. 507–517, 2005.

[196] E. Filipski, P. Subramanian, J. Carrière, C. Guettier, H. Barbason, and F. Lévi, "Circadian disruption accelerates liver carcinogenesis in mice," *Mutation Research—Genetic Toxicology and Environmental Mutagenesis*, vol. 680, no. 1-2, pp. 95–105, 2009.

[197] K. D. Bruce, D. Szczepankiewicz, K. K. Sihota et al., "Altered cellular redox status, sirtuin abundance and clock gene expression in a mouse model of developmentally primed NASH," *Biochimica et Biophysica Acta (BBA)—Molecular and Cell Biology of Lipids*, vol. 1861, no. 7, pp. 584–593, 2016.

[198] U. S. Udoh, J. A. Valcin, K. L. Gamble, and S. M. Bailey, "The molecular circadian clock and alcohol-induced liver injury," *Biomolecules*, vol. 5, no. 4, pp. 2504–2537, 2015.

[199] K. Honma, M. Hikosaka, K. Mochizuki, and T. Goda, "Loss of circadian rhythm of circulating insulin concentration induced by high-fat diet intake is associated with disrupted rhythmic expression of circadian clock genes in the liver," *Metabolism*, vol. 65, no. 4, pp. 482–491, 2016.

[200] F. W. Turek, C. Joshu, A. Kohsaka et al., "Obesity and metabolic syndrome in circadian Clock mutant mice," *Science*, vol. 308, no. 5724, pp. 1043–1045, 2005.

[201] K. L. Eckel-Mahan, V. R. Patel, S. de Mateo et al., "Reprogramming of the circadian clock by nutritional challenge," *Cell*, vol. 155, no. 7, pp. 1464–1478, 2013.

[202] K. Matsusue, T. Kusakabe, T. Noguchi et al., "Hepatic steatosis in leptin-deficient mice is promoted by the PPARγ target gene Fsp27," *Cell Metabolism*, vol. 7, no. 4, pp. 302–311, 2008.

[203] C. B. Green, N. Douris, S. Kojima et al., "Loss of Nocturnin, a circadian deadenylase, confers resistance to hepatic steatosis and diet-induced obesity," *Proceedings of the National Academy of Sciences of the United States of America*, vol. 104, no. 23, pp. 9888–9893, 2007.

[204] Y.-M. Lin, J. H. Chang, K.-T. Yeh et al., "Disturbance of circadian gene expression in hepatocellular carcinoma," *Molecular Carcinogenesis*, vol. 47, no. 12, pp. 925–933, 2008.

[205] B. Zhao, J. Lu, J. Yin et al., "A functional polymorphism in *PER3* gene is associated with prognosis in hepatocellular carcinoma," *Liver International*, vol. 32, no. 9, pp. 1451–1459, 2012.

[206] S. Ishibashi, S. Yamashita, H. Arai et al., "Effects of K-877, a novel selective PPARα modulator (SPPARMα), in dyslipidaemic patients: a randomized, double blind, active- and placebo-controlled, phase 2 trial," *Atherosclerosis*, vol. 249, pp. 36–43, 2016.

[207] S. Raza-Iqbal, T. Tanaka, M. Anai et al., "Transcriptome analysis of K-877 (A novel selective PPARα modulator (SPPARMα))-regulated genes in primary human hepatocytes and the mouse liver," *Journal of Atherosclerosis and Thrombosis*, vol. 22, no. 8, pp. 754–772, 2015.

[208] J. P. Taygerly, L. R. McGee, S. M. Rubenstein et al., "Discovery of INT131: a selective PPARγ modulator that enhances insulin sensitivity," *Bioorganic and Medicinal Chemistry*, vol. 21, no. 4, pp. 979–992, 2013.

[209] B. Cariou, R. Hanf, S. Lambert-Porcheron et al., "Dual peroxisome proliferator-activated receptor α/δ agonist gft505 improves hepatic and peripheral insulin sensitivity in abdominally obese subjects," *Diabetes Care*, vol. 36, no. 10, pp. 2923–2930, 2013.

[210] B. Cariou, Y. Zaïr, B. Staels, and E. Bruckert, "Effects of the new dual PPARα/δ agonist GFT505 on lipid and glucose homeostasis in abdominally obese patients with combined dyslipidemia or impaired glucose metabolism," *Diabetes Care*, vol. 34, no. 9, pp. 2008–2014, 2011.

[211] B. Staels, A. Rubenstrunk, B. Noel et al., "Hepatoprotective effects of the dual peroxisome proliferator-activated receptor alpha/delta agonist, GFT505, in rodent models of nonalcoholic fatty liver disease/nonalcoholic steatohepatitis," *Hepatology*, vol. 58, no. 6, pp. 1941–1952, 2013.

[212] V. Ratziu, S. A. Harrison, S. Francque et al., "Elafibranor, an agonist of the peroxisome proliferator–activated receptor–α and –δ, induces resolution of nonalcoholic steatohepatitis without fibrosis worsening," *Gastroenterology*, vol. 150, no. 5, pp. 1147.e5–1159.e5, 2016.

3

PPARδ as a Metabolic Initiator of Mammary Neoplasia and Immune Tolerance

Robert I. Glazer

Department of Oncology, Georgetown University Medical Center and the Lombardi Comprehensive Cancer Center, 3970 Reservoir Rd, NW, Washington, DC 20007, USA

Correspondence should be addressed to Robert I. Glazer; glazerr@georgetown.edu

Academic Editor: Stefano Caruso

PPARδ is a ligand-activated nuclear receptor that regulates the transcription of genes associated with proliferation, metabolism, inflammation, and immunity. Within this transcription factor family, PPARδ is unique in that it initiates oncogenesis in a metabolic and tissue-specific context, especially in mammary epithelium, and can regulate autoimmunity in some tissues. This review discusses its role in these processes and how it ultimately impacts breast cancer.

1. Introduction

The PPAR nuclear receptor family consists of the PPARα, PPARγ, and PPARδ/β isotypes, which function as heterodimeric partners with RXR with specificity dictated by high-affinity binding of PPAR ligands and coactivators [1]. Similar to other nuclear receptors, PPARs contain an N-terminal transactivation domain, a DNA-binding domain, a ligand-binding domain, and a C-terminal ligand-dependent transactivation region [2]. PPARs bind to a DR-1 response element (PPRE) with the consensus sequence AGG(T/A)CA that is recognized specifically by the PPAR heterodimeric partner [3]. Ligand-activated PPARs interact with coactivators CEBPA/B and NCOA3 and in the unliganded state with corepressor NCOR2 [4–7]. Of the three isotypes, PPARδ plays a dominant role in regulating fatty acid β-oxidation, glucose utilization, cholesterol transport, and energy balance [8–10] but also modulates the cell cycle, apoptosis, angiogenesis, inflammation, and cell lineage specification [11–14]. These multifaceted functions indicate that PPARδ has a critical homeostatic role in normal physiology and that its aberrant expression can impact the initiation and promotion of oncogenesis. This review discusses recent advances pertaining to the involvement of PPARδ in these processes primarily as they relate to mammary tumorigenesis.

2. PPARδ and Tumorigenesis

The role of PPARδ in tumorigenesis has been investigated for almost two decades, and whether it exerts an oncogenic or antioncogenic role depends in large part on the targeted tissue and the gene targeting strategy utilized [14–16]. In the context of the mammary gland, however, most animal models confirm that PPARδ exerts an oncogenic effect. This can be envisioned to result in part from competition between the tumor promoting effects of PPARδ and the tumor suppressor effects of PPARγ. PPARγ agonists reduce mammary carcinogenesis [17–19], which correlates with induction of PTEN [20, 21] and BRCA1 [22] tumor suppressor activity, as well as reduction of inflammation via the Cox2/Ptgs2 pathway [23]. Conversely, PPARγ haploinsufficiency [23] or expression of a dominant-negative Pax8-PPARγ transgene [24] and direct or indirect inhibition of PPARγ [21, 25] enhance DMBA mammary carcinogenesis. In MMTV-Pax8-PPARγ mice, the increased rate of carcinogenesis correlates with enhanced Wnt, Ras/Erk, and PDK1/Akt signaling, reduced PTEN expression, and a more stem cell-like phenotype [24]. The respective Yin/Yang functions of PPARδ and PPARγ are consistent with the ability of PPARδ to enhance survival through the PI3K and PDK1 pathways in response to wound healing [26, 27], as well as with the proliferative and

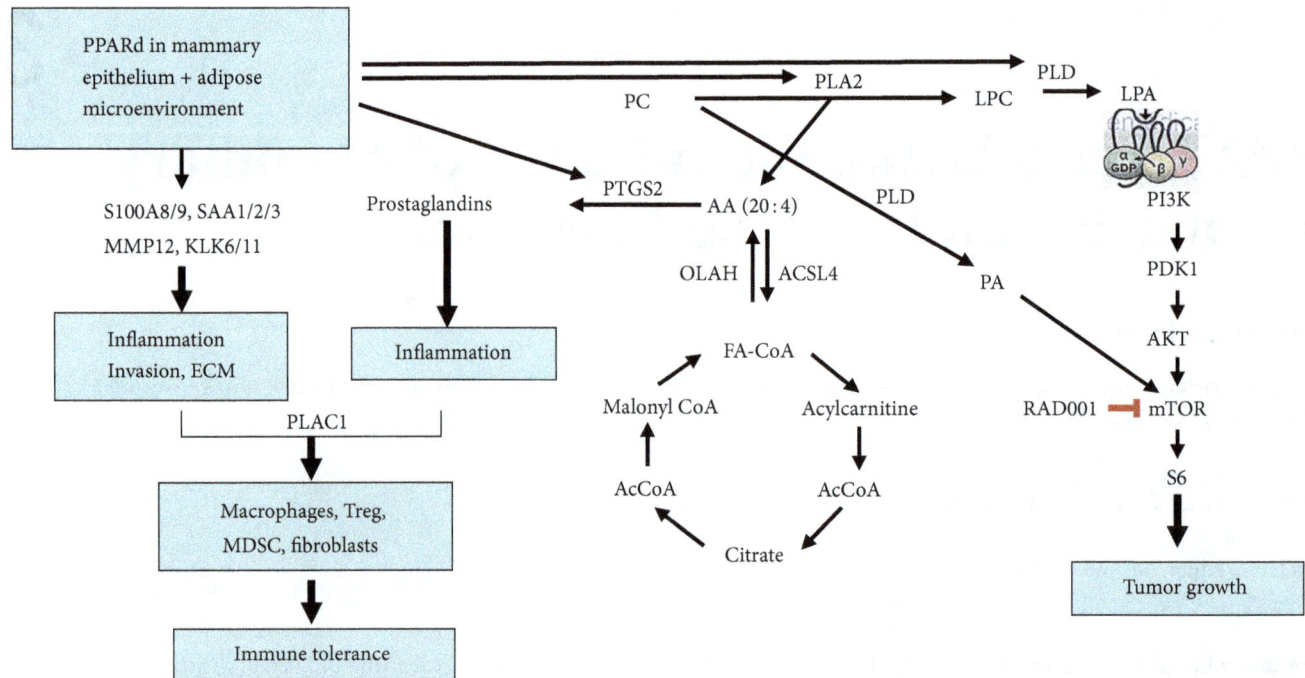

FIGURE 1: Interactions between inflammation, metabolism, and mTOR signaling in the mammary gland of MMTV-PPARδ mice. PPARδ activates PPRE-containing genes associated with metabolism (Olah, Ptgs2, Pla2, and Pld), invasion (Mmp12, Klk6), and inflammation (S100a8/9, Saa1/2/3). Arachidonic acid (AA) is a substrate for Ptgs2 and is a constituent of phosphatidylcholine (PC) required for prostaglandin synthesis. Lysophosphatidylcholine (LPC) is generated from PC by phospholipase A2 (Pla2), and lysophosphatidic acid (LPA) and phosphatidic acid (PA) are generated by phospholipase D (Pld). LPA stimulates mTOR through a G protein-coupled receptor, and PA directly activates mTOR. The mTOR inhibitor RAD001 (everolimus) inhibits tumorigenesis in this animal model. The net result is an increase in inflammation, extracellular matrix remodeling, immune suppression, and neoplasia. Adapted from [31].

angiogenic response of breast cancer and endothelial cells to conditional activation of PPARδ [28]. The induction of PDK1 signaling by the PPARδ agonist GW501516 in DMBA-treated wild-type mice [19], the increased expression of PPARδ in GW501516-treated MMTV-PDK1 mice [29], and reduction of mammary tumorigenesis in MMTV-Cox2 mice crossed into a PPARδ null background [30] further support its oncogenic potential. This outcome was ultimately proven by the generation of MMTV-PPARδ mice, which developed infiltrating mammary adenocarcinomas and whose progression was accelerated by, but not dependent on, agonist stimulation [31]. From a clinical perspective, this result is concordant with the increased expression of PPARδ in invasive breast cancer [12, 32] and by manifestation of a PPARδ signaling network that predicts poor survival in this disease [33].

A signature feature of MMTV-PPARδ mice is the development of ER+/PR+/ErbB2− tumors resembling the luminal B subtype of breast cancer [31], which is denoted by lower ER expression, higher Ki-67 staining, and a higher histologic grade [34]. Since ER mRNA is relatively low in these mice in comparison to immunohistochemical staining, it suggests that PPARδ may affect ER stability posttranslationally, for example, phosphorylation of ER Ser167 by mTOR/S6K [35], a pathway activated in this mouse model (Figure 1). The development of ER+ tumors in MMTV-PPARδ mice is similar to what was observed in DMBA-treated MMTV-Pax8-PPARγ mice [24] and DMBA-treated wild-type mice administered

the irreversible PPARγ inhibitor, GW9662 [25]. These findings support the notion that PPARγ and PPARδ, either by direct competition [36], cofactor competition [37], and/or ligand-dependent activation [38] have opposing actions that affect expansion of the ER+ lineage tumor subtype. Interestingly, ER+ tumors also arose in MMTV-NCOA3 mice [39, 40], but not in other MMTV-driven transgenic models [41], suggesting that it is the PPARδ coactivator complex itself, rather than the MMTV promoter that drives expansion of the ER+ lineage. This conclusion is also supported by the similarities between MMTV-NCOA3 and MMTV-PPARδ mice for activation of the mTOR signaling axis [39, 40], suggesting its importance in ER+ luminal tumor specification.

Another intriguing feature of MMTV-PPARδ mice is the association between the onset of neoplasia and the upregulation of Plac1 [31], a microvillous membrane protein expressed primarily in trophoblasts, but not in most somatic tissues [42] (Figure 1). Plac1 is reexpressed in several malignancies [43–45], and reduction of Plac1 in breast cancer cells inhibits proliferation and invasion [43]. These findings suggest that Plac1 may serve as a diagnostic biomarker as shown by the more favorable prognosis of colorectal cancer patients expressing Plac1 autoantibodies [46]. Analysis of a limited set of paired breast cancer specimens indicates that Plac1 expression is elevated in the majority of biopsies, but not in adjacent normal tissue (Isaacs and Glazer, unpublished results), which is consistent with the presence of circulating Plac1 RNA in the majority of breast cancer subjects [43, 44]. The high level of expression of Plac1 in MMTV-PPARδ mice also suggests that Plac1 may be under the transcriptional control of PPARδ as demonstrated by its dependence on the PPARδ coactivators CEBPA and CEBPB [47] and the presence of PPREs in the promoter regions of mouse and human *Plac1* (http://www.genecards.org/cgi-bin/carddisp.pl?gene=PLAC1 &keywords=plac1).

3. PPARδ and Inflammation

One of the earliest recognized functions of PPARδ was its antiapoptotic, chemotactic, and inflammatory actions mediated through the Akt and Rho pathways in response to wound healing in keratinocytes [26, 27, 48]. This was the first indication that PPARδ might be a contributing factor to inflammatory disorders, such as psoriasis [49], and tumorigenesis. It had been previously shown that inflammatory molecules, such as eicosanoids, could serve as endogenous PPARδ ligands [50–52]. In colon tumorigenesis and colitis, Ptgs2 and prostaglandin synthesis are dependent on PPARδ [53, 54], whereas inhibition of tumorigenesis by NSAIDs results from induction of the endogenous PPARδ antagonist, 13-S-hydroxyoctadecadienoic acid [55]. Of note is that a similar Ptgs2/prostaglandin phenotype is expressed in MMTV-PPARδ mice (Figure 1) [31], which is consistent with the induction of mammary tumorigenesis in MMTV-Ptgs2 mice [56], but not in PPARδ-null mice [30]. These findings suggest a feed-forward mechanism, whereby transactivation of the prostaglandin E2 receptor, Ptger4, by PPARδ [57], coupled with the generation of arachidonic acid by phospholipase A2 [58] and the biosynthesis of prostaglandin E_2 (PGE_2) via Pges2, elicits a self-sustaining inflammatory response.

In addition to activation of the prostaglandin axis, PPARδ increases expression of the acute phase proteins Saa1, Saa2, S100a8, and S100a9, as well as several members of the kallikrein gene family [31], all of which are elevated in ER^+ breast cancer [59, 60] and whose promoter regions contain PPREs. S100a8 and S100a9 are ligands for Ager (advanced glycation end-product receptor), another PPAR-dependent gene that mediates acute and chronic inflammation, tumor development, and metastasis in several types of cancer and proliferative disorders [61, 62], including gastric carcinogenesis [63] and psoriasis [49]. Thus, there is strong evidence to implicate PPARδ in driving multiple inflammatory pathways implicated in tumorigenesis.

4. PPARδ and Metabolism

PPARδ is one of the primary regulators of intermediary metabolism, including fatty acid synthesis and β-oxidation, particularly in adipose and muscle tissue [13, 64]. In MMTV-PPARδ mice, PPARδ functions as an integrator of metabolism and tumorigenesis via the biosynthesis of lysophosphatidic acid (LPA), a metabolite that promotes mammary tumorigenesis [65, 66], and phosphatidic acid (PA), a metabolite that directly activates mTOR [67] (Figure 1). The LPA/PA signaling pathway is also coupled to expression of Pdk4, a PPARδ-regulated inhibitor of pyruvate

oxidation that increases unsaturated fatty acid, arachidonic acid, LPA, and PA biosynthesis in MMTV-PDK1 mice [29, 31] and is in accordance with the capacity of long chain unsaturated fatty acids to serve as endogenous PPARδ ligands [50–52]. Additionally, PPARδ upregulates the fatty acid-binding protein (FABP) gene family [68], which facilitate fatty acid transport and potentiate EGFR- and ErbB2-mediated proliferation [69, 70] and invasion [71]. Lastly, PPARδ and fatty acid oxidation are required to maintain asymmetric stem cell division [72], an area that may be linked to ER^+ tumor specification and one unexplored thus far in mammary tumorigenesis.

5. PPARs and Immune Tolerance

One of the primary mechanisms associated with cancer progression is the coopting of immune tolerance to produce an immunologically permissive tumor microenvironment [73]. This can occur through several mechanisms associated with adaptive immunity, including expansion of tumor infiltrating regulatory T cells (Tregs), myeloid-derived suppressor cells (MDSC), and tumor-associated macrophages (TAM) [74, 75] (Figure 2). Tregs contribute to immune escape by activation of the programmed cell death protein-1 (PD-1) receptor through immune and tumor cell expression of its ligand, PD-L1 (not shown), which results in suppression of effector T cell function mediated by $CD4^+$ helper T cells and $CD8^+$ cytotoxic T cells. MDSC also differentiate into TAM with similar T cell inhibitory properties [76], a process driven by inflammatory Th2 cytokines, which ultimately leads to tumor progression. Although there are numerous studies of these pathways in immune tolerance, the role of PPARδ in this process has not been examined in mammary tumor models. Nevertheless, a clue as to its functional role in adaptive immunity may be gleaned from studies in diabetic obese mice. In liver and adipose tissue, PPARδ is required to maintain insulin sensitivity via Th2 cytokines, which promote M2 macrophage polarization [77, 78] that have the characteristics of TAMs, and promotes tolerance to "self" recognition [79] to prevent diabetes. This suggests that PPARδ may play a similar role in tumorigenesis, but with a decidedly different outcome. As discussed in Section 2, PPARδ regulates the inflammatory Saa1/2/3 and S100a8/9 pathways, which in tumor-bearing mice are associated with MDSC expansion [80] and metastasis [81]. Immune tolerance mediated by Tregs, MDSC, and TAM are dependent on PGE_2 synthesis, reactive oxygen species generated by NADPH oxidase (NOX1), and tryptophan depletion by indoleamine 2,3 dioxygenase (IDO) [74] (Figure 2), all of which are under the transcriptional control of PPARδ. MDSC and Treg infiltration of mammary tumors is dependent on PGE_2 synthesis and IDO activation [82], and inhibition of $CD8^+$ T cell activation via the PD-1/PD-L1 axis is dependent on mTOR activation [83], a pathway that is activated in MMTV-PPARδ mice [31]. Since the transcriptions of ARG1, IDO2, inducible nitric oxide synthetase (NOS2), Ptgs2, Ptger4, and NOX1 are all regulated by the coactivators CEBPA/B, which also function in this capacity with PPARδ, this suggests a mechanism whereby PPARδ may control adaptive immunity

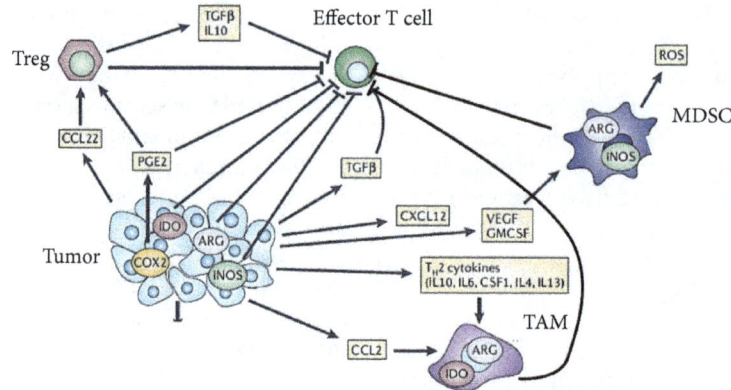

FIGURE 2: Metabolic interactions between tumor, stromal, and immune cells in the tumor microenvironment. Tumor and stromal cells express ARG, IDO, Cox2/Ptgs2, and iNOS/NOS2, which produce reactive oxygen species (ROS), chemokines, and Th2 cytokines that recruit Tregs, MDSC, and tumor-associated macrophages (TAM) to block effector T cell activation. Adapted from [84].

metabolically within the tumor microenvironment. This conclusion is also consistent with our recent finding that Plac1, which is overexpressed in MMTV-PPARδ mice, mediates immune tolerance in murine breast cancer cells by upregulating the expression of chemokines necessary for MDSC-mediated activation of Tregs (H. Yuan and R. I. Glazer, unpublished results). Thus, there is compelling evidence, although circumstantial in some instances, which suggests that PPARδ through its ability to regulate metabolic and inflammatory gene expression acts as a rheostat to control autoimmunity in normal tissues and immune tolerance during tumorigenesis.

6. Conclusions

Both genetic and pharmacological manipulation of PPARδ expression provide strong evidence for its role in regulating metabolism, inflammation, and immunity in a concerted fashion to ultimately impact mammary tumorigenesis. This conclusion suggests possible novel targets for drug development that may control this process and complement current approaches to develop immunotherapies for the treatment of cancer.

Competing Interests

The author declares that there are no competing interests.

Acknowledgments

The author acknowledges support from the National Cancer Institute, NIH, Avon Foundation for Women, and a Cancer Center Support Grant awarded to the Lombardi Comprehensive Cancer Center, Georgetown University.

References

[1] C. Grommes, G. E. Landreth, and M. T. Heneka, "Antineoplastic effects of peroxisome proliferator-activated receptor γ agonists," *Lancet Oncology*, vol. 5, no. 7, pp. 419–429, 2004.

[2] J. M. Olefsky and A. R. Saltiel, "PPARγ and the treatment of insulin resistance," *Trends in Endocrinology and Metabolism*, vol. 11, no. 9, pp. 362–368, 2000.

[3] J. Berger and J. A. Wagner, "Physiological and therapeutic roles of peroxisome proliferator-activated receptors," *Diabetes Technology and Therapeutics*, vol. 4, no. 2, pp. 163–174, 2002.

[4] J. Direnzo, M. Söderström, R. Kurokawa et al., "Peroxisome proliferator-activated receptors and retinoic acid receptors differentially control the interactions of retinoid X receptor heterodimers with ligands, coactivators, and corepressors," *Molecular and Cellular Biology*, vol. 17, no. 4, pp. 2166–2176, 1997.

[5] R. M. Lavinsky, K. Jepsen, T. Heinzel et al., "Diverse signaling pathways modulate nuclear receptor recruitment of N- CoR and SMRT complexes," *Proceedings of the National Academy of Sciences of the United States of America*, vol. 95, no. 6, pp. 2920–2925, 1998.

[6] R. T. Nolte, G. B. Wisely, S. Westin et al., "Ligand binding and co-activator assembly of the peroxisome proliferator-activated receptor-γ," *Nature*, vol. 395, no. 6698, pp. 137–143, 1998.

[7] Y. Yin, H. Yuan, C. Wang et al., "3-Phosphoinositide-dependent protein kinase-1 activates the peroxisome proliferator-activated receptor- and promotes adipocyte differentiation," *Molecular Endocrinology*, vol. 20, no. 2, pp. 268–278, 2006.

[8] J. P. Berger, T. E. Akiyama, and P. T. Meinke, "PPARs: therapeutic targets for metabolic disease," *Trends in Pharmacological Sciences*, vol. 26, no. 5, pp. 244–251, 2005.

[9] R. M. Evans, G. D. Barish, and Y.-X. Wang, "PPARs and the complex journey to obesity," *Nature Medicine*, vol. 10, no. 4, pp. 355–361, 2004.

[10] M. Lehrke and M. A. Lazar, "The many faces of PPARγ," *Cell*, vol. 123, no. 6, pp. 993–999, 2005.

[11] L. Michalik, B. Desvergne, and W. Wahli, "Peroxisome-proliferator-activated receptors and cancers: complex stories," *Nature Reviews Cancer*, vol. 4, no. 1, pp. 61–70, 2004.

[12] R. I. Glazer, H. Yuan, Z. Xie, and Y. Yin, "PPARγ and PPARδ as modulators of neoplasia and cell fate," *PPAR Research*, vol. 2008, Article ID 247379, 8 pages, 2008.

[13] K.-D. Wagner and N. Wagner, "Peroxisome proliferator-activated receptor beta/delta (PPARβ/δ) acts as regulator of metabolism linked to multiple cellular functions," *Pharmacology and Therapeutics*, vol. 125, no. 3, pp. 423–435, 2010.

[14] J. M. Peters, Y. M. Shah, and F. J. Gonzalez, "The role of peroxisome proliferator-activated receptors in carcinogenesis and chemoprevention," *Nature Reviews Cancer*, vol. 12, no. 3, pp. 181–195, 2012.

[15] M. Xu, X. Zuo, and I. Shureiqi, "Targeting peroxisome proliferator-activated receptor-β/δ in colon cancer: how to aim?" *Biochemical Pharmacology*, vol. 85, no. 5, pp. 607–611, 2013.

[16] J. M. Peters, P. L. Yao, and F. J. Gonzalez, "Targeting peroxisome proliferator-activated receptor-β/Δ (PPARβ/Δ) for cancer chemoprevention," *Current Pharmacology Reports*, vol. 1, no. 2, pp. 121–128, 2015.

[17] G. M. Pighetti, W. Novosad, C. Nicholson et al., "Therapeutic treatment of DMBA-induced mammary tumors with PPAR ligands," *Anticancer Research*, vol. 21, no. 2, pp. 825–830, 2001.

[18] N. Suh, Y. Wang, C. R. Williams et al., "A new ligand for the peroxisome proliferator-activated receptor-γ (PPAR-γ), GW7845, inhibits rat mammary carcinogenesis," *Cancer Research*, vol. 59, no. 22, pp. 5671–5673, 1999.

[19] Y. Yin, R. G. Russell, L. E. Dettin et al., "Peroxisome proliferator-activated receptor delta and γ agonists differentially alter tumor differentiation and progression during mammary carcinogenesis," *Cancer Research*, vol. 65, pp. 3950–3957, 2005.

[20] L. Patel, I. Pass, P. Coxon, C. P. Downes, S. A. Smith, and C. H. Macphee, "Tumor suppressor and anti-inflammatory actions of PPARγ agonists are mediated via upregulation of PTEN," *Current Biology*, vol. 11, no. 10, pp. 764–768, 2001.

[21] H. Yuan, G. Upadhyay, Y. Yin, L. Kopelovich, and R. I. Glazer, "Stem cell antigen-1 deficiency enhances the chemopreventive effect of peroxisome proliferator–activated receptorγ activation," *Cancer Prevention Research*, vol. 5, no. 1, pp. 51–60, 2012.

[22] M. Pignatelli, C. Cocca, A. Santos, and A. Perez-Castillo, "Enhancement of BRCA1 gene expression by the peroxisome proliferator-activated receptor γ in the MCF-7 breast cancer cell line," *Oncogene*, vol. 22, pp. 5446–5450, 2003.

[23] A. J. Apostoli, J. M. Roche, M. M. Schneider et al., "Opposing roles for mammary epithelial-specific PPARγ signaling and activation during breast tumour progression," *Molecular Cancer*, pp. 1–14, 2015.

[24] Y. Yin, H. Yuan, X. Zeng, L. Kopelovich, and R. I. Glazer, "Inhibition of peroxisome proliferator-activated receptor γ increases estrogen receptor-dependent tumor specification," *Cancer Research*, vol. 69, no. 2, pp. 687–694, 2009.

[25] H. Yuan, L. Kopelovich, Y. Yin, J. Lu, and R. I. Glazer, "Drug-targeted inhibition of peroxisome proliferator-activated receptor-gamma enhances the chemopreventive effect of antiestrogen therapy," *Oncotarget*, vol. 3, no. 3, pp. 345–356, 2012.

[26] N. Di-Po, N. S. Tan, L. Michalik, W. Wahli, and B. Desvergne, "Antiapoptotic role of PPARβ in keratinocytes via transcriptional control of the Akt1 signaling pathway," *Molecular Cell*, vol. 10, no. 4, pp. 721–733, 2002.

[27] N. Di-Poï, L. Michalik, N. S. Tan, B. Desvergne, and W. Wahli, "The anti-apoptotic role of PPARβ contributes to efficient skin wound healing," *Journal of Steroid Biochemistry and Molecular Biology*, vol. 85, no. 2–5, pp. 257–265, 2003.

[28] R. L. Stephen, M. C. U. Gustafsson, M. Jarvis et al., "Activation of peroxisome proliferator-activated receptor δ stimulates the proliferation of human breast and prostate cancer cell lines," *Cancer Research*, vol. 64, no. 9, pp. 3162–3170, 2004.

[29] C. B. Pollock, Y. Yin, H. Yuan et al., "PPARδ activation acts cooperatively with 3-phosphoinositide-dependent protein kinase-1 to enhance mammary tumorigenesis," *PLoS ONE*, vol. 6, no. 1, Article ID e16215, 2011.

[30] M. Ghosh, Y. Ai, K. Narko, Z. Wang, J. M. Peters, and T. Hla, "PPARδ is pro-tumorigenic in a mouse model of COX-2-induced mammary cancer," *Prostaglandins and Other Lipid Mediators*, vol. 88, no. 3-4, pp. 97–100, 2009.

[31] H. Yuan, J. Lu, J. Xiao et al., "PPARδ induces estrogen receptor-positive mammary neoplasia through an inflammatory and metabolic phenotype linked to mTOR activation," *Cancer Research*, vol. 73, no. 14, pp. 4349–4361, 2013.

[32] A. Abdollahi, C. Schwager, J. Kleeff et al., "Transcriptional network governing the angiogenic switch in human pancreatic cancer," *Proceedings of the National Academy of Sciences of the United States of America*, vol. 104, no. 31, pp. 12890–12895, 2007.

[33] R. Kittler, J. Zhou, S. Hua et al., "A Comprehensive Nuclear Receptor Network for Breast Cancer Cells," *Cell Reports*, vol. 3, no. 2, pp. 538–551, 2013.

[34] C. Sotiriou and L. Pusztai, "Gene-expression signatures in breast cancer," *New England Journal of Medicine*, vol. 360, no. 8, pp. 752–800, 2009.

[35] R. L. Yamnik and M. K. Holz, "mTOR/S6K1 and MAPK/RSK signaling pathways coordinately regulate estrogen receptor α serine 167 phosphorylation," *FEBS Letters*, vol. 584, no. 1, pp. 124–128, 2010.

[36] Y. Shi, M. Hon, and R. M. Evans, "The peroxisome proliferator-activated receptor δ, an integrator of transcriptional repression and nuclear receptor signaling," *Proceedings of the National Academy of Sciences of the United States of America*, vol. 99, no. 5, pp. 2613–2618, 2002.

[37] M. C. U. Gustafsson, D. Knight, and C. N. A. Palmer, "Ligand modulated antagonism of PPARγ by genomic and non-genomic actions of PPARδ," *PLoS ONE*, vol. 4, no. 9, Article ID e7046, 2009.

[38] T. Adhikary, K. Kaddatz, F. Finkernagel et al., "Genomewide analyses define different modes of transcriptional regulation by peroxisome proliferator-activated receptor-β/δ (PPARβ/δ)," *PLoS ONE*, vol. 6, no. 1, Article ID e16344, 2011.

[39] M. I. Torres-Arzayus, J. Yuan, J. L. DellaGatta, H. Lane, A. L. Kung, and M. Brown, "Targeting the AIB1 oncogene through mammalian target of rapamycin inhibition in the mammary gland," *Cancer Research*, vol. 66, no. 23, pp. 11381–11388, 2006.

[40] M. I. Torres-Arzayus, J. Font de Mora, J. Yuan et al., "High tumor incidence and activation of the PI3K/AKT pathway in transgenic mice define AIB1 as an oncogene," *Cancer Cell*, vol. 6, no. 3, pp. 263–274, 2004.

[41] J. I. Herschkowitz, K. Simin, V. J. Weigman et al., "Identification of conserved gene expression features between murine mammary carcinoma models and human breast tumors," *Genome Biology*, vol. 8, no. 5, article no. R76, 2007.

[42] M. Fant, A. Farina, R. Nagaraja, and D. Schlessinger, "PLAC1 (Placenta-specific 1): a novel, X-linked gene with roles in reproductive and cancer biology," *Prenatal Diagnosis*, vol. 30, no. 6, pp. 497–502, 2010.

[43] M. Koslowski, U. Sahin, R. Mitnacht-Kraus, G. Seitz, C. Huber, and Ö. Türeci, "A placenta-specific gene ectopically activated in many human cancers is essentially involved in malignant cell processes," *Cancer Research*, vol. 67, no. 19, pp. 9528–9534, 2007.

[44] W. A. Silva Jr., S. Gnjatic, E. Ritter et al., "PLAC1, a trophoblast-specific cell surface protein, is expressed in a range of human tumors and elicits spontaneous antibody responses," *Cancer Immunity*, vol. 7, article 18, 2007.

[45] X.-Y. Dong, J.-R. Peng, Y.-J. Ye et al., "PLAC1 is a tumor-specific antigen capable of eliciting spontaneous antibody responses in

human cancer patients," *International Journal of Cancer*, vol. 122, no. 9, pp. 2038–2043, 2008.

[46] F.-F. Liu, X.-Y. Dong, X.-W. Pang et al., "The specific immune response to tumor antigen CP1 and its correlation with improved survival in colon cancer patients," *Gastroenterology*, vol. 134, no. 4, pp. 998–1006, 2008.

[47] L. Brunelli, K. A. Cieslik, J. L. Alcorn, M. Vatta, and A. Baldini, "Peroxisome proliferator-activated receptor-δ upregulates 14-3-3ε in human endothelial cells via CCAAT/enhancer binding protein-β," *Circulation Research*, vol. 100, no. 5, pp. e59–e71, 2007.

[48] N. S. Tan, G. Icre, A. Montagner, B. Bordier-ten-Heggeler, W. Wahli, and L. Michalik, "The nuclear hormone receptor peroxisome proliferator-activated receptor β/δ potentiates cell chemotactism, polarization, and migration," *Molecular and Cellular Biology*, vol. 27, no. 20, pp. 7161–7175, 2007.

[49] M. Romanowska, L. Reilly, C. N. A. Palmer, M. C. U. Gustafsson, and J. Foerster, "Activation of PPARβ/δ causes a psoriasis-like skin disease in vivo," *PLoS ONE*, vol. 5, no. 3, Article ID e9701, 2010.

[50] S. A. Kliewer, S. S. Sundseth, S. A. Jones et al., "Fatty acids and eicosanoids regulate gene expression through direct interactions with peroxisome proliferator-activated receptors α and γ," *Proceedings of the National Academy of Sciences of the United States of America*, vol. 94, no. 9, pp. 4318–4323, 1997.

[51] B. M. Forman, J. Chen, and R. M. Evans, "Hypolipidemic drugs, polyunsaturated fatty acids, and eicosanoids are ligands for peroxisome proliferator-activated receptors α and δ," *Proceedings of the National Academy of Sciences of the United States of America*, vol. 94, no. 9, pp. 4312–4317, 1997.

[52] H. E. Xu, M. H. Lambert, V. G. Montana et al., "Molecular recognition of fatty acids by peroxisome proliferator- activated receptors," *Molecular Cell*, vol. 3, no. 3, pp. 397–403, 1999.

[53] R. A. Gupta, J. Tan, W. F. Krause et al., "Prostacyclin-mediated activation of peroxisome proliferator-activated receptor δ in colorectal cancer," *Proceedings of the National Academy of Sciences of the United States of America*, vol. 97, no. 24, pp. 13275–13280, 2000.

[54] D. Wang, L. Fu, W. Ning et al., "Peroxisome proliferator-activated receptor δ promotes colonic inflammation and tumor growth," *Proceedings of the National Academy of Sciences of the United States of America*, vol. 111, no. 19, pp. 7084–7089, 2014.

[55] I. Shureiqi, W. Jiang, X. Zuo et al., "The 15-lipoxygenase-1 product 13-S-hydroxyoctadecadienoic acid down-regulates PPAR-δ to induce apoptosis in colorectal cancer cells," *Proceedings of the National Academy of Sciences of the United States of America*, vol. 100, no. 17, pp. 9968–9973, 2003.

[56] C. H. Liu, S.-H. Chang, K. Narko et al., "Overexpression of cyclooxygenase-2 is sufficient to induce tumorigenesis in transgenic mice," *Journal of Biological Chemistry*, vol. 276, no. 21, pp. 18563–18569, 2001.

[57] S. Han, J. D. Ritzenthaler, B. Wingerd, and J. Roman, "Activation of peroxisome proliferator-activated receptor β/δ (PPARβ/δ) increases the expression of prostaglandin E$_2$ receptor subtype EP4: the roles of phosphatidylinositol 3-kinase and CCAAT/enhancer-binding protein β," *The Journal of Biological Chemistry*, vol. 280, no. 39, pp. 33240–33249, 2005.

[58] L. Xu, C. Han, K. Lim, and T. Wu, "Cross-talk between peroxisome proliferator-activated receptor δ and cytosolic phospholipase A$_2\alpha$/cyclooxygenase-2/prostaglandin E$_2$ signaling pathways in human hepatocellular carcinoma cells," *Cancer Research*, vol. 66, no. 24, pp. 11859–11868, 2006.

[59] J. Eswaran, D. Cyanam, P. Mudvari et al., "Transcriptomic landscape of breast cancers through mRNA sequencing," *Scientific Reports*, vol. 2, article 264, 2012.

[60] B. L. Pierce, R. Ballard-Barbash, L. Bernstein et al., "Elevated biomarkers of inflammation are associated with reduced survival among breast cancer patients," *Journal of Clinical Oncology*, vol. 27, no. 21, pp. 3437–3444, 2009.

[61] C. Gebhardt, J. Németh, P. Angel, and J. Hess, "S100A8 and S100A9 in inflammation and cancer," *Biochemical Pharmacology*, vol. 72, no. 11, pp. 1622–1631, 2006.

[62] S. Ghavami, S. Chitayat, M. Hashemi et al., "S100A8/A9: a Janus-faced molecule in cancer therapy and tumorgenesis," *European Journal of Pharmacology*, vol. 625, no. 1–3, pp. 73–83, 2009.

[63] C. B. Pollock, O. Rodriguez, P. L. Martin et al., "Induction of metastatic gastric cancer by peroxisome proliferator-activated receptorδ activation," *PPAR Research*, vol. 2010, Article ID 571783, 12 pages, 2010.

[64] G. D. Barish, V. A. Narkar, and R. M. Evans, "PPARδ: a dagger in the heart of the metabolic syndrome," *Journal of Clinical Investigation*, vol. 116, no. 3, pp. 590–597, 2006.

[65] J. Jonkers and W. H. Moolenaar, "Mammary tumorigenesis through LPA receptor signaling," *Cancer Cell*, vol. 15, no. 6, pp. 457–459, 2009.

[66] N. Panupinthu, H. Y. Lee, and G. B. Mills, "Lysophosphatidic acid production and action: critical new players in breast cancer initiation and progression," *British Journal of Cancer*, vol. 102, no. 6, pp. 941–946, 2010.

[67] D. A. Foster, "Phosphatidic acid signaling to mTOR: signals for the survival of human cancer cells," *Biochimica et Biophysica Acta (BBA)—Molecular and Cell Biology of Lipids*, vol. 1791, no. 9, pp. 949–955, 2009.

[68] J. Storch and A. E. Thumser, "Tissue-specific functions in the fatty acid-binding protein family," *The Journal of Biological Chemistry*, vol. 285, no. 43, pp. 32679–32683, 2010.

[69] P. Kannan-Thulasiraman, D. D. Seachrist, G. H. Mahabeleshwar, M. K. Jain, and N. Noy, "Fatty acid-binding protein 5 and PPARβ/δ are critical mediators of epidermal growth factor receptor-induced carcinoma cell growth," *Journal of Biological Chemistry*, vol. 286, no. 41, pp. 19106–19115, 2011.

[70] L. Levi, G. Lobo, M. K. Doud et al., "Genetic ablation of the fatty acid-binding protein FABP5 suppresses HER2-induced mammary tumorigenesis," *Cancer Research*, vol. 73, no. 15, pp. 4770–4780, 2013.

[71] K. M. Nieman, H. A. Kenny, C. V. Penicka et al., "Adipocytes promote ovarian cancer metastasis and provide energy for rapid tumor growth," *Nature Medicine*, vol. 17, no. 11, pp. 1498–1503, 2011.

[72] K. Ito, A. Carracedo, D. Weiss et al., "A PML-PPAR-δ pathway for fatty acid oxidation regulates hematopoietic stem cell maintenance," *Nature Medicine*, vol. 18, no. 9, pp. 1350–1358, 2012.

[73] L. M. Coussens, L. Zitvogel, and A. K. Palucka, "Neutralizing tumor-promoting chronic inflammation: a magic bullet?" *Science*, vol. 339, no. 6117, pp. 286–291, 2013.

[74] D. I. Gabrilovich and S. Nagaraj, "Myeloid-derived suppressor cells as regulators of the immune system," *Nature Reviews Immunology*, vol. 9, no. 3, pp. 162–174, 2009.

[75] D. M. Pardoll, "The blockade of immune checkpoints in cancer immunotherapy," *Nature Reviews Cancer*, vol. 12, no. 4, pp. 252–264, 2012.

[76] A. Sica and V. Bronte, "Altered macrophage differentiation and immune dysfunction in tumor development," *The Journal of Clinical Investigation*, vol. 117, no. 5, pp. 1155–1166, 2007.

[77] K. Kang, S. M. Reilly, V. Karabacak et al., "Adipocyte-derived Th2 cytokines and myeloid PPARδ regulate macrophage polarization and insulin sensitivity," *Cell Metabolism*, vol. 7, no. 6, pp. 485–495, 2008.

[78] J. I. Odegaard, R. R. Ricardo-Gonzalez, A. Red Eagle et al., "Alternative M2 activation of Kupffer cells by PPARδ ameliorates obesity-induced insulin resistance," *Cell Metabolism*, vol. 7, no. 6, pp. 496–507, 2008.

[79] L. Mukundan, J. I. Odegaard, C. R. Morel et al., "PPAR-δ senses and orchestrates clearance of apoptotic cells to promote tolerance," *Nature Medicine*, vol. 15, no. 11, pp. 1266–1272, 2009.

[80] P. Cheng, C. A. Corzo, N. Luetteke et al., "Inhibition of dendritic cell differentiation and accumulation of myeloid-derived suppressor cells in cancer is regulated by S100A9 protein," *Journal of Experimental Medicine*, vol. 205, no. 10, pp. 2235–2249, 2008.

[81] S. Hiratsuka, A. Watanabe, Y. Sakurai et al., "The S100A8-serum amyloid A3-TLR4 paracrine cascade establishes a premetastatic phase," *Nature Cell Biology*, vol. 10, no. 11, pp. 1349–1355, 2008.

[82] P. Sinha, V. K. Clements, A. M. Fulton, and S. Ostrand-Rosenberg, "Prostaglandin E2 promotes tumor progression by inducing myeloid-derived suppressor cells," *Cancer Research*, vol. 67, no. 9, pp. 4507–4513, 2007.

[83] C.-H. Chang, J. Qiu, D. O'Sullivan et al., "Metabolic competition in the tumor microenvironment is a driver of cancer progression," *Cell*, vol. 162, no. 6, pp. 1229–1241, 2015.

[84] A. J. Muller and P. A. Scherle, "Targeting the mechanisms of tumoral immune tolerance with small-molecule inhibitors," *Nature Reviews Cancer*, vol. 6, no. 8, pp. 613–625, 2006.

4

Caffeoylquinic Acid-Rich Extract of *Aster glehni* F. Schmidt Ameliorates Nonalcoholic Fatty Liver through the Regulation of PPARδ and Adiponectin in ApoE KO Mice

Yong-Jik Lee,[1] Yoo-Na Jang,[1] Yoon-Mi Han,[1,2] Hyun-Min Kim,[1,2] Jong-Min Jeong,[1,2] Min Jeoung Son,[3] Chang Bae Jin,[3] Hyoung Ja Kim,[3] and Hong Seog Seo[1,2]

[1]*Cardiovascular Center, Korea University, Guro Hospital, 148 Gurodong-ro, Guro-gu, Seoul 08308, Republic of Korea*
[2]*Department of Medical Science, Korea University College of Medicine (BK21 Plus KUMS Graduate Program), Main Building 6F Room 655, 73 Inchon-ro (Anam-dong 5-ga), Seongbuk-gu, Seoul 136-705, Republic of Korea*
[3]*Molecular Recognition Research Center, Materials and Life Science Research Division, Korea Institute of Science and Technology, Hwarangno 14 Gil 5, Seoul 136-791, Republic of Korea*

Correspondence should be addressed to Hyoung Ja Kim; khj@kist.re.kr and Hong Seog Seo; mdhsseo@unitel.co.kr

Academic Editor: Henrike Sell

Aster glehni is well known for its therapeutic properties. This study was performed to investigate the effects of *A. glehni* on nonalcoholic fatty liver disease (NAFLD) in atherosclerotic condition, by determining the levels of biomarkers related to lipid metabolism and inflammation in serum, liver, and adipose tissue. Body and abdominal adipose tissue weights and serum triglyceride level decreased in all groups treated with *A. glehni*. Serum adiponectin concentration and protein levels of peroxisome proliferator-activated receptor δ, 5′ adenosine monophosphate-activated protein kinase, acetyl-CoA carboxylase, superoxide dismutase, and PPARγ coactivator 1-alpha in liver tissues increased in the groups treated with *A. glehni*. Conversely, protein levels of ATP citrate lyase, fatty acid synthase, tumor necrosis factor α, and 3-hydroxy-3-methylglutaryl-CoA reductase and the concentrations of interleukin 6 and reactive oxygen species decreased upon *A. glehni*. Triglyceride concentration in the liver was lower in mice treated with *A. glehni* than in control mice. Lipid accumulation in HepG2 and 3T3-L1 cells decreased upon *A. glehni* treatment; this effect was suppressed in the presence of the PPARδ antagonist, GSK0660. Our findings suggest that *A. glehni* extracts may ameliorate NAFLD through regulation of PPARδ, adiponectin, and the related subgenes.

1. Introduction

Nonalcoholic fatty liver disease (NAFLD), characterized by the accumulation of triglyceride in hepatocytes, is one of the most common diseases today. Metabolic disorders such as obesity, diabetes mellitus, and hyperlipidemia are major risk factors for NAFLD and nonalcoholic steatohepatitis (NASH), which is a more severe form of NAFLD [1, 2]. Furthermore, NAFLD can be used as a representative clinical index of hypertension, cardiovascular disease, and diabetic complications [3, 4]. Adiponectin is an adipocytokine consisting of 244 amino acid residues and is specifically and highly expressed in adipose tissues [5]. Its expression is closely related to various metabolic diseases such as obesity,

type 2 diabetes, atherosclerosis, and cardiovascular disease [6, 7]. In addition, soybean embryo ameliorates nonalcoholic fatty liver through adiponectin mediated 5′ adenosine monophosphate-activated protein kinase α (AMPK α) pathway [8]. AMPK normalizes lipid homeostasis through several mechanisms. It downregulates cholesterol and fatty acid syntheses by inactivating the enzymes 3-hydroxy-3-methylglutaryl-CoA reductase (HMGCR) and fatty acid synthase (FASN), respectively. Further, AMPK upregulates fatty acid oxidation by inhibiting acetyl-CoA carboxylase (ACC) [9–11].

Throughout human history, many plants have been consumed not only as food, but also for preventing or even curing certain diseases. For instance, *Aster glehni* has been used in cooking and as traditional medicine for hundreds of years in Korea. In the *Dongui Bogam*, a Korean traditional medical encyclopedia, it is recorded that *A. glehni* exhibits antipyretic and analgesic activities and reduces phlegm and coughing. In addition, various therapeutic functions of *A. glehni* extract such as antiobesity, antioxidation, anti-inflammation, and antiwrinkle activities have been recently reported [12–14]. These studies suggest the potential antiadipogenesis and antiobesity effects of *A. glehni* and its therapeutic potential in treating obesity-related diseases.

Hitherto, there are few studies on the effects of *A. glehni* on metabolic diseases. Because many studies have reported a close correlation between NAFLD and cardiovascular diseases such as hypertension and atherosclerosis, we investigated the effect of *A. glehni* on nonalcoholic fatty liver in atherosclerotic mice and it was conducted with focusing on PPARδ. The present findings can be beneficial in further understanding the role of phytomedicines in treating atherosclerosis and fatty liver disease.

2. Materials and Methods

2.1. Plant Material. Parboiled and dried *A. glehni* F. Schmidt (family Compositae) were purchased from Ulleung Island, Gyeongsangbuk-do, Korea, in November 2012 and identified by Professor Chang-Soo Yook (Department of Pharmacognosy, Kyung Hee University, Seoul, Korea). Voucher specimens (971-12A-P) were deposited in the herbarium of the Korea Institute of Science and Technology.

2.2. Extraction Procedure. Chopped leaves and stem of *A. glehni* (12 kg) were extracted three times with methanol (70 L) at room temperature to give a methanol-soluble extract. The dried extract residue (2.6 kg) was suspended in water and partitioned with ethyl acetate. The ethyl acetate fraction was evaporated under reduced pressure to yield 41.0 g of residue. Organic solvents used in the extraction procedure were purchased from Sigma-Aldrich (St. Louis, MO, USA).

2.3. High-Performance Liquid Chromatography (HPLC) Analysis for Ethyl Acetate Extract of A. glehni. The ethyl acetate extract of *A. glehni* was analyzed using reverse-phase high-performance liquid chromatography (Waters 1500 Series System), with a 2998 PDA Detector (Waters, Worcester, MA, USA). Separation was performed using a Luna C18 column (5 μm, 250 × 4.6 mm, Phenomenex, Torrance, CA, USA) at 25°C with a sample injection volume of 10 μL. The mobile phase was a gradient of methanol and 1% acetic acid. The following gradient was used: 30% methanol (0 min), 40% methanol (0~10 min), 60% methanol (10~20 min), 80% methanol (20~30 min), and 100% methanol (30~40 min). The flow rate of the mobile phase was 1.0 ml/min. Organic solvents used in HPLC analysis were purchased from Sigma-Aldrich.

2.4. Cell Culture. HepG2 cells were cultured in Dulbecco's modified Eagle's medium (DMEM) containing 10% fetal bovine serum (FBS) and 1% antibiotic-antimycotic solution at 37°C in a 5% CO_2 incubator. The medium was replaced every 48–72 h. HepG2 cells within 95~110 passages were plated at a density of 5 × 10^4 cells per well in 24-well culture dishes or 1 × 10^6 cells per well in a 6-well culture plate in DMEM containing 10% FBS and 1% antibiotic-antimycotic solution. Cells were cultured for 24 to 48 h at 37°C in a 5% CO_2 incubator, and the media were changed to DMEM containing 1% FBS. Thereafter, cells were treated in high fatty acid (0.1 mM palmitate) and high cholesterol (0.2 mM) condition, with *A. glehni* extract (25 μg/mL) and the peroxisome proliferator-activated receptor δ (PPARδ) antagonist, GSK0660 (50 μM), for 24 h. HepG2 cells were also treated with dorsomorphin (AMPK antagonist, compound C) of 10 uM for 24 h. 3T3-L1 preadipocytes were cultured in DMEM containing 10% calf serum and 1% antibiotic-antimycotic solution at 37°C in a 5% CO_2 incubator. The medium was replaced every 48–72 h. 3T3-L1 cells within 8~18 passages were plated at a density of 5 × 10^4 cells per well in 24-well culture dishes in DMEM containing 10% calf serum and 1% antibiotic-antimycotic solution. When 3T3-L1 cells reached confluence, differentiation media were applied to cells, together with *A. glehni* extract and PPARδ antagonist. The differentiation media contained 0.0125 uM dexamethasone, 12.5 uM 3-isobutyl-1-methylxanthine, 10 μg/mL insulin, and 10% FBS. After differentiation for two days, the media were replaced with insulin media which contained 10 μg/mL insulin and 10% FBS. After incubation in insulin media for 2~4 days, the media were changed to maintenance media which contained only 10% FBS. All the concentrations of chemicals are final treatment concentrations. HepG2 and 3T3-L1 cell lines were purchased from the Korean Cell Line Bank (Seoul, Korea). All reagents for cell culture were purchased from Welgene Inc. (Daegu, Korea). Palmitate, cholesterol, GSK0660, compound C, and reagents for 3T3-L1 cell differentiation were purchased from Sigma-Aldrich.

2.5. Animal Study. In total, forty male apolipoprotein E knock-out (ApoE KO) mice were used in this study. Mice (six weeks of age) were adapted to the diet for seven days. Mice were fed diet containing 0.15% cholesterol and were divided into the following four groups: group (1), fed only cholesterol diet; group (2), fed cholesterol diet and 100 mg/kg/day *A. glehni* extract; group (3), fed cholesterol diet and 300 mg/kg/day *A. glehni* extract; and group (4), fed cholesterol diet and 500 mg/kg/day *A. glehni* extract. The extracts of all concentrations were administered through drinking water. All mice were sacrificed after four weeks. The administered amounts of *A. glehni* extracts were determined as follows: first, body weights of animals were estimated every week during whole experimental period, and then the administering amounts of *A. glehni* extracts were calculated on the basis of mean body weight per experimental group and general mean water drinking amount per mouse.

Animal experiments were performed according to the Animal Experiment Ethics Guide of Guro Hospital, Korea University. The experiments complied with the Korea University Animal Research Rules and Regulations, and the protocols were approved by the Korea University Institutional Animal Care and Use Committee (approval number:

KUIACUC-2014-40). The ApoE KO mice and 0.15% cholesterol diet were supplied by Doo Yeol Biotech (Seoul, Korea). The cholesterol diet was made by Doo Yeol Biotech adding 0.15% cholesterol to Teklad Global 18% Protein Rodent Diet. Ingredient composition for 0.15% cholesterol diet is described in Table 1.

2.6. Estimation of Triglyceride, Total Cholesterol, High-Density Lipoprotein (HDL) Cholesterol, Low-Density Lipoprotein (LDL) Cholesterol, Adiponectin, Interleukin 6 (IL6), and Reactive Oxygen Species (ROS) Concentrations in Serum or the Liver. Concentrations of triglyceride and cholesterols in serum were estimated by using enzymatic colorimetric assay kits (Kyowa Medex Co., Ltd., Tokyo, Japan) in the Department of Laboratory Medicine (Diagnostic Tests), Korea University, Guro Hospital (Seoul, Korea).

Enzymatic colorimetric assay kit (Cayman Chemical, Ann Arbor, MI, USA) was used to measure triglyceride concentrations in the liver tissues, according to the manufacturer's instructions. Sample preparation procedures were as follows. Liver tissue was rinsed in ice-cold PBS to remove excess blood. The minced liver tissue of 300 mg was homogenized in the diluted standard diluent of 2 ml. The extract was centrifuged at 10,000 ×g for 10 min at 4°C, and then the supernatant was transferred to another tube. The supernatant sample was diluted by the ratio of 1 : 5 before use. Standard and sample solutions (10 μL) were added to the wells, and the diluted enzyme buffer solution (150 μL) was added to each well. Afterward, the plate was carefully shaken for a few seconds, covered with a sealing tape, and incubated for 15 min at room temperature. The absorbance at 540 nm was measured using a microplate reader. Triglyceride concentrations in the samples were determined by interpolation from a standard curve prepared using the standard solutions, and expressed in mg/dL.

Adiponectin concentration in serum samples was assayed using an enzyme-linked immunosorbent assay (ELISA) kit that can detect both globular domain and full-length adiponectin from Abcam (Cambridge, UK). Experimental procedures were as follows. The 50 μL of adiponectin standard or sample added to each well of 96 well plates, and after covering wells with a sealing tape, was incubated for 1 hr at room temperature. After washing 5 times with 1x wash buffer of 200 μL, 1x biotinylated adiponectin antibody of 50 μL was added to each well, and it was incubated for 1 hr. After washing 5 times with 1x wash buffer of 200 μL, 1x streptavidin-peroxidase conjugate of 50 μL was added to each well, and it was incubated for 30 min. After washing 5 times with 1x wash buffer of 200 μL, chromogen substrate of 50 μL was added to each well, and it was incubated till the optimal blue color density develops. Stop solution of 50 μL was added to each well, and then, the absorbance was estimated with a microplate reader at a wavelength of 450 nm. Adiponectin concentration in the samples was determined by interpolation from a standard curve prepared with standard samples supplied by the manufacturer, and expressed in ng/mL.

IL6 concentration in the liver tissues was assayed using an enzyme-linked immunosorbent assay (ELISA) kit

TABLE 1: Ingredients of cholesterol diet.

	Unit	Amount
Macronutrients		
Crude protein	%	18.6
Fat (ether extract)	%	6.2
Carbohydrate (available)	%	44.2
Crude fiber	%	3.5
Neutral detergent fiber	%	14.7
Ash	%	5.3
Minerals		
Calcium	%	1.0
Phosphorus	%	0.7
Non-phytate phosphorus	%	0.4
Sodium	%	0.2
Potassium	%	0.6
Chloride	%	0.4
Magnesium	%	0.2
Zinc	mg/kg	70
Manganese	mg/kg	100
Copper	mg/kg	15
Iodine	mg/kg	6
Iron	mg/kg	200
Selenium	mg/kg	0.23
Amino acids		
Aspartic acid	%	1.4
Glutamic acid	%	3.4
Alanine	%	1.1
Glycine	%	0.8
Threonine	%	0.7
Proline	%	1.6
Serine	%	1.1
Leucine	%	1.8
Isoleucine	%	0.8
Valine	%	0.9
Phenylalanine	%	1.0
Tyrosine	%	0.6
Methionine	%	0.4
Cystine	%	0.3
Lysine	%	0.9
Histidine	%	0.4
Arginine	%	1.0
Tryptophan	%	0.2
Vitamins		
Vitamin A	IU/g	15.0
Vitamin D3	IU/g	1.5
Vitamin E	IU/kg	110
Vitamin K3	mg/kg	50
Vitamin B1	mg/kg	17
Vitamin B2	mg/kg	15
Niacin	mg/kg	70
Vitamin B6	mg/kg	18

Table 1: Continued.

	Unit	Amount
Pantothenic acid	mg/kg	33
Vitamin B12	mg/kg	0.08
Biotin	mg/kg	0.40
Folate	mg/kg	4
Choline	mg/kg	1200
Fatty acids		
C16:0 palmitic	%	0.7
C18 0 stearic	%	0.2
C18:1ω9 oleic	%	1.2
C18:2ω6 linoeic	%	3.1
C18:3ω3 linolenic	%	0.3
Total saturated	%	0.9
Total monounsaturated	%	1.3
Total polyunsaturated	%	3.4
Supplement		
Cholesterol	%	0.15

(Mybiosource, CA, USA). Sample preparation procedures were as follows. Liver tissue was rinsed in ice-cold PBS to remove excess blood. The minced liver tissue of 300 mg was homogenized in the diluted standard diluent of 2 ml. The extract was centrifuged at 5,000 ×g for 5 min at 4°C, and then the supernatant was transferred to another tube. The supernatant sample was diluted by the ratio of 1 : 30 before use. Standard and sample solutions (100 μL) were added to the wells, covered with the plate sealer, and incubated for 2 hr at 37°C. After removing the liquid in each well, detection reagent A of 100 μL was added to each well, and the sealed plate was incubated for 1 hr at 37°C. After aspirating the liquid in each well, wells were washed three times with 1x wash buffer, and detection B of 100 μL was added to each well, and the sealed plate was incubated for 2 hr at 37°C. After aspirating and washing, substrate solution of 90 μL was added to each well, and the sealed plate was incubated for 30 min at 37°C. Stop solution of 50 μL was added to each well, and then, the absorbance was estimated with a microplate reader at a wavelength of 450 nm. IL6 concentration in the samples was determined by interpolation from a standard curve prepared with standard samples supplied by the manufacturer, and expressed in ng/mL.

ROS concentration in the liver tissues was assayed using an enzyme-linked immunosorbent assay (ELISA) kit (Mybiosource, CA, USA). Liver tissue was rinsed in ice-cold PBS to remove excess blood. The minced liver tissue of 300 mg was homogenized in the diluted standard diluent of 2 ml. The extract was centrifuged at 10,000 rpm for 10 min at 4°C, and then the supernatant was transferred to another tube. Experimental procedures were as follows. Standard and sample solutions (100 μL) were added to the wells, covered with the plate sealer, and incubated for 2 hr at 37°C. After removing the liquid in each well, detection reagent A of 100 μL was added to each well, and the sealed plate was incubated for 90 min at 37°C. After aspirating the liquid in each well, wells were washed two times with 1x wash buffer,

and biotinylated mouse ROS antibody solution of 100 μL was added to each well, and the sealed plate was incubated for 1 hr at 37°C. After aspirating and washing, enzyme-conjugate solution of 100 μL was added to each well (excepting blank wells), and the sealed plate was incubated for 30 min at 37°C. Color reagent liquid of 100 μL and color reagent C were added to each well sequentially, and the absorbance was estimated with a microplate reader at a wavelength of 450 nm in 10 min. ROS concentration in the samples was determined by interpolation from a standard curve prepared with standard samples supplied by the manufacturer, and expressed in unit/mL.

2.7. Semiquantitative Reverse Transcription Polymerase Chain Reaction (RT-PCR). Total RNA was extracted by the TRIzol reagent® according to manual. Complementary DNA was synthesized by power cDNA synthesis kit from total RNA, and polymerase chain reactions for PPARδ, AMPKα1 subunit, interleukin 6 (IL6), tumor necrosis factor α (TNFα), and β-actin were administered with PCR Premix kit. The primer sequences used were as follows: forward 5$'$-GGCAGAGTTGCTAGGGTTCC-3$'$ and reward 5$'$-CAA-GGAACACCCCAAGACCT-3$'$ for mouse PPARδ (PCR product size is 294 bp); forward 5$'$-CCTGCTTGATGC-ACACACATGA-3$'$ and reward 5$'$-TCATCAAAAGGG-AGGGTTCC-3$'$ for mouse AMPKα1 subunit (PCR product size is 213 bp); forward 5$'$-TTCACAGAGGATACCACTCC-3$'$ and reward 5$'$-AAGTGCATCATCGTTGTTCA-3$'$ for mouse IL6 (PCR product size is 147 bp); forward 5$'$-CTACTC-CTCAGAGCCCCCAG-3$'$ and reward 5$'$-CAGGTCACT-GTCCCAGCATC-3$'$ for mouse TNFα (PCR product size is 126 bp); forward 5$'$-CTAGGCACCAGGGTGTGATG-3$'$ and reward 5$'$-CTACGTACATGGCTGGGGTG-3$'$ for mouse β-actin (PCR product size is 291 bp). The reaction mixture containing cDNA was preheated for 5 minutes at 95°C as an initial denaturation step. Polymerase chain reaction consisted of denaturation step for 20 seconds at 95°C, annealing step for 55°C at 10 seconds, extension step for 30 seconds at 72°C, and final extension step for 5 minutes at 72°C.

TRIzol reagent was purchased from Invitrogen (Carlsbad, California, USA). Maxime PCR Premix kit, cDNA synthesis kit, and PCR Premix were obtained from iNtRON Biotechnology (Gyeonggi-do, Korea).

2.8. Estimation of Succinate Dehydrogenase (SDH) Activity in the Liver. Tissue samples were homogenized in phosphate-buffered saline (PBS) containing 1% protease inhibitor. The homogenized extracts were centrifuged at 13,000 rpm, 4°C for 5 min. The supernatants were transferred into new tubes and mixed with incubation solution containing 1 mol/L phosphate buffer (25 μL), 0.2 mol/L sodium succinate (125 μL), 10 mg/mL nitroblue tetrazolium (NBT; 25 μL), and distilled water (235 μL). The mixture was incubated for 20 min at 37°C in a temperature-controlled chamber. Sodium succinate, nitroblue tetrazolium, and protease inhibitor were purchased from Sigma-Aldrich. An enzyme solution (90 μL) was added to prewarmed incubation solution (410 μL) and incubated at 37°C. After the reaction is complete, the absorbance of the reaction mixture was measured at a wavelength of 550 nm.

Enzyme activity was calculated using the following formula: enzyme activity = absorbance of enzyme reaction mixture − absorbance of diluted enzyme solution.

2.9. Immunohistochemistry. Tissue slides were soaked in xylene to remove paraffin and then sequentially soaked in 100~75% ethanol solutions for dehydration. Deparaffinized and dehydrated slides were reacted with 3% H_2O_2 solution for 10 min and washed. The slides were then blocked with normal serum solution for 1 h. The slides were then treated with primary antibodies for 1 h and washed with Tris-buffered saline containing 0.05% Tween 20 (TBS-T). Primary antibodies for superoxide dismutase (SOD) were obtained from Novus (Littleton, CO, USA) and for HMGCR from Santa Cruz Biotechnology, Inc., and TNFα and 4-hydroxynonenal (4-HNE) antibodies from Abcam. Secondary antibodies were reacted to the slides for 30 min. After washing with TBS-T, premixed Vectastain® ABC reagent was reacted with the slides for 30 min. The slides were then washed with TBS-T and reacted with 3,3′-diaminobenzidine substrate solution until a change in color was observed. After washing with tap water for 5 min, the slides were counterstained with hematoxylin. The slides were again washed with tap water, air-dried, and finally mounted. Immunohistochemistry kit (containing secondary antibody) was purchased from Vector Laboratories (Burlingame, CA, USA).

2.10. Oil Red O Staining. Cells in 24-well culture plates were fixed in 4% formaldehyde solution for 30 min and then washed with PBS for 5 min. The cells were stained with Oil Red O solution (Sigma-Aldrich) for 1 h. After a 40% isopropyl alcohol wash for 30 s, cells were washed twice with PBS for 5 min. The cells were observed with an optical microscope and photographed. Absolute isopropyl alcohol (1 mL) was added to each well, and the eluted Oil Red O was quantified with Spectramax plus 384 microplate reader (Molecular Devices LLC, Sunnyvale, CA, USA) at a wavelength of 530 nm.

2.11. Western Blot Analysis. Protein concentration was estimated by the Bradford method. Extracted proteins (10 μg) were loaded onto 10% sodium dodecyl sulfate (SDS) polyacrylamide gels and protein blotting on nitrocellulose membranes was performed for 90 min. The membranes were blocked overnight with 5% skim milk and washed three times for 10 min with TBS-T. Primary antibodies were bound to the membranes at room temperature for 2 h. Primary antibodies for total and phosphorylated forms of AMPK, ACC, and ATP citrate lyase (ACLY) were supplied by Cell Signaling Technology, Inc. (Danvers, MA, USA). Primary antibodies for peroxisome proliferator-activated receptor gamma coactivator 1-alpha (PGC-1α), PPARδ, PPARα, and FASN were purchased from Abcam. Primary antibody for β-actin was procured from Santa Cruz Biotechnology, Inc. Dilution conditions for primary antibodies were as follows: PPARδ was 1:500, AMPK, p-AMPK (at Thr172), ACC, p-ACC (at Ser79), ACLY, p-ACLY (at Ser455), FASN, PPARα, and PGC-1α were 1:1000, and β-actin was 1:800. After washing three times with TBS-T for 10 min, secondary antibodies (Santa

Cruz Biotechnology, Inc.) were bound to the membranes at room temperature for 1 h. Dilution conditions for secondary antibodies were as follows: anti-rabbit IgG antibodies for PPARδ, PPARα, AMPK, p-AMPK, ACC, p-ACC, ACLY, p-ACLY, FASN, and PGC-1α were 1:5000, and anti-mouse IgG antibody for β-actin was 1:5000. After three washes with TBS-T for 10 min and a single TBS wash for another 10 min, chemiluminescent substrate and enhancer solution (Bio-Rad, Hercules, CA, USA) were applied to membranes to determine the protein expression rate. Images were processed manually with Kodak GBX developer and fixer reagents (Carestream Health, Inc., Rochester, NY, USA) and analyzed using Image J program. β-Actin was used as the internal control to normalize the loaded proteins.

2.12. Hematoxylin and Eosin (H&E) Staining. The liver tissue of each mouse was harvested and fixed in 4% paraformaldehyde. The samples were embedded in paraffin, cut into 4~5 μm thick sections using a microtome, and stained with H&E (Sigma-Aldrich). The sections were visualized using an optical microscope (BX51; Olympus, Tokyo, Japan) and photographed.

2.13. Immunocytochemistry. Cells in chamber slide were fixed with ice-cold methanol for 15 min. The intrinsic peroxidase activity in cells was get rid of by treatment of PBS containing 0.3% H_2O_2 and 0.3% normal serum. After PBS washing for 5 min, PBS containing 0.25% Triton X-100 was added to cells and incubated for 10 min. After PBS washing for 5 min, the cells were incubated for 20 min with normal blocking serum which was diluted in PBS as ratio of 1:100. After removing blocking serum, the cells were incubated for 1 hr with primary antibody solution (PPARγ primary antibody was purchased from Abcam). After PBS washing for 5 min, secondary antibody solution was added to cells and incubated 30 min. After PBS washing for 5 min, Vectastain® ABC reagent was added to the cells and incubated for 30 min. After PBS washing for 5 min, 3,3′-diaminobenzidine (DAB) substrate solution was added and incubated until proper color change appeared. After washing three times with PBS, the cells were counterstained with hematoxylin. After washing with distilled water, the cells in chamber slide were dried, covered with glass, and then observed with optical microscope. Immunohistochemistry kit (containing secondary antibody) was purchased from Vector Laboratories.

2.14. Statistics. Data are presented as mean ± SEM (standard error of mean). Statistically significant differences between two groups were calculated by the unpaired *t*-test, and one way ANOVA test was used to compare means of three or more groups. The *p* value of <0.05 was considered significant.

3. Results

3.1. HPLC Analysis Profile of Ethyl Acetate Extract of A. glehni Showed That the Extract Contains Mainly Caffeoylquinic Acids. Ethyl acetate extract of *A. glehni* contains mainly caffeoylquinic acids of six kinds, and they are as follows: 5-caffeoylquinic acid, 3,4-dicaffeoylquinic acid, 3,5-dicaffeoylquinic acid, 4,5-dicaffeoylquinic acid, methyl 3,4-dicaffeoylquinic acid, and methyl 4,5-dicaffeoylquinic acid (Figure 1).

3.2. Weight of Body and Abdominal (Epididymal) Fat and Concentrations of Triglyceride, Total Cholesterol, HDL Cholesterol, LDL Cholesterol, and Adiponectin in the Serum of ApoE KO Mice Treated with 0.15% Cholesterol Diet and A. glehni Extracts Were Normalized by the Extracts.

The diet intake amount was not significantly different among experimental groups except for A. glehni extract treated group of 500 mg/kg/day (Figure 2(a)). Likewise, the drinking water intake amount was not different among all experimental groups (Figure 2(b)).

Body and abdominal (epididymal) adipose tissue weights of mice treated with A. glehni extract were significantly lower than those of control mice (Figures 2(c) and 2(d)). So the correlation between diet intake amount and body weight was not obvious.

The concentration of triglyceride in serum decreased in a concentration-dependent manner and significant differences were observed in groups treated with 300 and 500 mg/kg/day A. glehni extract (Figure 2(e)). Adiponectin is a glycosylated adipokine that is selectively secreted by adipocytes. It has been reported to improve insulin sensitization, stimulate fatty acid oxidation, reduce inflammation, and inhibit atherosclerosis [15]. Adiponectin level increased upon A. glehni extract treatment at all concentrations (Figure 2(f)). On the other hand, cholesterol levels changed according to the concentration of A. glehni administered: total cholesterol level decreased significantly after treatment with 500 mg/kg/day of the extract (Figure 2(g)), HDL cholesterol level increased after the same treatment (Figure 2(h)), and LDL cholesterol level decreased after treatment with 300 mg/kg/day of the extract (Figure 2(i)).

3.3. Semiquantitative RT-PCR Results for PPARδ, AMPKα1, IL6, and TNFα in the Liver of ApoE KO Mice Treated with 0.15% Cholesterol Diet and A. glehni Extracts Showed the Elevation of PPARδ and AMPKα1 and the Decrease of IL6 and TNFα.

The mRNA level for PPARδ was increased by A. glehni extracts of all concentrations (Figure 3(a)), and the expression of AMPKα1 catalytic subunit was significantly elevated with the extract treatment of 100 mg/kg/day concentration (Figure 3(b)). The mRNA levels for IL6 and TNFα which are involved in inflammation were lowered by the extracts of all concentrations (Figures 3(c) and 3(d)).

3.4. Western Blot Analyses of PPARδ, AMPK, ACC, ACLY, PGC-1α, and FASN Expression in the Liver of ApoE KO Mice Treated with 0.15% Cholesterol Diet and A. glehni Extracts Showed the Activation of Fatty Acid Oxidation and the Inhibition of Fatty Acid Synthesis by the Extracts.

Phosphorylated AMPK (P-AMPK) is the active form of the enzyme and regulates the activation of ACC. Once ACC is phosphorylated, it becomes inactivated and no longer catalyzes the production of malonyl-CoA—an essential component in fatty acid synthesis [16]. The function of ACLY is to link glucose and lipid metabolisms. In its active form, phosphorylated ACLY transforms citrate into acetyl-CoA, which can be used as a

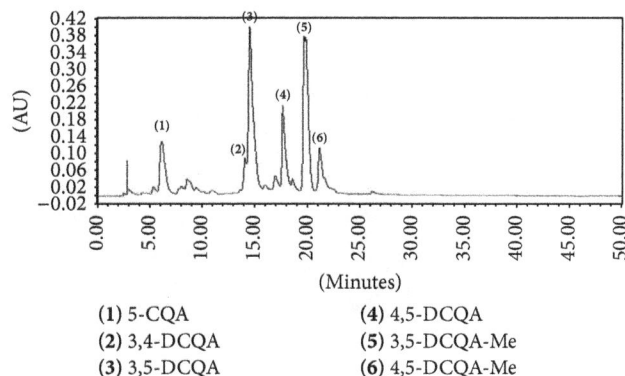

FIGURE 1: HPLC profile for ethyl acetate extract of Aster glehni. Separated phytochemicals are as follows: (1) 5-CQA: 5-caffeoylquinic acid, (2) 3,4-DCQA: 3,4-dicaffeoylquinic acid, (3) 3,5-DCQA: 3,5-dicaffeoylquinic acid, (4) 4,5-DCQA: 4,5-dicaffeoylquinic acid, (5) 3,5-DCQA-Me: methyl 3,4-dicaffeoylquinic acid, and (6) 4,5-DCQA-Me: methyl 4,5-dicaffeoylquinic acid.

substrate in the mevalonate and fatty acid synthesis pathways [17, 18]. The transcriptional coactivator PGC-1α coordinately increases mitochondrial biogenesis and respiration rates, as well as the uptake and utilization of substrates for energy production [19].

The protein level of PPARδ increased significantly in the liver of experimental groups treated with 300 and 500 mg/kg/day A. glehni extracts (Figure 4(a)). Similarly, the expression of P-AMPK increased significantly in the experimental group treated with 300 mg/kg/day A. glehni extract (Figure 4(b)). The expression of phosphorylated ACC (P-ACC) was significantly elevated in the groups treated with 300 mg/kg/day A. glehni extract (Figure 4(c)). Conversely, the expression of phosphorylated ACLY (P-ACLY) decreased significantly in all the groups given 100, 300, and 500 mg/kg/day A. glehni extracts (Figure 4(d)). Protein level of PGC-1α increased in groups treated with 300 and 500 mg/kg/day A. glehni extracts (Figure 4(e)), whereas that of FASN decreased in all groups treated with A. glehni extracts (Figure 4(f)).

3.5. Immunohistochemistry Analyses of TNFα, SOD, HMGCR, and 4-HNE Expression in Liver Sections of ApoE KO Mice Treated with 0.15% Cholesterol Diet and A. glehni Extracts Showed the Decreases of TNFα and HMGCR and the Increase of SOD.

It is generally known that hyperlipidemia aggravates inflammation and stimulates the generation of reactive oxygen species [20, 21]. The level of inflammation in the body can be estimated by the level of inflammatory cytokines such as TNFα; in this study, the level of TNFα decreased in all groups treated with A. glehni extracts. On the contrary, the expression of SOD, an enzyme that converts O_2^- into either molecular oxygen (O_2) or hydrogen peroxide (H_2O_2), increased in all groups treated with A. glehni extracts. The expression of HMGCR in the control group was clearly evident; however, its expression was attenuated in experimental groups treated with A. glehni extracts.

4-Hydroxynonenal (4-HNE) is generally known with a product of lipid peroxidation and an inducer of oxidative stress, and it was reported to accelerate the lipid accumulation

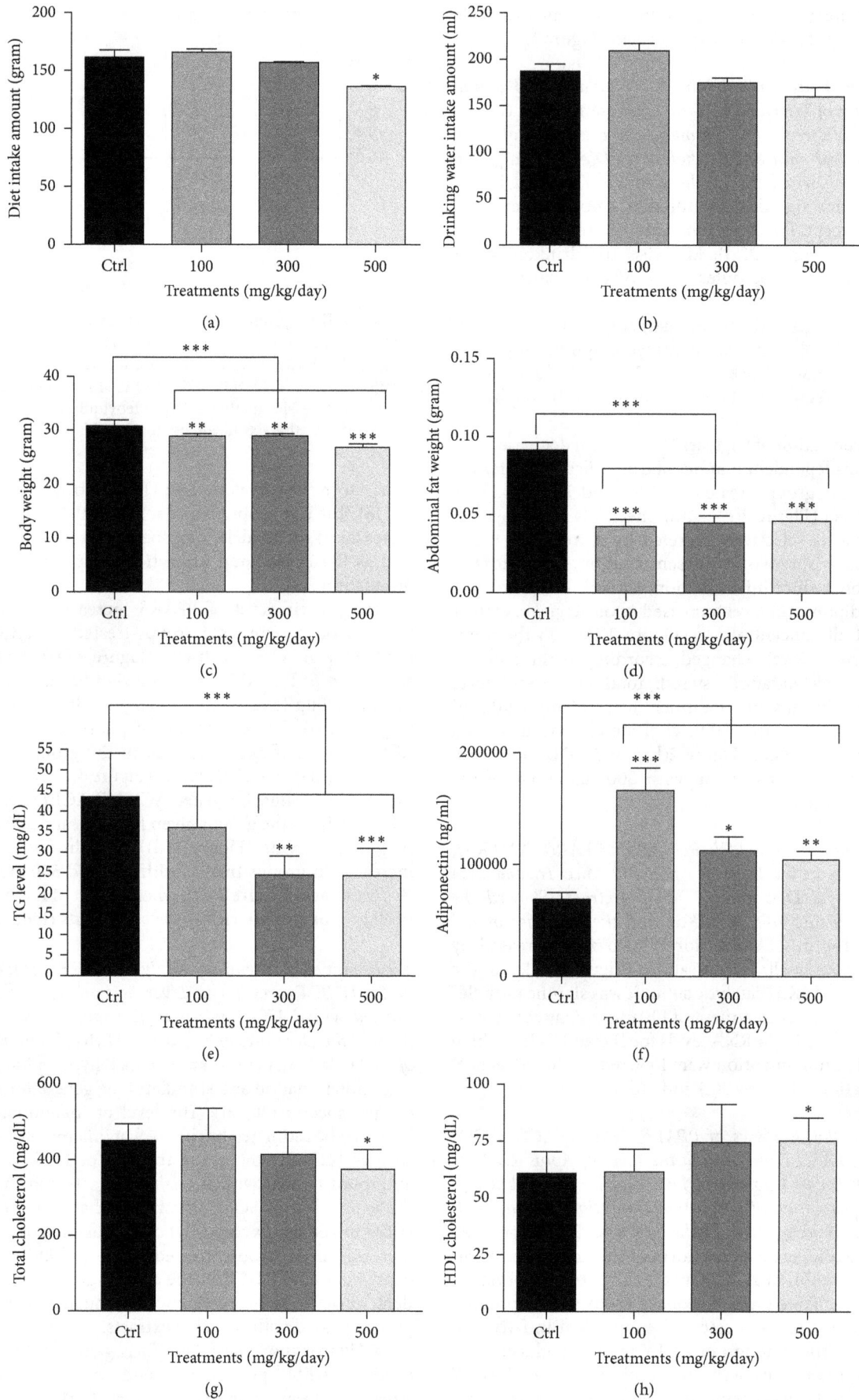

(a)

(b)

(c)

(d)

(e)

(f)

(g)

(h)

FIGURE 2: Continued.

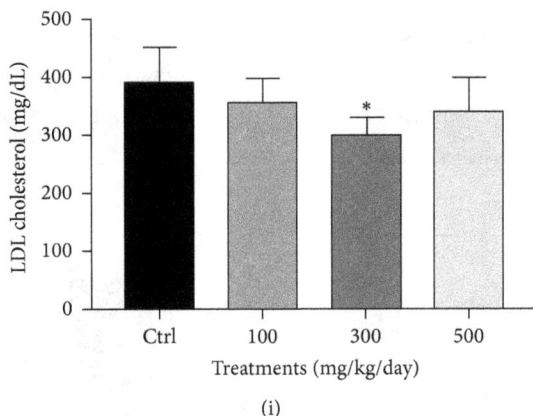

(i)

FIGURE 2: Effects of *Aster glehni* extract on diet intake amount, drinking water intake amount, body weight, abdominal adipose tissue weight, serum triglyceride, and serum adiponectin, total cholesterol, high-density lipoprotein (HDL) cholesterol, low-density lipoprotein (LDL) cholesterol in ApoE KO mice administered with 0.15% cholesterol diet. ((a) and (b)) Diet and drinking water intake amounts were estimated for four weeks. (c) Body weight of mice was estimated just prior to sacrifice. (d) Abdominal adipose tissue was removed from sacrificed mice and weighed. (e) Triglyceride concentration in serum was estimated with triglyceride colorimetric assay kit. (f) Adiponectin concentration in serum was estimated with mouse adiponectin enzyme-linked immunosorbent assay (ELISA) kit. (g, h, and i) Levels of cholesterols were estimated with triglyceride colorimetric assay kit. The results are expressed as means ± SEM. Values were statistically analyzed by unpaired t-test and one way ANOVA. All experiments were repeated three times. $^{*}p < 0.05$ versus control, $^{**}p < 0.01$ versus control, and $^{***}p < 0.001$ versus control.

in hepatocytes [22]. In addition, 4-HNE protein expression was decreased by AMPK agonist, 5-aminoimidazole-4-carboxamide-1-beta-D-ribofuranoside (AICAR) in alcohol induced fatty liver [23]. The 4-HNE expression was decreased with *A. glehni* extracts (Figure 5).

3.6. In the Liver of ApoE KO Mice Treated with 0.15% Cholesterol Diet and A. glehni Extracts, Succinate Dehydrogenase Activity Was Increased, Concentrations of Triglyceride, IL6, and ROS Were Decreased, and the Morphology of Hepatocytes Was Improved in the Group Treated with the Extract of 300 mg/kg/day. Succinate dehydrogenase catalyzes the reaction that converts succinate and flavin adenine dinucleotide (FAD) into fumarate and FADH2 in the citric acid cycle, also it participates in the electron transport chain known. In addition, the SDH is known as a biomarker of mitochondrial biogenesis, together with PGC-1α [24]. In this study, SDH activity increased only in mice treated with 300 mg/kg/day *A. glehni* (Figure 6(a)). Triglyceride concentration in the liver decreased significantly in the experimental group treated with 300 mg/kg/day *A. glehni* (Figure 6(b)). Ballooning of hepatocytes is an important index for the histological diagnosis of NASH [25]. IL6 concentration in the liver decreased in the experimental groups treated with *A. glehni* extracts of 300 and 500 mg/kg/day concentrations (Figure 6(c)). Also the concentration of reactive oxygen species (ROS) was decreased in experimental groups treated with *A. glehni* extracts of all concentrations (Figure 6(d)).

Balloon-like cell morphology was observed in all experimental groups except for the group treated with 300 mg/kg/day *A. glehni*, which exhibited liver morphology that was most similar to that of a normal liver (Figure 6(e)). These results suggested that a 300 mg/kg/day dosage of *A. glehni* was most effective in preventing and ameliorating fatty liver in ApoE KO mice given 0.15% cholesterol diet.

3.7. Oil Red O Staining and Western Blot Analyses for PPARδ, AMPK, and PGC-1α in HepG2 Cells Treated with A. glehni Extract and GSK0660 in High Fatty Acid and High Cholesterol Condition Showed the Direct Decrease of Lipid Accumulation and the Increases of Biomarkers Related to Lipid Oxidation. While the lipid content in HepG2 cells increased to 77.6% upon the cotreatment of palmitate and cholesterol compared to control, the elevated lipid level decreased significantly in cotreating condition of palmitate, cholesterol, and *A. glehni* extract. But the effect of *A. glehni* was inhibited by the cotreatment of PPARδ antagonist, GSK0660 (Figures 7(a) and 7(b)). Protein levels of PPARδ, P-AMPK, and PGC-1α increased upon *A. glehni* extract treatment compared with their levels in the control group. However, this effect of *A. glehni* extract was suppressed by the action of the PPARδ antagonist, GSK0660 (Figures 7(c)–7(e)).

3.8. Protein Expression Levels for PPARγ and PPARα Were Not Changed with A. glehni Extract in HepG2 Cells in High Fatty Acid and High Cholesterol Condition: AMPK Antagonist, Compound C, Did Not Affect the Protein Level of PPARδ. Aster glehni extract did not change the protein expression levels for PPARγ and PPARα in HepG2 cells treated with high fatty acid and high cholesterol (Figures 8(a) and 8(b)). The AMPK antagonist (compound C) did not reduce the PPARδ protein level (Figure 8(c)).

3.9. Oil Red O Staining of Differentiated 3T3-L1 Cells Treated with A. glehni Extract and GSK0660 in High Fatty Acid and High Cholesterol Condition Showed the Antiadipogenic Effect of the Extract, and Protein Levels for PPARδ, AMPK, and PGC-1α in Abdominal Fat Tissues from ApoE KO Mice Given 0.15% Cholesterol Diet Were Mainly Increased in the Group Treated with the Extract of 500 mg/kg/day. The lipid content in differentiated 3T3-L1 cells, which was increased by

(a)

(b)

(c)

(d)

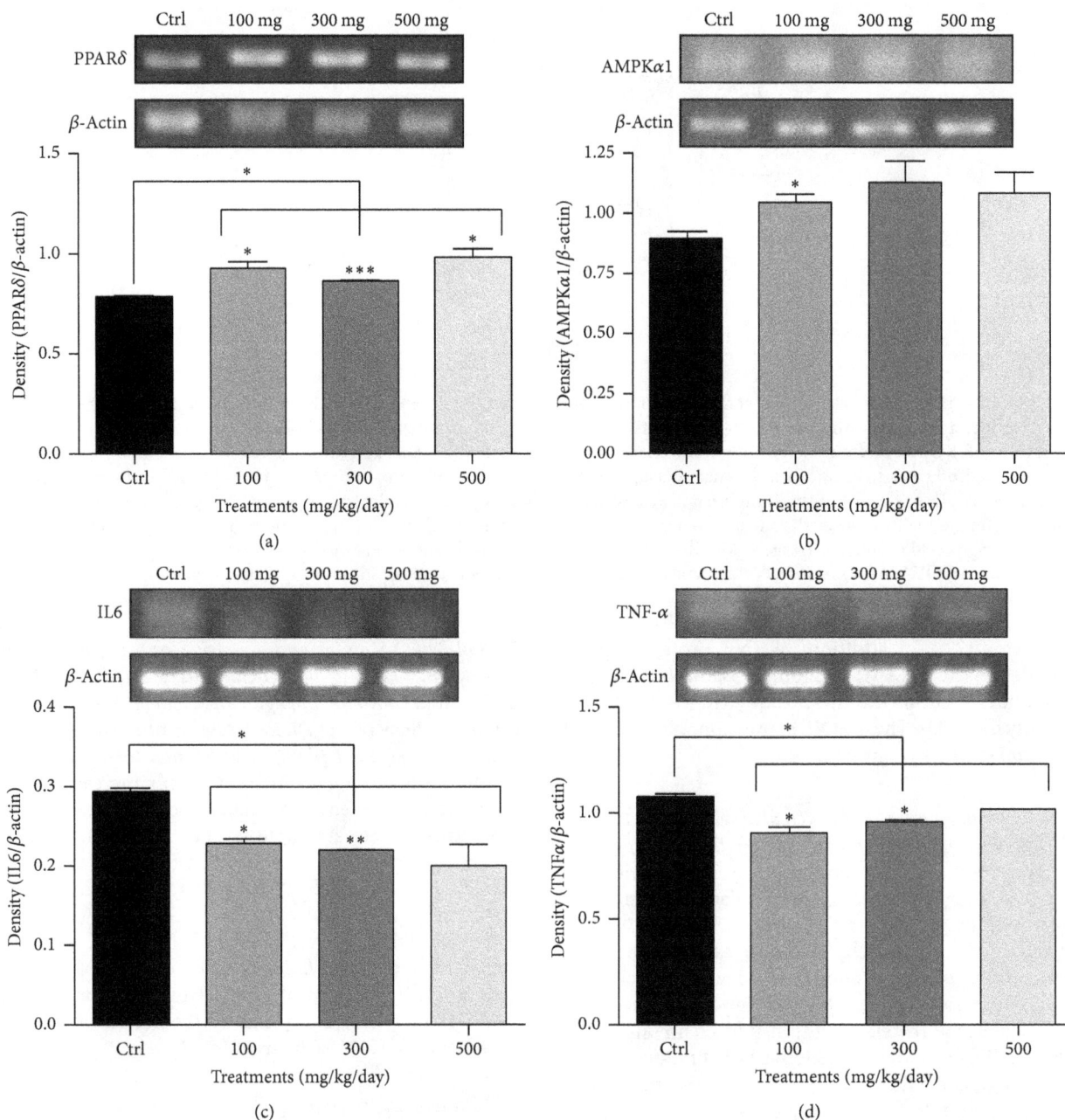

FIGURE 3: The mRNA levels of peroxisome proliferator-activated receptor delta (PPARδ), 5′ adenosine monophosphate-activated protein kinase α1 (AMPKα1), interleukin 6 (IL6), and tumor necrosis factor α (TNFα) in liver of ApoE KO mice treated with 0.15% cholesterol diet and *Aster glehni* extract. Total RNA was extracted by Trisol reagent from liver tissues of ApoE KO mice, and complementary DNA was synthesized by cDNA synthesis kit from the total RNA. Polymerase chain reaction (PCR) was done with cDNA, primers, and PCR Premix solution. The PCR image density was analyzed with Image J program. The results are expressed as means ± SEM. Values were statistically analyzed by unpaired t-test and one way ANOVA. All experiments were repeated three times. $^{*}p < 0.05$ versus control, $^{**}p < 0.01$ versus control, and $^{***}p < 0.001$ versus control.

palmitate and cholesterol treatment, decreased upon treatment with *A. glehni*, and the effect of *A. glehni* on these cells was also suppressed by the cotreatment of GSK0660 (Figures 9(a) and 9(b)). Protein levels for PPARδ, P-AMPK, and PGC-1α were highest in abdominal fat from mice treated with 500 mg/kg/day *A. glehni* compared to control (Figures 9(c)–9(e)).

4. Discussion

The liver has many essential physiological functions such as hematopoiesis, secretion of bile, eradication of foreign material and bacteria by Kupffer cells, and maintaining energy homeostasis of the body [26]. Many studies have reported that abnormal lipid metabolism in the liver is

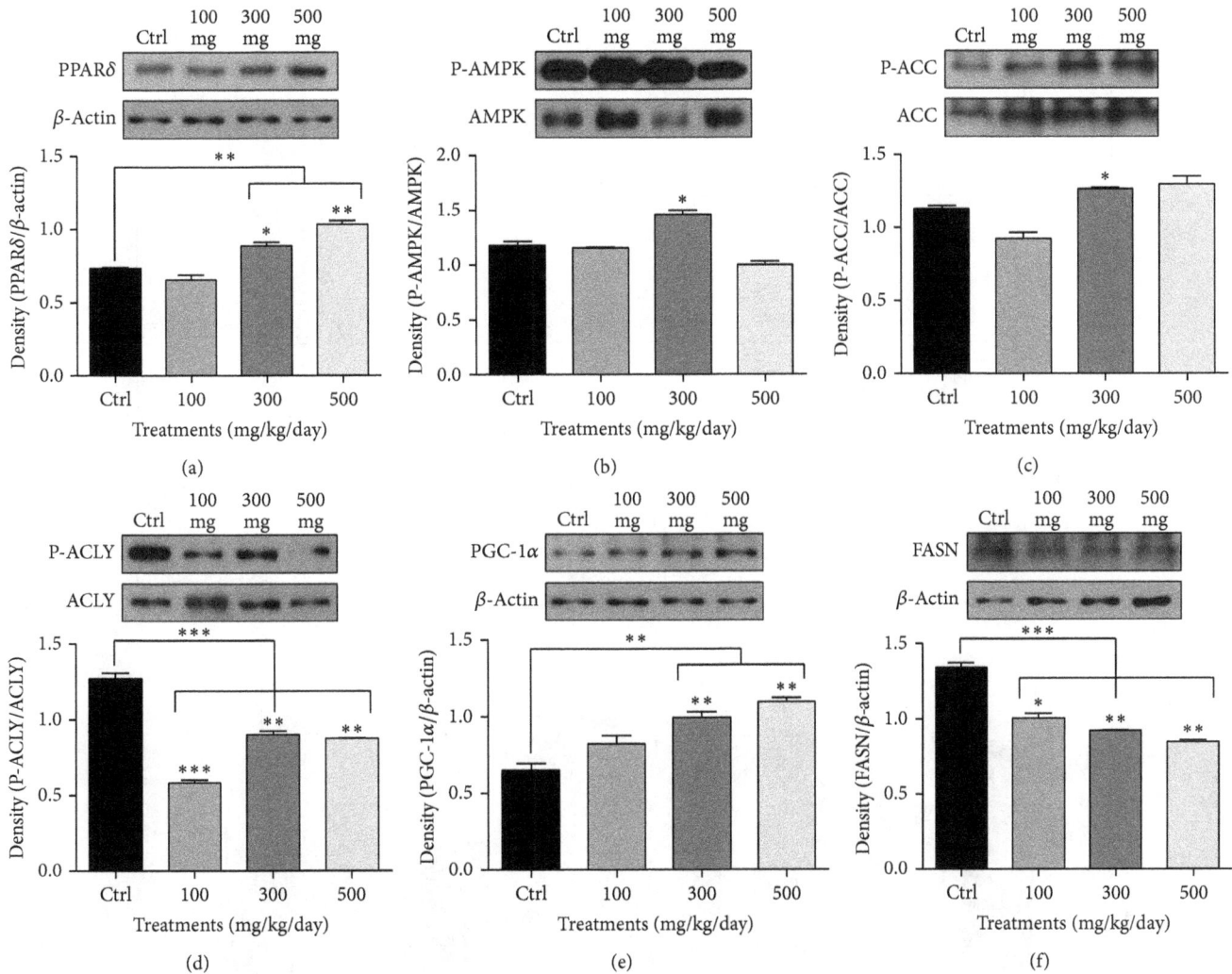

FIGURE 4: The protein levels of peroxisome proliferator-activated receptor delta (PPARδ), 5′ adenosine monophosphate-activated protein kinase (AMPK), acetyl-CoA carboxylase (ACC), ATP citrate lyase (ACLY), peroxisome proliferator-activated receptor gamma coactivator 1-alpha (PGC-1α), and fatty acid synthase (FASN) in liver of ApoE KO mice treated with 0.15% cholesterol diet and Aster glehni extract. Protein extracts were electrophoresed in 10% polyacrylamide gel and blotted to nitrocellulose membrane. The nitrocellulose membrane was bound with primary and secondary antibodies sequentially, and then the chemiluminescence was exposed to X-ray film. The density for bands on X-ray film was analyzed with Image J program. The results are expressed as means ± SEM. Values were statistically analyzed by unpaired t-test and one way ANOVA. All experiments were repeated three times. $^{*}p < 0.05$ versus control, $^{**}p < 0.01$ versus control, and $^{***}p < 0.001$ versus control.

related to various metabolic diseases such as atherosclerosis, obesity, type 2 diabetes, and hypertension. For instance, it has been reported that the risk of hypertension and type II diabetes is higher in patients with NAFLD than in those in the non-NAFLD group [27–30]. Moreover, carotid intima-media thickness is greater in patients with NAFLD than in the normal healthy population [31]. In obese persons, excess intrahepatic triglyceride is a strong indicator of metabolic abnormalities and is independent from other metabolic measurements like body mass index, percent body fat, and visceral fat mass [32]. Hence, metabolic functions of the liver are vital to maintain metabolic homeostasis and the overall health of the body.

In our study for the effect and the mechanism of Aster glehni on NAFLD in ApoE KO mice, the concentration of

adiponectin in serum was significantly higher in the experimental groups treated with A. glehni extracts than that of the control group. Moreover, the concentration of triglyceride in serum, the weight of abdominal adipose tissue, and the weight of body were lower in the A. glehni treated groups than in the untreated group. And A. glehni extract sequentially regulated genes involved in fatty acid metabolism. For instance, upregulation of adiponectin and PPARδ by A. glehni induced AMPK activation, which consequently increased the levels of PGC-1α and p-ACC; this in turn elevated SDH activity and decreased FASN expression. In addition, A. glehni suppressed protein levels of p-ACLY and HMGCR. Hence, the final outcome of A. glehni action is the decrease of triglyceride level in the liver (Figures 6 and 10). From the data for TG level and SDH (Figure 6), the most effective treatment

(a)

(b) Image density

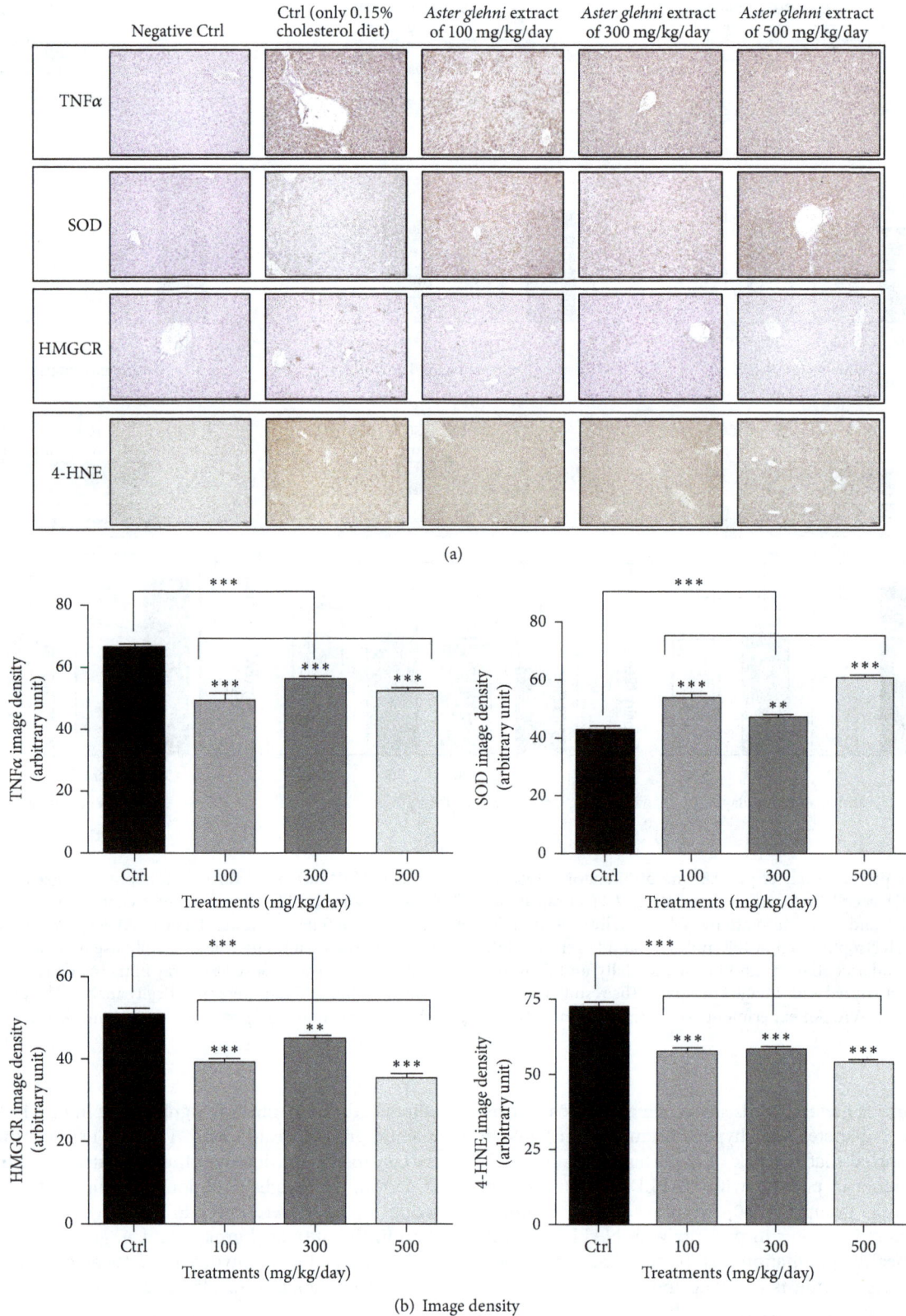

FIGURE 5: Immunohistochemistry for TNFα, SOD, HMGCR, and 4-HNE on frozen sectioned slides of liver in ApoE KO mice treated with 0.15% cholesterol diet and *Aster glehni* extract. (a) Liver tissue slides of ApoE KO mice were fixed and immunohistochemically stained with antibodies of TNFα, SOD, HMGCR, and 4-HNE. Images were taken at 200x magnification. (b) Densities for images were analyzed with Image J program. The results are expressed as means ± SEM. Values were statistically analyzed by unpaired t-test and one way ANOVA. All experiments were repeated three times. ** $p < 0.01$ versus control and *** $p < 0.001$ versus control.

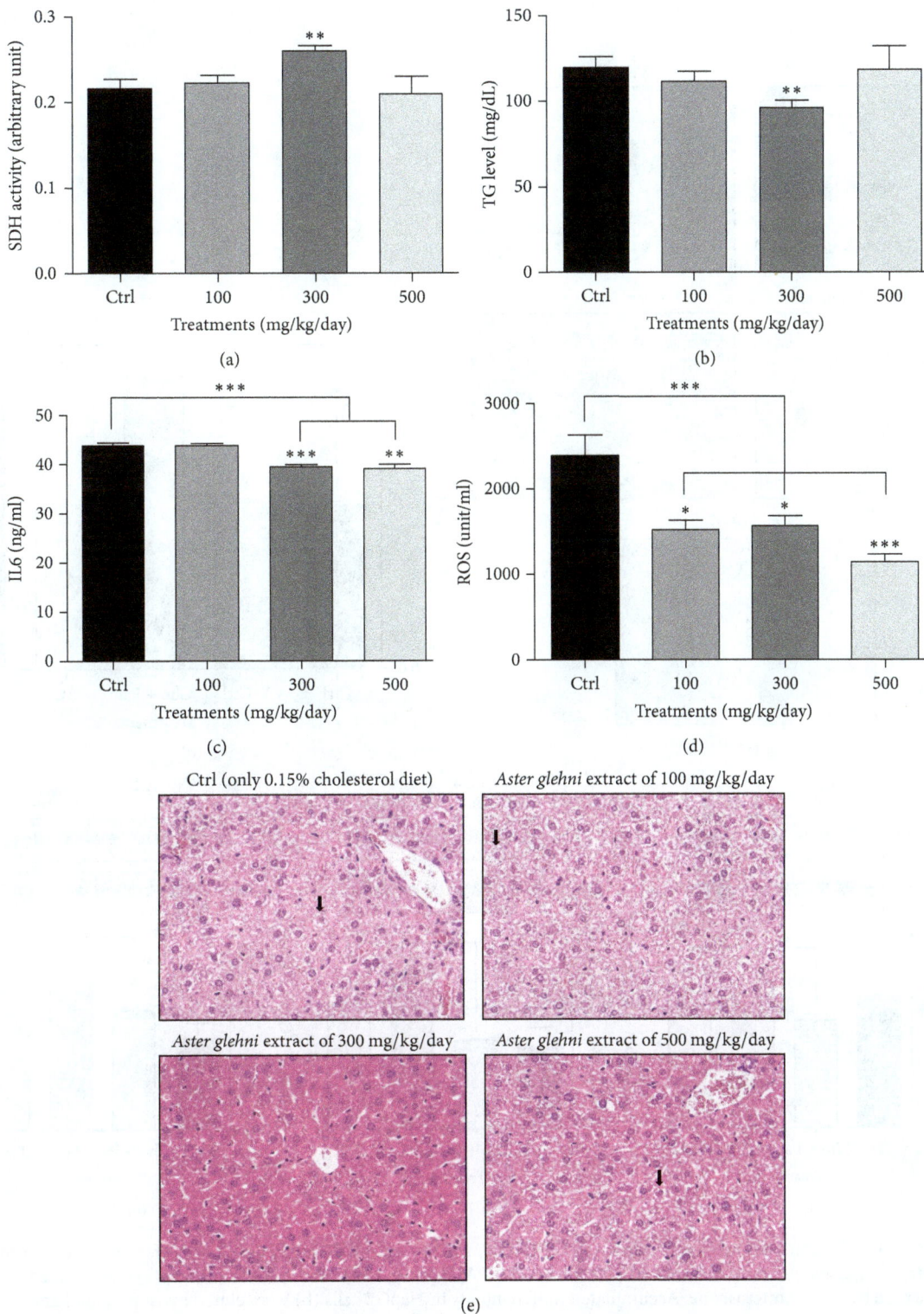

(a)

(b)

(c)

(d)

Ctrl (only 0.15% cholesterol diet)

Aster glehni extract of 100 mg/kg/day

Aster glehni extract of 300 mg/kg/day

Aster glehni extract of 500 mg/kg/day

(e)

FIGURE 6: Succinate dehydrogenase activity, triglyceride, interleukin 6 (IL6), and reactive oxygen species (ROS) concentrations, and hematoxylin and eosin staining in liver of ApoE KO mice treated with 0.15% cholesterol diet and *Aster glehni* extract. (a) Succinate dehydrogenase (SDH) activity in liver protein extracts of ApoE KO mice was estimated with colorimetric method containing nitroblue tetrazolium reagents. (b) Triglyceride (TG) contents in liver extracts of ApoE KO mice were estimated with triglyceride colorimetric assay kit. (c, d) IL6 and ROS contents in liver extracts of ApoE KO mice were estimated with IL6 and ROS colorimetric assay kits. (e) Liver tissue slides of ApoE KO mice were fixed and stained by hematoxylin and eosin reagents. Magnification is 200 times. The results are expressed as means ± SEM. Values were statistically analyzed by unpaired t-test and one way ANOVA. All experiments were repeated three times. Liver cells having representative ballooning morphology were indicated by arrow marks (↓). $^*p < 0.05$ versus control, $^{**}p < 0.01$ versus control, and $^{***}p < 0.001$ versus control.

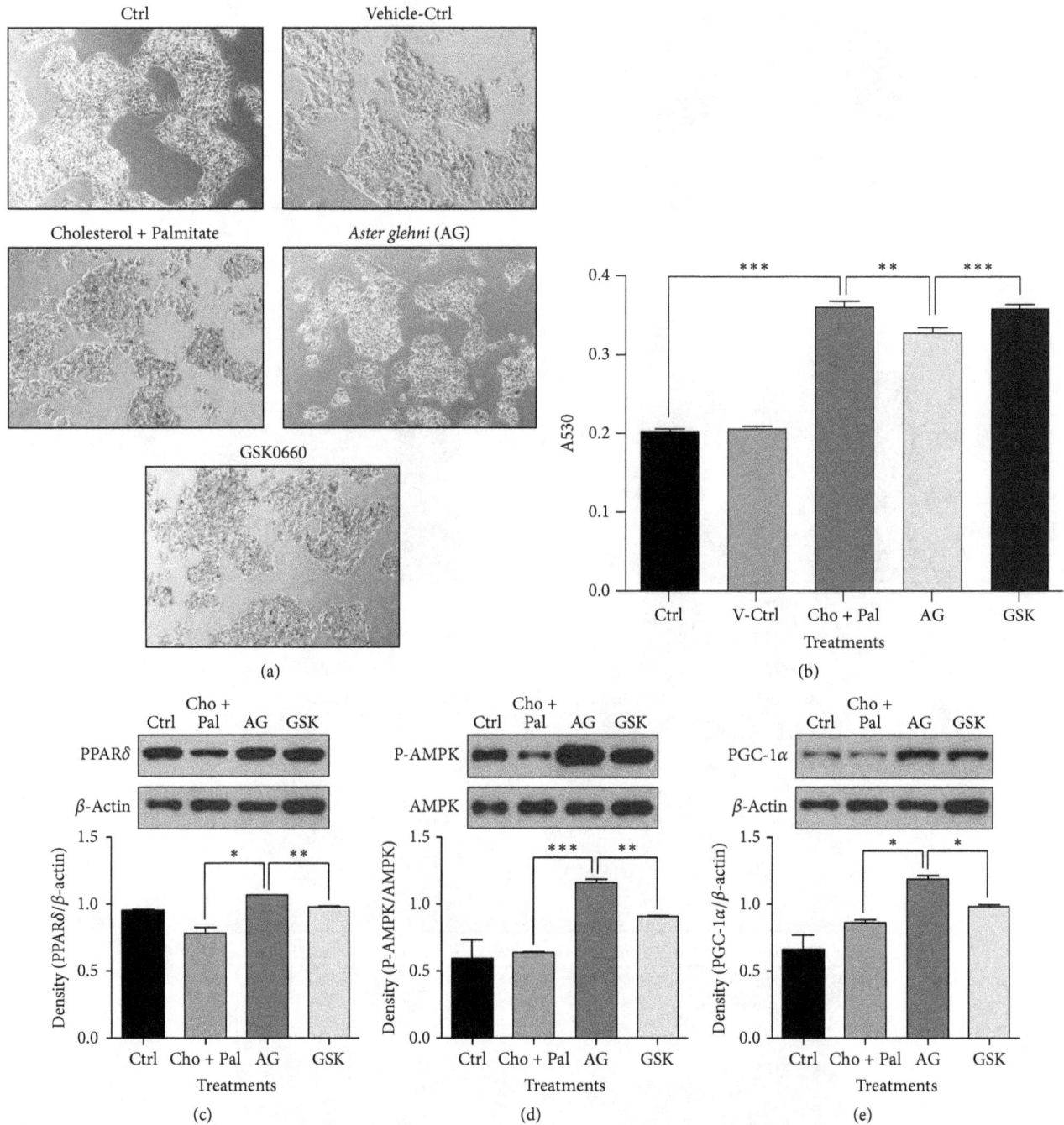

(a)

(b)

(c)   (d)   (e)

FIGURE 7: Oil Red O staining result and the protein levels of PPARδ, AMPK and PGC-1α in HepG2 cells treated with 0.2 mM cholesterol, 0.1 mM palmitate, 50 ug *Aster glehni* extract, and 50 uM GSK0660 (PPARδ antagonist). The lipids in HepG2 (a) were stained with Oil Red O reagent and observed by optical microscope. Accumulated lipid contents in HepG2 cells (b) were eluted by isopropanol and the absorbance of eluted Oil Red O was estimated with ELISA reader at the wave length of 530 nm. Magnification is 200 times. Meaning of indications: Ctrl is an untreated control group, V-Ctrl is a vehicle control group, Cho + Pal is a cholesterol and palmitate treated group, AG is a cholesterol, palmitate, and *A. glehni* treated group, and GSK is a cholesterol, palmitate, *A. glehni*, and GSK0660 treated group. Protein extracts were electrophoresed in 10% polyacrylamide gel and blotted to nitrocellulose membrane. The nitrocellulose membrane was bound with primary and secondary antibodies sequentially, and then the chemiluminescence was exposed to X-ray film. The density for bands on X-ray film was analyzed with Image J program (c, d, e). The results are expressed as means ± SEM. Values were statistically analyzed by unpaired t-test and one way ANOVA. All experiments were repeated three times. $^{*}p < 0.05$, $^{**}p < 0.01$, and $^{***}p < 0.001$.

(a)

(b)

(c)

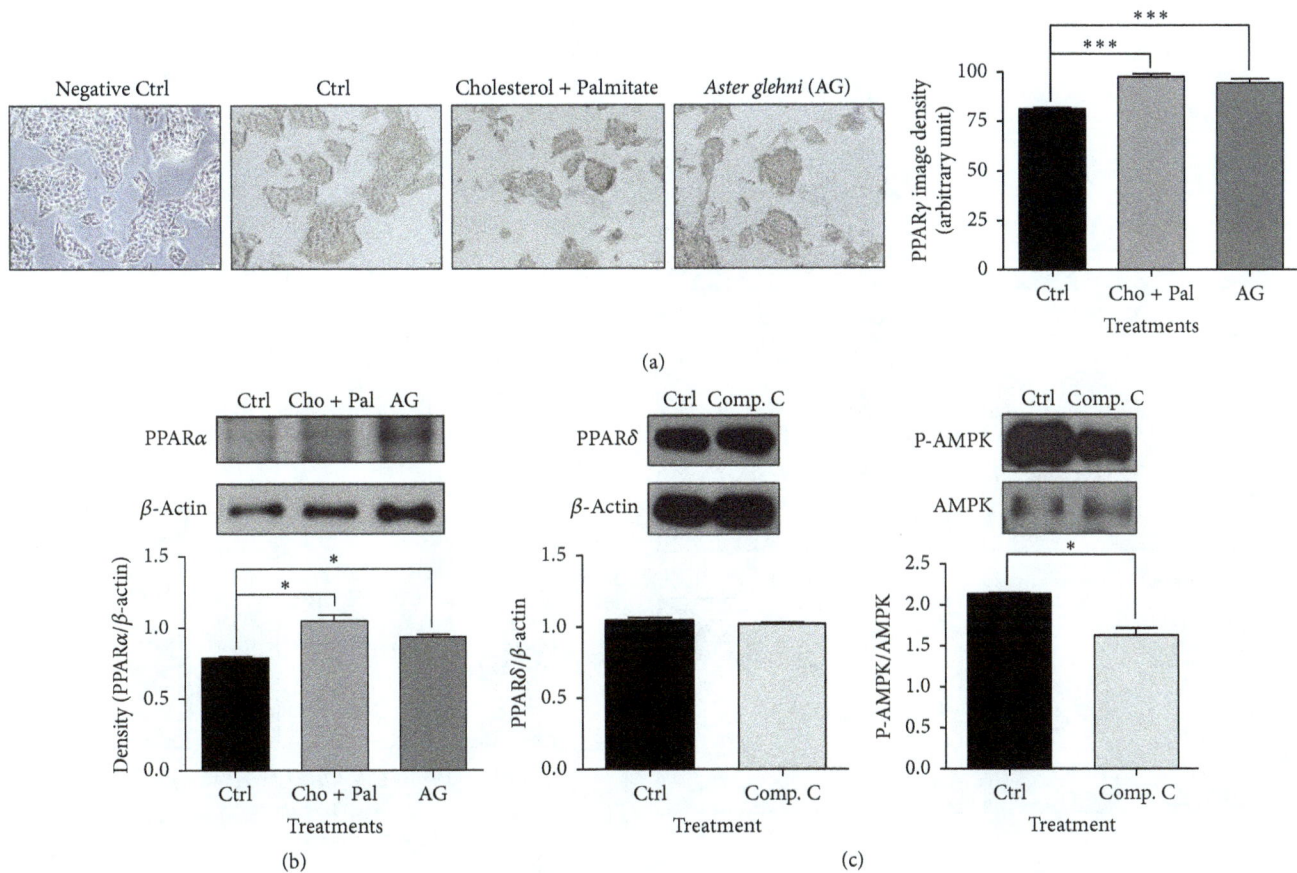

FIGURE 8: The protein levels of PPARγ and PPARα in HepG2 cells treated with 0.2 mM cholesterol, 0.1 mM palmitate, and 50 ug *Aster glehni* extract, and PPARδ and AMPK protein levels in HepG2 cells treated with 10 uM compound C (AMPK antagonist). (a) Liver tissue slides of ApoE KO mice were fixed and immunohistochemically stained with antibody of PPARγ. Images were taken at 200x magnification. (b, c) Protein extracts were electrophoresed in 10% polyacrylamide gel and blotted to nitrocellulose membrane. The nitrocellulose membrane was bound with primary and secondary antibodies sequentially, and then the chemiluminescence was exposed to X-ray film. The density for bands on X-ray film was analyzed with Image J program. The results are expressed as means ± SEM. Values were statistically analyzed by unpaired t-test and one way ANOVA. All experiments were repeated three times. $^*p < 0.05$ and $^{***}p < 0.001$.

concentration of *Aster glehni* extract to prevent NAFLD in atherosclerotic condition is supposed to be 300 mg/kg/day. But the *A. glehni* extract showed minus effects at the concentration over 300 mg/kg/day in liver lipid metabolism, and it is supported by the following result: the TG level in liver showed an elevated tendency in the group treated with extract of 500 mg/kg/day concentration compared to group treated with the extract of 300 mg/kg/day concentration. So, it can be postulated that the *A. glehni* extract of high concentration has negative effects in the liver lipid metabolism of ApoE KO mice.

A. glehni treatment may additionally ameliorate NAFLD via regulation of SOD, TNFα, 4-HNE, IL6, and ROS (Figures 5, 6, and 10). In this study, the cause for the reduction of body weight and abdominal adipose tissue mass by the treatment of *A. glehni* extract can be explained from the elevation of biomarkers related to fatty acid oxidative metabolism and the downregulation of biomarkers involved in lipid synthesis and inflammation. The PPARδ antagonist (GSK0660) offset the effects of *A. glehni* stimulating protein expression of PPARδ, p-AMPK, and PGC-1α in HepG2 cells (Figure 7)

and reversed its effect of lowering lipid accumulation in HepG2 and differentiated 3T3-L1 cells (Figures 7 and 9). These results indicate that PPARδ regulates AMPK and PGC-1α. In addition, the *A. glehni* extract did not affect protein expression for PPARα and PPARγ in the condition of cholesterol and palmitate cotreatment (Figures 8(a) and 8(b)), so it can be supposed that *A. glehni* extract specifically regulates PPARδ compared to PPARα and PPARγ. In addition, PPARδ antagonist (GSK0660) decreased the protein level of P-AMPK (Figure 7(d)), but the AMPK antagonist (compound C) did not change the PPARδ protein level (Figure 8(c)). So these results mean that PPARδ is an upper regulator against AMPK.

Our results are almost consistent with the results of other papers as follows.

In adipose tissues, inflammatory proteins such as C-reactive protein and TNFα are negatively regulated by adiponectin; adiponectin also suppresses TNFα production in cardiac cells [33]. Furthermore, it specifically suppresses TNFα-induced activation of inhibitor of κB- (IκB-) α/nuclear factor κB (NF-κB) through the cAMP-dependent pathway in human aortic endothelial cells [34]. Adiponectin level in

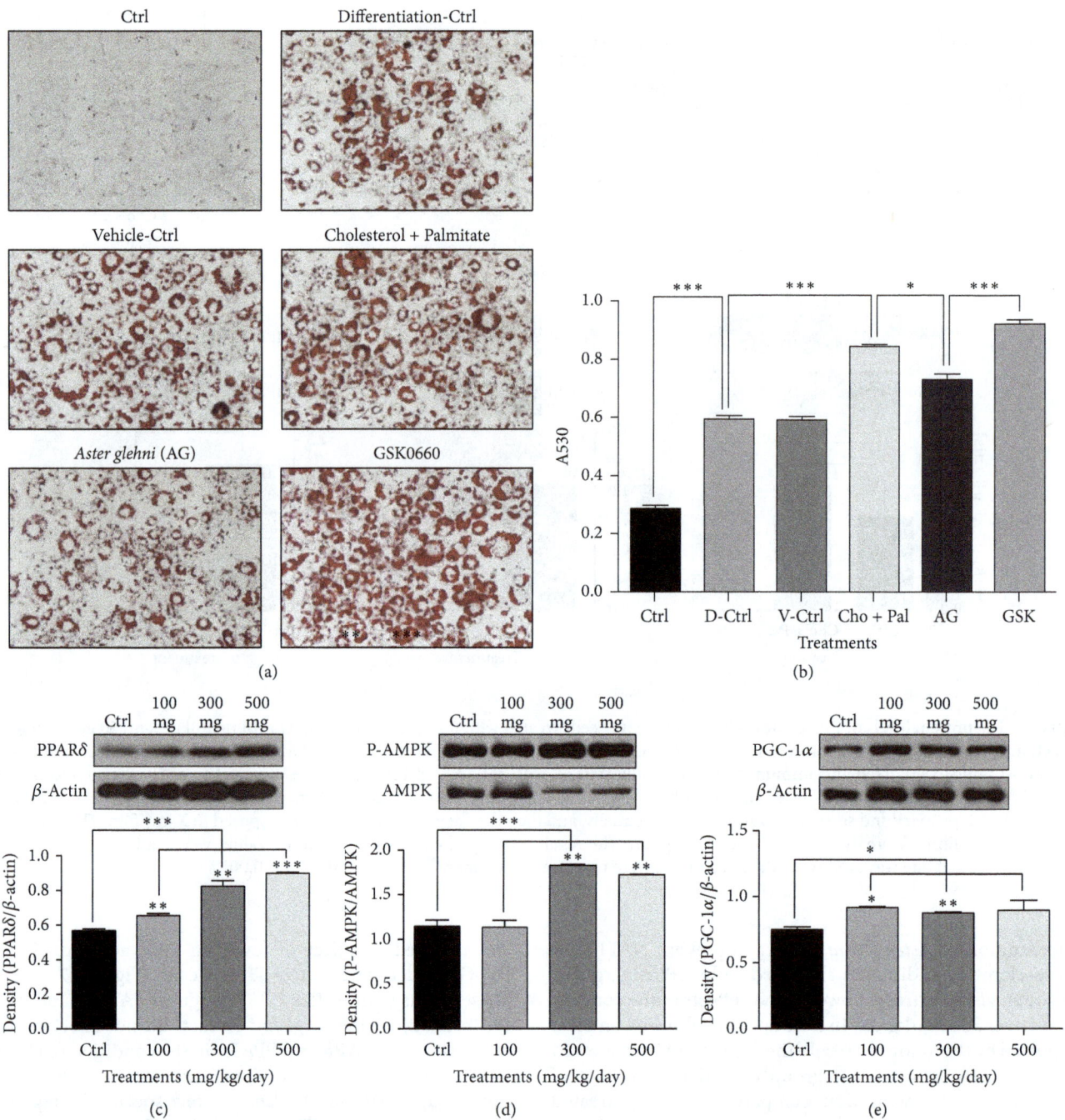

(a)

(b)

(c)

(d)

(e)

FIGURE 9: Oil Red O staining results in differentiated 3T3-L1 cells treated with 0.2 mM cholesterol, 0.1 mM palmitate, 50 ug *Aster glehni* extract, and 50 uM GSK0660 (PPARδ antagonist) and the protein levels of PPARδ, AMPK, and PGC-1α in abdominal fat tissues of ApoE KO mice treated with 0.15% cholesterol diet and *Aster glehni* extract. The lipids in differentiated 3T3-L1 cells (a) were stained with Oil Red O reagent and observed by optical microscope. Accumulated lipid contents in differentiated 3T3-L1 cells (b) were eluted by isopropanol and the absorbance of eluted Oil Red O was estimated with ELISA reader at the wave length of 530 nm. Magnification is 200 times. Meaning of indications: Ctrl is an untreated control group, D-Ctrl is a differentiation control group, V-Ctrl is a vehicle control group, Cho + Pal is a cholesterol and palmitate treated group, AG is a cholesterol, palmitate, and *A. glehni* treated group, and GSK is a cholesterol, palmitate, *A. glehni*, and GSK0660 treated group. Protein extracts were electrophoresed in 10% polyacrylamide gel and blotted to nitrocellulose membrane. The nitrocellulose membrane was bound with primary and secondary antibodies sequentially, and then the chemiluminescence was exposed to X-ray film. The density for bands on X-ray film was analyzed with Image J program (c, d, e). The results are expressed as means ± SEM. Values were statistically analyzed by unpaired t-test and one way ANOVA. All experiments were repeated three times. $^{*}p < 0.05$, $^{**}p < 0.01$, and $^{***}p < 0.001$.

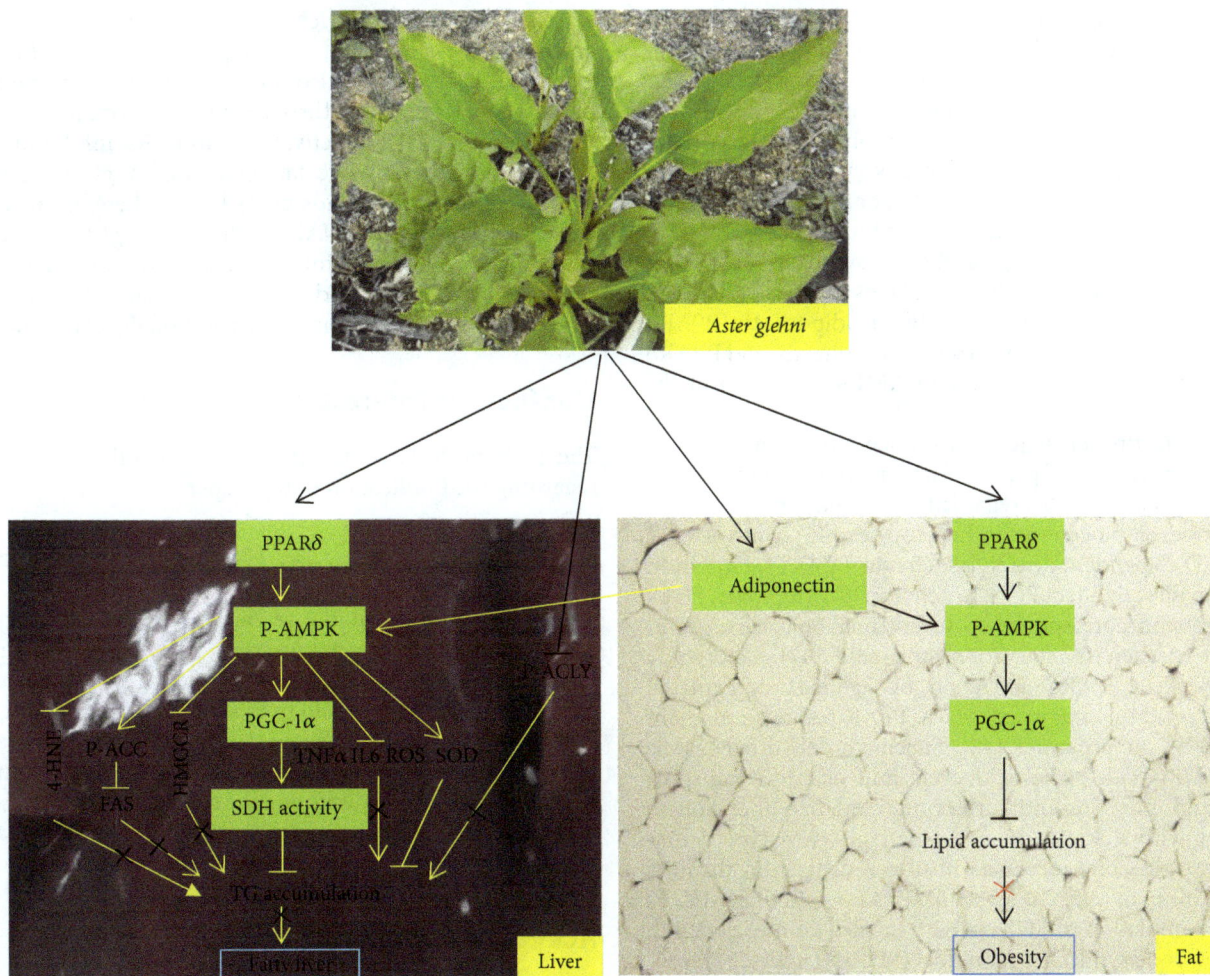

FIGURE 10: Schematic diagram for the functional mechanism of *Aster glehni* extract. Amelioration of nonalcoholic fatty liver by *Aster glehni* is mainly accomplished with catabolic activation such as the sequential regulation of PPARδ/adiponectin→P-AMPK→PGC-1α→SDH, also it is done by other pathway of P-AMPK→P-ACC which inhibits fatty acid synthesis. *Aster glehni* additionally lowers triglyceride accumulation in liver by inhibiting P-ACLY, also its anti-TG accumulation effect is done through the regulation of TNFα and SOD by P-AMPK. In addition, the extract may prevent obesity via PPARδ/adiponectin→P-AMPK→PGC pathway. Meaning of symbols: arrow means activation, up and horizontal line means inhibition, and × means blocking. Photograph of *Aster glehni* was quoted from Korea Rural Development Administration Genebank information center (PCV0039).

plasma of patients with metabolic diseases such as hypertension, type 2 diabetes, and obesity is lower than that of healthy subjects [35–37]. Adiponectin activates AMPK via phosphorylation. In turn, activated AMPK inactivates ACC by phosphorylation and decreases the production of malonyl-CoA, which is required in de novo fatty acid synthesis [16]. Also many studies in which PPARδ regulates AMPK activation were reported as follows: the activated PPARδ induced AMPK activation and affected glucose transport in skeletal muscle cells [38], PPARδ activation by agonist induced the normalization of p-AMPK and PGC-1α levels lowered in liver of mice given high fat diet [39], and angiotensin II receptor blocker, telmisartan, decreased the weight gain and elevated the running endurance through the regulation of PPARδ-AMPK pathway in which the activation of AMPK depends on PPARδ [40]. The role of AMPK in regulating lipid metabolism has been described extensively. For

example, intracellular triglyceride accumulation induced by TNFα decreased with administration of AMPK agonists such as metformin and 5-aminoimidazole-4-carboxamide-1-β-D-ribofuranoside (AICAR) in HepG2 cells. In addition, these AMPK agonists suppressed mechanistic target of rapamycin (mTOR) and p70S6K phosphorylation and reduced the levels of sterol regulatory element-binding protein-1 (SREBP-1) and FASN [41]. So it can be supposed that AMPK can lower the expression of inflammatory proteins such as TNFα as well as other proteins involved in fatty acid synthesis. Recently, Zhou et al. [42] demonstrated that the antiadipogenic effects of alpha-linolenic acid were dependent on AMPK and that its effects were abolished in AMPKα1 and AMPKα2 KO mice. In addition, the activation of AMPK by AICAR and metformin increases the activity of SOD. On the other hand, AMPK antagonist like compound C decreases the activity of SOD [43]. Moreover, resveratrol was shown to increase

SOD level through an AMPK-dependent mechanism in vascular endothelial cells that were subjected to high glucose-induced oxidative stress conditions [43]. However, it was reported that constitutive activation of endothelial AMPKα1 promoted vascular inflammation and obesity-induced fatty liver, largely via induction of cyclooxygenase-2 [44]. In cholesterol metabolism, AMPK activation by AICAR inhibited the expression of SREBP-2 and its target genes, HMGCR and 3-hydroxy-3-methylglutaryl-CoA synthase (HMGCS), which are key enzymes in cholesterol biosynthesis [45]. Based on these studies on the relation between adiponectin/PPARδ and lipid metabolism, it appears that adiponectin and PPARδ regulate lipid metabolism through AMPK activation in the liver.

Adiponectin deficiency can induce NASH through decreased expression of genes related to mitochondrial biogenesis such as PGC-1α, regarded as the master regulator of mitochondrial biogenesis, in hepatocytes [46]. Both AMPK and NAD-dependent deacetylase sirtuin-1 (SIRT1) have been shown to directly affect PGC-1α activity [19]. Moreover, PGC-1α expression corresponds to severe metabolic changes as a result of exercise, starvation, and cold [47]. One study reported that PPARδ activation by agonists upregulated PGC-1α mRNA expression via a PPAR-response element in the PGC-1α promoter [48]. Succinate dehydrogenase is involved in both citric acid cycle and electron transport chain and plays essential roles in oxidative metabolism together with PGC-1α. In obese patients with type 2 diabetes, rosiglitazone increased insulin sensitization through upregulation of mRNA levels of PPARδ and PGC-1α, as well as stimulation of SDH activity in skeletal muscles [49]. In a metabolic syndrome rat model (SHR/NDmcr-cp) representing characteristics of hypertension and obesity, exercise normalized the activity of SDH and the mRNA expression of PPARδ and PGC-1α [50]. Therefore, it can be supposed that the stimulation of PPARδ, PGC-1α, and SDH induces the activation of catabolic metabolism causing energy expenditure, as well as a decrease in triglyceride and increase in adiponectin levels in serum. Furthermore, succinate treatment increased protein levels of α-smooth muscle actin and G protein-coupled receptor 91, which are essential markers of fibrogenesis in human hepatic stellate cells [51], suggesting the significance of SDH in improving liver diseases like cirrhosis.

Consequently, our results suggest that A. glehni extract improves abnormal metabolic profiles in serum and liver through accelerating energy expenditure and stimulating of lipid catabolism by PPARδ and adiponectin and it can additionally ameliorate obesity through adiponectin/PPARδ-AMPK-PGC-1α pathway (Figure 10). Because body and abdominal fat weights were significantly lowered at all treatment concentrations, the decrease of diet intake at high dose (500 mg/kg/day) may be due to the strong taste of Aster glehni; however, the exact mechanism will be explained by further study. In our research, the relation between PPARδ and other biomarkers was relatively well studied; however, the reaction mechanism of adiponectin on lipid metabolism is deficient compared to PPARδ. So in the following study, additional experiments for adiponectin are necessary.

Caffeoylquinic acid-rich Pandanus tectorius fruit extract ameliorates dyslipidemia and hyperglycemia via the activation of AMPK [52]. Also 5-caffeoylquinic acid improved obesity and fatty liver through the amelioration of lipid metabolism by PPARα activation and LXRα inhibition [53]. In our study, the ethyl acetate extract of A. glehni contains mainly caffeoylquinic acids of six kinds. Therefore it can be supposed that the anti-NAFLD effect of A. glehni extract is dependent on caffeoylquinic acids. So in our following study, the anti-NAFLD effect and mechanism of caffeoylquinic acids purified from A. glehni should be additionally experimented.

Conflicts of Interest

The authors declare that there are no conflicts of interest regarding the publication of this paper.

Authors' Contributions

Yong-Jik Lee designed the research, performed all experiments, and wrote the manuscript. Yoo-Na Jang, Yoon-Mi Han, Hyun-Min Kim, and Jong-Min Jeong were involved in animal and molecular biology experiments. Min Jeoung Son and Chang Bae Jin contributed to extraction and preparation of experimental plant samples. Hong Seog Seo and Hyoung Ja Kim were involved in designing the research and set the study direction. All authors have read and agreed to the publication of the manuscript.

Acknowledgments

This research was supported by an intramural grant from the Korea Institute of Science and Technology (2E26990), a grant from the National Research Foundation of Korea (NRF-2016R1A2B3013825), a Korea University grant, a Korea University Guro Hospital Grant (O1600121), and a grant from BK21 Plus Korea University Medical Science Graduate Program. The authors thank Yoon Namkung for proofreading the manuscript and Tae Woo Jung for helping in experimental preparation.

References

[1] A. Kotronen, J. Westerbacka, R. Bergholm, K. H. Pietiläinen, and H. Yki-Järvinen, "Liver fat in the metabolic syndrome," Journal of Clinical Endocrinology and Metabolism, vol. 92, no. 9, pp. 3490–3497, 2007.

[2] P. Paschos and K. Paletas, "Non alcoholic fatty liver disease and metabolic syndrome," Hippokratia, vol. 13, no. 1, pp. 9–19, 2009.

[3] A. N. Mavrogiannaki and I. N. Migdalis, "Nonalcoholic fatty liver disease, diabetes mellitus and cardiovascular disease: newer data," International Journal of Endocrinology, vol. 2013, Article ID 450639, 8 pages, 2013.

[4] J.-H. Ryoo, Y. J. Suh, H. C. Shin, Y. K. Cho, J.-M. Choi, and S. K. Park, "Clinical association between non-alcoholic fatty liver disease and the development of hypertension," Journal of Gastroenterology and Hepatology (Australia), vol. 29, no. 11, pp. 1926–1931, 2014.

[5] K. Maeda, K. Okubo, I. Shimomura, T. Funahashi, Y. Matsuzawa, and K. Matsubara, "cDNA cloning and expression of a novel adipose specific collagen-like factor, apM1 (adipose most abundant gene transcript 1)," *Biochemical and Biophysical Research Communications*, vol. 221, no. 2, pp. 286–289, 1996.

[6] H. Ekmekci and O. B. Ekmekci, "The role of adiponectin in atherosclerosis and thrombosis," *Clinical and Applied Thrombosis/Hemostasis*, vol. 12, no. 2, pp. 163–168, 2006.

[7] T. A. Hopkins, N. Ouchi, R. Shibata, and K. Walsh, "Adiponectin actions in the cardiovascular system," *Cardiovascular Research*, vol. 74, no. 1, pp. 11–18, 2007.

[8] J. Hong, S. Kim, and H.-S. Kim, "Hepatoprotective effects of soybean embryo by enhancing adiponectin-mediated AMP-activated protein kinase α pathway in high-fat and high-cholesterol diet-induced nonalcoholic fatty liver disease," *Journal of Medicinal Food*, vol. 19, no. 6, pp. 549–559, 2016.

[9] P. R. Clarke and D. G. Hardie, "Regulation of HMG-CoA reductase: identification of the site phosphorylated by the AMP-activated protein kinase in vitro and in intact rat liver," *The EMBO Journal*, vol. 9, no. 8, pp. 2439–2446, 1990.

[10] M. Foretz, D. Carling, C. Guichard, P. Ferre, and F. Foufelle, "Amp-activated protein kinase inhibits the glucose-activated expression of fatty acid synthase gene in rat hepatocytes," *Journal of Biological Chemistry*, vol. 273, no. 24, pp. 14767–14771, 1998.

[11] A. Woods, D. Azzout-Marniche, M. Foretz et al., "Characterization of the role of AMP-activated protein kinase in the regulation of glucose-activated gene expression using constitutively active and dominant negative forms of the kinase," *Molecular and Cellular Biology*, vol. 20, no. 18, pp. 6704–6711, 2000.

[12] H.-H. Kim, G.-H. Park, K.-S. Park, J.-Y. Lee, and B.-J. An, "Anti-oxidant and anti-inflammation activity of fractions from Aster glehni Fr. Schm.," *Korean Journal of Microbiology and Biotechnology*, vol. 38, no. 4, pp. 434–441, 2010.

[13] H. H. Kim, G. H. Park, K. S. Park, J. Y. Lee, T. H. Kim, and B. J. An, "The effect of Aster glehni Fr. Schm. extracts on whitening and anti-wrinkle," *Journal of Life Science*, vol. 20, no. 7, pp. 1034–1040, 2010.

[14] H.-M. Lee, G. Yang, T.-G. Ahn et al., "Antiadipogenic effects of Aster glehni extract: in vivo and in vitro effects," *Evidence-Based Complementary and Alternative Medicine*, vol. 2013, Article ID 859624, 10 pages, 2013.

[15] A. Xu, Y. Wang, and K. S. L. Lam, "Adiponectin," in *Adipose Tissue and Adipokines on Health and Disease*, G. Fantuzzi and T. Mazzone, Eds., pp. 47–57, Humana Press Inc, 2007.

[16] J. P. Wen, C. E. Liu, Y. T. Hu, G. Chen, and L. X. Lin, "Globular adiponectin regulates energy homeostasis through AMP-activated protein kinase-acetyl-CoA carboxylase (AMPK/ACC) pathway in the hypothalamus," *Molecular and Cellular Biochemistry*, vol. 344, no. 1-2, pp. 109–115, 2010.

[17] M. Chypre, N. Zaidi, and K. Smans, "ATP-citrate lyase: A mini-review," *Biochemical and Biophysical Research Communications*, vol. 422, no. 1, pp. 1–4, 2012.

[18] G. Hatzivassiliou, F. Zhao, D. E. Bauer et al., "ATP citrate lyase inhibition can suppress tumor cell growth," *Cancer Cell*, vol. 8, no. 4, pp. 311–321, 2005.

[19] C. Cantó and J. Auwerx, "PGC-1α, SIRT1 and AMPK, an energy sensing network that controls energy expenditure," *Current Opinion in Lipidology*, vol. 20, no. 2, pp. 98–105, 2009.

[20] Y. S. Bhalodia, N. R. Sheth, J. D. Vaghasiya, and N. P. Jivani, "Hyperlipidemia enhanced oxidative stress and inflammatory response evoked by renal ischemia/reperfusion injury," *International Journal of Pharmacology*, vol. 6, no. 1, pp. 25–30, 2010.

[21] X.-L. Cao, J. Du, Y. Zhang, J.-T. Yan, and X.-M. Hu, "Hyperlipidemia exacerbates cerebral injury through oxidative stress, inflammation and neuronal apoptosis in MCAO/reperfusion rats," *Experimental Brain Research*, vol. 233, no. 10, pp. 2753–2765, 2015.

[22] S. Kim, S. Park, B. Kim, and J. Kwon, "Toll-like receptor 7 affects the pathogenesis of non-alcoholic fatty liver disease," *Scientific Reports*, vol. 6, Article ID 27849, 2016.

[23] K. Tomita, G. Tamiya, S. Ando et al., "AICAR, an AMPK activator, has protective effects on alcohol-induced fatty liver in rats," *Alcoholism: Clinical and Experimental Research*, vol. 29, no. 12, 2005.

[24] A. R. Konopka, M. K. Suer, C. A. Wolff, and M. P. Harber, "Markers of human skeletal muscle mitochondrial biogenesis and quality control: Effects of age and aerobic exercise training," *Journals of Gerontology - Series A Biological Sciences and Medical Sciences*, vol. 69, no. 4, pp. 371–378, 2014.

[25] E. M. Brunt and D. G. Tiniakos, "Histopathology of nonalcoholic fatty liver disease," *World Journal of Gastroenterology*, vol. 16, no. 42, pp. 5286–5296, 2010.

[26] M. Bilzer, F. Roggel, and A. L. Gerbes, "Role of Kupffer cells in host defense and liver disease," *Liver International*, vol. 26, no. 10, pp. 1175–1186, 2006.

[27] K. Cusi, "Nonalcoholic fatty liver disease in type 2 diabetes mellitus," *Current Opinion in Endocrinology, Diabetes and Obesity*, vol. 16, no. 2, pp. 141–149, 2009.

[28] N. C. Leite, G. F. Salles, A. L. E. Araujo, C. A. Villela-Nogueira, and C. R. L. Cardoso, "Prevalence and associated factors of non-alcoholic fatty liver disease in patients with type-2 diabetes mellitus," *Liver International*, vol. 29, no. 1, pp. 113–119, 2009.

[29] A. López-Suárez, J. M. R. Guerrero, J. Elvira-González, M. Beltrán-Robles, F. Cañas-Hormigo, and A. Bascuñana-Quirell, "Nonalcoholic fatty liver disease is associated with blood pressure in hypertensive and nonhypertensive individuals from the general population with normal levels of alanine aminotransferase," *European Journal of Gastroenterology and Hepatology*, vol. 23, no. 11, pp. 1011–1017, 2011.

[30] G. Targher, L. Bertolini, R. Padovani et al., "Prevalence of nonalcoholic fatty liver disease and its association with cardiovascular disease among type 2 diabetic patients," *Diabetes Care*, vol. 30, no. 5, pp. 1212–1218, 2007.

[31] J. Cai, S. Zhang, and W. Huang, "Association between nonalcoholic fatty liver disease and carotid atherosclerosis: A meta-analysis," *International Journal of Clinical and Experimental Medicine*, vol. 8, no. 5, pp. 7673–7678, 2015.

[32] E. Fabbrini, S. Sullivan, and S. Klein, "Obesity and nonalcoholic fatty liver disease: biochemical, metabolic, and clinical implications," *Hepatology*, vol. 51, no. 2, pp. 679–689, 2010.

[33] N. Ouchi and K. Walsh, "Adiponectin as an anti-inflammatory factor," *Clinica Chimica Acta*, vol. 380, no. 1-2, pp. 24–30, 2007.

[34] N. Ouchi, S. Kihara, Y. Arita et al., "Adiponectin, an adipocyte-derived plasma protein, inhibits endothelial NF-κB signaling through a cAMP-dependent pathway," *Circulation*, vol. 102, no. 11, pp. 1296–1301, 2000.

[35] M. Adamczak, A. Więcek, T. Funahashi, J. Chudek, F. Kokot, and Y. Matsuzawa, "Decreased plasma adiponectin concentration in patients with essential hypertension," *American Journal of Hypertension*, vol. 16, no. 1, pp. 72–75, 2003.

[36] K. M. Choi, J. Lee, K. W. Lee et al., "Serum adiponectin concentrations predict the developments of type 2 diabetes and the metabolic syndrome in elderly Koreans," *Clinical Endocrinology*, vol. 61, no. 1, pp. 75–80, 2004.

[37] R. Weiss, S. Dufour, A. Groszmann et al., "Low adiponectin levels in adolescent obesity: a marker of increased intramyocellular lipid accumulation," *Journal of Clinical Endocrinology and Metabolism*, vol. 88, no. 5, pp. 2014–2018, 2003.

[38] D. K. Krämer, L. Al-Khalili, S. Perrini et al., "Direct activation of glucose transport in primary human myotubes after activation of peroxisome proliferator—activated receptor δ," *Diabetes*, vol. 54, no. 4, pp. 1157–1163, 2005.

[39] E. Barroso, R. Rodríguez-Calvo, L. Serrano-Marco et al., "The PPARβ/δ activator GW501516 prevents the down-regulation of AMPK caused by a high-fat diet in liver and amplifies the PGC-1α-lipin 1-PPARα pathway leading to increased fatty acid oxidation," *Endocrinology*, vol. 152, no. 5, pp. 1848–1859, 2011.

[40] X. Feng, Z. Luo, L. Ma et al., "Angiotensin II receptor blocker telmisartan enhances running endurance of skeletal muscle through activation of the PPAR-δ/AMPK pathway," *Journal of Cellular and Molecular Medicine*, vol. 15, no. 7, pp. 1572–1581, 2011.

[41] Q. Lv, Q. Zhen, L. Liu et al., "AMP-kinase pathway is involved in tumor necrosis factor alpha-induced lipid accumulation in human hepatoma cells," *Life Sciences*, vol. 131, pp. 23–29, 2015.

[42] X. Zhou, W. Wu, J. Chen, X. Wang, and Y. Wang, "AMP-activated protein kinase is required for the anti-adipogenic effects of alpha-linolenic acid," *Nutrition and Metabolism*, vol. 12, no. 1, article no. 10, 2015.

[43] T. M. D. Nguyen, F. Seigneurin, P. Froment, Y. Combarnous, and E. Blesbois, "The 5′-AMP-activated protein kinase (AMPK) is involved in the augmentation of antioxidant defenses in cryopreserved chicken sperm," *PLoS ONE*, vol. 10, no. 7, Article ID e0134420, 2015.

[44] Y. Liang, B. Huang, E. Song, B. Bai, and Y. Wang, "Constitutive activation of AMPK α1 in vascular endothelium promotes high-fat diet-induced fatty liver injury: Role of COX-2 induction," *British Journal of Pharmacology*, vol. 171, no. 2, pp. 498–508, 2014.

[45] S. Liu, F. Jing, C. Yu, L. Gao, Y. Qin, and J. Zhao, "AICAR-induced activation of AMPK inhibits TSH/SREBP-2/HMGCR pathway in liver," *PLoS ONE*, vol. 10, no. 5, Article ID e0124951, 2015.

[46] P. Handa, B. D. Maliken, J. E. Nelson et al., "Reduced adiponectin signaling due to weight gain results in nonalcoholic steatohepatitis through impaired mitochondrial biogenesis," *Hepatology*, vol. 60, no. 1, pp. 133–145, 2014.

[47] A. Meirhaeghe, V. Crowley, C. Lenaghan et al., "Characterization of the human, mouse and rat PGC1β (peroxisomeproliferator-activated receptor-γ co-activator 1β) gene in vitro and in vivo," *Biochemical Journal*, vol. 373, no. 1, pp. 155–165, 2003.

[48] E. Hondares, I. Pineda-Torra, R. Iglesias, B. Staels, F. Villarroya, and M. Giralt, "PPARδ, but not PPARα, activates PGC-1α gene transcription in muscle," *Biochemical and Biophysical Research Communications*, vol. 354, no. 4, pp. 1021–1027, 2007.

[49] M. Mensink, M. K. C. Hesselink, A. P. Russell, G. Schaart, J.-P. Sels, and P. Schrauwen, "Improved skeletal muscle oxidative enzyme activity and restoration of PGC-1α and PPARβ/δ gene expression upon rosiglitazone treatment in obese patients with type 2 diabetes mellitus," *International Journal of Obesity*, vol. 31, no. 8, pp. 1302–1310, 2007.

[50] F. Nagatomo, H. Fujino, H. Kondo et al., "The effects of running exercise on oxidative capacity and PGC-1α mRNA levels in the soleus muscle of rats with metabolic syndrome," *Journal of Physiological Sciences*, vol. 62, no. 2, pp. 105–114, 2012.

[51] Y. H. Li, S. H. Woo, D. H. Choi, and E.-H. Cho, "Succinate causes α-SMA production through GPR91 activation in hepatic stellate cells," *Biochemical and Biophysical Research Communications*, vol. 463, no. 4, pp. 853–858, 2015.

[52] C. Wu, X. Zhang, X. Zhang et al., "The caffeoylquinic acid-rich Pandanus tectorius fruit extract increases insulin sensitivity and regulates hepatic glucose and lipid metabolism in diabetic db/db mice," *Journal of Nutritional Biochemistry*, vol. 25, no. 4, pp. 412–419, 2014.

[53] K. Huang, X.-C. Liang, Y.-L. Zhong, W.-Y. He, and Z. Wang, "5-Caffeoylquinic acid decreases diet-induced obesity in rats by modulating PPARα and LXRα transcription," *Journal of the Science of Food and Agriculture*, vol. 95, no. 9, pp. 1903–1910, 2015.

5

PPARγ and its Role in Cardiovascular Diseases

Mini Chandra, Sumitra Miriyala, and Manikandan Panchatcharam

Department of Cellular Biology and Anatomy, Louisiana State University Health Sciences Center, Shreveport, USA

Correspondence should be addressed to Manikandan Panchatcharam; mpanch@lsuhsc.edu

Academic Editor: Richard P. Phipps

Peroxisome proliferator-activated receptor Gamma (PPARγ), a ligand-activated transcription factor, has a role in various cellular functions as well as glucose homeostasis, lipid metabolism, and prevention of oxidative stress. The activators of PPARγ are already widely used in the treatment of diabetes mellitus. The cardioprotective effect of PPARγ activation has been studied extensively over the years making them potential therapeutic targets in diseases associated with cardiovascular disorders. However, they are also associated with adverse cardiovascular events such as congestive heart failure and myocardial infarction. This review aims to discuss the role of PPARγ in the various cardiovascular diseases and summarize the current knowledge on PPARγ agonists from multiple clinical trials. Finally, we also review the new PPARγ agonists under development as potential therapeutics with reduced or no adverse effects.

1. Introduction

Peroxisome proliferation-activated receptor gamma (PPARγ) is a ligand-activated transcription factor from the nuclear receptor family of peroxisome proliferator-activated receptors (PPARs). They contain a ligand binding domain which is hydrophobic and a type II zinc finger DNA-binding domain [1]. PPARs bind as heterodimers with the retinoid X receptor (RXRα) which is 9-cis retinoic acid receptor. PPAR RXR heterodimers transactivate genes by binding specific sequences in the promotor regions of these genes. When a ligand activates PPARγ it results in subsequent activation of target genes as well as inhibition of the inflammatory response of transcription factors. In the absence of ligands, this PPAR RXR heterodimer binds to co-repressors and in turn suppresses the target genes [2, 3]. There are four isoforms of PPARγ detected in humans, PPARγ1, PPARγ2, PPARγ3 and PPARγ4 [4]. Out of these isoforms PPARγ 1, 3 and 4 encode the same protein whereas PPARγ2 is expressed in adipose tissue only [5]. The location of human PPARγ gene has been identified as chromosome 3p25 [6]. In mice, the location is on chromosome 6 [7].

PPARγ is activated by both natural and synthetic ligands such as derivatives of prostaglandins like 15-deoxy-Delta12, 14-prostaglandin J2 [8], derivatives of fatty acid oxidation hydroxy octadecadienoic acid (HODE) which are components of oxidized low density lipoproteins (LDL) [9], lysophosphatidic acid (LPA) [10], Thiazolidinediones (TZD) like pioglitazone and rosiglitazone [8] and natural dietary substances found in the food [11].

PPARγ is highly expressed in adipocytes [12], vascular smooth muscle cells (VSMCs) [13], macrophages [14], cardiomyocytes [15] and endothelial cells. PPARγ activation serves a role in glucose homeostasis and adipogenesis in subcutaneous fat [16], regulating the metabolism of lipid in adipocytes, keeping oxidative stress in check as well as inhibiting apoptosis and maintaining endothelial function, cell proliferation and cell differentiation [17]. It also has a role against inflammation [18]. PPARγ activation results in reduced expression of factors such as TNF-alpha, IL-1 and resistin which are insulin resistance-inducing adipokines. In macrophages, PPARγ suppresses the inducible nitric oxide synthase (iNOS) upregulation and reactive oxygen species (ROS) production. These roles serve to benefit against many

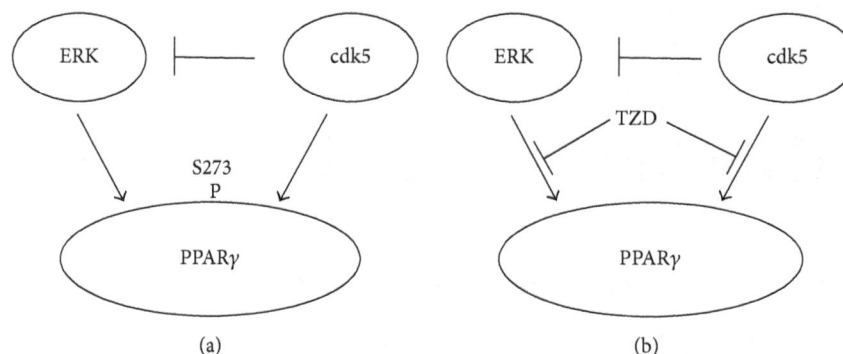

FIGURE 1: (a) Phosphorylation of PPARγ by ERK and CDK5 which also suppresses ERK Kinase. (b) TZD blocking the access of ERK and CDK5.

diseases which are risk factors for cardiovascular disorders such as atherosclerosis, diabetes, hypertension, obesity and dyslipidemia.

2. PPARγ and Insulin Resistance

Insulin resistance such as seen in Type 2 diabetes, impaired glucose tolerance, and metabolic syndrome is a well-established risk factor for cardiovascular disease. PPARγ controls the genes encoding peptides or proteins involved in insulin resistance. PPARγ activators are commonly used in the treatment of type 2 diabetes showing certain abnormalities which are associated with the risk of cardiovascular disease such as increased glucose, insulin and triglyceride levels along with reduced levels of high-density lipoprotein cholesterol (HDL-C) and adiponectin levels [19], a hormone produced in white adipose tissue which has antioxidative, anti-inflammatory and vasodilator effects [20] and has been linked to cardiovascular diseases, insulin resistance states and obesity [21]. Other abnormalities include increased circulating levels of non-esterified fatty acids (NEFA) which are implicated in oxidative stress and induction of inflammatory response in the endothelium. They are associated with endothelial dysfunction and hypertension. High NEFA levels may also predispose cardiomyocytes to a ventricular arrhythmia [22].

PPARγ redistributes triacylglycerol from the subcutaneous fat and visceral fat [23] where the activators of PPARγ move the fat from the visceral adipose tissue, liver and muscles towards subcutaneous tissue by increasing insulin sensitivity in the peripheral and hepatic tissue thereby lowering the concentrations of plasma fatty acid [24]. There also occurs an improvement in the glycemic control. There also occurs improvement in the above-mentioned risk factors of diabetes-related risk of cardiovascular diseases such as lowering of triglycerides and plasma NEFA through its effect on the macrophages along with the increased HDL-C and adiponectin [25].

The most common activators of PPARγ are Thiazolidinedione (TZD) such as pioglitazone and rosiglitazone which are synthetic agonist ligands of PPARγ. One of the mechanisms of action of TZD is the prevention of the phosphorylation

of PPARγ. High-fat diet activates the protein kinase cyclin-dependent kinase 5 (CDK5) activity which leads to the subsequent phosphorylation of PPARγ decreasing its insulin sensitizing effect. For the development of diabetes, PPARγ gets phosphorylated by CDK5 at serine 273 leading to alterations in many genes in the adipose tissue resulting in increased insulin resistance [26]. Recently, the role of CDK5 and extracellular signal-regulated kinases (ERK) was demonstrated in the phosphorylation of PPARγ by Banks et al. They created CDK5 knockout mice in the adipose tissue and demonstrated that in the absence of CDK5, there still occurs an increase in the phosphorylation of PPARγ at serine 273 due to direct effect of ERK. In the presence of CDK5, ERK is suppressed due to its action on ERK kinase (MEK) [27] (Figure 1(a)). TZDs block the phosphorylation of PPARγ by both CDK5 and ERK (Figure 1(b)).

Their data sheds new light to the regulation of PPARγ and another alternative to the treatment of Type 2 Diabetes.

TZDs are already used in the treatment of type 2 diabetes [28]. They are used as monotherapy or as add-on therapy and result in improved insulin sensitivity demonstrating reduced insulin concentrations along with a decrease in the hemoglobin A1c (HbA1c) and fasting blood glucose [25, 29]. TZD also has been shown to increase serum levels of HDL-cholesterol and decrease triglycerides and LDL-cholesterol levels [30]. The decrease in NEFA is observed in both fasting and postprandial levels with decrease becoming apparent as early as 4 weeks of starting treatment [31], with the two TZDs rosiglitazone and pioglitazone showing similar reductions but greater when compared to treatments with metformin, sulfonylureas or statins [32]. TZD treatment doubles the concentration of circulating adiponectin produced by adipose tissue in insulin resistant states [21]. In the diabetic heart, Rosiglitazone demonstrates a protective role, by decreasing cardiac fibrosis and protection against apoptosis as well as improvement in the left ventricular diastolic dysfunction [33, 34]. Similarly, Pioglitazone showed an improvement in the worsening of ischemic preconditioning in the diabetic myocardium [35]. Though the role of TZDs as an insulin-sensitizing treatment conferring benefit to the cardiovascular system would, in theory, be of advantage in future treatments of cardiovascular events associated with high insulin resistance states, clinical trials have not been able to support it. In the BARI-2D (Bypass Angioplasty Revascularization Investigation 2 Diabetes) trial which hypothesized that insulin-sensitizing treatment using TZD would result in greater cardiovascular benefit, lower mean HbA1c and fasting insulin levels was shown although it did not show decreased the occurrence of myocardial infarction (MI) or death upon follow-up 5 years later [36]. It is, however, notable that in the trial the use of multiple glycemic control agents makes it impossible to comment on the efficacy of the TZDs. As mentioned previously, the demonstration by Banks et al. of the involvement of ERK pathway in the phosphorylation of PPARγ in mice model [27] may offer an alternative to increasing the sensitivity of insulin as well lowering the occurrence of cardiovascular events by adding a kinase inhibitor thus increasing the effectiveness of TZDs.

3. Atherosclerosis, Vascular Disease and PPARγ

The proliferation of vascular smooth muscle cells and damage to endothelial cells resulting in the expression of adhesion molecules and ultimately leukocyte adhesion are important events in the development of atherosclerosis. Insulin resistance is implicated in the development of atherosclerosis [37]. There are many studies which demonstrate the beneficial role of PPARγ in limiting the progression of atherosclerosis as well as the acceleration of atherosclerosis with the knockout of PPARγ in macrophages [25]. PPARγ ligands are expressed in the atherosclerotic plaques [38] and have an effect on both these cells. Ligands of PPARγ decrease cytokines such as nitric oxide synthase, IL-6, and tumor necrosis factor α [14] thereby reducing the inflammatory response associated with atherosclerosis. The secretion of metalloproteinases (MMPs) especially MMP-9, by macrophages is responsible for the rupture of atherosclerotic plaques by degrading the extracellular matrix. PPARγ in both vascular smooth muscle cells and macrophages reduces the expression of MMP thereby hindering the migration of vascular smooth muscle cells thus preventing the plaques from becoming vulnerable to rupture [13, 14]. In 2000, Li et al. demonstrated the inhibition of atherosclerosis progression in LDL receptor-deficient mice using rosiglitazone. The reduction in the atherosclerotic lesion was seen in male mice but did not show similar results in female mice [39]. This highlights the importance of conducting more gender specific studies for actions of PPARγ. To determine whether the improvement seen by Li et al. was due to effect of TZD on the artery itself or on the metabolic system, Collins et al. used LDL receptor-deficient male mice and fed them two different diets, one group was fed high-fat diet and the other group was on high fructose diet, along with 3 months treatment with troglitazone, a PPARγ agonist. The results showed a decrease of the lesion in both groups but only the high-fat diet group of mice showed an increase in insulin sensitivity. Thus the conclusion can be made that the role of TZD in decreasing insulin resistance and decreasing atherosclerotic plaques are independent of each other [40]. In 2009, Nakaya et al. reported prevention of atherosclerotic progression with pioglitazone treatment

though the existing lesion was not reversed nor was any improvement seen in advanced atherosclerotic lesions in mice models of LDLR receptor deficiency (LDLR$^{-/-}$) [41]. In 2011, reduction in lesion inflammation was demonstrated in rabbits given pioglitazone treatment for 3 months [42].

Insulin resistance is associated with the development of atherosclerosis. The risk of occurrence of an atherosclerotic event is related to the severity of hyperglycemia as observed by the HbA1c levels [43]. Though in clinical trials such as the PROACTIVE (Prospective Pioglitazone Clinical Trial in Macrovascular Events) a PPARγ activator such as pioglitazone did not show a correlation between its effect on HbA1c and risk of development of cardiovascular disease [44].

Effects of PPARγ agonist on carotid atherosclerosis has been varied. A double blind study done on patients with normal glucose tolerance and stable coronary artery disease showed TZD, pioglitazone stimulates the production of endothelial progenitor cells in vascular injury promoting endothelial repair [45]. The STARR (Study of Atherosclerosis with Ramipril and Rosiglitazone) study compared the carotid artery medial thickness progression in rosiglitazone group compared with placebo. After a study period of 3 years there was a trend towards less carotid artery intimal thickness progression in the rosiglitazone group, however, it was not statistically significant [46]. Another trial comparing carotid artery intimal thickness between two study groups on pioglitazone verses glimepiride (Chicago trial) showed stable carotid artery intimal thickness in pioglitazone group, however, progression of intimal thickness was seen in the glimepiride group which was statistically significant [47]. One long-term study of pioglitazone compared with glimepiride has shown the reversal of carotid atheroma volume in the pioglitazone group. In contrast, the carotid artery atheroma showed progression in the glimepiride group (PERISCOPE trial; Pioglitazone Effect on Regression of Intravascular Sonographic Coronary Obstruction Prospective Evaluation) [48]. Though not conclusive, these studies taken together do point towards the beneficial effect of TZDs. Statins, which are used in the treatment of atherosclerosis result in an increase in PPARγ activity by activating extracellular signal-regulated kinase (ERK) 1/2 and p38 mitogen-activated protein kinase (MAPK) pathways [49]. Lobeglitazone is a new PPARγ agonist shown to have anti-atherosclerotic properties. It can be used in the treatment of patients with a cardiovascular disease associated with diabetes. A significant decrease in the atherosclerotic lesion was observed in apolipoprotein E gene knockout mice (Apo$^{-/-}$) on high cholesterol and high-fat diet with the use of Lobeglitazone, as well as reduced formation of neointima after balloon injury to the carotid artery [50].

Endothelial PPARγ regulates the gene expressions of NADPH oxidase, superoxide dismutase and catalase thus increasing vasodilation [51]. The treatment with TZD resultant activation of PPARγ in adipocytes and inflammatory cells in the adipose tissue inhibits release of inflammatory mediators along with the reduction in local inflammation [52]. ROS can lead to alteration of vascular function [53] thus playing a role in the development of cardiovascular

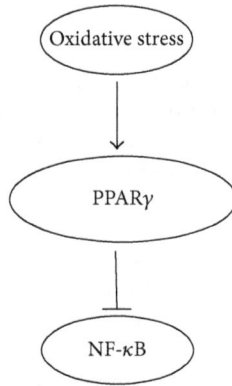

FIGURE 2: PPARγ suppresses the activation of NF-κB decreasing its inflammatory effects.

disorders. Oxidative stress reduces the expression of PPARγ in the vascular endothelial cells [54]. In turn, PPARγ has a protective effect on the cardiomyocytes by upregulation of the antiapoptotic Bcl-2 protein against oxidative stress [55].

It is worth noting that the direct effect of PPARγ on the heart leads to heart failure. This was demonstrated in transgenic mice models of PPARγ created by Son et al., which expressed PPARγ1 in the heart. An increase in triglyceride uptake and increased fatty acid oxidation was observed and the mice developed dilated cardiomyopathy with the production of damaged mitochondria [56] when treated with PPARγ agonist TZD rosiglitazone.

4. Ischemia-Reperfusion Injury and PPARγ

Previous studies using rat models of ischemia-reperfusion injury have demonstrated a reduction in myocardial damage with the use of TZDs [57]. The TZDs rosiglitazone, pioglitazone, and ciglitazone, all resulted in a decrease of myocardial infarct size.

Rosiglitazone has a cardio protective effect in both non-diabetic and diabetic rats limiting the damage to the heart following ischemia/reperfusion injury via inhibition of Jun NH (2)-terminal kinase phosphorylation [58]. Another mechanism by which Rosiglitazone provides cardioprotection is by selective overexpression of angiotensin type 2 along with the inhibition of p42/44 MAPK pathway. This effect was demonstrated to be separate from the insulin-sensitizing effect of Rosiglitazone [59]. Yet another mechanism for reduction of heart injury due to ischemia was observed in hypercholesterolaemic rats. Rosiglitazone reduced the increased activity of myeloperoxidase induced by hypercholesterolemia thus resulting in a decrease in infarct size [60]. The TZD ciglitazone results in decreased myocardial damage, infiltration of neutrophils and cytokine production by increasing DNA binding of PPARγ and decreasing the activation of nuclear factor κB (Figure 2) [61]. Pioglitazone also has protective effect against MI, exhibiting reduced infarct size in rabbit model via activation of PPARγ, PI-3 kinases, eNOS and Akt pathways [62].

5. Limitation of PPARγ as a Therapeutic Measure in Cardiovascular Disease

Though treatment with activators of PPARγ seems to have a favorable effect on the risk factors for cardiovascular disease, it also has adverse effects on the cardiovascular system which mitigates its beneficial effects thus limiting their widespread use in patients with cardiovascular risk.

In humans, the treatment with PPARγ agonist TZD leads to increase the risk of developing edema and congestive heart failure which is thought to be due to the retention of salt and water (Rubenstrunk, Hanf et al. 2007). The mechanism by which TZD causes fluid retention may be due to the increased transcription of SGK1 (Serum/Glucocorticoid-Regulated Kinase-1) which activates the renal epithelial sodium channels [63]. Currently, the increase in vascular permeability due to increased levels of vascular endothelial growth factor in these patients is known [64]. In a study by Tang et al., no association was observed between severity of heart failure and risk of fluid retention [65], though much research still needs to be conducted before making use of TZDs in clinical settings. PPARγ are also responsible for weight gain due to increase in the adipose tissue mass [66], may increase low-density lipoproteins cholesterol concentration [67], promote the onset of ventricular fibrillation in severe ischemia [68], and modify cardiac ion channels promoting arrhythmia [69]. Even though it has been shown to decrease the progression of atherosclerosis [70], pioglitazone has also been shown to develop plaque necrosis [71] in advanced atherosclerosis in a study done on LDL receptor-deficient mice. It has been reported that treatment with rosiglitazone is linked with an increase in MI in humans [72, 73]. Though in the RECORD (Rosiglitazone evaluated for cardiovascular outcomes in oral agent combination therapy for type 2 diabetes) trial, rosiglitazone was shown to be linked with risk of heart failure and not MI [74]. Unlike rosiglitazone, pioglitazone does not induce cardiac hypertrophy as seen in mice [75]. Pioglitazone has a more positive effect than rosiglitazone on lipid profile with improvement in LDL and triglycerides in patients with diabetes and dyslipidemia [67]. It has also shown a positive effect on the endothelial progenitor cells by increasing their number in patients with coronary artery disease which help in improving vascular function [45]. Due to the possibility of developing cardiac dysfunction with the use of TZD in patients with congestive heart failure, their use in these patients is avoided.

Patients with congestive heart failure are prone to develop heart failure following PPARγ therapy as a result of increased plasma volume. It is notable however that in both animal and clinical studies the resultant heart failure has not been linked to the effect of TZD on left ventricular systolic function [76]. More recently, TZD has been associated with bone loss [77], with the use rosiglitazone shown to be responsible for an increase in fractures in diabetic patients [78].

6. Clinical Trials to Determine the Efficacy of PPARγ Activators

6.1. IRIS Trial. The IRIS (insulin resistance intervention after stroke) trial is a randomized trial to determine the efficacy of pioglitazone in patients with no history of heart failure, who are insulin resistant and non-diabetic, having a history of recent transient ischemic attack or ischemic stroke. Insulin resistance criteria was an HOMA-IR (Homeostatic Model Assessment-Insulin Resistance) index higher than 3. The hypothesis of this trial was that Pioglitazone will decrease the rate of myocardial infarction and stroke in the selected group. The results of this trial are demonstrated lowered rates of myocardial infarction, stroke, and death in patients receiving pioglitazone. These subjects showed improvement in blood pressure, improved levels of triglycerides, HDL cholesterol and insulin sensitivity. Moreover, the rate of heart failure in the pioglitazone group was not higher than the placebo group. This trial provides information which may be of great importance due to the fact that this trial is in patients who are not diabetic thereby reducing the chances of confounding results by multiple diabetic therapies. This study also determines whether the use of pioglitazone in patients on statins is beneficial.

7. PROACTIVE

PROACTIVE (Prospective Pioglitazone Clinical Trial in Macrovascular Events) trial compared pioglitazone with a placebo in the type 2 diabetic patients with HbA1c greater than 6.5% who were also suffering from the atherosclerotic disease in a double-blind study, with a mean follow-up of 34.5 months. It sought to determine the effect of pioglitazone in reducing the incidence of macrovascular complications. Pioglitazone did not have a significant effect on the primary and main secondary endpoints in the patients treated with insulin though there was a lowering in the mean insulin dose in patients on pioglitazone as compared to those on placebo with discontinuation of insulin in 9% pioglitazone patients as compared to 2% placebo patients [79]. Furthermore, in a subgroup analysis done previously, pioglitazone significantly reduced the occurrence of MI by 28% in patients with prior history of MI [80]. Although pioglitazone did significantly reduce the risk of myocardial infarction, it also increased the risk of edema in the subjects. These studies demonstrate a positive efficacy of pioglitazone in cardiovascular disease but a loner observation would be more conclusive. Also, due to the use of other treatments for diabetes in an imbalanced manner in terms of frequency and dosage may also have affected the outcome of study if they also affect the cardiovascular system. Another point of note in these trials is the use of statin in only half of the patients studied. The risk of death was reduced only by 5% in patients treated with a statin and given pioglitazone but was 25% in patients not on statin [44].

8. RECORD Trial

RECORD trial tested the use of rosiglitazone as an add-on therapy in patients with type 2 diabetes not controlled by sulfonylurea or metformin alone with mean HbA1c of 7.9%. The group treated with rosiglitazone exhibited higher levels of LDL-C, HDL-C and weight and lower levels. After a mean follow-up of 5.5 years, the group with rosiglitazone had a higher frequency of heart failure. The higher use of statins and diuretics in patients on rosiglitazone as well as the lower event rate and subsequent low statistical power due to lack of follow-up are limitations of this trial [81]. The RECORD results do not show a significant difference between metformin/sulfonylurea group and rosiglitazone group in terms of myocardial infarction, stroke or cardiovascular death. Although the risk of heart failure is relatively small, it is nevertheless an important concern. This reinforces the importance of not using TZDs in patients with heart failure.

9. DREAM Trial

The DREAM (Diabetes Reduction Assessment with Ramipril and rosiglitazone Medication) trial was done to determine the effect of 8 mg per day rosiglitazone and/or Ramipril on patients with impaired glucose tolerance or impaired fasting glucose but with no history of cardiovascular disease. Follow-up after 3 years showed a significant reduction in the development of new onset diabetes in patients on rosiglitazone although it was also associated with increased development of heart failure as compared to patients on Ramipril [82]. This study demonstrates a positive role of rosiglitazone in reducing or even eliminating the risk of developing diabetes in obese subjects. However, the short follow-up period of this trial, as well as exclusion of cardiovascular disease history in subjects, limit the conclusions that can be drawn about rosiglitazone and its cardiovascular effects. The heart failure observed in the patients receiving rosiglitazone may be due to the effect of the drug on the kidney resulting in fluid overload a subsequent heart failure in some individuals.

10. ACT NOW Trial

The ACT NOW (Actos Now for the prevention of Diabetes) trial sought to determine the effect of pioglitazone in the prevention of new-onset diabetes in patients with impaired glucose tolerance. Patients either received placebo or 45 mg of pioglitazone. After a 2.2-year mean follow-up, a significant reduction in the fasting glucose levels was observed in the pioglitazone group, as well as reduced levels of HbA1c and increase in the levels of HDL-C. 5% of people progressed to diabetes in the pioglitazone group as compared to 16.7% seen in the placebo group. However, the pioglitazone group did have the adverse effect of increased incidence of edema and weight gain [83]. Therefore, in patients with impaired glucose tolerance, pioglitazone reduced the risk of diabetes, improved HDL cholesterol levels and liver enzymes but was associated with edema and weight gain.

11. ADOPT Trial

A Diabetes Outcome Progression Trial (ADOPT) used patients with newly diagnosed type 2 diabetes to determine the glycemic durability of three drugs to be used as first-line treatment namely, rosiglitazone, metformin, and glyburide. Treatment was for a median of 4 years with primary outcome set as the failure of monotherapy with fasting blood glucose level more than 10 mmol/L after 6 weeks of treatment. Follow-up at 5 years revealed a lower number of failure in rosiglitazone-treated patients (15%) with low HbA1c and high insulin sensitivity though again was associated with weight gain and edema [84]. This study was significant because it demonstrates that rosiglitazone maintained targeted sugar level for a longer period when compared to metformin and glyburide.

12. Metanalysis of Clinical Trials

The meta-analysis of controlled trials of pioglitazone shows a reduction in the risk of MI, stroke or death in patients with type 2 diabetes mellitus [85, 86]. On the other hand, a meta-analysis of trials with rosiglitazone, it has been linked to an increased risk of MI though the associated mortality is still low [87]. Due to this reason, rosiglitazone use is limited in the United States whereas it is not used in Europe [88].

13. Comparative Analysis

No randomized trial has been conducted to compare the two TZDs pioglitazone and rosiglitazone although it has been compared in cohort studies, treatment with rosiglitazone is associated with higher rates of cardiovascular events [89–91]. Upon meta-analysis of observational studies, rosiglitazone was associated with higher incidence of adverse cardiovascular events such as congestive heart failure, MI, and death [92].

These trials have been very important in providing evidence to support the decisions made in choosing therapy. Studies like ADOPT which compare a TZD with commonly used antidiabetic drugs provide valuable new information to help guide future treatments. Although rosiglitazone is associated with the adverse effect of edema and weight gain, metformin and glyburide are also associated with gastrointestinal effects and weight gain respectively. However, it was shown that hyperglycemia associated with diabetes can be slowed using TZD.

Despite such positive effects, the contradictory results of trials, as well as the adverse effects of TZDs, most important being development of congestive heart failure, have limited the use of TZDs. On one hand, TZDs has a role in increasing the incidence of heart failure due to fluid retention. On the other hand, studies like PROACTIVE also suggest a beneficial role of TZDs in reducing cardiovascular disease. Similarly, DREAM trial showed an increase in heart failure but ADOPT trial showed no difference in the incidence of heart failure between rosiglitazone and other antidiabetic drugs.

14. New PPARγ Activators and Future Therapeutic Measures

Dual PPAR alpha and γ activators are being developed to combine the HDL-C raising and triglyceride lowering effect of PPAR alpha with the insulin sensitivity increasing the effect of PPARγ. PPARα activation upregulates the genes responsible for fatty acid transport and activation. Ligands for PPARα are used to treat hyperlipidemia. In this regard, Glitazar class of drugs were developed which activated both the isoforms of PPAR but the increased incidence of adverse effects prevented further research [93, 94]. Another dual activator by the name of aleglitazar has completed phase III trials [95]. The study SYNCHRONY, a phase II randomized trial to determine the cardiovascular disease risk of aleglitazar in type 2 diabetic patients [96], demonstrated a significant decrease in levels of HbA1c as well as on levels of triglyceride and LDL. In addition, an increase in HDL cholesterol was also found. However, in the phase III study known as ALECARDIO, a randomized clinical trial to determine the protective effect of aleglitazar in type 2 diabetic patients who have suffered an acute coronary syndrome did not find a reduction in the incidence of myocardial infarction or cardiovascular death with the use of aleglitazar. On the contrary, an increase in the risk of heart failure, bone fractures, gastrointestinal hemorrhage and renal function was observed.

Currently, the development of partial PPARγ agonists is underway in the hopes that unlike TZDs which are full PPARγ agonists, selective partial agonists will be associated with lesser adverse effects such as fluid retention, heart failure, and so forth while retaining the insulin sensitizing effects. New specific PPARγ agonist S26948, displays a reduction in atherosclerotic lesions along with anti-diabetic effects [97]. INT-131 besylate is another selective peroxisome proliferator activated receptor γ modulator (SPPARM) evaluated in a study to determine its safety and efficacy in type 2 diabetes mellitus. A reduction in the fasting plasma glucose was observed without fluid retention or weight gain when compared to a similar model of rosiglitazone. At a dosage of 1 mg the fasting glucose reduced from 163 to 142 mg/dL without any change in the levels of NEFA, adiponectin or fasting glucose. Upon increasing the dose to 10 mg the reduction in glucose was from 183 to 137 mg/dL with significant lowering of NEFA, adiponectin, and insulin. However, an increase in weight gain and edema, as well as decrease in hematocrit levels, was also observed a phase II study using the 10 mg dosage, therefore, the advantage of using partial PPARγ activators is yet to be determined with further studies [98]. SR1664 is a new anti-diabetic compound without the side effects of fluid retention and weight gain. Similar to rosiglitazone it blocked the phosphorylation of PPARγ via CDK5 and is classified as a non-agonist inhibitor of CDK5 without adipogenic function in vitro [99].

The effect of a new TZD, Rivoglitazone, on the control of lipids and glucose has been compared to pioglitazone in a double-blind randomized control trial in Chinese patients with type 2 diabetes. It has been reported to be a safe and efficacious TZD-associated with improvement in glycemic control but further studies are still to be conducted [100].

Another new TZD PPARγ partial agonist, balaglitazone is currently under evaluation in phase III clinical trial in US and Europe which shows glycemic control as an add-on to insulin therapy with a lower incidence of fat accumulation and fluid retention when compared to pioglitazone [101]. A new dual PPARα and PPARγ agonist known as Saroglitazar, with a higher activity for PPARα and moderate PPARγ activity, has been approved for the treatment of type 2 diabetes in India in order to control diabetic dyslipidemia [102]. However, further studies are still to be conducted before any conclusions can be made on its effect on the cardiovascular system.

15. Conclusions

PPARγ plays an important role in cardiovascular diseases but much research is still needed to establish its function in the cardiovascular system. PPARγ agonists confer benefits in diabetes and atherosclerosis, known risk factors associated with cardiovascular disease. They are beneficial as therapeutic agents resulting in improved insulin resistance, reduced glucose levels in the blood as well as reduced inflammation. However, they also have deleterious effects such as increased higher risk incidence of congestive heart failure. Therefore, their use is limited in clinical settings. At present, the use of PPARγ agonists among patients is at the discretion of the physicians. Further research on PPAR physiology and pharmacology, as well the knowledge gained by the use of PPARγ agonists, both known and under development, should assist in the development of newer and safer therapeutic agents.

Competing Interests

The authors declare that they have no competing interests.

References

[1] A. Abbas, J. Blandon, J. Rude, A. Elfar, and D. Mukherjee, "PPAR- γ agonist in treatment of diabetes: cardiovascular safety considerations," *Cardiovascular and Hematological Agents in Medicinal Chemistry*, vol. 10, no. 2, pp. 124–134, 2012.

[2] D. J. Mangelsdorf and R. M. Evans, "The RXR heterodimers and orphan receptors," *Cell*, vol. 83, no. 6, pp. 841–850, 1995.

[3] S. Ogawa, J. Lozach, K. Jepsen et al., "A nuclear receptor corepressor transcriptional checkpoint controlling activator protein 1-dependent gene networks required for macrophage activation," *Proceedings of the National Academy of Sciences of the United States of America*, vol. 101, no. 40, pp. 14461–14466, 2004.

[4] N. Wang, R. Yin, Y. Liu, G. Mao, and F. Xi, "Role of peroxisome proliferator-activated receptor-γ in atherosclerosis: an update," *Circulation Journal*, vol. 75, no. 3, pp. 528–535, 2011.

[5] M. Lehrke and M. A. Lazar, "The many faces of PPARγ," *Cell*, vol. 123, no. 6, pp. 993–999, 2005.

[6] M. E. Greene, B. Blumberg, O. W. McBride et al., "Isolation of the human peroxisome proliferator activated receptor gamma cDNA: expression in hematopoietic cells and chromosomal mapping," *Gene Expression*, vol. 4, no. 4-5, pp. 281–299, 1995.

[7] P. S. Jones, R. Savory, P. Barratt et al., "Chromosomal localisation, inducibility, tissue-specific expression and strain differences in three murine peroxisome-proliferator-activated-receptor genes," *European Journal of Biochemistry*, vol. 233, no. 1, pp. 219–226, 1995.

[8] R. M. Touyz and E. L. Schiffrin, "Peroxisome proliferator-activated receptors in vascular biology-molecular mechanisms and clinical implications," *Vascular Pharmacology*, vol. 45, no. 1, pp. 19–28, 2006.

[9] L. Nagy, P. Tontonoz, J. G. A. Alvarez, H. Chen, and R. M. Evans, "Oxidized LDL regulates macrophage gene expression through ligand activation of PPARγ," *Cell*, vol. 93, no. 2, pp. 229–240, 1998.

[10] T. M. McIntyre, A. V. Pontsler, A. R. Silva et al., "Identification of an intracellular receptor for lysophosphatidic acid (LPA): LPA is a transcellular PPARγ agonist," *Proceedings of the National Academy of Sciences of the United States of America*, vol. 100, no. 1, pp. 131–136, 2003.

[11] A. Majdalawieh and H.-S. Ro, "PPARgamma1 and LXRalpha face a new regulator of macrophage cholesterol homeostasis and inflammatory responsiveness, AEBP1," *Nuclear receptor signaling*, vol. 8, p. e004, 2010.

[12] M. Adams, C. T. Montague, J. B. Prins et al., "Activators of peroxisome proliferator-activated receptor γ have depot-specific effects on human preadipocyte differentiation," *The Journal of Clinical Investigation*, vol. 100, no. 12, pp. 3149–3153, 1997.

[13] N. Marx, U. Schönbeck, M. A. Lazar, P. Libby, and J. Plutzky, "Peroxisome proliferator-activated receptor gamma activators inhibit gene expression and migration in human vascular smooth muscle cells," *Circulation Research*, vol. 83, no. 11, pp. 1097–1103, 1998.

[14] M. Ricote, A. C. Li, T. M. Willson, C. J. Kelly, and C. K. Glass, "The peroxisome proliferator-activated receptor-γ is a negative regulator of macrophage activation," *Nature*, vol. 391, no. 6662, pp. 79–82, 1998.

[15] H. Takano, T. Nagai, M. Asakawa et al., "Peroxisome proliferator-activated receptor activators inhibit lipopolysaccharide-induced tumor necrosis factor-α expression in neonatal rat cardiac myocytes," *Circulation Research*, vol. 87, no. 7, pp. 596–602, 2000.

[16] B. M. Spiegelman, "Peroxisome proliferator-activated receptor gamma: a key regulator of adipogenesis and systemic insulin sensitivity," *European journal of medical research*, vol. 2, no. 11, pp. 457–464, 1997.

[17] R. Kapadia, J.-H. Yi, and R. Vemuganti, "Mechanisms of anti-inflammatory and neuroprotective actions of PPAR-gamma agonists," *Frontiers in Bioscience*, vol. 13, no. 5, pp. 1813–1826, 2008.

[18] P. Tontonoz and B. M. Spiegelman, "Fat and beyond: the diverse biology of PPARγ," *Annual Review of Biochemistry*, vol. 77, pp. 289–312, 2008.

[19] K. B. Doshi, S. R. Kashyap, D. M. Brennan, B. M. Hoar, L. Cho, and B. J. Hoogwerf, "All-cause mortality risk predictors in a preventive cardiology clinic cohort-examining diabetes and individual metabolic syndrome criteria: a PRECIS database study," *Diabetes, Obesity and Metabolism*, vol. 11, no. 2, pp. 102–108, 2009.

[20] X. Hui, K. S. Lam, P. M. Vanhoutte, and A. Xu, "Adiponectin and cardiovascular health: an update," *British Journal of Pharmacology*, vol. 165, no. 3, pp. 574–590, 2012.

[21] N. Riera-Guardia and D. Rothenbacher, "The effect of thia-zolidinediones on adiponectin serum level: a meta-analysis," *Diabetes, Obesity and Metabolism*, vol. 10, no. 5, pp. 367–375, 2008.

[22] J. S. Charnock, "Lipids and cardiac arrhythmia," *Progress in Lipid Research*, vol. 33, no. 4, pp. 355–385, 1994.

[23] W. T. Festuccia, P.-G. Blanchard, V. Turcotte et al., "Depot-specific effects of the PPARγ agonist rosiglitazone on adipose tissue glucose uptake and metabolism," *Journal of Lipid Research*, vol. 50, no. 6, pp. 1185–1194, 2009.

[24] A. B. Mayerson, R. S. Hundal, S. Dufour et al., "The effects of rosiglitazone on insulin sensitivity, lipolysis, and hepatic and skeletal muscle triglyceride content in patients with type 2 diabetes," *Diabetes*, vol. 51, no. 3, pp. 797–802, 2002.

[25] J. V. Huang, C. R. Greyson, and G. G. Schwartz, "PPAR-γ as a therapeutic target in cardiovascular disease: evidence and uncertainty," *Journal of Lipid Research*, vol. 53, no. 9, pp. 1738–1754, 2012.

[26] J. H. Choi, A. S. Banks, J. L. Estall et al., "Anti-diabetic drugs inhibit obesity-linked phosphorylation of PPARγ by Cdk5," *Nature*, vol. 466, no. 7305, pp. 451–456, 2010.

[27] A. S. Banks, F. E. McAllister, J. P. G. Camporez et al., "An ERK/Cdk5 axis controls the diabetogenic actions of PPARγ," *Nature*, vol. 517, no. 7534, pp. 391–395, 2015.

[28] J. M. Lehmann, L. B. Moore, T. A. Smith-Oliver, W. O. Wilkison, T. M. Willson, and S. A. Kliewer, "An antidiabetic thiazolidine-dione is a high affinity ligand for peroxisome proliferator-activated receptor γ (PPARγ)," *Journal of Biological Chemistry*, vol. 270, no. 22, pp. 12953–12956, 1995.

[29] G. Perriello, S. Pampanelli, C. Di Pietro, and P. Brunetti, "Comparison of glycaemic control over 1 year with pioglitazone or gliclazide in patients with type 2 diabetes," *Diabetic Medicine*, vol. 23, no. 3, pp. 246–252, 2006.

[30] A. Komatsu and K. Node, "Effects of PPARgamma agonist on dyslipidemia and atherosclerosis," *Nippon Rinsho*, vol. 68, no. 2, pp. 294–298, 2010.

[31] F. Abbasi, N. K. C. Lima, and G. M. Reaven, "Relationship between changes in insulin sensitivity and associated cardiovascular disease risk factors in thiazolidinedione-treated, insulin-resistant, nondiabetic individuals: pioglitazone versus rosiglitazone," *Metabolism*, vol. 58, no. 3, pp. 373–378, 2009.

[32] F. Abbasi, Y.-D. I. Chen, H. M. F. Farin, C. Lamendola, and G. M. Reaven, "Comparison of three treatment approaches to decreasing cardiovascular disease risk in nondiabetic insulin-resistant dyslipidemic subjects," *The American Journal of Cardiology*, vol. 102, no. 1, pp. 64–69, 2008.

[33] A. Baraka and H. AbdelGawad, "Targeting apoptosis in the heart of streptozotocin-induced diabetic rats," *Journal of Cardiovascular Pharmacology and Therapeutics*, vol. 15, no. 2, pp. 175–181, 2010.

[34] S.-H. Ihm, K. Chang, H.-Y. Kim et al., "Peroxisome proliferator-activated receptor-γ activation attenuates cardiac fibrosis in type 2 diabetic rats: the effect of rosiglitazone on myocardial expression of receptor for advanced glycation end products and of connective tissue growth factor," *Basic Research in Cardiology*, vol. 105, no. 3, pp. 399–407, 2010.

[35] H. Sasaki, K. Ogawa, M. Shimizu et al., "The insulin sensitizer pioglitazone improves the deterioration of ischemic preconditioning in type 2 diabetes mellitus rats," *International Heart Journal*, vol. 48, no. 5, pp. 623–635, 2007.

[36] R. L. Frye, P. August, M. M. Brooks et al., "A randomized trial of therapies for type 2 diabetes and coronary artery disease," *The New England Journal of Medicine*, vol. 360, no. 24, pp. 2503–2515, 2009.

[37] A. D'Souza, M. Hussain, F. C. Howarth, N. M. Woods, K. Bidasee, and J. Singh, "Pathogenesis and pathophysiology of accelerated atherosclerosis in the diabetic heart," *Molecular and Cellular Biochemistry*, vol. 331, no. 1-2, pp. 89–116, 2009.

[38] N. Marx, G. Sukhova, C. Murphy, P. Libby, and J. Plutzky, "Macrophages in human atheroma contain PPARγ: differentiation-dependent peroxisomal proliferator-activated receptor γ (PPARγ) expression and reduction of MMP-9 activity through PPARγ activation in mononuclear phagocytes in vitro," *American Journal of Pathology*, vol. 153, no. 1, pp. 17–23, 1998.

[39] A. C. Li, K. K. Brown, M. J. Silvestre, T. M. Willson, W. Palinski, and C. K. Glass, "Peroxisome proliferator-activated receptor γ ligands inhibit development of atherosclerosis in LDL receptor-deficient mice," *The Journal of Clinical Investigation*, vol. 106, no. 4, pp. 523–531, 2000.

[40] A. R. Collins, W. P. Meehan, U. Kintscher et al., "Troglitazone inhibits formation of early atherosclerotic lesions in diabetic and nondiabetic low density lipoprotein receptor-deficient mice," *Arteriosclerosis, Thrombosis, and Vascular Biology*, vol. 21, no. 3, pp. 365–371, 2001.

[41] H. Nakaya, B. D. Summers, A. C. Nicholson, A. M. Gotto Jr., D. P. Hajjar, and J. Han, "Atherosclerosis in LDLR-knockout mice is inhibited, but not reversed, by the PPARγ ligand pioglitazone," *American Journal of Pathology*, vol. 174, no. 6, pp. 2007–2014, 2009.

[42] E. Vucic, S. D. Dickson, C. Calcagno et al., "Pioglitazone modulates vascular inflammation in atherosclerotic rabbits: noninvasive assessment with FDG-PET-CT and dynamic contrast-enhanced MR imaging," *JACC: Cardiovascular Imaging*, vol. 4, no. 10, pp. 1100–1109, 2011.

[43] I. M. Stratton, A. I. Adler, H. A. W. Neil et al., "Association of glycaemia with macrovascular and microvascular complications of type 2 diabetes (UKPDS 35): prospective observational study," *British Medical Journal*, vol. 321, no. 7258, pp. 405–412, 2000.

[44] E. Ferrannini, D. J. Betteridge, J. A. Dormandy et al., "High-density lipoprotein-cholesterol and not HbA1c was directly related to cardiovascular outcome in PROactive," *Diabetes, Obesity and Metabolism*, vol. 13, no. 8, pp. 759–764, 2011.

[45] C. Werner, C. H. Kamani, C. Gensch, M. Böhm, and U. Laufs, "The peroxisome proliferator–activated receptor-γ agonist pioglitazone increases number and function of endothelial progenitor cells in patients with coronary artery disease and normal glucose tolerance," *Diabetes*, vol. 56, no. 10, pp. 2609–2615, 2007.

[46] E. M. Lonn, H. C. Gerstein, P. Sheridan et al., "Effect of ramipril and of rosiglitazone on carotid intima-media thickness in people with impaired glucose tolerance or impaired fasting glucose: STARR (STudy of Atherosclerosis with Ramipril and Rosiglitazone)," *Journal of the American College of Cardiology*, vol. 53, no. 22, pp. 2028–2035, 2009.

[47] M. H. Davidson, C. A. Beam, S. Haffner, A. Perez, R. Dagostino, and T. Mazzone, "Pioglitazone versus glimepiride on coronary artery calcium progression in patients with type 2 diabetes mellitus: a secondary end point of the CHICAGO study," *Arteriosclerosis, Thrombosis, and Vascular Biology*, vol. 30, no. 9, pp. 1873–1876, 2010.

[48] S. E. Nissen, S. J. Nicholls, K. Wolski et al., "Comparison of pioglitazone vs glimepiride on progression of coronary atherosclerosis in patients with type 2 diabetes: the PERISCOPE

randomized controlled trial," *JAMA*, vol. 299, no. 13, pp. 1561–1573, 2008.

[49] M. Yano, T. Matsumura, T. Senokuchi et al., "Statins activate peroxisome proliferator-activated receptor γ through extracellular signal-regulated kinase 1/2 and p38 mitogen-activated protein kinase-dependent cyclooxygenase-2 expression in macrophages," *Circulation Research*, vol. 100, no. 10, pp. 1442–1451, 2007.

[50] S. Lim, K.-S. Lee, J. E. Lee et al., "Effect of a new PPAR-gamma agonist, lobeglitazone, on neointimal formation after balloon injury in rats and the development of atherosclerosis," *Atherosclerosis*, vol. 243, no. 1, pp. 107–119, 2015.

[51] P. Ketsawatsomkron and C. D. Sigmund, "Molecular mechanisms regulating vascular tone by peroxisome proliferator activated receptor gamma," *Current Opinion in Nephrology and Hypertension*, vol. 24, no. 2, pp. 123–130, 2015.

[52] A. Foryst-Ludwig, M. Hartge, M. Clemenz et al., "PPARgamma activation attenuates T-lymphocyte-dependent inflammation of adipose tissue and development of insulin resistance in obese mice," *Cardiovascular Diabetology*, vol. 9, article no. 64, 2010.

[53] A. San Martín, P. Du, A. Dikalova et al., "Reactive oxygen species-selective regulation of aortic inflammatory gene expression in Type 2 diabetes," *American Journal of Physiology—Heart and Circulatory Physiology*, vol. 292, no. 5, pp. H2073–H2082, 2007.

[54] C. Blanquicett, B.-Y. Kang, J. D. Ritzenthaler, D. P. Jones, and C. M. Hart, "Oxidative stress modulates PPARγ in vascular endothelial cells," *Free Radical Biology and Medicine*, vol. 48, no. 12, pp. 1618–1625, 2010.

[55] Y. Ren, C. Sun, Y. Sun et al., "PPAR gamma protects cardiomyocytes against oxidative stress and apoptosis via Bcl-2 upregulation," *Vascular Pharmacology*, vol. 51, no. 2-3, pp. 169–174, 2009.

[56] N. Son, T. Park, H. Yamashita et al., "Cardiomyocyte expression of PPARγ leads to cardiac dysfunction in mice," *Journal of Clinical Investigation*, vol. 117, no. 10, pp. 2791–2801, 2007.

[57] N. S. Wayman, Y. Hattori, M. C. Mcdonald et al., "Ligands of the peroxisome proliferator-activated receptors (PPAR-γ and PPAR-α) reduce myocardial infarct size," *The FASEB Journal*, vol. 16, no. 9, pp. 1027–1040, 2002.

[58] N. Khandoudi, P. Delerive, I. Berrebi-Bertrand, R. E. Buckingham, B. Staels, and A. Bril, "Rosiglitazone, a peroxisome proliferator-activated receptor-γ, inhibits the Jun NH 2-terminal kinase/activating protein 1 pathway and protects the heart from ischemia/reperfusion injury," *Diabetes*, vol. 51, no. 5, pp. 1507–1514, 2002.

[59] B. Molavi, J. Chen, and J. L. Mehta, "Cardioprotective effects of rosiglitazone are associated with selective overexpression of type 2 angiotensin receptors and inhibition of p42/44 MAPK," *American Journal of Physiology—Heart and Circulatory Physiology*, vol. 291, no. 2, pp. H687–H693, 2006.

[60] H.-R. Liu, L. Tao, E. Gao et al., "Rosiglitazone inhibits hypercholesterolaemia-induced myeloperoxidase upregulation—a novel mechanism for the cardioprotective effects of PPAR agonists," *Cardiovascular Research*, vol. 81, no. 2, pp. 344–352, 2009.

[61] B. Zingarelli, P. W. Hake, P. Mangeshkar et al., "Diverse cardioprotective signaling mechanisms of peroxisome proliferator-activated receptor-γ ligands, 15-deoxy-Δ12,14-prostaglandin J2 and ciglitazone, in reperfusion injury: role of nuclear factor-κB, heat shock factor 1, and Akt," *Shock*, vol. 28, no. 5, pp. 554–563, 2007.

[62] S. Yasuda, H. Kobayashi, M. Iwasa et al., "Antidiabetic drug pioglitazone protects the heart via activation of PPAR-γ receptors, PI3-kinase, Akt, and eNOS pathway in a rabbit model of myocardial infarction," *American Journal of Physiology—Heart and Circulatory Physiology*, vol. 296, no. 5, pp. H1558–H1565, 2009.

[63] F. Artunc, D. Sandulache, O. Nasir et al., "Lack of the serum and glucocorticoid-inducible kinase SGK1 attenuates the volume retention after treatment with the PPARγ agonist pioglitazone," *Pflugers Archiv European Journal of Physiology*, vol. 456, no. 2, pp. 425–436, 2008.

[64] K. B. Sotiropoulos, A. Clermont, Y. Yasuda et al., "Adipose-specific effect of rosiglitazone on vascular permeability and protein kinase C activation: novel mechanism for PPARgamma agonist's effects on edema and weight gain," *The FASEB Journal*, vol. 20, no. 8, pp. 1203–1205, 2006.

[65] W. H. W. Tang, G. S. Francis, B. J. Hoogwerf, and J. B. Young, "Fluid retention after initiation of thiazolidinedione therapy in diabetic patients with established chronic heart failure," *Journal of the American College of Cardiology*, vol. 41, no. 8, pp. 1394–1398, 2003.

[66] Y. Miyazaki, A. Mahankali, M. Matsuda et al., "Effect of pioglitazone on abdominal fat distribution and insulin sensitivity in type 2 diabetic patients," *Journal of Clinical Endocrinology and Metabolism*, vol. 87, no. 6, pp. 2784–2791, 2002.

[67] R. B. Goldberg, D. M. Kendall, M. A. Deeg et al., "A comparison of lipid and glycemic effects of pioglitazone and rosiglitazone in patients with type 2 diabetes and dyslipidemia," *Diabetes Care*, vol. 28, no. 7, pp. 1547–1554, 2005.

[68] L. Lu, M. J. Reiter, Y. Xu, A. Chicco, C. R. Greyson, and G. G. Schwartz, "Thiazolidinedione drugs block cardiac KATP channels and may increase propensity for ischaemic ventricular fibrillation in pigs," *Diabetologia*, vol. 51, no. 4, pp. 675–685, 2008.

[69] J. C. Hancox, "Cardiac ion channel modulation by the hypoglycaemic agent rosiglitazone," *British Journal of Pharmacology*, vol. 163, no. 3, pp. 496–498, 2011.

[70] N. Marx, H. Duez, J.-C. Fruchart, and B. Staels, "Peroxisome proliferator-activated receptors and atherogenesis: regulators of gene expression in vascular cells," *Circulation Research*, vol. 94, no. 9, pp. 1168–1178, 2004.

[71] E. Thorp, G. Kuriakose, Y. M. Shah, F. J. Gonzalez, and I. Tabas, "Pioglitazone increases macrophage apoptosis and plaque necrosis in advanced atherosclerotic lesions of nondiabetic low-density lipoprotein receptor-null mice," *Circulation*, vol. 116, no. 19, pp. 2182–2190, 2007.

[72] S. E. Nissen and K. Wolski, "Effect of rosiglitazone on the risk of myocardial infarction and death from cardiovascular causes," *New England Journal of Medicine*, vol. 356, no. 24, pp. 2457–2471, 2007.

[73] S. Singh, Y. K. Loke, and C. D. Furberg, "Long-term risk of cardiovascular events with rosiglitazone: a meta-analysis," *Journal of the American Medical Association*, vol. 298, no. 10, pp. 1189–1195, 2007.

[74] K. W. Mahaffey, G. Hafley, S. Dickerson et al., "Results of a reevaluation of cardiovascular outcomes in the RECORD trial," *American Heart Journal*, vol. 166, no. 2, pp. 240.e1–249.e1, 2013.

[75] S. Z. Duan, C. Y. Ivashchenko, M. W. Russell, D. S. Milstone, and R. M. Mortensen, "Cardiomyocyte-specific knockout and agonist of peroxisome proliferator-activated receptor-gamma both induce cardiac hypertrophy in mice," *Circulation Research*, vol. 97, no. 4, pp. 372–379, 2005.

[76] N. Narang, S. I. Armstead, A. Stream et al., "Assessment of cardiac structure and function in patients without and with peripheral oedema during rosiglitazone treatment," *Diabetes and Vascular Disease Research*, vol. 8, no. 2, pp. 101–108, 2011.

[77] T. P. Burris, S. A. Busby, and P. R. Griffin, "Targeting orphan nuclear receptors for treatment of metabolic diseases and autoimmunity," *Chemistry and Biology*, vol. 19, no. 1, pp. 51–59, 2012.

[78] W. Wei, X. Wang, M. Yang, L. C. Smith, and P. C. Dechow, "PGC1beta mediates PPARgamma activation of osteoclastogenesis and rosiglitazone-induced bone loss," *Cell Metabolism*, vol. 11, no. 6, pp. 503–516, 2010.

[79] B. Charbonnel, R. DeFronzo, J. Davidson et al., "Pioglitazone use in combination with insulin in the prospective pioglitazone clinical trial in macrovascular events study (PROactive19)," *Journal of Clinical Endocrinology and Metabolism*, vol. 95, no. 5, pp. 2163–2171, 2010.

[80] E. Erdmann, J. A. Dormandy, B. Charbonnel, M. Massi-Benedetti, I. K. Moules, and A. M. Skene, "The effect of pioglitazone on recurrent myocardial infarction in 2,445 patients with type 2 diabetes and previous myocardial infarction. results from the PROactive (PROactive 05) Study," *Journal of the American College of Cardiology*, vol. 49, no. 17, pp. 1772–1780, 2007.

[81] P. D. Home, S. J. Pocock, H. Beck-Nielsen et al., "Rosiglitazone evaluated for cardiovascular outcomes in oral agent combination therapy for type 2 diabetes (RECORD): a multicentre, randomised, open-label trial," *The Lancet*, vol. 373, no. 9681, pp. 2125–2135, 2009.

[82] H. C. Gerstein, S. Yusuf, R. R. Holman et al., "Effect of rosiglitazone on the frequency of diabetes in patients with impaired glucose tolerance or impaired fasting glucose: a randomised controlled trial," *The Lancet*, vol. 368, no. 9541, pp. 1096–1105, 2006.

[83] R. A. DeFronzo, D. Tripathy, D. C. Schwenke et al., "Pioglitazone for diabetes prevention in impaired glucose tolerance," *The New England Journal of Medicine*, vol. 364, no. 12, pp. 1104–1115, 2011.

[84] S. E. Kahn, S. M. Haffner, M. A. Heise et al., "Glycemic durability of rosiglitazone, metformin, or glyburide monotherapy," *New England Journal of Medicine*, vol. 355, no. 23, pp. 2427–2443, 2006.

[85] A. M. Lincoff, K. Wolski, S. J. Nicholls, and S. E. Nissen, "Pioglitazone and risk of cardiovascular events in patients with type 2 diabetes mellitus: a meta-analysis of randomized trials," *The Journal of the American Medical Association*, vol. 298, no. 10, pp. 1180–1188, 2007.

[86] E. Mannucci, M. Monami, C. Lamanna, G. F. Gensini, and N. Marchionni, "Pioglitazone and cardiovascular risk. A comprehensive meta-analysis of randomized clinical trials," *Diabetes, Obesity and Metabolism*, vol. 10, no. 12, pp. 1221–1238, 2008.

[87] S. E. Nissen and K. Wolski, "Rosiglitazone revisited: an updated meta-analysis of risk for myocardial infarction and cardiovascular mortality," *Archives of Internal Medicine*, vol. 170, no. 14, pp. 1191–1201, 2010.

[88] J. Woodcock, J. M. Sharfstein, and M. Hamburg, "Regulatory action on rosiglitazone by the U.S. food and drug administration," *New England Journal of Medicine*, vol. 363, no. 16, pp. 1489–1491, 2010.

[89] N. Ziyadeh, A. T. McAfee, C. Koro, J. Landon, and K. Arnold Chan, "The thiazolidinediones rosiglitazone and pioglitazone and the risk of coronary heart disease: a retrospective cohort study using a US health insurance database," *Clinical Therapeutics*, vol. 31, no. 11, pp. 2665–2677, 2009.

[90] F.-Y. Hsiao, W.-F. Huang, Y.-W. Wen, P.-F. Chen, K. N. Kuo, and Y.-W. Tsai, "Thiazolidinediones and cardiovascular events in patients with type 2 diabetes mellitus: a retrospective cohort study of over 473000 patients using the national health insurance database in Taiwan," *Drug Safety*, vol. 32, no. 8, pp. 675–690, 2009.

[91] Z. A. Habib, L. Tzogias, S. L. Havstad et al., "Relationship between thiazolidinedione use and cardiovascular outcomes and all-cause mortality among patients with diabetes: a time-updated propensity analysis," *Pharmacoepidemiology and Drug Safety*, vol. 18, no. 6, pp. 437–447, 2009.

[92] Y. K. Loke, C. S. Kwok, and S. Singh, "Comparative cardiovascular effects of thiazolidinediones: systematic review and meta-analysis of observational studies," *BMJ*, vol. 342, no. 7799, Article ID d1309, p. 692, 2011.

[93] P. Balakumar, M. Rose, S. S. Ganti, P. Krishan, and M. Singh, "PPAR dual agonists: are they opening Pandora's Box?" *Pharmacological Research*, vol. 56, no. 2, pp. 91–98, 2007.

[94] L. M. Younk, L. Uhl, and S. N. Davis, "Pharmacokinetics, efficacy and safety of aleglitazar for the treatment of type 2 diabetes with high cardiovascular risk," *Expert Opinion on Drug Metabolism and Toxicology*, vol. 7, no. 6, pp. 753–763, 2011.

[95] B. C. Hansen, X. T. Tigno, A. Bénardeau, M. Meyer, E. Sebokova, and J. Mizrahi, "Effects of aleglitazar, a balanced dual peroxisome proliferator-activated receptor α/γ agonist on glycemic and lipid parameters in a primate model of the metabolic syndrome," *Cardiovascular Diabetology*, vol. 10, article no. 7, 2011.

[96] R. R. Henry, A. M. Lincoff, S. Mudaliar, M. Rabbia, C. Chognot, and M. Herz, "Effect of the dual peroxisome proliferator-activated receptor-α/γ agonist aleglitazar on risk of cardiovascular disease in patients with type 2 diabetes (SYNCHRONY): a phase II, randomised, dose-ranging study," *The Lancet*, vol. 374, no. 9684, pp. 126–135, 2009.

[97] M. C. Carmona, K. Louche, B. Lefebvre et al., "S 26948: a new specific peroxisome proliferator-activated receptor γ modulator with potent antidiabetes and antiatherogenic effects," *Diabetes*, vol. 56, no. 11, pp. 2797–2808, 2007.

[98] F. L. Dunn, L. S. Higgins, J. Fredrickson, and A. M. Depaoli, "Selective modulation of PPARγ activity can lower plasma glucose without typical thiazolidinedione side-effects in patients with Type 2 diabetes," *Journal of Diabetes and its Complications*, vol. 25, no. 3, pp. 151–158, 2011.

[99] J. H. Choi, A. S. Banks, T. M. Kamenecka et al., "Antidiabetic actions of a non-agonist PPARγ ligand blocking Cdk5-mediated phosphorylation," *Nature*, vol. 477, no. 7365, pp. 477–481, 2011.

[100] A. P. S. Kong, A. Yamasaki, R. Ozaki et al., "A randomized-controlled trial to investigate the effects of rivoglitazone, a novel PPAR gamma agonist on glucose-lipid control in type 2 diabetes," *Diabetes, Obesity and Metabolism*, vol. 13, no. 9, pp. 806–813, 2011.

[101] R. Agrawal, P. Jain, and S. N. Dikshit, "Balaglitazone: a second generation peroxisome proliferator-activated receptor (PPAR) gamma (γ) agonist," *Mini-Reviews in Medicinal Chemistry*, vol. 12, no. 2, pp. 87–97, 2012.

[102] R. Agrawal, "The first approved agent in the Glitazar's class: Saroglitazar," *Current Drug Targets*, vol. 15, no. 2, pp. 151–155, 2014.

6

Commonalities in the Association between PPARG and Vitamin D Related with Obesity and Carcinogenesis

Borja Bandera Merchan,[1] **Francisco José Tinahones,**[1,2] **and Manuel Macías-González**[1,2]

[1] *Unidad de Gestión Clínica Endocrinología y Nutrición, Instituto de Investigación Biomédica de Málaga (IBIMA),*
 Complejo Hospitalario de Málaga (Virgen de la Victoria), Universidad de Málaga, 29010 Malaga, Spain
[2] *CIBER Pathophysiology of Obesity and Nutrition (CB06/03), 28029 Madrid, Spain*

Correspondence should be addressed to Francisco José Tinahones; fjtinahones@hotmail.com
and Manuel Macías-González; mmacias.manuel@gmail.com

Academic Editor: Daniele Fanale

The PPAR nuclear receptor family has acquired great relevance in the last decade, which is formed by three different isoforms (PPARα, PPARβ/δ, and PPAR Y). Those nuclear receptors are members of the steroid receptor superfamily which take part in essential metabolic and life-sustaining actions. Specifically, PPARG has been implicated in the regulation of processes concerning metabolism, inflammation, atherosclerosis, cell differentiation, and proliferation. Thus, a considerable amount of literature has emerged in the last ten years linking PPARG signalling with metabolic conditions such as obesity and diabetes, cardiovascular disease, and, more recently, cancer. This review paper, at crossroads of basic sciences, preclinical, and clinical data, intends to analyse the last research concerning PPARG signalling in obesity and cancer. Afterwards, possible links between four interrelated actors will be established: PPARG, the vitamin D/VDR system, obesity, and cancer, opening up the door to further investigation and new hypothesis in this fascinating area of research.

1. Introduction

There are three subtypes of PPARG, known as PPARG1, PPARG2, and PPARG3. It has been established that PPARG2 leads in potency as a transcription factor [1]. PPARG performs its functions mainly through PPARG1 and PPARG2 [2]. Moreover, it shares lots of additional features with its other counterparts. Concerning that, the parallelism found between the PPARG system and the vitamin D/vitamin D receptor (VD/VDR) system will be further explored later on.

In order to modulate gene expression, the PPAR NRs family, and specifically the PPARG, after binding with either natural or synthetic ligands, heterodimerizes with the Retinoid X Receptor (RXR) as vitamin D receptor (VDR) does.

Later on, the complex PPARG-RXR translocates to the nucleus in order to get attached to PPREs (PPAR Response Elements), genome nucleotides sequences wherefrom the PPARs will coordinate the expression or repression of some genes involved in metabolism, immunity, differentiation, or cellular proliferation, to cite some [3–6].

Once in the nucleus, several molecules known as corepressors and coactivators, which show histone modifying activities by themselves [7], bind the PPARG-RXR complex, showing some control over the genetic expression-repression interplay. Some known corepressors are SMRT or NCOR. When it comes to coactivators, we can mention p300/CRRB-binding protein (CBP) or SRC/p160 [8]. Importantly, differential recruitment of coactivators implies different gene expression patterns [9], wherefrom it can be deduced that the corepressors and coactivators comprise another gene expression regulatory point which is worth studying. PPREs are normally found in the promoter of those genes, which is regulated by PPARG activity [3]. The direct nucleotide sequences which PPARG-RXR will be bound to are known as DR-1 motifs (direct hexanucleotide repeats) of PPRE [8]. Some PPARG target genes are those codifying CD36, FABP4 (Fatty Acid Binding Protein 4), adiponectin, or the CCAAT/enhancer binding protein α [10], all being genes involved in adipose tissue homeostasis. However, afar of its adipose functions PPARG is also vital for development of some important organs such as heart and the placenta [11].

2. The PPARG Physiology

PPARG behaves as a transcription factor, as many other nuclear receptors (NRs) do. Then, it modulates the expression and repression of a myriad of genes involved in metabolic homeostasis, regulating energy expenditure and storage [12, 13]. Some PPARG target genes are those codifying CD36, FABP4 (Fatty Acid Binding Protein 4), adiponectin, or the CCAAT/enhancer binding protein α [10], all being genes involved in adipose tissue homeostasis. However, afar of its adipose functions PPARG is also vital for development of some important organs such as heart and the placenta [11]. Although most research on PPARG has been focused on its metabolic action, some of them are neurogenesis, osteogenesis, cancer, or cardiovascular disease [14]. Such pleiotropism of actions gives us a clue of the relevance of this transcription factor regarding health and disease. We know for instance that universal PPARG deletion and life are not compatible [11].

The considerable host of actions performed by PPARG can be compared to those of vitamin D and VDR [15], which has been implicated in neurologic disorders [16–18], autoimmune pathologies [19–21], cardiovascular disease [22], diabetes mellitus [23, 24], psoriasis [15] or infectious disease [25, 26], and, above all of what is mentioned, cancer [27, 28].

3. PPARG and Obesity

Much has been already written about PPARG signalling and its role in conditions such as obesity or diabetes. In obesity, PPARG orchestrates adipocyte maturation and differentiation, harmonising the role of many other players in that process [29]. Remarkably, it is the only known factor, which is completely necessary and sufficient for the adipocyte differentiation process to occur [11, 30]. This nuclear receptor acts, then, as a master regulator of adipogenesis.

In addition, it is widely known that PPARG has an important whole-body insulin-sensitizer role. For example, muscle-PPARG knocked-out mice are insulin resistant [31]. In adipose tissue, PPARG deletion leads to increases in bone mass, lipoatrophy, and insulin resistance (IR) [32]. In the same fashion, PPARG induces the proliferation of adipocytes progenitors into mature adipocytes and diminishes the osteoblasts population likewise [33].

The specific deletion of PPARG in liver conduces to IR and decrease of hepatic fat depots [34]. Even in macrophages, the presence of PPARG is important to keep adequate insulin sensitivity levels throughout the body [35, 36]. It is then easy to deduce that one of the main objectives of PPARG activity is the insulin sensitivity maintenance through different tissues.

Thiazolidinediones (TZD), a family of synthetic PPARG agonist widely used in diabetes treatment, show clear improvements in insulin sensitivity, enhanced adipocyte differentiation, reduction of leptin levels, and upregulation of adiponectin [37].

Contrary to the catabolic actions elicited by the PPARα and PPARδ, the PPARG is in charge of anabolic functions. As we have already addressed, adipogenesis and lipid storage are some of them. Illustrating this, a high-fat feeding augments PPARG expression while fasting diminishes it [38].

Remarkably, PPARG performs different functions in metabolically sick rodents and metabolically healthy ones. In disease, PPARG activation seems to improve metabolic parameters, but in the healthy population its downregulation shows antiobesity effects [39].

In the same way, more different effects have been described in metabolic health and disease regarding PPARG expression. For instance, in healthy subjects a high-fat meal greatly induced the expression of PPARG while the same high-fat feeding diminished PPARG expression in a group of morbidly obese patients [40].

In like manner, an indirect correlation between IR and PPARG expression, measured by glucose status, HOMA-IR index, and insulin levels, can be set in morbidly obese persons, whose visceral adipose and muscle tissues show less PPARG expression as IR increases [40].

During placentation and intrauterine development, the PPARG gene methylation patterns could be altered by maternal nutrition, which actually exerts long-term effects upon the receptor status in the offspring, as indicated very recently by Lendvai et al. [41]. This is preliminary evidence about the early programming of our lifelong metabolism set points through nutritional inputs, which could easily leave us susceptible to obesity and metabolic disease in later stages of life.

4. PPARG and Cancer

PPARG is highly expressed in lung, prostate, colorectal, bladder, and breast tumours [42]. Furthermore, we can find in the literature compelling evidence for PPARG having antineoplastic actions in colon, prostate, breast, and lung cancers [43, 44], which happen to be the most prevalent forms of cancer in occident (Figure 1).

Solid evidence backs up that epigenetic events frequently found in cancer can hamper nuclear receptors responsiveness toward their ligands. In that respect, increased levels of corepressor NCOR in prostate cancer can silence the expression of target genes and constitute a potential epigenetic lesion, which selectively distorts the actions of PPARG/PPARα [45].

In the same line, PPARG promoter methylation in colorectal carcinoma (CRC) is associated with poor prognosis [46]. This transcriptional silencing of PPARG is operated through HDAC1 (Histone Deacetylase 1), EZH2 (Enhancer of Zeste 2 Polycomb Repressive Complex 2 Subunit), and MeCP2 (Methyl CpG Binding Protein 2) recruitment, leading to repressive chromatin states that eventually increase cell proliferation and invasive potential [46]. Correspondingly, APC$^{\text{min}/+}$ mice which have undergone PPARG genetic ablation demonstrate increased colon tumour growth [47].

In the literature, some mutations and variations in PPARG expression have been associated with cancer in our specie [48, 49]. Beyond that, its expression comprises an independent prognostic factor in CRC [50, 51].

Apart from epigenetics, we should not lose sight of the fact that metabolic syndrome, insulin resistance, obesity,

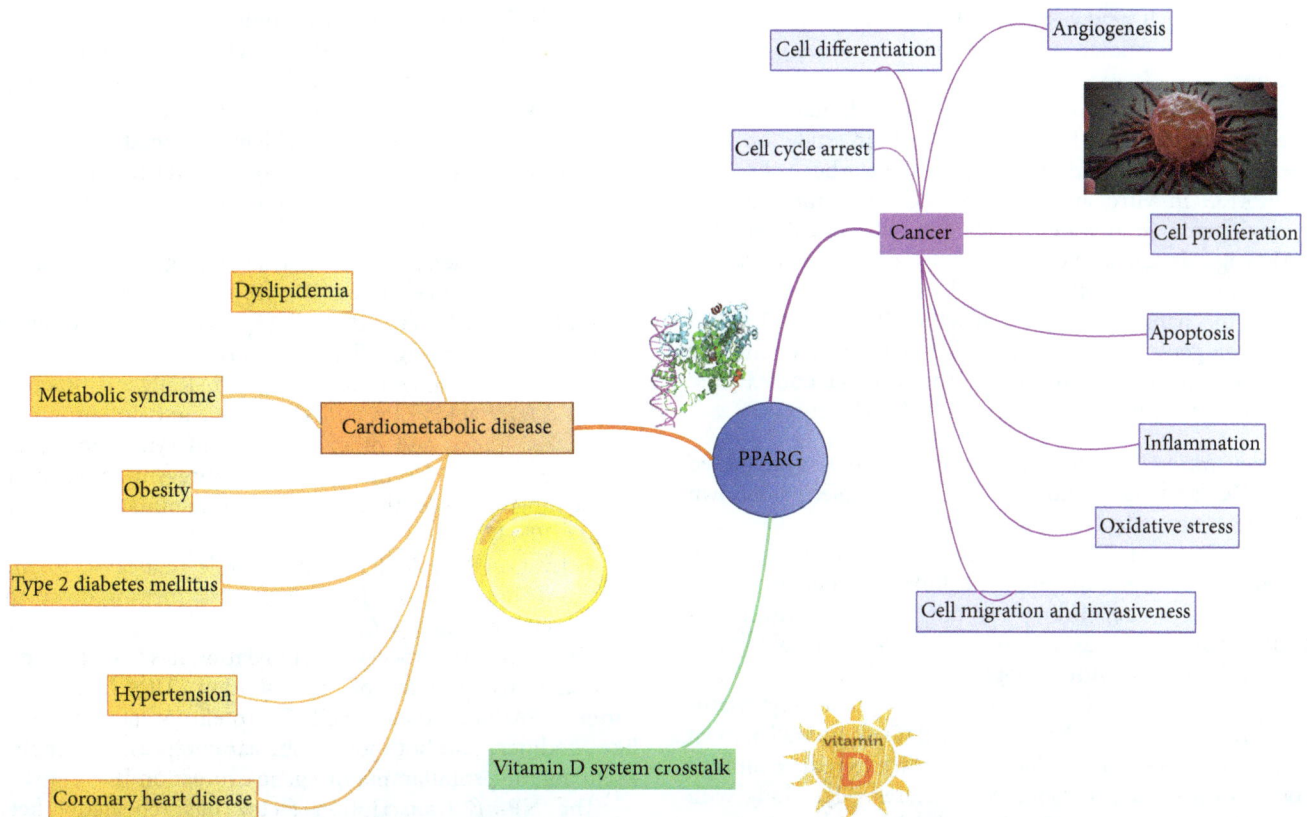

FIGURE 1: PPARG actions: PPARG plays an important role in cardiometabolic disease and cancer. The noteworthy crosstalk between vitamin D system and PPARG is also considered. Arrow's width exemplifies the level of consistency found in the literature regarding each association in the mind picture.

and inflammation, importantly interrelated conditions in which PPARG has modifying and regulatory actions, increase cancer risk [52–59], which adds weight to PPARG and cancer research (Figure 1).

There is some evidence linking PPARG agonist's actions to better cancer treatment responsiveness as well. PPARG agonist Rosiglitazone, in this phase II clinical trial, raised the radioiodine uptake in differentiated thyroid cancer [60].

IFN-β treated pancreatic cancer cells were more affected when Troglitazone was added to the therapy, showing synergistic effects between IFN-β and TGZ [61]. But it is necessary to be careful in some studies, in which PPARG agonist like Rosiglitazone acts as a great promoter of hydroxybutyl nitrosamine-induced urinary bladder cancers [62].

In the following paragraphs, we will review what we know about the specific molecular actions of PPARG in cancer biology. Cell cycle arrest, cell differentiation, angiogenesis, proliferation, invasiveness, migration capacity, apoptosis, inflammation, and oxidative stress should be evaluated.

4.1. Cell Cycle Arrests.
Some evidence suggests that PPARG and its agonists have the ability to interfere with the cellular cycle and then, likely, with malignancies development.

In renal cell carcinoma, Troglitazone (TGZ) was able to induce G2/M cell cycle arrest via activation of p38 MAPK (Mitogen-Activated Protein Kinase) [63].

In human pancreatic cancer cells the same phenomenon is observed: PPARG is able to trigger cell cycle arrest of the malignant cells through activation by thiazolidinediones [64].

Through PPARG activation, its ligands increase the expression of the cyclin-dependent kinase inhibitors p21 [64, 65] and p27 [65–69], enhance the turnover of β-catenin, and downregulate the expression of cyclin D1 [70–74].

4.2. Differentiation.
In vitro activation of PPARG by its ligands correlates with increased expression of carcinoembryonic antigen (CEA), E-cadherin, developmentally regulated GTP-binding protein 1 (DRG), alkaline phosphatase, or keratins, all of them being molecules expressed in well differentiated cells, opposing to the undifferentiated cell state commonly found in most cancers [48, 64, 75–77].

Tontonoz et al. gave us the first evidence about the effectiveness of PPARG ligands inducing differentiation in human cancer cells, concretely in liposarcoma cancer cells [75]. Again, in human liposarcoma, treatment with Troglitazone raised the level of differentiation of its cells [78].

More evidence that PPARG enhances terminal differentiation in cells is reviewed in papers of Grommes et al. and Koeffler, respectively [43, 44].

4.3. Angiogenesis.
It is common knowledge that angiogenesis is a vital step in malignant development. The complex

process by which new vessels are formed, angiogenesis, has been feverishly studied as a new possible target in cancer treatment.

In vitro and in vivo angiogenesis-modulating functions have been described for PPARG [79]. In spite of that, differential effects regarding angiogenesis have been observed for PPARG in vitro and in vivo, showing either pro- or antiangiogenic actions dependent on cell context [80–85]. PPARG agonist can also enhance VEGF expression in cancer cells, as some studies reveal [86, 87].

The mechanisms deciding whether PPARG will act as a proangiogenic factor or as an antiangiogenic one are still elusive to us, but we believe that cellular context and environment are likely the controllers of such process.

4.4. Proliferation. Antiproliferative actions are also attributed to PPARG and its ligands. TZD, for example, has shown antiproliferative effects [88, 89].

Modulation of PPARG can have differential effects on carcinogenesis depending on the cellular microenvironment [90]. Therefore, depending on the cellular environment PPARG can behave as a proliferative or antiproliferative factor, as happened with angiogenesis.

Tumour cells are frequently in shortage of polyunsaturated fatty acids. Docosahexaenoic acid (DHA), a well-known ligand of the PPAR family, has been shown to reduce tumour proliferation in lung tumour cell cultures [91]. Along with that, DHA in breast cancer cells diminishes proliferation and increases apoptosis [92, 93].

In prostate cancer, PPARG ligand activation effect was assessed in a phase II clinical trial. The results showed a hampered cancer cell growth [94].

Eukaryotic initiation factor 2 is a target of inhibition for PPARG agonists (i.e., thiazolidinediones). Such factor inhibition, which is mediated in a PPARG-independent way, truncates the translation process [95].

In liposarcoma patients, treatment with Rosiglitazone increased the necessary time to double tumour volume in this clinical trial [96]. In other studies, however, Troglitazone (another member of the thiazolidinedione family) had low or no effects in prostate cancer [97] or breast or colorectal cancer [98, 99].

4.5. Apoptosis. The combined effect of an RXR agonist and Troglitazone curtailed gastric cancer cells proliferation in vitro by enhancing apoptotic mechanisms [100].

PPARG agonists increased the expression of PTEN [101–105], BAX, BAD [106, 107], and the turnover of the FLICE inhibitory protein (FLIP) [108, 109], known for its antiapoptotic role.

Conversely, PPARG agonists can inhibit BCL-X$_L$ and BCL-2 expression [107, 110], PI3K activity, and AKT phosphorylation [101, 111, 112] and restrain the activation of JUN N-terminal protein kinase [107]. It is worth mentioning that many of those actions were elicited in a PPARG-independent manner. The exact mechanisms by which these effects are performed are still unknown.

4.6. Inflammation. Nowadays, it is common knowledge in the scientific community that chronic inflammation promotes

cancer. The milieu found in chronic inflammation acts as a facilitator for carcinogenesis and cancer development [52, 113]. This has been shown in colorectal, liver, bladder, lung, and gastric neoplasms [114, 115] and investigated in several more. The range of processes in which inflammation partakes in carcinogenesis goes from cell growth and survival, metastasis and cell invasion, treatment response, angiogenesis, and tumour immunity [115, 116].

There is evidence of PPARG having anti-inflammatory activity in several cell lines [117, 118]. In models of experimentally induced colitis PPARG expressed in macrophages is capable of inhibiting inflammation [119].

It is widely known that some PPAR ligands such as omega-3 fatty acids EPA and DHA have anti-inflammatory properties. Those and other natural and synthetic ligands could be used in the future as chemopreventive agents in a vast range of conditions linked to inflammation, that is, cancer [105, 120, 121].

Activation of PPARG by its ligands reduces cytokines such as TNFα and NF-$\kappa\beta$ in monocytes, turning down the inflammatory milieu [120, 122].

The epigenetic process of sumoylation has been linked to PPARG transrepression of inflammation. After ligand activation, PPARG binds to a SUMO protein (Small Ubiquitin-like Modifier) and both join a nuclear corepressor complex, reducing the proinflammatory gene expression [123].

The NF-$\kappa\beta$ transcription factor has repeatedly been associated with tumour development and thriving [52]. Interacting with this factor, PPARG inhibits the genesis of proinflammatory molecules such as IL-6, TNF, and MCP1 through transrepression [3, 117].

Again, a word of caution must be said due to the seemingly tumour-promoting effects of PPARG found sporadically [124–127]. Therefore, it seems as if the effects carried on by the cell depend of cell context and environment. Environment is, usually, at the helm of cellular functions.

4.7. Oxidative Stress. PPARG has demonstrated an antioxidant effect [128, 129]. SOD (Superoxide Dismutase) expression might well be regulated by PPAR because a PPRE is found in the Cu/Zn-SOD promoter [40].

IR found in diabetes mellitus and metabolic disease is certainly correlated with increased oxidative stress, which eventually could lead to an increased risk of cancer through nongenomic carcinogenesis [130–133].

In macrophages, PPARG mediates some notable abilities: uptake and reverse transport of cholesterol, macrophage subtype specification (enhancing the M2 macrophage phenotype, which is associated with higher insulin sensitivity and lower inflammation levels), and anti-inflammation properties [36, 134, 135].

Postprandial hypertriglyceridemia is associated with lower PPARG expression in metabolic syndrome patients while in healthy subjects the same "insult" leads to overexpression of PPARG [136]. We could hypothesize that since the PPARG system is injured in the metabolically ill patients, after an oxidative stress insult (a high-fat feeding), it cannot respond, leaving us more susceptible to oxidative actions and its consequences (hypothesis coined as "*nuclear receptor exhaustion theory*"). In the healthy group, the PPARG would perfectly be capable of managing the lipid storage and would act as an oxidative stress buffer.

4.8. Cell Migration and Invasiveness. Less evidence is available with respect to invasiveness and PPARG. However, we should pay attention to some preliminary data.

The PPARG gene modulates the invasion of cytotrophoblast into uterine tissue, which could be a novel indicator of some invasion-related function of PPARG [137].

Going further, this study by Yoshizumi et al. showed how PPARG ligand thiazolidinedione (TZD) is able to inhibit growth and metastasis of HT-29 human colon cancer cells, via the induction of cell differentiation. The use of the TZD drives to G1 arrest, in association with a great increase in p21Waf-1, Drg-1, and E-cadherin expression [77].

Paradoxically, molecules with PPARG antagonist actions are able to inhibit invasiveness and proliferation of some cancer cell lines [26, 138–140]. Again, one nuclear receptor can exert one or just the opposite function depending on the cellular environment and ligand exposure.

5. Connecting the Dots: PPARG, Vitamin D System, Obesity, and Cancer

Often in biology and medicine research, we tend to focus on the individualities of separated molecules or molecule systems in order to explain their functions, forgetting the intermolecular communication, which is ever-present in every biological system. More frequent than not, that separateness gives us a rather limited perspective of the matter at hand. For instance, the interconnectedness of biology systems and the emerging properties of such interconnectedness should be further examined and taken into account.

The crosstalk between different NRs, the "dance" and messages they give one another, is recently becoming an exciting new area which will be explored. This is the case of the VDR/VD and the PPARG system, in which both have been shown to be involved in some relationship we do not utterly understand yet.

5.1. PPARG and VDR/VD System: Commonalities in Cancer. Noteworthy, great parallelism exists between PPARG and the VDR/VD system regarding its protective role in carcinogenesis. There are a vast number of studies describing the anticancer properties of vitamin D. The majority of them are brilliantly analysed in this review by Feldman et al. [28].

Vitamin D has been extensively associated with anti-inflammatory actions [141–143], apoptotic mechanisms [144–150], antiproliferative functions [151–159], prodifferentiation effects [160–166], antiangiogenic properties [167–171], a potential role-managing invasion and metastasis [172–184], microRNA modulation [185–189], and even some role in the Hedgehog signalling pathway modulation [190]. Remarkably, most of those actions have been attributed to PPARG signalling in a somewhat lesser extent, as reviewed in this work. Such similarity and overlap in anticancer actions are worth studying.

Moreover, there is enough evidence to assert that epigenetic events can influence both PPARG and VDR/VD systems behaviour.

In this study, Fujiki et al. showed that in a diabetic mouse model PPARG promoter methylation levels are higher than those of the control mice [191], along with the possibility of methylation reversal when the animals were exposed to 5AZA (5′-aza-cytidine). At least three messages can be drawn from this study: (1) the PPARG system is susceptible to epigenetic regulation, (2) diabetes and other metabolic conditions could alter the PPARG epigenetic landscape and then disrupt its proper functioning, and (3) this disruption can be reversed by drug-induced changes or, likely, by lifestyle changes.

The vitamin D system is likewise susceptible to epigenetic regulation [192–195] and, interestingly, in cancer this epigenetic repression of the vitamin D system is almost always present [196–204], which compellingly leaves the door opened to the possibility of the same phenomena happening in the PPARG system.

In fact, PPARG promoter hypermethylation is a prognostic factor of adverse outcome in colorectal cancer [46, 205]. Higher levels of PPARG promoter methylation were found in advanced tumour stages while earlier stages showed lower methylation levels. This suggests that as happens with vitamin D, advanced cancer stages can epigenetically repress PPARG expression and then nullify its antineoplastic actions.

5.2. The PPARG/VDR Crosstalk: What an Interesting Conversation! Some studies have clearly shown the existence of some communication between PPARG and VD/VDR. Interestingly, potent VDRE (Vitamin D Response Elements) have been discovered in human PPARδ promoter, which opens the door to VDR/VD influence over the PPAR system [206]. In the opposite direction, some studies have demonstrated the ability of PPARG to bind VDR and inhibit vitamin D-mediated transactivation [207]. This data might be an indicator of bidirectional or reciprocal actions of both systems influencing each other, which have deep implications and introduce new and interesting questions to ponder upon.

Even between PPAR subtypes some modulation of expression have been found: PPARδ could repress PPARα and PPARG gene expression [208], illustrating the complexity of PPAR system regulation.

In the adipocyte cell, the VD/VDR system has shown anti-PPARG activity, inhibiting its expression and then adipogenesis [209, 210], which is contradictory with the commonly found proadipogenesis effects of vitamin D [211], at least in human. The factors leading to either pro- or antiadipogenesis effects are completely uncharted.

In melanoma cell lines, administration of calcitriol and several PPAR ligands modified the expression of both PPARG and VDR, demonstrating again this intriguing connection [212]. Sertznig et al. conclude in this article that calcitriol and some PPAR ligands can inhibit proliferation of the human melanoma cell line MeWo [213].

5.3. PPARG and VD/VDR System: Metabolic Commonalities. We are about to discuss the metabolic effects of vitamin D and their analogy with those of PPARG, establishing again the parallelism.

As contradictory as it seems, VDR or CYP27B1 knocked-out mice show great fat mass loss [211] while obesity in humans is commonly associated with poor vitamin D plasmatic levels [214]. Actually, an indirect relationship between Body Mass Index (BMI) and 25OHD3 has been amply described in the literature [215].

In addition, low plasmatic vitamin D levels are associated with increased risk of type 2 diabetes mellitus (T2DM) independently of BMI [24] and with hypertension, dyslipidemia (DLP), and metabolic syndrome (MS) [216, 217]. Besides, vitamin D deficiency predisposes to diabetes in animal models, while its supplementation prevents the disease [214]. Concerning PPARG, we have extensively discussed before in the review its orchestrating actions regarding adipogenesis and adipocyte metabolism. Both calcitriol (the active form of vitamin D) and PPARG seem to oppose metabolic homeostasis disruption.

Another paradoxical event is found in the fact that in humans calcitriol enhances adipogenesis while in mice the same hormone diminishes it via downregulation of C/EBPβ mRNA and upregulation of CBFA2T1 (a corepressor) [218, 219]. With reference to PPARG, it enhances adipogenesis [10].

In human subcutaneous preadipocytes, calcitriol elicits actions impressively similar to those of PPARG in adipocyte maturation and differentiation. For instance, calcitriol is able to increase the expression of the enzyme Fatty Acid Synthase (FASN) increasing lipogenesis in like manner as PPARG [210].

The *storage capacity theory* introduces the idea that lipid storage capacity and the ability of PPARG to manage the processes leading to lipid storage are limited. As to that, when the organism reaches a lipid level threshold lipotoxicity shows up, PPARG is no more capable of lipid handling, and the harmful hormonal environment of obesity starts to spread through the organism [220].

Transferring the same concept of *"nuclear receptor exhaustion"* to VD/VDR anticancer actions we could establish a parallelism. It has shown that the VD/VDR is epigenetically downregulated in late cancer stages but overexpressed or normally expressed in early stages [221, 222]. As the aforementioned studies show, in those later stages epigenetic downregulation of the VD system molecules occurs, leaving it unable to exert its antineoplastic functions properly. Is obesity, as cancer does with vitamin D, acting as a negative epigenetic driver when it comes to PPARG signalling? That could answer why in most morbidly obese patients expression of PPARG is greatly lower in comparison to healthy subjects.

Accordingly, PPARG1 and PPARG2 expression in visceral adipose tissue (VAT) from morbidly obese (MO) subjects is significantly downregulated when compared to metabolically healthy subjects [223]. Not only that, in insulin resistant MO subjects PPARG expression is even lower [220] compared with noninsulin resistant MO patients, whichever interestingly correlates with the lower vitamin D levels found in MO with IR compared to their insulin sensitive counterparts [24]. Somehow, the metabolic impairment caused by insulin resistance is able to deteriorate both PPARG and VD/VDR

system. The underlying mechanism behind this deterioration should be further studied.

A disrupted VDR/VD system leads mice to loss of fat deposits and great increase of energy expenditure. In relation to that, VDR$^{-/-}$ mice increase the expression of UCP1 (uncoupling protein 1 or Thermogenin) twenty-five-fold [211], with the consequent energy consumption. Is vitamin D, along with PPARG, an energy-conserving and metabolic homeostasis-maintaining hormone?

However, adipose tissue is not the only one affected by disruption of the VD system. A shortage of calcitriol in rats was related with increased skeletal muscle ubiquitination and loss of total muscle mass [224]. On the PPARG side, its activation through TZD in growing pigs increased muscle fiber oxidative capacity independently of fiber type [225]. Overexpression of PPARδ in mice almost doubles the animal endurance and exercise capacity [226]. We should not lose sight of the important role the muscle has in obesity and metabolic disease pathogenesis, being a potential target for calcitriol and PPAR modulating actions.

Taken all data together, the vitamin D system seems to team up with PPARG in order to maintain proper metabolic homeostasis. Notwithstanding, in some occasions this love relationship breaks apart and both partners seem to bother one another in ways that we utterly ignore but, likely, have something to do with epigenetic regulation.

6. Conclusions

The PPARG transcription factor has been classically associated with metabolic homeostasis and lipid storage functions. Recently, newfound anticancer actions are assigned to this nuclear receptor.

However, its anticancer actions are not always consistent; in some studies some oncogenic effects have been described. We believe that cellular environment is the guiding factor behind PPARG actions and cells are controlled "from outside in." In alignment with this, the PPARG and other nuclear receptors would only be "cellular effectors," carriers of outside messages of health or disease.

When a "disease threshold" is reached, in either obesity or cancer, PPARG and VDR expression, respectively, diminishes. However, in early stages of those diseases, the expression of those nuclear receptors is higher than normal. Derived from these observations, we have coined the so-called *"nuclear receptor exhaustion theory,"* by which, in an early disease stage, nuclear receptors PPARG and VDR counterbalance the harmful effects that obesity and cancer exert upon the organism, their expression being high. However, sadly, if disease progresses, it generates epigenetic silencing mechanisms upon both transcription factors, whose expression decreases radically. This silencing leaves us increasingly susceptible to disease. The positive side is that through drugs or, better yet, lifestyle changes reversal of epigenetic changes is possible.

There is an exciting function overlap between PPARG and VDR/VD system, both of which wield oncoprotective and metabolic actions. Actually, parallel metabolic and anticancer actions are described in the literature, suggesting that they team up to keep at bay those diseases. Maybe the detailed

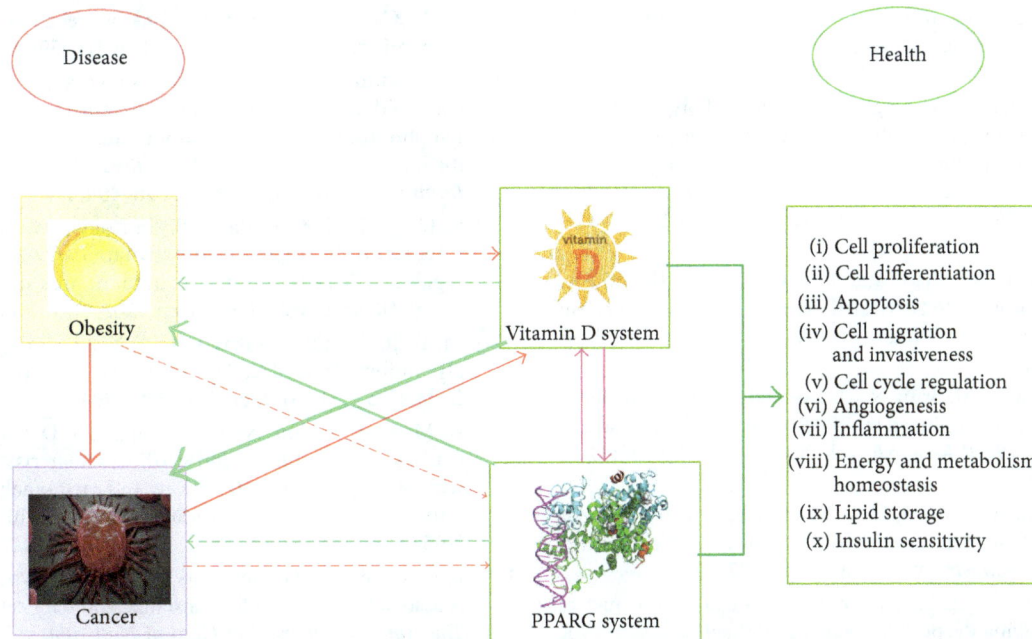

FIGURE 2: The four players: this figure shows the interrelation between the four players: obesity, cancer, vitamin D system, and PPARG. Red arrow: harmful effects, which contribute to disease. Green arrow:positive effects, which contribute to health. Disease perpetuates itself damaging both nuclear receptors. Arrow's width is in proportion with the strength and consistency of each association found in the literature. Dashed line: yet-to-be determined, preliminary, or hypothetical effects. Continuous line: in vitro/in vivo demonstrated effects. Right box: in green, actions mainly attributed to vitamin D, and in purple, actions classically attributed to PPARG. However, it is known that both agents exert every action illustrated in this box, in a higher or lower extent.

study of this overlap could give us clues in respect to the molecular pathogenesis of important conditions as metabolic disease and cancer. Further study in this new area is necessary to elucidate those questions.

Obesity, a first-order problem in our society, is linked with increased risk of cancer incidence and progression. The debatable factors behind this risk are an increment in oxidative stress, chronic inflammation, poorer vitamin D status, hormone misbalance, and, arguably, PPARG silencing through unknown mechanisms. As we know, PPARG and the vitamin D system play conjunctly a yet-to-elucidate role in cancer, so it is not surprising at all that their hypothetical epigenetic repression in obesity could be another mechanism linking this metabolic disorder to malignancies.

It has been shown, both in vitro and in vitro, that the tumours are capable of epigenetically silencing both the vitamin D and the PPARG system. This silencing could lead to the deterioration of their anticancer and metabolic actions.

Finally, a worse known crosstalk between the two NRs exists. Its usefulness, purpose, and message are (almost) utterly unexplored to us and should be studied more diligently. The interrelation, reciprocity, and interdependence of all four actors examined here might be the starting point of new fascinating research linking epigenetic signalling and two of the most hurtful diseases of our time (Figure 2).

Additional Points

Design is literature review across preclinical studies, descriptive studies, analytic studies, and reference lists of selected studies. The author focused mainly on systematic and narrative reviews. Data sources are medline (Pubmed), Jábega 2.0 (Málaga University Search Engine Software), Gerión search engine, and screening of citations and references. Regarding eligibility criteria, we focused on papers published in magazines considered to be in the first impact factor quartile without restrictions regarding publishing date. Keywords are PPARG; Obesity; Transcription factor; Vitamin D; Calcitriol; Vitamin D Receptor; Epigenetics; Nuclear Receptor; Cancer; Methylation.

Competing Interests

The authors declare that there are no competing interests.

Acknowledgments

This study was supported by "Centros de Investigación En Red" (CIBER, CB06/03/0018), the "Instituto de Salud Carlos III" (ISCIII), and grants from ISCIII (PI11/01661) and from Consejería de Innovacion, Ciencia y Empresa de la Junta de Andalucía (PI11-CTS-8181) and cofinanced by the European Regional Development Fund (FEDER). M. Macías-González was recipient of the Nicolas Monarde program from the Servicio Andaluz de Salud, Junta de Andalucía, Spain (C0029-2014).

References

[1] J. N. Feige, L. Gelman, L. Michalik, B. Desvergne, and W. Wahli, "From molecular action to physiological outputs: peroxisome

proliferator-activated receptors are nuclear receptors at the crossroads of key cellular functions," *Progress in Lipid Research*, vol. 45, no. 2, pp. 120–159, 2006.

[2] Y. Zhu, C. Qi, J. R. Korenberg et al., "Structural organization of mouse peroxisome proliferator-activated receptor γ (mPPARγ) gene: alternative promoter use and different splicing yield two mPPARγ isoforms," *Proceedings of the National Academy of Sciences of the United States of America*, vol. 92, no. 17, pp. 7921–7925, 1995.

[3] J. M. Peters, Y. M. Shah, and F. J. Gonzalez, "The role of peroxisome proliferator-activated receptors in carcinogenesis and chemoprevention," *Nature Reviews Cancer*, vol. 12, no. 3, pp. 181–195, 2012.

[4] A. Rogue, C. Spire, M. Brun, N. Claude, and A. Guillouzo, "Gene expression changes induced by PPAR γ agonists in animal and human liver," *PPAR Research*, vol. 2010, Article ID 325183, 16 pages, 2010.

[5] T. M. Willson, P. J. Brown, D. D. Sternbach, and B. R. Henke, "The PPARs: from orphan receptors to drug discovery," *Journal of Medicinal Chemistry*, vol. 43, no. 4, pp. 527–550, 2000.

[6] M. Schupp and M. A. Lazar, "Endogenous ligands for nuclear receptors: digging deeper," *Journal of Biological Chemistry*, vol. 285, no. 52, pp. 40409–40415, 2010.

[7] S. C. Wu and Y. Zhang, "Minireview: role of protein methylation and demethylation in nuclear hormone signaling," *Molecular Endocrinology*, vol. 23, no. 9, pp. 1323–1334, 2009.

[8] S. Sugii and R. M. Evans, "Epigenetic codes of PPARγ in metabolic disease," *FEBS Letters*, vol. 585, no. 13, pp. 2121–2128, 2011.

[9] Y. Kodera, K.-I. Takeyama, A. Murayama, M. Suzawa, Y. Masuhiro, and S. Kato, "Ligand type-specific interactions of peroxisome proliferator-activated receptor γ with transcriptional coactivators," *The Journal of Biological Chemistry*, vol. 275, no. 43, pp. 33201–33204, 2000.

[10] P. Tontonoz and B. M. Spiegelman, "Fat and beyond: the diverse biology of PPARγ," *Annual Review of Biochemistry*, vol. 77, pp. 289–312, 2008.

[11] Y. Barak, M. C. Nelson, E. S. Ong et al., "PPARγ is required for placental, cardiac, and adipose tissue development," *Molecular Cell*, vol. 4, no. 4, pp. 585–595, 1999.

[12] J. Berger and D. E. Moller, "The mechanisms of action of PPARs," *Annual Review of Medicine*, vol. 53, no. 1, pp. 409–435, 2002.

[13] E. Boitier, J.-C. Gautier, and R. Roberts, "Advances in understanding the regulation of apoptosis and mitosis by peroxisome-proliferator activated receptors in pre-clinical models: relevance for human health and disease," *Comparative Hepatology*, vol. 2, article 3, 2003.

[14] J.-H. Kim, J. Song, and K. W. Park, "The multifaceted factor peroxisome proliferator-activated receptor γ (PPARγ) in metabolism, immunity, and cancer," *Archives of Pharmacal Research*, vol. 38, no. 3, pp. 302–312, 2015.

[15] S. Nagpal, S. Na, and R. Rathnachalam, "Noncalcemic actions of vitamin D receptor ligands," *Endocrine Reviews*, vol. 26, no. 5, pp. 662–687, 2005.

[16] N. J. Groves, J. J. McGrath, and T. H. J. Burne, "Vitamin D as a neurosteroid affecting the developing and adult brain," *Annual Review of Nutrition*, vol. 34, pp. 117–141, 2014.

[17] J. W. London, "Low Vitamin D is linked to faster cognitive decline in older adults," *The British Medical Journal*, vol. 351, Article ID h4916, 2015.

[18] M. McCarthy, "Study supports link between low vitamin D and dementia risk," *BMJ*, vol. 349, Article ID g5049, 2014.

[19] T. Koizumi, Y. Nakao, T. Matsui et al., "Effects of corticosteroid and 1,24R-dihydroxy-vitamin D₃ administration on lymphoproliferation and autoimmune disease in MRL/MP-lpr/lpr mice," *International Archives of Allergy and Applied Immunology*, vol. 77, no. 4, pp. 396–404, 1985.

[20] S. Gregori, N. Giarratana, S. Smiroldo, M. Uskokovic, and L. Adorini, "A 1α,25-dihydroxyvitamin D₃ analog enhances regulatory T-cells and arrests autoimmune diabetes in NOD mice," *Diabetes*, vol. 51, no. 5, pp. 1367–1374, 2002.

[21] M. Tsuji, K. Fujii, T. Nakano, and Y. Nishii, "1α-hydroxyvitamin D₃ inhibits Type II collagen-induced arthritis in rats," *FEBS Letters*, vol. 337, no. 3, pp. 248–250, 1994.

[22] A. Manousopoulou, N. M. Al-Daghri, S. D. Garbis, and G. P. Chrousos, "Vitamin D and cardiovascular risk among adults with obesity: a systematic review and meta-analysis," *European Journal of Clinical Investigation*, vol. 45, no. 10, pp. 1113–1126, 2015.

[23] B. J. Boucher, W. G. John, and K. Noonan, "Hypovitaminosis D is associated with insulin resistance and beta cell dysfunction," *The American Journal of Clinical Nutrition*, vol. 80, no. 6, pp. 1666–1667, 2004.

[24] M. Clemente-Postigo, A. Muñoz-Garach, M. Serrano et al., "Serum 25-hydroxyvitamin D and adipose tissue vitamin D receptor gene expression: relationship with obesity and type 2 diabetes," *The Journal of Clinical Endocrinology & Metabolism*, vol. 100, no. 4, pp. E591–E595, 2015.

[25] G. Bakdash, T. M. M. van Capel, L. M. K. Mason, M. L. Kapsenberg, and E. C. de Jong, "Vitamin D3 metabolite calcidiol primes human dendritic cells to promote the development of immunomodulatory IL-10-producing T cells," *Vaccine*, vol. 32, no. 47, pp. 6294–6302, 2014.

[26] K. Takahashi, "Influence of bacteria on epigenetic gene control," *Cellular and Molecular Life Sciences*, vol. 71, no. 6, pp. 1045–1054, 2014.

[27] Y. Ma, C. S. Johnson, and D. L. Trump, *Mechanistic Insights of Vitamin D Anticancer Effects*, 2016.

[28] D. Feldman, A. V. Krishnan, S. Swami, E. Giovannucci, and B. J. Feldman, "The role of vitamin D in reducing cancer risk and progression," *Nature Reviews Cancer*, vol. 14, no. 5, pp. 342–357, 2014.

[29] A. G. Cristancho and M. A. Lazar, "Forming functional fat: a growing understanding of adipocyte differentiation," *Nature Reviews Molecular Cell Biology*, vol. 12, no. 11, pp. 722–734, 2011.

[30] E. D. Rosen and B. M. Spiegelman, "Molecular regulation of adipogenesis," *Annual Review of Cell and Developmental Biology*, vol. 16, pp. 145–171, 2000.

[31] A. L. Hevener, W. He, Y. Barak et al., "Muscle-specific Pparg deletion causes insulin resistance," *Nature Medicine*, vol. 9, no. 12, pp. 1491–1497, 2003.

[32] F. Wang, S. E. Mullican, J. R. DiSpirito, L. C. Peed, and M. A. Lazar, "Lipoatrophy and severe metabolic disturbance in mice with fat-specific deletion of PPARγ," *Proceedings of the National Academy of Sciences of the United States of America*, vol. 110, no. 46, pp. 18656–18661, 2013.

[33] K. Won Park, D. S. Halperin, and P. Tontonoz, "Before they were fat: adipocyte progenitors," *Cell Metabolism*, vol. 8, no. 6, pp. 454–457, 2008.

[34] K. Matsusue, M. Haluzik, G. Lambert et al., "Liver-specific disruption of PPARγ in leptin-deficient mice improves fatty

liver but aggravates diabetic phenotypes," *Journal of Clinical Investigation*, vol. 111, no. 5, pp. 737–747, 2003.

[35] A. L. Hevener, J. M. Olefsky, D. Reichart et al., "Macrophage PPARγ is required for normal skeletal muscle and hepatic insulin sensitivity and full antidiabetic effects of thiazolidine-diones," *Journal of Clinical Investigation*, vol. 117, no. 6, pp. 1658–1669, 2007.

[36] J. I. Odegaard, R. R. Ricardo-Gonzalez, M. H. Goforth et al., "Macrophage-specific PPARγ controls alternative activation and improves insulin resistance," *Nature*, vol. 447, no. 7148, pp. 1116–1120, 2007.

[37] Z. Ament, M. Masoodi, and J. L. Griffin, "Applications of metabolomics for understanding the action of peroxisome proliferator-activated receptors (PPARs) in diabetes, obesity and cancer," *Genome Medicine*, vol. 4, no. 4, article 32, 2012.

[38] A. Vidal-Puig, M. Jimenez-Liñan, B. B. Lowell et al., "Regulation of PPAR γ gene expression by nutrition and obesity in rodents," *The Journal of Clinical Investigation*, vol. 97, no. 11, pp. 2553–2561, 1996.

[39] M. U. Imam, M. Ismail, H. Ithnin, Z. Tubesha, and A. R. Omar, "Effects of germinated brown rice and its bioactive compounds on the expression of the peroxisome proliferator-activated receptor gamma gene," *Nutrients*, vol. 5, no. 2, pp. 468–477, 2013.

[40] E. Garcia-Fuentes, M. Murri, L. Garrido-Sanchez et al., "PPARγ expression after a high-fat meal is associated with plasma superoxide dismutase activity in morbidly obese persons," *Obesity*, vol. 18, no. 5, pp. 952–958, 2010.

[41] Á. Lendvai, M. J. Deutsch, T. Plösch, and R. Ensenauer, "The peroxisome proliferator-activated receptors under epigenetic control in placental metabolism and fetal development," *American Journal of Physiology-Endocrinology And Metabolism*, vol. 310, no. 10, pp. E797–E810, 2016.

[42] M. J. Campbell, C. Carlberg, and H. P. Koeffler, "A role for the PPARγ in cancer therapy," *PPAR Research*, vol. 2008, Article ID 314974, 17 pages, 2008.

[43] C. Grommes, G. E. Landreth, and M. T. Heneka, "Antineoplastic effects of peroxisome proliferator-activated receptor γ agonists," *Lancet Oncology*, vol. 5, no. 7, pp. 419–429, 2004.

[44] H. P. Koeffler, "Peroxisome proliferator-activated receptor γ and cancers," *Clinical Cancer Research*, vol. 9, no. 1, pp. 1–9, 2003.

[45] S. Battaglia, O. Maguire, J. L. Thorne et al., "Elevated NCOR1 disrupts PPARα/γ signaling in prostate cancer and forms a targetable epigenetic lesion," *Carcinogenesis*, vol. 31, no. 9, pp. 1650–1660, 2010.

[46] M. Pancione, L. Sabatino, A. Fucci et al., "Epigenetic silencing of peroxisome proliferator-activated receptor γ is a biomarker for colorectal cancer progression and adverse patients' outcome," *PLoS ONE*, vol. 5, no. 12, Article ID e14229, 2010.

[47] C. A. McAlpine, Y. Barak, I. Matise, and R. T. Cormier, "Intestinal-specific PPARγ deficiency enhances tumorigenesis in Apc^Min/+ mice," *International Journal of Cancer*, vol. 119, no. 10, pp. 2339–2346, 2006.

[48] P. Sarraf, E. Mueller, W. M. Smith et al., "Loss-of-function mutations in PPARγ associated with human colon cancer," *Molecular Cell*, vol. 3, no. 6, pp. 799–804, 1999.

[49] D. Capaccio, A. Ciccodicola, L. Sabatino et al., "A novel germline mutation in Peroxisome Proliferator-Activated Receptor γ gene associated with large intestine polyp formation and dyslipidemia," *Biochimica et Biophysica Acta-Molecular Basis of Disease*, vol. 1802, no. 6, pp. 572–581, 2010.

[50] M. Pancione, N. Forte, L. Sabatino et al., "Reduced β-catenin and peroxisome proliferator-activated receptor-γ expression levels are associated with colorectal cancer metastatic progression: correlation with tumor-associated macrophages, cyclooxygenase 2, and patient outcome," *Human Pathology*, vol. 40, no. 5, pp. 714–725, 2009.

[51] S. Ogino, K. Shima, Y. Baba et al., "Colorectal cancer expression of peroxisome proliferator-activated receptor γ (PPARG, PPARγ) is associated with good prognosis," *Gastroenterology*, vol. 136, no. 4, pp. 1242–1250, 2009.

[52] A. Mantovani, P. Allavena, A. Sica, and F. Balkwill, "Cancer-related inflammation," *Nature*, vol. 454, no. 7203, pp. 436–444, 2008.

[53] S. Tsugane and M. Inoue, "Insulin resistance and cancer: epidemiological evidence," *Cancer Science*, vol. 101, no. 5, pp. 1073–1079, 2010.

[54] I. Bilic, "Obesity and cancer," *Periodicum Biologorum*, vol. 116, no. 4, pp. 355–359, 2014.

[55] M. J. Khandekar, P. Cohen, and B. M. Spiegelman, "Molecular mechanisms of cancer development in obesity," *Nature Reviews Cancer*, vol. 11, no. 12, pp. 886–895, 2011.

[56] A. G. Renehan, "Obesity and cancer," in *Adipose Tissue in Health and Disease*, pp. 369–384, 2010.

[57] E. E. Calle and R. Kaaks, "Overweight, obesity and cancer: epidemiological evidence and proposed mechanisms," *Nature Reviews Cancer*, vol. 4, no. 8, pp. 579–591, 2004.

[58] K. Y. Wolin, K. Carson, and G. A. Colditz, "Obesity and cancer," *Oncologist*, vol. 15, no. 6, pp. 556–565, 2010.

[59] C. A. Gonzá Lez Svatetz and A. Goday Arnó, "Obesidad y cáncer," *Medicina Clínica*, vol. 145, no. 1, pp. 24–30, 2015.

[60] E. Kebebew, M. Peng, E. Reiff et al., "A phase II trial of rosiglitazone in patients with thyroglobulin-positive and radioiodine-negative differentiated thyroid cancer," *Surgery*, vol. 140, no. 6, pp. 960–967, 2006.

[61] G. Vitale, S. Zappavigna, M. Marra et al., "The PPAR-γ agonist troglitazone antagonizes survival pathways induced by STAT-3 in recombinant interferon-β treated pancreatic cancer cells," *Biotechnology Advances*, vol. 30, no. 1, pp. 169–184, 2012.

[62] R. A. Lubet, S. M. Fischer, V. E. Steele, M. M. Juliana, R. Desmond, and C. J. Grubbs, "Rosiglitazone, a PPAR γ agonist: potent promoter of hydroxybutyl(butyl)nitrosamine-induced urinary bladder cancers," *International Journal of Cancer*, vol. 123, no. 10, pp. 2254–2259, 2008.

[63] M. Fujita, T. Yagami, M. Fujio et al., "Cytotoxicity of troglitazone through PPARγ-independent pathway and p38 MAPK pathway in renal cell carcinoma," *Cancer Letters*, vol. 312, no. 2, pp. 219–227, 2011.

[64] A. Elnemr, T. Ohta, K. Iwata et al., "PPARgamma ligand (thiazolidinedione) induces growth arrest and differentiation markers of human pancreatic cancer cells," *International Journal of Oncology*, vol. 17, no. 6, pp. 1157–1164, 2000.

[65] H. Koga, S. Sakisaka, M. Harada et al., "Involvement of p21^WAF1/Cip1, p27^Kip1, and p18^INK4c in troglitazone-induced cell-cycle arrest in human hepatoma cell lines," *Hepatology*, vol. 33, no. 5, pp. 1087–1097, 2001.

[66] F. Chen and L. E. Harrison, "Ciglitazone-induced cellular anti-proliferation increases p27 kip1 protein levels through both increased transcriptional activity and inhibition of proteasome degradation," *Cellular Signalling*, vol. 17, no. 7, pp. 809–816, 2005.

[67] F. Chen, E. Kim, C.-C. Wang, and L. E. Harrison, "Ciglitazone-induced p27 gene transcriptional activity is mediated through

Sp1 and is negatively regulated by the MAPK signaling pathway," *Cellular Signalling*, vol. 17, no. 12, pp. 1572–1577, 2005.

[68] W. Motomura, T. Okumura, N. Takahashi, T. Obara, and Y. Kohgo, "Activation of peroxisome proliferator-activated receptor gamma by troglitazone inhibits cell growth through the increase of p27KiP1 in human. Pancreatic carcinoma cells," *Cancer Research*, vol. 60, no. 19, pp. 5558–5564, 2000.

[69] A. Itami, G. Watanabe, Y. Shimada et al., "Ligands for peroxisome proliferator-activated receptor γ inhibit growth of pancreatic cancers both in vitro and in vivo," *International Journal of Cancer*, vol. 94, no. 3, pp. 370–376, 2001.

[70] H. Lapillonne, M. Konopleva, T. Tsao et al., "Activation of peroxisome proliferator-activated receptor gamma by a novel synthetic triterpenoid 2-cyano-3,12-dioxooleana-1,9-dien-28-oic acid induces growth arrest and apoptosis in breast cancer cells," *Cancer Research*, vol. 63, no. 18, pp. 5926–5939, 2003.

[71] J.-W. Huang, C.-W. Shiau, Y.-T. Yang et al., "Peroxisome proliferator-activated receptor γ-independent ablation of cyclin D1 by thiazolidinediones and their derivatives in breast cancer cells," *Molecular Pharmacology*, vol. 67, no. 4, pp. 1342–1348, 2005.

[72] C. Qin, R. Burghardt, R. Smith, M. Wormke, J. Stewart, and S. Safe, "Peroxisome proliferator-activated receptor γ agonists induce proteasome-dependent degradation of cyclin D1 and estrogen receptor α in MCF-7 breast cancer cells," *Cancer Research*, vol. 63, no. 5, pp. 958–964, 2003.

[73] C. Wang, M. Fu, M. D'Amico et al., "Inhibition of cellular proliferation through IκB kinase-independent and peroxisome proliferator-activated receptor γ-dependent repression of cyclin D1," *Molecular and Cellular Biology*, vol. 21, no. 9, pp. 3057–3070, 2001.

[74] F. Yin, S. Wakino, Z. Liu et al., "Troglitazone inhibits growth of MCF-7 breast carcinoma cells by targeting G1 cell cycle regulators," *Biochemical and Biophysical Research Communications*, vol. 286, no. 5, pp. 916–922, 2001.

[75] P. Tontonoz, S. Singer, B. M. Forman et al., "Terminal differentiation of human liposarcoma cells induced by ligands for peroxisome proliferator-activated receptor γ and the retinoid X receptor," *Proceedings of the National Academy of Sciences of the United States of America*, vol. 94, no. 1, pp. 237–241, 1997.

[76] R. A. Gupta, J. A. Brockman, P. Sarraf, T. M. Willson, and R. N. DuBois, "Target genes of peroxisome proliferator-activated receptor γ in colorectal cancer cells," *The Journal of Biological Chemistry*, vol. 276, no. 32, pp. 29681–29687, 2001.

[77] T. Yoshizumi, T. Ohta, I. Ninomiya et al., "Thiazolidinedione, a peroxisome proliferator-activated receptor-gamma ligand, inhibits growth and metastasis of HT-29 human colon cancer cells through differentiation-promoting effects," *International Journal of Oncology*, vol. 25, no. 3, pp. 631–639, 2004.

[78] G. D. Demetri, C. D. M. Fletcher, E. Mueller et al., "Induction of solid tumor differentiation by the peroxisome proliferator-activated receptor-γ ligand troglitazone in patients with liposarcoma," *Proceedings of the National Academy of Sciences of the United States of America*, vol. 96, no. 7, pp. 3951–3956, 1999.

[79] A. Margeli, G. Kouraklis, and S. Theocharis, "Peroxisome proliferator activated receptor-γ (PPAR-γ) ligands and angiogenesis," *Angiogenesis*, vol. 6, no. 3, pp. 165–169, 2003.

[80] F. Biscetti, E. Gaetani, A. Flex et al., "Selective activation of peroxisome proliferator-activated receptor (PPAR)α and PPARγ induces neoangiogenesis through a vascular endothelial growth factor-dependent mechanism," *Diabetes*, vol. 57, no. 5, pp. 1394–1404, 2008.

[81] K. Chu, S.-T. Lee, J.-S. Koo et al., "Peroxisome proliferator-activated receptor-γ-agonist, rosiglitazone, promotes angiogenesis after focal cerebral ischemia," *Brain Research*, vol. 1093, no. 1, pp. 208–218, 2006.

[82] P.-H. Huang, M. Sata, H. Nishimatsu, M. Sumi, Y. Hirata, and R. Nagai, "Pioglitazone ameliorates endothelial dysfunction and restores ischemia-induced angiogenesis in diabetic mice," *Biomedicine and Pharmacotherapy*, vol. 62, no. 1, pp. 46–52, 2008.

[83] D. Bishop-Bailey and T. Hla, "Endothelial cell apoptosis induced by the peroxisome proliferator- activated receptor (PPAR) ligand 15-deoxy-Δ12,14-prostaglandin J2," *Journal of Biological Chemistry*, vol. 274, no. 24, pp. 17042–17048, 1999.

[84] X. Xin, S. Yang, J. Kowalski, and M. E. Gerritsen, "Peroxisome proliferator-activated receptor γ ligands are potent inhibitors of angiogenesis in vitro and in vivo," *The Journal of Biological Chemistry*, vol. 274, no. 13, pp. 9116–9121, 1999.

[85] A. Margeli, G. Kouraklis, and S. Theocharis, "Peroxisome proliferator activated receptor-γ (PPAR-γ) ligands and angiogenesis," *Angiogenesis*, vol. 6, no. 3, pp. 165–169, 2003.

[86] S. Fauconnet, I. Lascombe, E. Chabannes et al., "Differential regulation of vascular endothelial growth factor expression by peroxisome proliferator-activated receptors in bladder cancer cells," *Journal of Biological Chemistry*, vol. 277, no. 26, pp. 23534–23543, 2002.

[87] V. Chintalgattu, G. S. Harris, S. M. Akula, and L. C. Katwa, "PPAR-γ agonists induce the expression of VEGF and its receptors in cultured cardiac myofibroblasts," *Cardiovascular Research*, vol. 74, no. 1, pp. 140–150, 2007.

[88] R. M. Bambury, G. Iyer, and J. E. Rosenberg, "Specific PPAR gamma agonists may have different effects on cancer incidence," *Annals of Oncology*, vol. 24, no. 3, article 854, 2013.

[89] M. Terrasi, V. Bazan, S. Caruso et al., "Effects of PPARγ agonists on the expression of leptin and vascular endothelial growth factor in breast cancer cells," *Journal of Cellular Physiology*, vol. 228, no. 6, pp. 1368–1374, 2013.

[90] H. A. Elrod and S.-Y. Sun, "PPARγ and apoptosis in cancer," *PPAR Research*, vol. 2008, Article ID 704165, 12 pages, 2008.

[91] A. Trombetta, M. Maggiora, G. Martinasso, P. Cotogni, R. A. Canuto, and G. Muzio, "Arachidonic and docosahexaenoic acids reduce the growth of A549 human lung-tumor cells increasing lipid peroxidation and PPARs," *Chemico-Biological Interactions*, vol. 165, no. 3, pp. 239–250, 2007.

[92] I. J. Edwards, I. M. Berquin, H. Sun et al., "Differential effects of delivery of omega-3 fatty acids to human cancer cells by low-density lipoproteins versus albumin," *Clinical Cancer Research*, vol. 10, no. 24, pp. 8275–8283, 2004.

[93] H. Sun, I. M. Berquin, R. T. Owens, J. T. O'Flaherty, and I. J. Edwards, "Peroxisome proliferator-activated receptor γ-mediated up-regulation of syndecan-1 by n-3 fatty acids promotes apoptosis of human breast cancer cells," *Cancer Research*, vol. 68, no. 8, pp. 2912–2919, 2008.

[94] E. Mueller, M. Smith, P. Sarraf et al., "Effects of ligand activation of peroxisome proliferator-activated receptor γ in human prostate cancer," *Proceedings of the National Academy of Sciences of the United States of America*, vol. 97, no. 20, pp. 10990–10995, 2000.

[95] S. S. Palakurthi, H. Aktas, L. M. Grubissich, R. M. Mortensen, and J. A. Halperin, "Anticancer effects of thiazolidinediones are independent of peroxisome proliferator-activated receptor γ and mediated by inhibition of translation initiation," *Cancer Research*, vol. 61, no. 16, pp. 6213–6218, 2001.

[96] G. Debrock, V. Vanhentenrijk, R. Sciot, M. Debiec-Rychter, R. Oyen, and A. Van Oosterom, "A phase II trial with rosiglitazone in liposarcoma patients," *British Journal of Cancer*, vol. 89, no. 8, pp. 1409–1412, 2003.

[97] M. R. Smith, J. Manola, D. S. Kaufman et al., "Rosiglitazone versus placebo for men with prostate carcinoma and a rising serum prostate-specific antigen level after radical prostatectomy and/or radiation therapy," *Cancer*, vol. 101, no. 7, pp. 1569–1574, 2004.

[98] H. J. Burstein, G. D. Demetri, E. Mueller, P. Sarraf, B. M. Spiegelman, and E. P. Winer, "Use of the peroxisome proliferator-activated receptor (PPAR) γ ligand troglitazone as treatment for refractory breast cancer: a phase II study," *Breast Cancer Research and Treatment*, vol. 79, no. 3, pp. 391–397, 2003.

[99] M. H. Kulke, G. D. Demetri, N. E. Sharpless et al., "A phase II study of troglitazone, an activator of the PPARγ receptor, in patients with chemotherapy-resistant metastatic colorectal cancer," *Cancer Journal*, vol. 8, no. 5, pp. 395–399, 2002.

[100] Y. Liu, Z.-A. Zhu, S.-N. Zhang et al., "Combinational effect of PPARγ agonist and RXR agonist on the growth of SGC7901 gastric carcinoma cells in vitro," *Tumor Biology*, vol. 34, no. 4, pp. 2409–2418, 2013.

[101] B. Farrow and B. M. Evers, "Activation of PPARγ increases PTEN expression in pancreatic cancer cells," *Biochemical and Biophysical Research Communications*, vol. 301, no. 1, pp. 50–53, 2003.

[102] W. Zhang, N. Wu, Z. Li, L. Wang, J. Jin, and X.-L. Zha, "PPARγ activator rosiglitazone inhibits cell migration via upregulation of PTEN in human hepatocarcinoma cell line BEL-7404," *Cancer Biology and Therapy*, vol. 5, no. 8, pp. 1008–1014, 2006.

[103] R. E. Teresi, C.-W. Shaiu, C.-S. Chen, V. K. Chatterjee, K. A. Waite, and C. Eng, "Increased PTEN expression due to transcriptional activation of PPARγ by Lovastatin and Rosiglitazone," *International Journal of Cancer*, vol. 118, no. 10, pp. 2390–2398, 2006.

[104] S. Y. Lee, G. Y. Hur, K. H. Jung et al., "PPAR-γ agonist increase gefitinib's antitumor activity through PTEN expression," *Lung Cancer*, vol. 51, no. 3, pp. 297–301, 2006.

[105] L. Patel, I. Pass, P. Coxon, C. P. Downes, S. A. Smith, and C. H. Macphee, "Tumor suppressor and anti-inflammatory actions of PPARγ agonists are mediated via upregulation of PTEN," *Current Biology*, vol. 11, no. 10, pp. 764–768, 2001.

[106] T. Zander, J. A. Kraus, C. Grommes et al., "Induction of apoptosis in human and rat glioma by agonists of the nuclear receptor PPARγ," *Journal of Neurochemistry*, vol. 81, no. 5, pp. 1052–1060, 2002.

[107] M.-A. Bae and B. J. Song, "Critical role of c-Jun N-terminal protein kinase activation in troglitazone-induced apoptosis of human HepG2 hepatoma cells," *Molecular Pharmacology*, vol. 63, no. 2, pp. 401–408, 2003.

[108] Y. Kim, N. Suh, M. Sporn, and J. C. Reed, "An inducible pathway for degradation of FLIP protein sensitizes tumor cells to TRAIL-induced apoptosis," *Journal of Biological Chemistry*, vol. 277, no. 25, pp. 22320–22329, 2002.

[109] K. Schultze, B. Böck, A. Eckert et al., "Troglitazone sensitizes tumor cells to TRAIL-induced apoptosis via down-regulation of FLIP and survivin," *Apoptosis*, vol. 11, no. 9, pp. 1503–1512, 2006.

[110] C.-W. Shiau, C.-C. Yang, S. K. Kulp et al., "Thiazolidenediones mediate apoptosis in prostate cancer cells in part through inhibition of Bcl-xL/Bcl-2 functions independently of PPARγ," *Cancer Research*, vol. 65, no. 4, pp. 1561–1569, 2005.

[111] K. Y. Kim, S. S. Kim, and H. G. Cheon, "Differential anti-proliferative actions of peroxisome proliferator-activated receptor-γ agonists in MCF-7 breast cancer cells," *Biochemical Pharmacology*, vol. 72, no. 5, pp. 530–540, 2006.

[112] K.-H. Yan, C.-J. Yao, H.-Y. Chang, G.-M. Lai, A.-L. Cheng, and S.-E. Chuang, "The synergistic anticancer effect of troglitazone combined with aspirin causes cell cycle arrest and apoptosis in human lung cancer cells," *Molecular Carcinogenesis*, vol. 49, no. 3, pp. 235–246, 2010.

[113] F. Colotta, P. Allavena, A. Sica, C. Garlanda, and A. Mantovani, "Cancer-related inflammation, the seventh hallmark of cancer: links to genetic instability," *Carcinogenesis*, vol. 30, no. 7, pp. 1073–1081, 2009.

[114] T. Atsumi, R. Singh, L. Sabharwal et al., "Inflammation amplifier, a new paradigm in cancer biology," *Cancer Research*, vol. 74, no. 1, pp. 8–14, 2014.

[115] N. Gagliani, B. Hu, S. Huber, E. Elinav, and R. A. Flavell, "The fire within: microbes inflame tumors," *Cell*, vol. 157, no. 4, pp. 776–783, 2014.

[116] C. I. Diakos, K. A. Charles, D. C. McMillan, and S. J. Clarke, "Cancer-related inflammation and treatment effectiveness," *The Lancet Oncology*, vol. 15, no. 11, pp. e493–e503, 2014.

[117] C. K. Glass and K. Saijo, "Nuclear receptor transrepression pathways that regulate inflammation in macrophages and T cells," *Nature Reviews Immunology*, vol. 10, no. 5, pp. 365–376, 2010.

[118] D. S. Straus and C. K. Glass, "Anti-inflammatory actions of PPAR ligands: new insights on cellular and molecular mechanisms," *Trends in Immunology*, vol. 28, no. 12, pp. 551–558, 2007.

[119] Y. M. Shah, K. Morimura, and F. J. Gonzalez, "Expression of peroxisome proliferator-activated receptor-γ in macrophage suppresses experimentally induced colitis," *American Journal of Physiology—Gastrointestinal and Liver Physiology*, vol. 292, no. 2, pp. G657–G666, 2007.

[120] D. S. Straus, G. Pascual, M. Li et al., "15-Deoxy-$\Delta^{12,14}$-prostaglandin J$_2$ inhibits multiple steps in the NF-κB signaling pathway," *Proceedings of the National Academy of Sciences of the United States of America*, vol. 97, no. 9, pp. 4844–4849, 2000.

[121] R. Kapadia, J.-H. Yi, and R. Vemuganti, "Mechanisms of anti-inflammatory and neuroprotective actions of PPAR-gamma agonists," *Frontiers in Bioscience*, vol. 13, no. 5, pp. 1813–1826, 2008.

[122] A. M. Sharma and B. Staels, "Review: peroxisome proliferator-activated receptor gamma and adipose tissue—understanding obesity-related changes in regulation of lipid and glucose metabolism," *The Journal of Clinical Endocrinology & Metabolism*, vol. 92, no. 2, pp. 386–395, 2007.

[123] G. Pascual, A. L. Fong, S. Ogawa et al., "A SUMOylation-dependent pathway mediates transrepression of inflammatory response genes by PPAR-γ," *Nature*, vol. 437, no. 7059, pp. 759–763, 2005.

[124] A. M. Lefebvre, I. Chen, P. Desreumaux et al., "Activation of the peroxisome proliferator-activated receptor γ promotes the development of colon tumors in C57BL/6J-APCMin/+ mice," *Nature Medicine*, vol. 4, no. 9, pp. 1053–1057, 1998.

[125] M. V. Pino, M. F. Kelley, and Z. Jayyosi, "Promotion of colon tumors in C57BL/6J-APC(min)/+ mice by thiazolidinedione PPARγ agonists and a structurally unrelated PPARγ agonist," *Toxicologic Pathology*, vol. 32, no. 1, pp. 58–63, 2004.

[126] E. Saez, P. Tontonoz, M. C. Nelson et al., "Activators of the nuclear receptor PPARγ enhance colon polyp formation," *Nature Medicine*, vol. 4, no. 9, pp. 1058–1061, 1998.

[127] K. Yang, K.-H. Fan, S. A. Lamprecht et al., "Peroxisome proliferator-activated receptor γ agonist troglitazone induces colon tumors in normal C57BL/6J mice and enhances colonic carcinogenesis in Apc1638 N/+ Mlh1+/- double mutant mice," *International Journal of Cancer*, vol. 116, no. 4, pp. 495–499, 2005.

[128] Z. Bagi, A. Koller, and G. Kaley, "PPARγ activation, by reducing oxidative stress, increases NO bioavailability in coronary arterioles of mice with Type 2 diabetes," *American Journal of Physiology—Heart and Circulatory Physiology*, vol. 286, no. 2, pp. H742–H748, 2004.

[129] I. Inoue, S.-I. Goto, T. Matsunaga et al., "The ligands/activators for peroxisome proliferator-activated receptor α (PPARα) and PPARγ increase Cu^{2+},Zn^{2+}-superoxide dismutase and decrease p22phox message expressions in primary endothelial cells," *Metabolism: Clinical and Experimental*, vol. 50, no. 1, pp. 3–11, 2001.

[130] F. J. Tinahones, M. Murri-Pierri, L. Garrido-Sánchez et al., "Oxidative stress in severely obese persons is greater in those with insulin resistance," *Obesity*, vol. 17, no. 2, pp. 240–246, 2009.

[131] S. O. Olusi, "Obesity is an independent risk factor for plasma lipid peroxidation and depletion of erythrocyte cytoprotectic enzymes in humans," *International Journal of Obesity and Related Metabolic Disorders*, vol. 26, no. 9, pp. 1159–1164, 2002.

[132] F. Giacco and M. Brownlee, "Oxidative stress and diabetic complications," *Circulation Research*, vol. 107, no. 9, pp. 1058–1070, 2010.

[133] J. W. Baynes, "Role of oxidative stress in development of complications in diabetes," *Diabetes*, vol. 40, no. 4, pp. 405–412, 1991.

[134] J. M. Olefsky and C. K. Glass, "Macrophages, inflammation, and insulin resistance," *Annual Review of Physiology*, vol. 72, no. 1, pp. 219–246, 2010.

[135] K. J. Moore, M. L. Fitzgerald, and M. W. Freeman, "Peroxisome proliferator-activated receptors in macrophage biology: friend or foe?" *Current Opinion in Lipidology*, vol. 12, no. 5, pp. 519–527, 2001.

[136] M. Macias-Gonzalez, F. Cardona, M. Queipo-Ortuño, R. Bernal, M. Martin, and F. J. Tinahones, "PPARγ mRNA expression is reduced in peripheral blood mononuclear cells after fat overload in patients with metabolic syndrome," *Journal of Nutrition*, vol. 138, no. 5, pp. 903–907, 2008.

[137] M. Bilban, P. Haslinger, J. Prast et al., "Identification of novel trophoblast invasion-related genes: heme oxygenase-1 controls motility via peroxisome proliferator-activated receptor γ," *Endocrinology*, vol. 150, no. 2, pp. 1000–1013, 2009.

[138] J. D. Burton, M. E. Castillo, D. M. Goldenberg, and R. D. Blumenthal, "Peroxisome proliferator-activated receptor-γ antagonists exhibit potent antiproliferative effects versus many hematopoietic and epithelial cancer cell lines," *Anti-Cancer Drugs*, vol. 18, no. 5, pp. 525–534, 2007.

[139] K. L. Schaefer, K. Wada, H. Takahashi et al., "Peroxisome proliferator-activated receptor γ inhibition prevents adhesion to the extracellular matrix and induces anoikis in hepatocellular carcinoma cells," *Cancer Research*, vol. 65, no. 6, pp. 2251–2259, 2005.

[140] M. A. Lea, M. Sura, and C. Desbordes, "Inhibition of cell proliferation by potential peroxisome proliferator-activated receptor (PPAR) gamma agonists and antagonists," *Anticancer Research*, vol. 24, no. 5A, pp. 2765–2771, 2004.

[141] L. Nonn, L. Peng, D. Feldman, and D. M. Peehl, "Inhibition of p38 by vitamin D reduces interleukin-6 production in normal prostate cells via mitogen-activated protein kinase phosphatase 5: implications for prostate cancer prevention by vitamin D," *Cancer Research*, vol. 66, no. 8, pp. 4516–4524, 2006.

[142] B.-Y. Bao, J. Yao, and Y.-F. Lee, "1α, 25-dihydroxyvitamin D_3 suppresses interleukin-8-mediated prostate cancer cell angiogenesis," *Carcinogenesis*, vol. 27, no. 9, pp. 1883–1893, 2006.

[143] J. Moreno, A. V. Krishnan, S. Swami, L. Nonn, D. M. Peehl, and D. Feldman, "Regulation of prostaglandin metabolism by calcitriol attenuates growth stimulation in prostate cancer cells," *Cancer Research*, vol. 65, no. 17, pp. 7917–7925, 2005.

[144] N. Wagner, K.-D. Wagner, G. Schley, L. Badiali, H. Theres, and H. Scholz, "1,25-Dihydroxyvitamin D3-induced apoptosis of retinoblastoma cells is associated with reciprocal changes of Bcl-2 and bax," *Experimental Eye Research*, vol. 77, no. 1, pp. 1–9, 2003.

[145] S. Kizildag, H. Ates, and S. Kizildag, "Treatment of K562 cells with 1,25-dihydroxyvitamin D3 induces distinct alterations in the expression of apoptosis-related genes BCL2, BAX, BCLXL, and p21," *Annals of Hematology*, vol. 89, no. 1, pp. 1–7, 2010.

[146] M. Peterlik, W. B. Grant, and H. S. Cross, "Calcium, vitamin D and cancer," *Anticancer Research*, vol. 29, no. 9, pp. 3687–3698, 2009.

[147] G. E. Weitsman, R. Koren, E. Zuck, C. Rotem, U. A. Liberman, and A. Ravid, "Vitamin D sensitizes breast cancer cells to the action of H_2O_2: mitochondria as a convergence point in the death pathway," *Free Radical Biology and Medicine*, vol. 39, no. 2, pp. 266–278, 2005.

[148] A. Ravid and R. Koren, "The role of reactive oxygen species in the anticancer activity of vitamin D," in *Vitamin D Analogs in Cancer Prevention and Therapy*, vol. 164 of *Recent Results in Cancer Research*, pp. 357–367, Springer, Berlin, Germany, 2003.

[149] P. De Haes, M. Garmyn, H. Degreef, K. Vantieghem, R. Bouillon, and S. Segaert, "1,25-Dihydroxyvitamin D3 inhibits ultraviolet B-induced apoptosis, Jun kinase activation, and interleukin-6 production in primary human keratinocytes," *Journal of Cellular Biochemistry*, vol. 89, no. 4, pp. 663–673, 2003.

[150] R. Riachy, B. Vandewalle, E. Moerman et al., "1,25-Dihydroxyvitamin D_3 protects human pancreatic islets against cytokine-induced apoptosis via down-regulation of the Fas receptor," *Apoptosis*, vol. 11, no. 2, pp. 151–159, 2006.

[151] O. Flores, Z. Wang, K. E. Knudsen, and K. L. Burnstein, "Nuclear targeting of cyclin-dependent kinase 2 reveals essential roles of cyclin-dependent kinase 2 localization and cyclin E in vitamin D-mediated growth inhibition," *Endocrinology*, vol. 151, no. 3, pp. 896–908, 2010.

[152] S. S. Jensen, M. W. Madsen, J. Lukas, L. Binderup, and J. Bartek, "Inhibitory effects of 1α,25-dihydroxyvitamin D_3 on the G_1–S phase-controlling machinery," *Molecular Endocrinology*, vol. 15, no. 8, pp. 1370–1380, 2001.

[153] G. Hager, J. Kornfehl, B. Knerer, G. Weigel, and M. Formanek, "Molecular analysis of p21 promoter activity isolated from squamous carcinoma cell lines of the head and neck under the influence of 1,25(OH)$_2$ vitamin D3 and its analogs," *Acta Oto-Laryngologica*, vol. 124, no. 1, pp. 90–96, 2004.

[154] P. A. Hershberger, R. A. Modzelewski, Z. R. Shurin, R. M. Rueger, D. L. Trump, and C. S. Johnson, "1,25-dihydroxycholecalciferol (1,25-D3) inhibits the growth of squamous cell carcinoma and down-modulates p21(Waf1/Cip1) in vitro and in vivo," *Cancer Research*, vol. 59, no. 11, pp. 2644–2649, 1999.

[155] K. Colston, M. J. Colston, and D. Feldman, "1,25-Dihydroxyvitamin D_3 and malignant melanoma: the presence of receptors

and inhibition of cell growth in culture," *Endocrinology*, vol. 108, no. 3, pp. 1083–1086, 1981.

[156] B. J. Boyle, X.-Y. Zhao, P. Cohen, and D. Feldman, "Insulin-like growth factor binding protein-3 mediates $1\alpha,25$-dihydroxyvitamin D3 growth inhibition in the LNCaP prostate cancer cell line through p21/WAF1," *The Journal of Urology*, vol. 165, no. 4, pp. 1319–1324, 2001.

[157] J. Welsh, "Cellular and molecular effects of vitamin D on carcinogenesis," *Archives of Biochemistry and Biophysics*, vol. 523, no. 1, pp. 107–114, 2012.

[158] J. N. P. Rohan and N. L. Weigel, "$1\alpha,25$-dihydroxyvitamin D_3 reduces c-Myc expression, inhibiting proliferation and causing G_1 accumulation in C4-2 prostate cancer cells," *Endocrinology*, vol. 150, no. 5, pp. 2046–2054, 2009.

[159] X. Wang, S. Pesakhov, A. Weng et al., "ERK 5/MAPK pathway has a major role in $1\alpha,25$-(OH)2 vitamin D3-induced terminal differentiation of myeloid leukemia cells," *The Journal of Steroid Biochemistry and Molecular Biology*, vol. 144, pp. 223–227, 2014.

[160] N. Pendás-Franco, J. M. González-Sancho, Y. Suárez et al., "Vitamin D regulates the phenotype of human breast cancer cells," *Differentiation*, vol. 75, no. 3, pp. 193–207, 2007.

[161] E. Gocek and G. P. Studzinski, "Vitamin D and differentiation in cancer," *Critical Reviews in Clinical Laboratory Sciences*, vol. 46, no. 4, pp. 190–209, 2009.

[162] M. Liu, M.-H. Lee, M. Cohen, M. Bommakanti, and L. P. Freedman, "Transcriptional activation of the Cdk inhibitor p21 by vitamin D_3 leads to the induced differentiation of the myelomonocytic cell line U937," *Genes & Development*, vol. 10, no. 2, pp. 142–153, 1996.

[163] F. Pereira, M. J. Larriba, and A. Muñoz, "Vitamin D and colon cancer," *Endocrine-Related Cancer*, vol. 19, no. 3, pp. R51–R71, 2012.

[164] H. G. Pálmer, M. J. Larriba, J. M. García et al., "The transcription factor SNAIL represses vitamin D receptor expression and responsiveness in human colon cancer," *Nature Medicine*, vol. 10, no. 9, pp. 917–919, 2004.

[165] K. K. Deeb, D. L. Trump, and C. S. Johnson, "Vitamin D signalling pathways in cancer: potential for anticancer therapeutics," *Nature Reviews Cancer*, vol. 7, no. 9, pp. 684–700, 2007.

[166] S. Upadhyay, A. Verone, S. Shoemaker et al., "1,25-dihydroxyvitamin D_3 $(1,25(OH)_2D_3)$ signaling capacity and the epithelial-mesenchymal transition in non-small cell lung cancer (NSCLC): implications for use of $1,25(OH)_2D3$ in NSCLC treatment," *Cancers*, vol. 5, no. 4, pp. 1504–1521, 2013.

[167] R. Fukuda, B. Kelly, and G. L. Semenza, "Vascular endothelial growth factor gene expression in colon cancer cells exposed to prostaglandin E2 is mediated by hypoxia-inducible factor 1," *Cancer Research*, vol. 63, no. 9, pp. 2330–2334, 2003.

[168] N. I. Fernandez-Garcia, H. G. Palmer, M. Garcia et al., "$1_\alpha,25$-Dihydroxyvitamin D3 regulates the expression of Id1 and Id2 genes and the angiogenic phenotype of human colon carcinoma cells," *Oncogene*, vol. 24, no. 43, pp. 6533–6544, 2005.

[169] M. J. Levine and D. Teegarden, "$1\alpha,25$-dihydroxycholecalciferol increases the expression of vascular endothelial growth factor in C3H10T1/2 mouse embryo fibroblasts," *The Journal of Nutrition*, vol. 134, no. 9, pp. 2244–2250, 2004.

[170] R. Lin, N. Amizuka, T. Sasaki et al., "$1\alpha,25$-dihydroxyvitamin D3 promotes vascularization of the chondro-osseous junction by stimulating expression of vascular endothelial growth factor and matrix metalloproteinase 9," *Journal of Bone and Mineral Research*, vol. 17, no. 9, pp. 1604–1612, 2002.

[171] M. Grundmann, M. Haidar, S. Placzko et al., "Vitamin D improves the angiogenic properties of endothelial progenitor cells," *American Journal of Physiology—Cell Physiology*, vol. 303, no. 9, pp. C954–C962, 2012.

[172] M. J. Campbell, E. Elstner, S. Holden, M. Uskokovic, and H. P. Koeffler, "Inhibition of proliferation of prostate cancer cells by a 19-nor- hexafluoride vitamin D3 analogue involves the induction of p21(waf1) p27(kip1) and E-cadherin," *Journal of Molecular Endocrinology*, vol. 19, no. 1, pp. 15–27, 1997.

[173] Y. Ma, W.-D. Yu, B. Su et al., "Regulation of motility, invasion, and metastatic potential of squamous cell carcinoma by $1\alpha,25$-dihydroxycholecalciferol," *Cancer*, vol. 119, no. 3, pp. 563–574, 2013.

[174] J.-W. Hsu, S. Yasmin-Karim, M. R. King et al., "Suppression of prostate cancer cell rolling and adhesion to endothelium by $1\alpha,25$-dihydroxyvitamin D_3," *The American Journal of Pathology*, vol. 178, no. 2, pp. 872–880, 2011.

[175] J. M. González-Sancho, M. Alvarez-Dolado, and A. Muñoz, "1,25-dihydroxyvitamin D3 inhibits tenascin-C expression in mammary epithelial cells," *FEBS Letters*, vol. 426, no. 2, pp. 225–228, 1998.

[176] V. Sung and D. Feldman, "1,25-Dihydroxyvitamin D3 decreases human prostate cancer cell adhesion and migration," *Molecular and Cellular Endocrinology*, vol. 164, no. 1-2, pp. 133–143, 2000.

[177] H.-W. Lo, S.-C. Hsu, W. Xia et al., "Epidermal growth factor receptor cooperates with signal transducer and activator of transcription 3 to induce epithelial-mesenchymal transition in cancer cells via up-regulation of TWIST gene expression," *Cancer Research*, vol. 67, no. 19, pp. 9066–9076, 2007.

[178] N. J. Sullivan, A. K. Sasser, A. E. Axel et al., "Interleukin-6 induces an epithelial-mesenchymal transition phenotype in human breast cancer cells," *Oncogene*, vol. 28, no. 33, pp. 2940–2947, 2009.

[179] Y. Wu, J. Deng, P. G. Rychahou, S. Qiu, B. M. Evers, and B. P. Zhou, "Stabilization of snail by NF-κB is required for inflammation-induced cell migration and invasion," *Cancer Cell*, vol. 15, no. 5, pp. 416–428, 2009.

[180] K.-C. Chiang, C.-N. Yeh, J.-T. Hsu et al., "The vitamin D analog, MART-10, represses metastasis potential via downregulation of epithelial-mesenchymal transition in pancreatic cancer cells," *Cancer Letters*, vol. 354, no. 2, pp. 235–244, 2014.

[181] K.-C. Chiang, S.-F. Kuo, C.-H. Chen et al., "MART-10, the vitamin D analog, is a potent drug to inhibit anaplastic thyroid cancer cell metastatic potential," *Cancer Letters*, vol. 369, no. 1, pp. 76–85, 2015.

[182] K. Koli and J. Keski-Oja, "$1\alpha,25$-dihydroxyvitamin D_3 and its analogues down-regulate cell invasion-associated proteases in cultured malignant cells," *Cell Growth and Differentiation*, vol. 11, no. 4, pp. 221–229, 2000.

[183] B.-Y. Bao, S.-D. Yeh, and Y.-F. Lee, "1alpha,25-dihydroxyvitamin D3 inhibits prostate cancer cell invasion via modulation of selective proteases," *Carcinogenesis*, vol. 27, no. 1, pp. 32–42, 2006.

[184] A. A. Ajibade, J. S. Kirk, E. Karasik et al., "Early growth inhibition is followed by increased metastatic disease with vitamin D (Calcitriol) treatment in the TRAMP model of prostate cancer," *PLoS ONE*, vol. 9, no. 2, Article ID e89555, 2014.

[185] S. Alvarez-Díaz, N. Valle, G. Ferrer-Mayorga et al., "MicroRNA-22 is induced by vitamin D and contributes to its antiproliferative, antimigratory and gene regulatory effects in colon cancer cells," *Human Molecular Genetics*, vol. 21, no. 10, pp. 2157–2165, 2012.

[186] S. K. R. Padi, Q. Zhang, Y. M. Rustum, C. Morrison, and B. Guo, "MicroRNA-627 mediates the epigenetic mechanisms of vitamin d to suppress proliferation of human colorectal cancer cells and growth of xenograft tumors in mice," *Gastroenterology*, vol. 145, no. 2, pp. 437–446, 2013.

[187] X. Wang, E. Gocek, C.-G. Liu, and G. P. Studzinski, "MicroRNAs181 regulate the expression of p27Kip1 in human myeloid leukemia cells induced to differentiate by 1,25-dihydroxyvitamin D3," *Cell Cycle*, vol. 8, no. 5, pp. 736–741, 2009.

[188] E. Gocek, X. Wang, X. Liu, C.-G. Liu, and G. P. Studzinski, "MicroRNA-32 upregulation by 1,25-dihydroxyvitamin D 3in human myeloid leukemia cells leads to bim targeting and inhibition of AraC-induced apoptosis," *Cancer Research*, vol. 71, no. 19, pp. 6230–6239, 2011.

[189] H.-J. Ting, J. Messing, S. Yasmin-Karim, and Y.-F. Lee, "Identification of microRNA-98 as a therapeutic target inhibiting prostate cancer growth and a biomarker induced by vitamin D," *The Journal of Biological Chemistry*, vol. 288, no. 1, pp. 1–9, 2013.

[190] M. F. Bijlsma, C. A. Spek, D. Zivkovic, S. Van De Water, F. Rezaee, and M. P. Peppelenbosch, "Repression of smoothened by patched-dependent (pro-)vitamin D3 secretion," *PLoS Biology*, vol. 4, no. 8, pp. 1397–1410, 2006.

[191] K. Fujiki, F. Kano, K. Shiota, and M. Murata, "Expression of the peroxisome proliferator activated receptor gamma gene is repressed by DNA methylation in visceral adipose tissue of mouse models of diabetes," *BMC Biology*, vol. 7, article 38, 2009.

[192] S. A. Abedin, C. M. Banwell, K. W. Colston, C. Carlberg, and M. J. Campbell, "Epigenetic corruption of VDR signalling in malignancy," *Anticancer Research*, vol. 26, no. 4, pp. 2557–2566, 2006.

[193] J. Höbaus, I. S. Fetahu, M. Khorchide, T. Manhardt, and E. Kallay, "Epigenetic regulation of the 1,25-dihydroxyvitamin D3 24-hydroxylase (CYP24A1) in colon cancer cells," *Journal of Steroid Biochemistry and Molecular Biology*, vol. 136, no. 1, pp. 296–299, 2013.

[194] J. Höbaus, D. M. Hummel, U. Thiem et al., "Increased copy-number and not DNA hypomethylation causes overexpression of the candidate proto-oncogene CYP24A1 in colorectal cancer," *International Journal of Cancer*, vol. 133, no. 6, pp. 1380–1388, 2013.

[195] D. Karolchik, G. P. Barber, J. Casper et al., "The UCSC genome browser database: 2014 update," *Nucleic Acids Research*, vol. 42, no. 1, pp. D764–D770, 2014.

[196] R. Marik, M. Fackler, E. Gabrielson et al., "DNA methylation-related vitamin D receptor insensitivity in breast cancer," *Cancer Biology & Therapy*, vol. 10, no. 1, pp. 44–53, 2010.

[197] C. A. Godman, R. Joshi, B. R. Tierney et al., "HDAC3 impacts multiple oncogenic pathways in colon cancer cells with effects on Wnt and vitamin D signaling," *Cancer Biology & Therapy*, vol. 7, no. 10, pp. 1570–1580, 2014.

[198] H. Zhu, X. Wang, H. Shi et al., "A genome-wide methylation study of severe vitamin D deficiency in African American adolescents," *Journal of Pediatrics*, vol. 162, no. 5, pp. 1004–1009.e1, 2013.

[199] H. Shi, P. S. Yan, C.-M. Chen et al., "Expressed CpG island sequence tag microarray for dual screening of DNA hypermethylation and gene silencing in cancer cells," *Cancer Research*, vol. 62, no. 11, pp. 3214–3220, 2002.

[200] B. Novakovic, M. Sibson, H. K. Ng et al., "Placenta-specific methylation of the vitamin D 24-hydroxylase gene. Implications for feedback autoregulation of active vitamin D levels at the fetomaternal interface," *The Journal of Biological Chemistry*, vol. 284, no. 22, pp. 14838–14848, 2009.

[201] H. Shi, J. Guo, D. J. Duff et al., "Discovery of novel epigenetic markers in non-Hodgkin's lymphoma," *Carcinogenesis*, vol. 28, no. 1, pp. 60–70, 2007.

[202] M. Wjst, I. Heimbeck, D. Kutschke, and K. Pukelsheim, "Epigenetic regulation of vitamin D converting enzymes," *Journal of Steroid Biochemistry and Molecular Biology*, vol. 121, no. 1-2, pp. 80–83, 2010.

[203] J.-Y. Hsu, D. Feldman, J. E. McNeal, and D. M. Peehl, "Reduced 1α-hydroxylase activity in human prostate cancer cells correlates with decreased susceptibility to 25-hydroxyvitamin D_3-induced growth inhibition," *Cancer Research*, vol. 61, no. 7, pp. 2852–2856, 2001.

[204] M. Tannour-Louet, S. K. Lewis, J.-F. Louet et al., "Increased expression of CYP24A1 correlates with advanced stages of prostate cancer and can cause resistance to vitamin D3-based therapies," *The FASEB Journal*, vol. 28, no. 1, pp. 364–372, 2014.

[205] L. Sabatino, A. Fucci, M. Pancione, and V. Colantuoni, "PPARG epigenetic deregulation and its role in colorectal tumorigenesis," *PPAR Research*, vol. 2012, Article ID 687492, 12 pages, 2012.

[206] T. W. Dunlop, S. Väisänen, C. Frank, F. Molnár, L. Sinkkonen, and C. Carlberg, "The human peroxisome proliferator-activated receptor δ gene is a primary target of 1α,25-dihydroxyvitamin D3 and its nuclear receptor," *Journal of Molecular Biology*, vol. 349, no. 2, pp. 248–260, 2005.

[207] F. Alimirah, X. Peng, L. Yuan et al., "Crosstalk between the peroxisome proliferator-activated receptor γ (PPARγ) and the vitamin D receptor (VDR) in human breast cancer cells: PPARγ binds to VDR and inhibits 1α,25-dihydroxyvitamin D3 mediated transactivation," *Experimental Cell Research*, vol. 318, no. 19, pp. 2490–2497, 2012.

[208] Y. Shi, M. Hon, and R. M. Evans, "The peroxisome proliferator-activated receptor δ, an integrator of transcriptional repression and nuclear receptor signaling," *Proceedings of the National Academy of Sciences of the United States of America*, vol. 99, no. 5, pp. 2613–2618, 2002.

[209] R. J. Wood, "Vitamin D and adipogenesis: new molecular insights," *Nutrition Reviews*, vol. 66, no. 1, pp. 40–46, 2008.

[210] C. J. Narvaez, K. M. Simmons, J. Brunton, A. Salinero, S. V. Chittur, and J. E. Welsh, "Induction of STEAP4 correlates with 1,25-dihydroxyvitamin D3 stimulation of adipogenesis in mesenchymal progenitor cells derived from human adipose tissue," *Journal of Cellular Physiology*, vol. 228, no. 10, pp. 2024–2036, 2013.

[211] R. Bouillon, G. Carmeliet, L. Lieben et al., "Vitamin D and energy homeostasis—of mice and men," *Nature Reviews Endocrinology*, vol. 10, no. 2, pp. 79–87, 2014.

[212] P. Sertznig, T. Dunlop, M. Seifert, W. Tilgen, and J. Reichrath, "Cross-talk between Vitamin D Receptor (VDR)- and Peroxisome Proliferator-activated Receptor (PPAR)-signaling in melanoma cells," *Anticancer Research*, vol. 29, no. 9, pp. 3647–3658, 2009.

[213] P. Sertznig, M. Seifert, W. Tilgen, and J. Reichrath, "Peroxisome proliferator-activated receptor (PPAR) and vitamin D receptor (VDR) signaling pathways in melanoma cells: promising new therapeutic targets?" *Journal of Steroid Biochemistry and Molecular Biology*, vol. 121, no. 1-2, pp. 383–386, 2010.

[214] T. L. Van Belle, C. Gysemans, and C. Mathieu, "Vitamin D and diabetes: the odd couple," *Trends in Endocrinology and Metabolism*, vol. 24, no. 11, pp. 561–568, 2013.

[215] K. S. Vimaleswaran, D. J. Berry, C. Lu et al., "Causal relationship between obesity and vitamin D status: bi-directional mendelian randomization analysis of multiple cohorts," *PLoS Medicine*, vol. 10, no. 2, Article ID e1001383, 2013.

[216] J. Auwerx, R. Bouillon, and H. Kesteloot, "Relation between 25-hydroxyvitamin D3, apolipoprotein A-I, and high density lipoprotein cholesterol," *Arteriosclerosis, Thrombosis, and Vascular Biology*, vol. 12, no. 6, pp. 671–674, 1992.

[217] S. Kayaniyil, S. B. Harris, R. Retnakaran et al., "Prospective association of 25(OH)D with metabolic syndrome," *Clinical Endocrinology*, vol. 80, no. 4, pp. 502–507, 2014.

[218] Y. Yoon, "Anti-adipogenic effects of 1,25-dihydroxyvitamin D3 are mediated by the maintenance of the wingless-type MMTV integration site/β-catenin pathway," *International Journal of Molecular Medicine*, vol. 30, no. 5, pp. 1219–1224, 2012.

[219] J. M. Blumberg, I. Tzameli, I. Astapova, F. S. Lam, J. S. Flier, and A. N. Hollenberg, "Complex role of the vitamin D receptor and its ligand in adipogenesis in 3T3-L1 cells," *The Journal of Biological Chemistry*, vol. 281, no. 16, pp. 11205–11213, 2006.

[220] M. Macías-Gonzalez, I. Moreno-Santos, J. M. García-Almeida, F. J. Tinahones, and E. Garcia-Fuentes, "PPARγ2 protects against obesity by means of a mechanism that mediates insulin resistance," *European Journal of Clinical Investigation*, vol. 39, no. 11, pp. 972–979, 2009.

[221] J. B. Rawson, Z. Sun, E. Dicks et al., "Vitamin D intake is negatively associated with promoter methylation of the Wnt antagonist gene DKK1 in a large group of colorectal cancer patients," *Nutrition and Cancer*, vol. 64, no. 7, pp. 919–928, 2012.

[222] J. B. Rawson, M. Manno, M. Mrkonjic et al., "Promoter methylation of Wnt antagonists DKK1 and SFRP1 is associated with opposing tumor subtypes in two large populations of colorectal cancer patients," *Carcinogenesis*, vol. 32, no. 5, pp. 741–747, 2011.

[223] J. Hoffstedt, P. Arner, G. Hellers, and F. Lönnqvist, "Variation in adrenergic regulation of lipolysis between omental and subcutaneous adipocytes from obese and non-obese men," *Journal of Lipid Research*, vol. 38, no. 4, pp. 795–804, 1997.

[224] M. Bhat, R. Kalam, S. Syh Qadri, S. Madabushi, and A. Ismail, "Vitamin D deficiency-induced muscle wasting occurs through the ubiquitin proteasome pathway and is partially corrected by calcium in male rats," *Endocrinology*, vol. 154, no. 11, pp. 4018–4029, 2013.

[225] G. J. Hausman, S. P. Poulos, T. D. Pringle, and M. J. Azain, "The influence of thiazolidinediones on adipogenesis in vitro and in vivo: potential modifiers of intramuscular adipose tissue deposition in meat animals," *Journal of Animal Science*, vol. 86, no. 14, pp. E236–E243, 2008.

[226] Y.-X. Wang, C.-L. Zhang, R. T. Yu et al., "Regulation of muscle fiber type and running endurance by PPARδ," *PLoS Biology*, vol. 2, no. 10, article e294, 2004.

7

PPAR Agonists for the Prevention and Treatment of Lung Cancer

Sowmya P. Lakshmi,[1,2] **Aravind T. Reddy,**[1,2] **Asoka Banno,**[1] **and Raju C. Reddy**[1,2]

[1]*Department of Medicine, Division of Pulmonary, Allergy and Critical Care Medicine, University of Pittsburgh School of Medicine, Pittsburgh, PA 15213, USA*
[2]*Veterans Affairs Pittsburgh Healthcare System, Pittsburgh, PA 15240, USA*

Correspondence should be addressed to Raju C. Reddy; reddyrc@upmc.edu

Academic Editor: Valeria Amodeo

Lung cancer is the most common and most fatal of all malignancies worldwide. Furthermore, with more than half of all lung cancer patients presenting with distant metastases at the time of initial diagnosis, the overall prognosis for the disease is poor. There is thus a desperate need for new prevention and treatment strategies. Recently, a family of nuclear hormone receptors, the peroxisome proliferator-activated receptors (PPARs), has attracted significant attention for its role in various malignancies including lung cancer. Three PPARs, PPARα, PPARβ/δ, and PPARγ, display distinct biological activities and varied influences on lung cancer biology. PPARα activation generally inhibits tumorigenesis through its antiangiogenic and anti-inflammatory effects. Activated PPARγ is also antitumorigenic and antimetastatic, regulating several functions of cancer cells and controlling the tumor microenvironment. Unlike PPARα and PPARγ, whether PPARβ/δ activation is anti- or protumorigenic or even inconsequential currently remains an open question that requires additional investigation. This review of current literature emphasizes the multifaceted effects of PPAR agonists in lung cancer and discusses how they may be applied as novel therapeutic strategies for the disease.

1. Introduction

Approximately 1.8 million people were newly diagnosed with lung cancer and approximately 1.6 million died from it in 2012, making lung cancer the most common and most fatal malignancy in the world [1]. In the USA alone, 224,390 new cases and 158,080 deaths are estimated for 2016 [2]. A number of risk factors such as hereditary genetic mutations, occupational exposure to lung carcinogens, poor diet, and air pollution have been associated with lung cancer [3]. Chronic lung inflammation and certain pulmonary infections have also shown a positive association [3, 4]. Nevertheless, tobacco smoke is the single, major contributor to the pathogenesis of lung cancer, increasing the lifetime risk even in those who quit smoking. Lung cancer is categorized into two major histological subtypes, small cell lung cancer (SCLC) and non-small cell lung cancer (NSCLC). NSCLC accounts for as much as 85% of all lung cancers and includes adenocarcinoma,

squamous cell carcinoma, and large cell carcinoma, while the more aggressive, neuroendocrine tumor SCLC represents most of the rest [5, 6]. Because more than half of lung cancer patients are diagnosed in an advanced stage, with distant metastases [2] and a 5-year survival rate of approximately 2% [7], the overall 5-year relative survival rate for all lung cancer patients combined falls below 18% [2, 7]. This dire state stresses the need for novel approaches in prevention, early detection, and therapy for the disease.

A family of nuclear hormone receptors, the peroxisome proliferator-activated receptors (PPARs), has recently attracted interest as potential therapeutic targets for a variety of malignancies, including lung cancer [8]. Besides being key regulators of lipid and glucose metabolism [9, 10], PPARs, as ligand-activated transcription factors, are also involved in cellular processes including cell differentiation, proliferation, survival, apoptosis, and motility [11–13]. Since many tumors result from dysregulation of these cellular processes and metabolic disorders have been associated with increased cancer risk [14], the role of PPARs in cancer biology is not surprising. PPARs have indeed been implicated in the regulation of various solid cancers as well as leukemias [8, 12].

The PPAR family comprises three members, PPARα, PPARβ/δ, and PPARγ [15]. Each PPAR subtype is unique in its structure and function [10]. All three PPAR receptors are found in many cells and tissues throughout the body [16–18]. While sharing some common ligands, PPAR family members also respond to distinct repertoires of natural and synthetic ligands, as might be expected from their specific biological activities [13]. PPARα can be activated by fatty acids and eicosanoids (e.g., 8(S)-hydroxyeicosatetraenoic acid and leukotriene B_4) as well as synthetic fibric acid derivatives (e.g., clofibrate and fenofibrate) and pirinixic acid (WY-14,643) [13, 19]. Saturated and unsaturated fatty acids and eicosanoids such as prostacyclin can activate PPARβ/δ [13, 20]. In addition, synthetic compounds with higher affinities for the receptor have been developed [8, 13]. Natural PPARγ ligands include saturated and unsaturated fatty acids, eicosanoid derivatives such as 15-deoxy-$\Delta^{12,14}$-prostaglandin J_2 (15d-PGJ_2), and nitrated fatty acids such as nitrated linoleic acid and nitrated oleic acid [21–23]. Synthetic molecules, most notably thiazolidinediones (TZDs) such as pioglitazone, rosiglitazone, troglitazone, and ciglitazone, are potent PPARγ agonists [23]. Upon binding to their respective receptors, these agonists induce dissociation of corepressors that otherwise maintain PPARs in their inactive state [10]. Corepressor dissociation allows the receptors to heterodimerize with retinoid X receptors and initiate transcription by binding to specific PPAR response elements in the promoter regions of their target genes [10]. Emerging evidence suggests that each PPAR regulates tumorigenesis of different cancer types. Moreover, it has been reported that expression of all three isotypes is altered during lung carcinogenesis [24–26]. Thus, PPAR agonists hold potential as novel chemopreventive and therapeutic agents for lung cancer, warranting a review of current literature and further investigation.

2. PPARs in Lung Cancer

2.1. PPARα. PPARα was the first PPAR subtype to be identified [27]. Its primary function is to regulate energy homeostasis, controlling fatty acid catabolism and lipoprotein metabolism, especially in the liver, as well as metabolism of glucose and amino acids [10, 11, 14]. *In vitro* and *in vivo* studies have shown that PPARα agonists also play a regulatory role in inflammatory responses [10]. The function of PPARα during carcinogenesis has not been extensively defined, with most available studies focusing on its role in hepatocarcinogenesis in rodents. In this context, long-term PPARα activation leads to the development of tumors via induction of DNA replication and cell proliferation and suppression of apoptosis [11, 16]. Reactive oxygen species that are byproducts of fatty acid metabolism mediated by PPARα are also thought to contribute to tumorigenesis [11, 16]. Further supporting the involvement of PPARα in hepatocarcinogenesis is the finding

that mice lacking PPARα are resistant to the agonist WY-14,643-induced increase in DNA synthesis and formation of hepatic neoplasia [28]. Interestingly, epidemiological data suggest this tumorigenic effect of PPARα activation is absent in humans [11, 16], perhaps due to significantly lower expression of PPARα in human hepatocytes and/or inefficient ligand activation of human PPARα [11]. Another plausible explanation suggests that human PPARα does not exert carcinogenic effects, as activation of a humanized PPARα in transgenic mice does not induce hepatic tumors [14]. In sum, although the between-species variation in effects of PPARα activation on liver carcinogenesis requires further elucidation, humans appear to be protected from the harmful outcomes of PPARα agonists [11].

The involvement of PPARα in lung cancer biology has been extensively investigated within the past decade. A study using a mouse xenograft model showed that absence of PPARα expression in the host animals suppresses tumor growth of Lewis lung carcinoma (LLC) cells and lung and liver metastasis of B16 melanoma cells [29]. This suppression of tumorigenesis and metastasis reflects an increase in leukocyte infiltration of the tumor that is associated with host tissues' antitumor inflammatory responses as well as a reduction in tumor angiogenesis. Intriguingly, the same research group found that PPARα agonists such as fenofibrate and WY-14,643 have the same antitumorigenic and antiangiogenic effects via host PPARα [30]. Together, these two seemingly contradictory observations imply that the antitumor effect of PPARα may be two-pronged; complete absence of PPARα expression allows tumor clearance by the host's immune system while agonist-induced stimulation of PPARα prohibits the exaggerated inflammatory responses of the host that can aggravate tumor development [29, 30].

WY-14,643 has also demonstrated a similar antiangiogenic effect, consequently inhibiting tumor formation in a mouse xenograft model established with A549 NSCLC cells as well as in a mouse model of spontaneous NSCLC [31, 32]. In addition to suppressing primary tumor development, PPARα activation by WY-14,643 inhibits metastasis to the contralateral lung and to the liver in an orthotopic NSCLC model [32]. This negative effect of PPARα stimulation during carcinogenesis is directed toward proliferation of endothelial cells, rather than tumor cells, via suppression of epoxyeicosatrienoic acid biosynthesis [31, 32]. Epoxyeicosatrienoic acids have been shown by both *in vitro* and *in vivo* studies to be proangiogenic [32]. Lastly, fenofibrate treatment was found in mice to significantly abrogate neoplasia formation induced by the potent carcinogen 4-nitroquinoline 1-oxide [33]. These studies supporting the antitumorigenic effect of PPARα agonists, combined with clinical efficacy and safety of these molecules in treating hyperlipidemia, certainly warrant closer investigation of PPARα as a therapeutic target in lung cancer.

2.2. PPARβ/δ. PPARβ/δ is involved in a variety of physiological processes including embryonic development, lipid metabolism, wound healing, and inflammation [11, 14, 16, 34]. Its critical role in regulation of cellular functions such as adhesion, proliferation, differentiation, and survival has also been well characterized, especially in keratinocytes [11, 16, 34], strongly suggesting its involvement in carcinogenesis. The biological function of PPARβ/δ in cancer has perhaps been most studied in colon cancer. However, its effect during carcinogenesis remains highly controversial due to lack of consensus in clinical and experimental data. One controversy revolves around expression of PPARβ/δ, with some studies reporting enhanced expression in colon tumors compared to nontransformed colonic epithelium in which PPARβ/δ expression is normally high. However, most of these studies are associated with significant limitations such as small sample size, lack of appropriate controls, or inadequate experimental methods and thus need to be interpreted with some caution [14]. The most robust findings to date are provided by the recent retrospective clinical analysis of 141 subjects, showing that higher PPARβ/δ expression in primary colorectal tumors is associated with lower expression of a marker related to cell proliferation rate, more differentiated cells, reduced rate of lymph node metastasis, and better patient survival following radiation treatment [35]. This report supports the protective role of PPARβ/δ in human colorectal cancer. In contrast, an *in vivo* study using a colorectal cancer cell xenograft model found that PPARβ/δ deficiency in the grafted tumor cells suppresses tumor growth, suggesting a protumorigenic role [36]. However, when interpreting these expression data, it is important to note that PPARβ/δ expression does not indicate the receptor is functionally active; the receptor's activity can be modulated by a variety of factors such as ligand availability and the presence or absence of other proteins [14] as well as by posttranslational modifications. Thus, future studies should examine and compare activity state in addition to expression of PPARβ/δ in tumors and normal tissue counterparts.

Evidence regarding functional outcomes of PPARβ/δ activation is similarly contradictory; some studies show activated PPARβ/δ promotes tumor development by stimulating cell proliferation and preventing apoptosis while others propose receptor activation attenuates tumorigenesis by inducing differentiation and suppressing exaggerated inflammatory responses [14, 16]. Several molecular mechanisms have been proposed to underlie PPARβ/δ's effect on tumorigenesis. Two pathways implicated in its protumorigenic effect are increased expression of vascular endothelial growth factor (VEGF) and enhanced prosurvival signaling involving integrin linked kinase (ILK), 3-phosphoinositide-dependent-protein kinase 1 (PDPK1), phosphatase and tensin homolog deleted on chromosome 10 (PTEN), and AKT [14]. It has been shown that the antitumorigenic effect is mediated through enhanced activity of prodifferentiation genes and/or suppression of proinflammatory signals mediated primarily by the NF-κB pathway [14].

Similar discrepancies are present in cancers of other tissues, with the exception of skin cancer where there seems to be general agreement on the protective role of PPARβ/δ [14]. The involvement of PPARβ/δ in lung cancer was first reported in an *in vitro* study showing that the agonist L-165041 induces growth inhibition of A549 cells, as evidenced by decreased expression of the proliferation marker proliferating cell nuclear antigen (PCNA) [37]. The authors identified

induction of G_1 cell cycle arrest as a result of reduced cyclin D expression, rather than induction of apoptosis, as the underlying mechanism. This antiproliferative effect of PPARβ/δ activation parallels several *in vivo* observations. Although involvement of PPARβ/δ was not directly assessed and a PPARβ/δ-independent mechanism remains a viable possibility, one research group used multiple lung cancer models to demonstrate that lung tumorigenesis is suppressed by increased synthesis of the PPARβ/δ agonist prostacyclin [38, 39]. Mice lacking PPARβ/δ expression also display increased tumor incidence in a RAF-induced lung cancer model [40]. These *in vitro* and *in vivo* data suggest a protective role of PPARβ/δ against lung cancer.

It has also been postulated that PPARβ/δ may prevent lung cancer via its anti-inflammatory function, as it does with colorectal cancer. In two independent studies, one using a lipopolysaccharide-induced pulmonary inflammation model [41] and the other using a carrageenan-induced pleurisy model [42], the potent PPARβ/δ agonist GW0742 was shown to reduce neutrophil infiltration into the lungs and suppress expression of proinflammatory cytokines such as interleukin-6 (IL-6), IL-1β, and tumor necrosis factor-α (TNF-α) [41, 42]. Although these studies did not assess the effect of PPARβ/δ's anti-inflammatory activity on lung carcinogenesis, pulmonary inflammation has been implicated as a contributing factor [4, 12, 43]. The anti-inflammatory function of PPARβ/δ agonists in the context of lung cancer biology is therefore worthy of further investigation.

In contrast to these studies, however, others have provided evidence that PPARβ/δ activation promotes lung cancer; the agonist GW501516 stimulates proliferation, inhibits apoptosis, and supports anchorage-independent growth of A549, H157, and H23 NSCLC cells [25]. The proliferative effect is mediated through PDPK1 overexpression, increased AKT phosphorylation, and PTEN suppression, while resistance to apoptosis results from enhanced expression of B-cell lymphoma-extra large (Bcl-x$_L$) and cyclooxygenase-2 (COX-2). PPARβ/δ can potentiate tumor formation by modulation not only of cancer cells but also of nontransformed cells in the tumor microenvironment. In a mouse xenograft model with LLC cells, absence of PPARβ/δ in the host animals significantly reduced tumor volume and improved survival of the animals [44]. This suppression of LLC cell tumor growth in the PPARβ/δ-deficient mice is a consequence of dysregulated angiogenesis and reduced blood flow.

Other studies suggest that PPARβ/δ may not influence tumorigenesis at all. One such study observed that GW501516 or GW0742 had no effect on expression of PTEN or PDPK1, or on AKT phosphorylation, in A549 or H1838 NSCLC cells, implying that PPARβ/δ activation does not influence these cells' proliferation [45]. No change in the percentage of cells in each phase of the cell cycle was observed either. Likewise, the PPARβ/δ antagonist GSK3787 did not affect proliferation of A549 or H1838 cells [46].

Thus, based on our current knowledge, it is difficult to draw a definite conclusion regarding the biological effect of PPARβ/δ activation in lung cancer. There are several possible explanations for these discrepancies, however. First, the contradictory results may be related to PPARβ/δ's ability to repress as well as induce target gene expression; it has been observed that PPARβ/δ can repress the transcription of its target genes when not bound by its ligands, whereas ligand-bound PPARβ/δ induces expression [16]. Secondly, PPARβ/δ activity may be affected by the presence or absence of cofactors and repressors [16]. Therefore, it is conceivable that the between-study variability in cell culture conditions and genetic background of model animals creates differential cellular environments and thereby leads to the contradictory observations [16]. Finally, many PPAR ligands demonstrate PPAR-dependent and -independent activities, which makes data interpretation more challenging [16]. In summary, further careful analyses are required to delineate the complexities of PPARβ/δ expression and activation in lung cancer.

2.3. PPARγ. PPARγ is an established regulator of adipocyte differentiation, glucose metabolism, and lipid homeostasis [10, 23]. Its involvement in inflammation has also been recognized [10]. More recently, PPARγ's role in cancer has become apparent; PPARγ hinders tumor development and progression, in most cases by modulating differentiation, proliferation, apoptosis, and motility of cancer cells through a variety of molecular pathways [8, 17, 47, 48]. In addition to regulating the oncogenic activities of cancer cells, PPARγ can control the tumor microenvironment; the receptor creates a hostile environment for tumor growth and metastasis via multiple mechanisms [8, 17]. In the context of lung cancer, with general agreement on its role as a tumor suppressor, the biological effects of activated PPARγ are perhaps better defined than those of PPARα or PPARβ/δ [8]. As its influence on cancer cells has been extensively reviewed elsewhere [8, 17, 18], this review will focus on how the microenvironment may be affected by PPARγ's anti-inflammatory function.

Lung carcinogens such as tobacco smoke and inhaled asbestos are known to cause chronic pulmonary inflammation that is associated with lung carcinogenesis [4, 43]. Key players in the cancer-associated inflammatory responses are cellular constituents of the tumor microenvironment such as tumor-associated macrophages, neutrophils, and fibroblasts that secrete growth factors, cytokines, chemokines, reactive oxygen species, and matrix metalloproteinases (MMPs) [4]. The influence of the resulting inflammatory microenvironment on tumor formation and metastasis is multifold and often involves the NF-κB signaling pathway [4]. For instance, inflammation has been shown to increase the rate of genetic mutation within the adjacent epithelial cells and the proliferation of those mutated cells [4]. Tumor-associated macrophages can facilitate tumor angiogenesis, a process that supplies microscopic tumors with nutrients and provides cancer cells with ready access to the circulation required for metastasis [4, 49–51]. The cells mediating cancer-associated inflammatory responses also promote metastasis by contributing MMPs, the key regulator of extracellular matrix remodeling and disruption [4, 52].

PPARγ has been shown to affect multiple aspects of these cancer-associated inflammatory responses. Agonist activation of PPARγ, whose expression increases upon macrophage and monocyte activation [10], suppresses these leukocytes' production of inflammatory mediators such as inducible

nitric oxide synthase, MMP-9, scavenger receptor A, TNF-α, IL-1β, and IL-6 [53–55]. Importantly, these inflammatory molecules have been shown to promote tumorigenesis in several cancers [56]. The negative regulation of inflammatory responses is mediated by the inhibition of transcription factors, for example, NF-κB, activator protein-1 (AP-1), members of the signal transducer and activator of transcription (STAT) protein family, and nuclear factor of activated T cells (NFAT), often via a mechanism termed transrepression [17, 57]. During transrepression, PPARγ interacts with transcription factors and sequesters them from their response elements, preventing inflammatory responses [57]. PPARγ also regulates pathways essential to expression and activity of these transcription factors.

15d-PGJ$_2$, troglitazone, ciglitazone, and rosiglitazone [58, 59], as well as constitutively active PPARγ [59], also suppress differentiation of human lung fibroblasts into myofibroblasts [58, 59]. Myofibroblasts within the tumor microenvironment are the predominant source of tumor-supporting extracellular matrix and also produce molecules that facilitate tumor growth and progression [17, 60] and are considered more carcinogenic than normal fibroblasts [60]. PPARγ agonists also prevent the myofibroblast-associated increase in collagen secretion [58, 59] that can result in remodeling of the tumor microenvironment and facilitate cancer pathogenesis [61]. Furthermore, PPARγ agonists demonstrate suppressive effects on neutrophils' chemotactic response and neutrophil cytokine production [62]. As predicted by this concept, in a mouse model of pulmonary inflammation, endothelial cell PPARγ deficiency enhanced neutrophil infiltration into the lungs and exacerbated tissue injury [63]. These studies, providing a link between PPARγ, inflammation, and cancer, highlight the significance of inflammation-associated cells as a trigger of tumorigenesis as well as of PPARγ as a tumor suppressor acting via multiple mechanisms.

It may prove beneficial to pursue PPARγ activation as a novel chemopreventive strategy [64]. The chemopreventive effects of PPARγ agonists in lung cancer have been reported by several studies. Troglitazone and pioglitazone as well as sulindac sulfide, a nonsteroidal anti-inflammatory drug known to activate PPARγ, significantly reduce primary tumor formation by A549 cells in a xenograft mouse model [65, 66]. Pioglitazone also decreases tumor volume and significantly deters disease progression in mouse models of spontaneous lung adenocarcinoma and squamous cell carcinoma induced by vinyl carbamate and N-nitroso-tris-chloroethylurea, respectively [67]. These findings suggest that PPARγ agonists can inhibit epithelial cell transformation in the early stages of tumorigenesis. Most significantly, one epidemiologic analysis of diabetic patients from 10 Veterans Affairs medical centers, comparing 11,289 TZD users with 76,389 nonusers, observed a 33% reduction in subsequent lung cancer diagnosis in the former group [68], thus underscoring the chemopreventive potential of PPARγ agonists. A clinical trial (NCT00780234) designed to assess the ability of pioglitazone to prevent lung cancer in a more general, nondiabetic population has been initiated, and its results may provide additional justification for the application of PPARγ agonists as a chemopreventive strategy against lung cancer.

3. Therapeutic Application of PPAR Ligands for Lung Cancer

All three members of the PPAR family demonstrate involvement in carcinogenesis, although their mode of action differs. These receptors are therefore attractive targets for lung cancer prevention and treatment. Indeed, the therapeutic applicability of PPARγ agonists is evident in several studies. Besides experimental data supporting the use of PPARγ agonists as a monotherapy for lung cancer, as discussed above, multiple PPARγ agonists demonstrate synergy with commonly used traditional chemotherapeutic drugs such as cisplatin, carboplatin, and paclitaxel, inhibiting proliferation of multiple NSCLC cell lines and suppressing tumor growth in a xenograft lung cancer model [69, 70]. This synergistic effect has also been observed between PPARγ agonists and targeted therapies such as gefitinib, an epidermal growth factor receptor inhibitor, and lovastatin, an inhibitor of 3-hydroxy-3-methyl-glutaryl-coenzyme A reductase (HMG-CoA reductase) [71, 72]. These data substantiate the chemotherapeutic potential of PPARγ agonists. Unlike PPARγ agonists, however, the clinical applicability of PPARα and PPARβ/δ ligands in lung cancer has not been assessed. Nevertheless, the PPARα fibrate agonists have proven relatively safe and effective for treatment of dyslipidemia and cardiovascular disease [11] and clinical assessment of PPARβ/δ ligands should be starting soon. In this context, reported studies showing their physiological effects in lung cancer make a strong argument for further investigation of their chemopreventive and chemotherapeutic potentials.

Some PPAR agonists activate two or all three PPAR receptors [14, 73]. Recently, an intriguing concept has emerged suggesting that use of these dual- or pan-PPAR agonists may be more beneficial than using agents targeting a single PPAR subtype. For instance, one recent clinical trial observed bezafibrate, a pan-PPAR agonist, reduced development of new colon cancer by 53%, although there was no comparison to more selective PPAR agonists [74]. This finding can be interpreted as showing that lower-affinity pan-PPAR agonists may be useful as a novel chemopreventive strategy [14]. Simultaneous activation of PPARα and/or PPARβ/δ may also alleviate the known side effects of PPARγ agonists (weight gain and bone fractures) by stimulating lipid metabolism and bone formation [14, 73]. Thus, activation of more than one PPAR receptor should also be pursued as a new therapeutic approach in lung cancer.

4. Conclusions

Our understanding of PPARs in lung cancer remains incomplete. In particular, the effect of PPARβ/δ expression and activation on carcinogenesis has yet to be delineated and the controversy regarding its role must be resolved before the potential of its agonists/antagonists as therapeutic agents can be evaluated. Nevertheless, based on review of extensive experimental data, the involvement of all three PPAR receptors in lung cancer biology is undeniable. Therefore, with further investigation and additional clinical trials, PPAR modulators may become a valuable tool in the prevention and treatment of lung cancer.

Abbreviations

15d-PGJ$_2$:	15-Deoxy-$\Delta^{12,14}$-prostaglandin J$_2$
AP-1:	Activator protein-1
Bcl-x$_L$:	B-cell lymphoma-extra large
COX-2:	Cyclooxygenase-2
HMG-CoA reductase:	3-Hydroxy-3-methyl-glutaryl-coenzyme A reductase
IL:	Interleukin
ILK:	Integrin linked kinase
LLC:	Lewis lung carcinoma
MMP:	Matrix metalloproteinase
NFAT:	Nuclear factor of activated T cells
NSCLC:	Non-small cell lung cancer
PCNA:	Proliferating cell nuclear antigen
PDPK1:	3-Phosphoinositide-dependent-protein kinase 1
PPAR:	Peroxisome proliferator-activated receptor
PTEN:	Phosphatase and tensin homolog deleted on chromosome 10
SCLC:	Small cell lung cancer
STAT:	Signal transducer and activator of transcription
TNF-α:	Tumor necrosis factor-α
TZD:	Thiazolidinedione
VEGF:	Vascular endothelial growth factor.

Disclosure

The contents in this article do not represent the views of the US Department of Veterans Affairs or the United States Government.

Competing Interests

The authors declare that they have no conflict of interests.

Acknowledgments

This work was supported by a Merit Review Award from the US Department of Veterans Affairs and National Institutes of Health Grants HL093196 and AI125338 (RCR).

References

[1] J. Ferlay, I. Soerjomataram, R. Dikshit et al., "Cancer incidence and mortality worldwide: sources, methods and major patterns in GLOBOCAN 2012," International Journal of Cancer, vol. 136, no. 5, pp. E359–E386, 2015.

[2] R. L. Siegel, K. D. Miller, and A. Jemal, "Cancer statistics, 2016," CA Cancer Journal for Clinicians, vol. 66, no. 1, pp. 7–30, 2016.

[3] J. Malhotra, M. Malvezzi, E. Negri, C. La Vecchia, and P. Boffetta, "Risk factors for lung cancer worldwide," European Respiratory Journal, vol. 48, no. 3, pp. 889–902, 2016.

[4] L. Shi, L. Wang, J. Hou et al., "Targeting roles of inflammatory microenvironment in lung cancer and metastasis," *Cancer and Metastasis Reviews*, vol. 34, no. 2, pp. 319–331, 2015.

[5] G. P. Kalemkerian, W. Akerley, P. Bogner et al., "Small cell lung cancer," *Journal of the National Comprehensive Cancer Network*, vol. 11, no. 1, pp. 78–98, 2013.

[6] Y. Sekido, K. M. Fong, and J. D. Minna, "Progress in understanding the molecular pathogenesis of human lung cancer," *Biochimica et Biophysica Acta (BBA)—Reviews on Cancer*, vol. 1378, no. 1, pp. F21–F59, 1998.

[7] D. S. Ettinger, D. E. Wood, W. Akerley et al., "NCCN guidelines insights: non-small cell lung cancer, version 4.2016," *JNCCN Journal of the National Comprehensive Cancer Network*, vol. 14, no. 3, pp. 255–264, 2016.

[8] V. G. Keshamouni, S. Han, and J. Roman, "Peroxisome proliferator-activated receptors in lung cancer," *PPAR Research*, vol. 2007, Article ID 90289, 10 pages, 2007.

[9] P. E. Almeida, A. B. Carneiro, A. R. Silva, and P. T. Bozza, "PPARγ expression and function in mycobacterial infection: roles in lipid metabolism, immunity, and bacterial killing," *PPAR Research*, vol. 2012, Article ID 383829, 7 pages, 2012.

[10] R. B. Clark, "The role of PPARs in inflammation and immunity," *Journal of Leukocyte Biology*, vol. 71, no. 3, pp. 388–400, 2002.

[11] L. Michalik, B. Desvergne, and W. Wahli, "Peroxisome-proliferator-activated receptors and cancers: complex stories," *Nature Reviews Cancer*, vol. 4, no. 1, pp. 61–70, 2004.

[12] L. Michalik and W. Wahli, "PPARs mediate lipid signaling in inflammation and cancer," *PPAR Research*, vol. 2008, Article ID 134059, 15 pages, 2008.

[13] J. E. Ward and X. Tan, "Peroxisome proliferator activated receptor ligands as regulators of airway inflammation and remodelling in chronic lung disease," *PPAR Research*, vol. 2007, Article ID 14983, 12 pages, 2007.

[14] J. M. Peters, Y. M. Shah, and F. J. Gonzalez, "The role of peroxisome proliferator-activated receptors in carcinogenesis and chemoprevention," *Nature Reviews Cancer*, vol. 12, no. 3, pp. 181–195, 2012.

[15] B. P. Kota, T. H.-W. Huang, and B. D. Roufogalis, "An overview on biological mechanisms of PPARs," *Pharmacological Research*, vol. 51, no. 2, pp. 85–94, 2005.

[16] K. Tachibana, D. Yamasaki, K. Ishimoto, and T. Doi, "The role of PPARs in cancer," *PPAR Research*, vol. 2008, Article ID 102737, 15 pages, 2008.

[17] A. K. Reka, M. T. Goswami, R. Krishnapuram, T. J. Standiford, and V. G. Keshamouni, "Molecular cross-regulation between PPAR-γ and other signaling pathways: implications for lung cancer therapy," *Lung Cancer*, vol. 72, no. 2, pp. 154–159, 2011.

[18] M. Y. Li, T. W. Lee, A. P. Yim, and G. G. Chen, "Function of Pparγ and its ligands in lung cancer," *Critical Reviews in Clinical Laboratory Sciences*, vol. 43, no. 2, pp. 183–202, 2006.

[19] V. R. Narala, R. K. Adapala, M. V. Suresh, T. G. Brock, M. Peters-Golden, and R. C. Reddy, "Leukotriene B₄ is a physiologically relevant endogenous peroxisome proliferator-activated receptor-α agonist," *Journal of Biological Chemistry*, vol. 285, no. 29, pp. 22067–22074, 2010.

[20] R. A. Daynes and D. C. Jones, "Emerging roles of PPARs in inflammation and immunity," *Nature Reviews Immunology*, vol. 2, no. 10, pp. 748–759, 2002.

[21] Y. Li, J. Zhang, F. J. Schopfer et al., "Molecular recognition of nitrated fatty acids by PPARγ," *Nature Structural & Molecular Biology*, vol. 15, no. 8, pp. 865–867, 2008.

[22] A. T. Reddy, S. P. Lakshmi, Y. Zhang, and R. C. Reddy, "Nitrated fatty acids reverse pulmonary fibrosis by dedifferentiating myofibroblasts and promoting collagen uptake by alveolar macrophages," *The FASEB Journal*, vol. 28, no. 12, pp. 5299–5310, 2014.

[23] J. Berger and D. E. Moller, "The mechanisms of action of PPARs," *Annual Review of Medicine*, vol. 53, pp. 409–435, 2002.

[24] M.-Y. Li, H. Yuan, L. T. Ma et al., "Roles of peroxisome proliferator-activated receptor-α and -γ in the development of non-small cell lung cancer," *American Journal of Respiratory Cell and Molecular Biology*, vol. 43, no. 6, pp. 674–683, 2010.

[25] T. V. Pedchenko, A. L. Gonzalez, D. Wang, R. N. DuBois, and P. P. Massion, "Peroxisome proliferator-activated receptor β/δ expression and activation in lung cancer," *American Journal of Respiratory Cell and Molecular Biology*, vol. 39, no. 6, pp. 689–696, 2008.

[26] K.-I. Inoue, Y. Kawahito, Y. Tsubouchi et al., "Expression of peroxisome proliferator-activated receptor (PPAR)-γ in human lung cancer," *Anticancer Research*, vol. 21, no. 4A, pp. 2471–2476, 2001.

[27] I. Issemann and S. Green, "Activation of a member of the steroid hormone receptor superfamily by peroxisome proliferators," *Nature*, vol. 347, no. 6294, pp. 645–650, 1990.

[28] J. M. Peters, R. C. Cattley, and F. J. Gonzalez, "Role of PPARα in the mechanism of action of the nongenotoxic carcinogen and peroxisome proliferator Wy-14,643," *Carcinogenesis*, vol. 18, no. 11, pp. 2029–2033, 1997.

[29] A. Kaipainen, M. W. Kieran, S. Huang et al., "PPARα deficiency in inflammatory cells suppresses tumor growth," *PLOS ONE*, vol. 2, no. 2, article e260, 2007.

[30] D. Panigrahy, A. Kaipainen, S. Huang et al., "PPARα agonist fenofibrate suppresses tumor growth through direct and indirect angiogenesis inhibition," *Proceedings of the National Academy of Sciences of the United States of America*, vol. 105, no. 3, pp. 985–990, 2008.

[31] A. Pozzi, M. R. Ibanez, A. E. Gatica et al., "Peroxisomal proliferator-activated receptor-α-dependent inhibition of endothelial cell proliferation and tumorigenesis," *Journal of Biological Chemistry*, vol. 282, no. 24, pp. 17685–17695, 2007.

[32] N. Skrypnyk, X. Chen, W. Hu et al., "PPARα activation can help prevent and treat non-small cell lung cancer," *Cancer Research*, vol. 74, no. 2, pp. 621–631, 2014.

[33] T. Kuno, K. Hata, M. Takamatsu et al., "The peroxisome proliferator-activated receptor (PPAR) α agonist fenofibrate suppresses chemically induced lung alveolar proliferative lesions in male obese hyperlipidemic mice," *International Journal of Molecular Sciences*, vol. 15, no. 5, pp. 9160–9172, 2014.

[34] A. D. Burdick, D. J. Kim, M. A. Peraza, F. J. Gonzalez, and J. M. Peters, "The role of peroxisome proliferator-activated receptor-β/δ in epithelial cell growth and differentiation," *Cellular Signalling*, vol. 18, no. 1, pp. 9–20, 2006.

[35] L. Yang, H. Zhang, Z.-G. Zhou, H. Yan, G. Adell, and X.-F. Sun, "Biological function and prognostic significance of peroxisome proliferator-activated receptor δ in rectal cancer," *Clinical Cancer Research*, vol. 17, no. 11, pp. 3760–3770, 2011.

[36] B. H. Park, B. Vogelstein, and K. W. Kinzler, "Genetic disruption of PPARδ decreases the tumorigenicity of human colon cancer cells," *Proceedings of the National Academy of Sciences of the United States of America*, vol. 98, no. 5, pp. 2598–2603, 2001.

[37] K. Fukumoto, Y. Yano, N. Virgona et al., "Peroxisome proliferator-activated receptor δ as a molecular target to regulate lung

cancer cell growth," *FEBS Letters*, vol. 579, no. 17, pp. 3829–3836, 2005.

[38] R. L. Keith, Y. E. Miller, T. M. Hudish et al., "Pulmonary prostacyclin synthase overexpression chemoprevents tobacco smoke lung carcinogenesis in mice," *Cancer Research*, vol. 64, no. 16, pp. 5897–5904, 2004.

[39] R. L. Keith, Y. E. Miller, Y. Hoshikawa et al., "Manipulation of pulmonary prostacyclin synthase expression prevents murine lung cancer," *Cancer Research*, vol. 62, no. 3, pp. 734–740, 2002.

[40] S. Müller-Brüsselbach, S. Ebrahimsade, J. Jäkel et al., "Growth of transgenic RAF-induced lung adenomas is increased in mice with a disrupted PPARbeta/delta gene," *International Journal of Oncology*, vol. 31, no. 3, pp. 607–611, 2007.

[41] Z. Haskova, B. Hoang, G. Luo et al., "Modulation of LPS-induced pulmonary neutrophil infiltration and cytokine production by the selective PPARβ/δ ligand GW0742," *Inflammation Research*, vol. 57, no. 7, pp. 314–321, 2008.

[42] R. Di Paola, C. Crisafulli, E. Mazzon et al., "GW0742, a high-affinity PPAR -β/δ agonist, inhibits acute lung injury in mice," *Shock*, vol. 33, no. 4, pp. 426–435, 2010.

[43] D. R. Brenner, D. Scherer, K. Muir et al., "A review of the application of inflammatory biomarkers in epidemiologic cancer research," *Cancer Epidemiology Biomarkers and Prevention*, vol. 23, no. 9, pp. 1729–1751, 2014.

[44] S. Müller-Brüsselbach, M. Kömhoff, M. Rieck et al., "Deregulation of tumor angiogenesis and blockade of tumor growth in PPARβ-deficient mice," *EMBO Journal*, vol. 26, no. 15, pp. 3686–3698, 2007.

[45] P. He, M. G. Borland, B. Zhu et al., "Effect of ligand activation of peroxisome proliferator-activated receptor-β/δ (PPARβ/δ) in human lung cancer cell lines," *Toxicology*, vol. 254, no. 1-2, pp. 112–117, 2008.

[46] P. S. Palkar, M. G. Borland, S. Naruhn et al., "Cellular and pharmacological selectivity of the peroxisome proliferator-activated receptor-β/δ antagonist GSK3787," *Molecular Pharmacology*, vol. 78, no. 3, pp. 419–430, 2010.

[47] T.-H. Chang and E. Szabo, "Induction of differentiation and apoptosis by ligands of peroxisome proliferator-activated receptor γ in non-small cell lung cancer," *Cancer Research*, vol. 60, no. 4, pp. 1129–1138, 2000.

[48] Y. Tsubouchi, H. Sano, Y. Kawahito et al., "Inhibition of human lung cancer cell growth by the peroxisome proliferator-activated receptor-γ agonists through induction of apoptosis," *Biochemical and Biophysical Research Communications*, vol. 270, no. 2, pp. 400–405, 2000.

[49] W. Guo and F. G. Giancotti, "Integrin signalling during tumour progression," *Nature Reviews Molecular Cell Biology*, vol. 5, no. 10, pp. 816–826, 2004.

[50] G. Bergers and L. E. Benjamin, "Tumorigenesis and the angiogenic switch," *Nature Reviews Cancer*, vol. 3, no. 6, pp. 401–410, 2003.

[51] E. S. White, S. R. B. Strom, N. L. Wys, and D. A. Arenberg, "Non-small cell lung cancer cells induce monocytes to increase expression of angiogenic activity," *Journal of Immunology*, vol. 166, no. 12, pp. 7549–7555, 2001.

[52] H. Paz, N. Pathak, and J. Yang, "Invading one step at a time: the role of invadopodia in tumor metastasis," *Oncogene*, vol. 33, no. 33, pp. 4193–4202, 2014.

[53] M. Ricote, J. T. Huang, J. S. Welch, and C. K. Glass, "The peroxisome proliferator-activated receptor (PPARγ) as a regulator of monocyte/macrophage function," *Journal of Leukocyte Biology*, vol. 66, no. 5, pp. 733–739, 1999.

[54] M. Ricote, A. C. Li, T. M. Willson, C. J. Kelly, and C. K. Glass, "The peroxisome proliferator-activated receptor-γ is a negative regulator of macrophage activation," *Nature*, vol. 391, no. 6662, pp. 79–82, 1998.

[55] C. Jiang, A. T. Ting, and B. Seed, "PPAR-γ agonists inhibit production of monocyte inflammatory cytokines," *Nature*, vol. 391, no. 6662, pp. 82–86, 1998.

[56] J. A. Van Ginderachter, K. Movahedi, J. Van Den Bossche, and P. De Baetselier, "Macrophages, PPARs, and cancer," *PPAR Research*, vol. 2008, Article ID 169414, 11 pages, 2008.

[57] M. V. Schmidt, B. Brüne, and A. Von Knethen, "The nuclear hormone receptor PPARγ as a therapeutic target in major diseases," *TheScientificWorldJournal*, vol. 10, pp. 2181–2197, 2010.

[58] H. A. Burgess, L. E. Daugherty, T. H. Thatcher et al., "PPARγ agonists inhibit TGF-β induced pulmonary myofibroblast differentiation and collagen production: implications for therapy of lung fibrosis," *American Journal of Physiology—Lung Cellular and Molecular Physiology*, vol. 288, no. 6, pp. L1146–L1153, 2005.

[59] J. E. Milam, V. G. Keshamouni, S. H. Phan et al., "PPAR-γ agonists inhibit profibrotic phenotypes in human lung fibroblasts and bleomycin-induced pulmonary fibrosis," *American Journal of Physiology—Lung Cellular and Molecular Physiology*, vol. 294, no. 5, pp. L891–L901, 2008.

[60] M. Shimoda, K. T. Mellody, and A. Orimo, "Carcinoma-associated fibroblasts are a rate-limiting determinant for tumour progression," *Seminars in Cell and Developmental Biology*, vol. 21, no. 1, pp. 19–25, 2010.

[61] M. Fang, J. Yuan, C. Peng, and Y. Li, "Collagen as a double-edged sword in tumor progression," *Tumor Biology*, vol. 35, no. 4, pp. 2871–2882, 2014.

[62] T. J. Standiford, V. C. Keshamouni, and R. C. Reddy, "Peroxisome proliferator-activated receptor-γ as a regulator of lung inflammation and repair," *Proceedings of the American Thoracic Society*, vol. 2, no. 3, pp. 226–231, 2005.

[63] A. T. Reddy, S. P. Lakshmi, J. M. Kleinhenz, R. L. Sutliff, C. M. Hart, and R. C. Reddy, "Endothelial cell peroxisome proliferator-activated receptor γ reduces endotoxemic pulmonary inflammation and injury," *The Journal of Immunology*, vol. 189, no. 11, pp. 5411–5420, 2012.

[64] F. Ondrey, "Peroxisome proliferator-activated receptor γ pathway targeting in carcinogenesis: implications for chemoprevention," *Clinical Cancer Research*, vol. 15, no. 1, pp. 2–8, 2009.

[65] V. G. Keshamouni, R. C. Reddy, D. A. Arenberg et al., "Peroxisome proliferator-activated receptor-γ activation inhibits tumor progression in non-small-cell lung cancer," *Oncogene*, vol. 23, no. 1, pp. 100–108, 2004.

[66] M. Wick, G. Hurteau, C. Dessev et al., "Peroxisome proliferator-activated receptor-γ is a target of nonsteroidal anti-inflammatory drugs mediating cyclooxygenase-independent inhibition of lung cancer cell growth," *Molecular Pharmacology*, vol. 62, no. 5, pp. 1207–1214, 2002.

[67] Y. Wang, M. James, W. Wen et al., "Chemopreventive effects of pioglitazone on chemically induced lung carcinogenesis in mice," *Molecular Cancer Therapeutics*, vol. 9, no. 11, pp. 3074–3082, 2010.

[68] R. Govindarajan, L. Ratnasinghe, D. L. Simmons et al., "Thiazolidinediones and the risk of lung, prostate, and colon cancer in patients with diabetes," *Journal of Clinical Oncology*, vol. 25, no. 12, pp. 1476–1481, 2007.

[69] G. D. Girnun, E. Naseri, S. B. Vafai et al., "Synergy between PPARγ ligands and platinum-based drugs in cancer," *Cancer Cell*, vol. 11, no. 5, pp. 395–406, 2007.

[70] R. C. Reddy, A. Srirangam, K. Reddy et al., "Chemotherapeutic drugs induce PPAR-γ expression and show sequence-specific synergy with PPAR-γ ligands in inhibition of non-small cell lung cancer," *Neoplasia*, vol. 10, no. 6, pp. 597–603, 2008.

[71] S. Y. Lee, G. Y. Hur, K. H. Jung et al., "PPAR-γ agonist increase gefitinib's antitumor activity through PTEN expression," *Lung Cancer*, vol. 51, no. 3, pp. 297–301, 2006.

[72] C.-J. Yao, G.-M. Lai, C.-F. Chan, A.-L. Cheng, Y.-Y. Yang, and S.-E. Chuang, "Dramatic synergistic anticancer effect of clinically achievable doses of lovastatin and troglitazone," *International Journal of Cancer*, vol. 118, no. 3, pp. 773–779, 2006.

[73] K. Still, P. Grabowski, I. Mackie, M. Perry, and N. Bishop, "The peroxisome proliferator activator receptor alpha/delta agonists linoleic acid and bezafibrate upregulate osteoblast differentiation and induce periosteal bone formation in vivo," *Calcified Tissue International*, vol. 83, no. 4, pp. 285–292, 2008.

[74] A. Tenenbaum, V. Boyko, E. Z. Fisman et al., "Does the lipid-lowering peroxisome proliferator-activated receptors ligand bezafibrate prevent colon cancer in patients with coronary artery disease?" *Cardiovascular Diabetology*, vol. 7, article 18, 2008.

8

Deciphering the Roles of Thiazolidinediones and PPARγ in Bladder Cancer

Melody Chiu,[1] Lucien McBeth,[1] Puneet Sindhwani,[2] and Terry D. Hinds[1,2]

[1]Center for Hypertension and Personalized Medicine, Department of Physiology & Pharmacology,
University of Toledo College of Medicine, Toledo, OH 43614, USA
[2]Department of Urology, University of Toledo College of Medicine, Toledo, OH 43614, USA

Correspondence should be addressed to Terry D. Hinds; terry.hinds@utoledo.edu

Academic Editor: Stefano Caruso

The use of thiazolidinedione (TZD) therapy in type II diabetic patients has proven useful in the lowering of blood glucose levels. However, recent investigations have shown that there may be potential health concerns associated, including the risk of developing bladder cancer as well as complications in the cardiovasculature. TZDs are ligands for the nuclear receptor PPARγ, and activation causes lipid uptake and insulin sensitization, both of which are critical processes for diabetic patients whose bodies are unable to utilize insulin effectively. Several studies have shown that PPARγ/TZDs decrease IGF-1 levels and, thus, reduce cancer growth in carcinomas such as the pancreas, colon, liver, and prostate. However, other studies have shed light on the potential of the receptor as a biomarker for uroepithelial carcinomas, particularly due to its stimulatory effect on migration of bladder cancer cells. Furthermore, PPARγ may provide the tumor-promoting microenvironment by de novo synthesis of nutrients that are needed for bladder cancer development. In this review, we closely examine the TZD class of drugs and their effects on PPARγ in patient studies along with additional molecular factors that are positive modulators, such as protein phosphatase 5 (PP5), which may have considerable implications for bladder cancer therapy.

1. Introduction

The predominant type of bladder cancer diagnosed among individuals in the United States is urothelial (transitional cell) carcinoma [1]. Bladder cancer is the fourth most common type of cancer found among men in the United States and an important cause of death worldwide [2, 3]. In 2015 alone, the American Cancer Society predicted a total of 74,000 newly diagnosed cases and 16,000 deaths from bladder cancer in the United States [4]. The cause of bladder cancer appears to be multifactorial; both exogenous environmental and endogenous molecular factors may potentially play a role in cancer development [5, 6]. Environmental factors such as cigarette smoking and occupational exposure to chemical carcinogens are among the top risk factors; however, family history and genetics also increase the susceptibility to bladder carcinogenesis [7]. Moreover, evidence has suggested an association between diabetes mellitus and the increased risk of bladder cancer [8]. Rates of type II diabetes mellitus among

adults and children have been continuously rising. In the 2014 National Diabetes Statistics Report, the Centers for Disease Control and Prevention estimated that 29.1 million people (9.3% of the population) are diagnosed with diabetes in the United States [9]. Worldwide, an estimated 382 million adults were diagnosed with diabetes in 2013 [10], with type II diabetes accounting for nearly 90–95% of these diabetic individuals [11].

There has been increasing evidence showing that antidiabetic TZDs are linked to the risk of bladder cancer as well as other complications such as cardiovasculature (CVD) events. TZDs, such as pioglitazone and rosiglitazone, are synthetic ligands of peroxisome proliferator-activated receptors gamma (PPARγ) used in therapeutic treatments for patients diagnosed with type II diabetes mellitus [12, 13]. These ligands bind to PPARγ and play a role in metabolism through induction of genes that control glucose and lipid uptake [13]. Through a series of metabolic pathways, PPARγ also activates adipogenesis, which is the process of transforming a preadipocyte stem cell into fully mature adipocyte [14]. Eventually, this process reduces insulin resistance by assisting in glucose uptake [15]. Potentially, PPARγ signaling in bladder cancer cells may provide a tumor microenvironment that allows for de novo lipogenesis for the use of increasing tumor mass and energy usage. However, the role of PPARγ in bladder cells is unknown.

PPARγ is expressed in white and brown adipose tissues as well as in the urinary bladder [16, 17]. More notably, high levels of PPARγ are selectively expressed in the transitional epithelium of the ureter and urinary bladder, the area where bladder cancer typically arises. PPARα is another member of the PPAR family that is expressed in the ureter and bladder epithelium, but at a significantly lower level compared to PPARγ [17]. Despite the prominent differences between the two receptors, there has also been evidence depicting a degree of crosstalk between the receptors in urinary bladder epithelium. A combination of synthetic ligands, known as "dual-acting agonists," includes PPARα and PPARγ agonists and has been shown to have a carcinogenic impact in rodents, primarily affecting the bladder epithelium [18]. In this review, we discuss the functions of PPARγ and the effects of TZD therapy in the urinary bladder and to a lesser extent the role of PPARα.

2. PPARγ Function

The PPARγ gene is located on chromosome 3 in humans and is alternatively spliced to produce two major proteins; however, alternative usage of the promoter provides four different transcripts [19, 20]. The mRNAs of transcripts PPARγ1, PPARγ3, and PPARγ4 result in identical protein products that we refer to as PPARγ1. The protein product from the mRNA of PPARγ2 is comparable to that of PPARγ1; however, the product contains 30 additional amino acids located at the NH_2-terminal region (reviewed in [20]) [21]. Not surprisingly, the isoforms have varying expression levels in cells; PPARγ1 is expressed in nearly all cells, whereas PPARγ2 is principally expressed in adipocytes [22]. However, it is unknown whether there is a difference in PPARγ1 and PPARγ2 expression levels in bladder cancer cells. PPARγ is also involved in regulating inflammatory processes [23]. There is evidence that shows PPARγ activation in endothelial cells reduces systemic inflammation [24]. While the role in adipocytes and insulin sensitivity is well understood, the effects of PPARγ activation in many other cell types remain unclear including bladder cancer.

PPARs are ligand-activated transcription factors that belong to the nuclear receptor superfamily [22]. When a ligand binds to an isoform of the PPAR family, the receptor is activated, translocates to bind regulatory regions on DNA, and then combines with retinoid X receptors (RXRs) to form heterodimers (Figure 1). Consequently, these heterodimers serve as transcriptional activators for various genes by binding to specific PPAR response elements (PPREs) [13]. Of the PPARs, PPARγ is found to have the highest expression levels in adipose tissue. Once activated in adipocytes by TZDs or natural ligands, such as essential fatty acids and eicosanoids [25], PPARγ is involved in the secretion of adiponectin and leptin. These adipokines regulate insulin activity in peripheral tissues to maintain glucose sensitivity in the body. In addition, PPARγ regulates genes involved in fatty acid transport, release, and storage by increasing expression of genes involved in fatty acid import such as cluster of differentiation 36 (CD36) and adipocyte protein 2 (aP2) [21, 26]; therefore, PPARγ has a major role in lipid and carbohydrate metabolism.

TZDs have long been a common therapeutic method to treat patients with type II diabetes mellitus. TZDs are used to treat hyperglycemia and insulin resistance, lowering fasting blood glucose and insulin, as well as HbA1C levels [27]. Previously, up to 20% of antidiabetic medications prescribed in the USA were TZDs [28]. In the past, it has been shown that TZDs are effective in therapy as a second-line treatment after metformin, the current first-line agent in type II diabetes [27, 29]. They are high-affinity synthetic agonists of PPARγ [12], and PPARγ activation affects lipid metabolism and ultimately enhances lipid storage and promotes insulin sensitivity in adipose tissue, liver, and muscle [16, 23]. Despite many benefits, TZDs have also been shown to induce weight gain among diabetic patients on long-term therapy [30], which occurs from activation of adipogenesis and the expansion of fat cells. Of the TZD class, rosiglitazone and pioglitazone are the most prevalently used drugs in clinical settings [31]. Studies have reported the adverse health effects of these medications, including the possible risk of developing bladder cancer or cardiovascular events [12, 32, 33]. However, there is a conundrum for the effects of PPARγ and its ligands in cancer. Several cancers have shown reduced growth with PPARγ activation with the TZD troglitazone such as in carcinomas of the breast, kidney, liver, colon, pancreas, and prostate [34–39] as well as in non-small-cell lung cancer [40] and ACTH-secreting pituitary adenomas [41]. However, most of the antigrowth properties of TZDs have been with troglitazone and not pioglitazone or rosiglitazone. Rosiglitazone may be associated with a lower risk of breast cancer [42], thyroid cancer [43], and nonmelanoma skin cancer [44]. On the other hand, pioglitazone seems to be neutral or slightly (possibly not significant) associated with various cancers including bladder cancer [45], ovarian cancer [46], oral cancer [47], kidney cancer [48], and thyroid cancer [49]. Analysis of specific TZDs and their actions on growth and migration are important for understanding the impact they may have in a specific cancer.

Some TZDs have been shown to reduce levels of the insulin-like growth factor-1 (IGF-1) in the blood, which is a known growth factor that may induce cancer [50]. Plasma levels of IGF-1 and IGF binding protein-3 (IGFBP-3) have been shown to be an association with bladder cancer risk [51]. It is not known how PPARγ affects the expression of IGF-1, IGFBP-3, or the IGF receptor (IGFR) in the bladder or differences among the TZD drug class. The use of pioglitazone, and not rosiglitazone, has been associated with an increased risk of bladder cancer in a population-based cohort study, suggesting the risk is TZD specific and not a particular class [52]. Investigations on the consequences of troglitazone, rosiglitazone, and pioglitazone on the IGF system in uroepithelial carcinomas may reveal differences between the drugs.

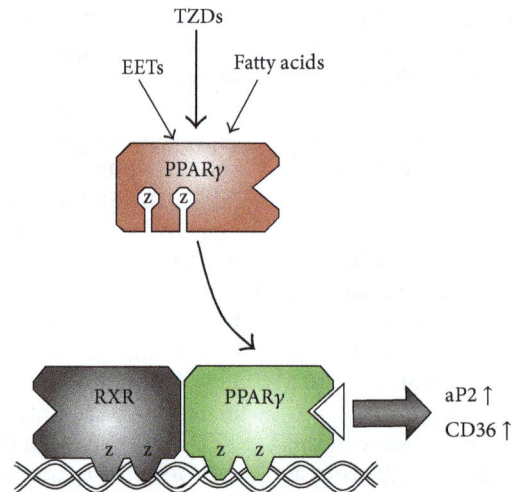

FIGURE 1: PPARγ heterodimerizes with RXR for transcriptional regulation. PPARγ ligands such as eicosanoids (EETs), fatty acids, or thiazolidinediones (TZDs) bind to PPARγ to cause transactivation resulting in the binding to regulatory regions on DNA. PPARγ combines with retinoid X receptors (RXRs) to form heterodimers, which together serve as transcriptional activators for various genes by binding to specific PPAR response elements (PPREs) in their promoters.

3. TZDs and Bladder Cancer

An interim longitudinal cohort study using the Kaiser Permanente Northern California Registry analyzed a sample size of 193,099 diabetic patients and observed a correlation between pioglitazone therapy and bladder cancer [12]. The increased dosage and duration of pioglitazone treatment show rises in bladder cancer incidence rates, with a 30% risk of developing bladder cancer among patients on pioglitazone therapy after 12–24 months. Furthermore, the risk increases to 50% for patients on pioglitazone therapy for 2 or more years [12]. In the 10-year follow-up, however, the statistical significance was not found while there was a numerical increased adjusted risk of 78% (0.93–3.4, 95% CI) for patients on pioglitazone treatment for 1.5–4 years [53]. Additionally, Hsiao et al. showed current users of both pioglitazone and rosiglitazone had increased risks of developing bladder cancer [32]. The correlation between pioglitazone and bladder cancer is consistent with the previous Kaiser cohort study. However, the use of rosiglitazone was not associated with an increased risk of bladder cancer in any analysis [52], but it has been linked to increased risk of cardiovascular events [54]. However, rosiglitazone was not increased in bladder cancer risk [55].

Pioglitazone may be the only TZD to enhance cases of bladder cancer, as results from the National Health Insurance Research Database (NHIRD) group also presented an association with uroepithelial carcinomas [32]. Through the NHIRD study, it was shown that increased exposure period to both pioglitazone and rosiglitazone is related to an increased risk of bladder cancer. Regardless of whether patients have been on pioglitazone or rosiglitazone treatment, the highest risk of bladder cancer is among diabetic patients with the longest exposure to either treatment. The NHIRD cohort showed the odds ratios for the risk of bladder cancer among diabetic patients on pioglitazone therapy in the exposure groups were 1.45 (<1 year), 1.74 (between 1 and 2 years), and

2.93 (2 or more years) [27]. Similarly, odds ratios for patients on rosiglitazone therapy were 0.98 (<1 year), 1.78 (between 1-2 years), and 2.00 (2 or more years) [31]. The increased duration of pioglitazone or rosiglitazone therapy is associated with increased risk of bladder cancer, with the highest risk among diabetic patients on therapy for 2 or more years [32]. However, this observation may only apply to specific TZDs and not all of them [29], as there appears to be a weaker association between bladder cancer and rosiglitazone.

There is some debate as to the association of TZDs with bladder cancer. Two meta-analyses show only moderate to no risk of developing bladder cancer. Monami et al. found that the overall risk of malignancies (regardless of location) was decreased by TZD treatments [56]. However, there was a numerical, but not statistically significant, increase in the risk of bladder cancer development from pioglitazone treatment (2.05 Mantel-Haenszel odds ratio, $p = 0.12$) but no association with rosiglitazone treatment (0.91, $p = 0.62$). Interestingly, the odds ratio was associated with a large confidence interval, 0.84–5.02, which the authors attributed to a small sample size, three studies, due to potential bias from incomplete disclosure of negative results. In addition, the second meta-analysis conducted by Bosetti et al. showed only a modest increased risk of developing bladder cancer when treated with TZDs for less than two years (relative risk 1.20, CI 1.07–1.34) [57]. There was a moderate increased risk for treatment longer than two years (relative risk 1.42, CI 1.17–1.72), which the authors led to claim that the short-term (less than two years) treatment with TZDs in type II diabetes mellitus might be worth the modest risk of developing bladder cancer.

4. PPARγ and Bladder Cancer

To provide a closer look at the impact of PPARγ on bladder cell progression, Yang et al. analyzed samples of both benign bladder and bladder cancer mucosal samples by fluorescence in situ hybridization (FISH) assay for expression of PPARγ, and the authors found 31% (8/21 samples) of the bladder cancer mucosal samples and 4.3% (1/23 samples) of benign bladder samples showed amplification [58]. In addition, lower levels of PPARγ amplification were detected in non-muscle-invasive bladder cancer samples compared to muscle-invasive samples (16.7% versus 46.7%, resp.) [58]. Yang et al. also observed different rates of cell migration and invasion in various bladder cancer cell lines that have PPARγ expression. The 5637 bladder cell line had a considerably higher mRNA and protein expression of PPARγ compared to other bladder cancer cell lines such as UMUC-3. Moreover, the 5637 cancer cell line displayed higher cell migration and invasion than the UMUC-3 cell line [58]. Another study showed that the T24 bladder cancer cell line expresses PPARγ and high levels of the nuclear receptor glucocorticoid receptor β (GRβ), which also showed higher migration rates than the UMUC-3 cells that have low PPARγ and GRβ expression [59]. These results suggest that PPARγ may be a potential biomarker of bladder cancer aggressiveness, where high levels of receptor expression correlate with higher rates of cancer cell migration and invasion.

Rosiglitazone treatments have been shown to have varying effects on 5637 and UMUC-3 cancer cells [58]. The 5637 bladder cancer cells display significantly enhanced cell migration and invasion with rosiglitazone treatment. On the other hand, there are minimal rates of cell migration and invasion in UMUC-3 cells, and rosiglitazone has less of an effect. The difference in the levels of PPARγ expression between the two cancer cell lines may account for this observation, as the 5637 cell line has a considerably higher PPARγ expression than UMUC-3 cell line [58]. Lubet et al. performed a series of experiments using rosiglitazone and hydroxybutyl(butyl)nitrosamine (OH-BBN), which is a carcinogen that is known to induce urinary bladder cancer in rats [13]. Interestingly, rats treated with rosiglitazone had 100% incidence of bladder cancer, while the untreated control group had a 57% incidence of bladder cancer. There were also increased levels of PPARγ expression in the presence of rosiglitazone treatment compared to those that were not treated. Furthermore, rats that were exposed to OH-BBN and treated with the highest dosage of rosiglitazone have the highest incidence of bladder cancer. Rats on rosiglitazone therapy had earlier cancer onsets and larger tumor sizes in the bladders, and a dose-dependent response existed between rosiglitazone and bladder cancer incidence. TZDs may not have an effect in the earlier stages but may promote cancer progression at the later stages of bladder cancer [13]. However, it is important to note that in humans rosiglitazone has not been associated with higher risk, but this has been observed with pioglitazone. Regardless, decreasing PPARγ expression may potentially alter bladder cancer migration and invasive abilities. Therefore, regulating levels of PPARγ expression in the urinary bladder may have implications for targeting bladder cancer, particularly regarding metastasis and cancer cell progression.

5. An Independent Microenvironment through PPARγ

In general, tumor development in the urinary bladder is dependent upon complex interactions with host molecular factors that are part of its surrounding microenvironment [60, 61]. Furthermore, there are signaling interactions of a certain level in the microenvironment that are capable of inducing malignant transformation of cells, such as factors that promote angiogenesis, abnormal development, and proliferation. Neoangiogenesis, or the formation of new blood vessels from preexisting vessels, is required for tumor growth, and vascular endothelial growth factor (VEGF) has been shown to play a critical role as a proangiogenic factor in bladder cancer progression [62]. VEGF-A is the primary proangiogenic factor that serves to maintain adequate levels of oxygen and nutrient supply in growing adipose tissue and is positively regulated by PPARγ [63]. The levels of VEGF found in the urine and bladder tissue are significantly elevated in patients diagnosed with urinary bladder carcinoma compared to cancer-free patients [64]. Additionally, it has been shown that VEGF-A is found in bladder tumors and is upregulated in patients with invasive bladder cancer [65]. Potentially, VEGF-A may also be enhanced by PPARγ in bladder tumor tissue consequently enhancing tumor growth and migration through angiogenesis. However, the specific TZDs that may enhance VEGF-A or if PPARγ induces VEGF-A in bladder are yet to be determined.

In order to continue to proliferate indefinitely, cancer cells require molecular factors that increase both glucose uptake and rates of glycolysis for energy. Elevated rates of glycolysis produce higher amounts of lactic acid, and this pathway enhances lipogenesis through fatty acid synthase (FAS). FAS is the key enzyme involved in de novo synthesis of fatty acids for lipid storage, and high expression levels are frequently limited in tissues with lipogenic activity, such as adipose tissue and liver [66]. However, it has been shown that FAS is overexpressed in numerous human cancers, including bladder cancer, and its expression level is positively correlated with tumor progression [67]. Similar to FAS, fatty acid binding proteins (FABPs) are involved in lipid metabolism and facilitate the transfer of lipids, including lipid droplets for storage, across various cellular membranes and compartments [68–70]. Adipocyte-type FABP (A-FABP), also known as adipocyte protein 2 (aP2) and fatty acid binding protein 4 (FABP4), binds to long chain fatty acids and PPARγ agonists [69]. These ligands bind and activate A-FABPs in the cytosol, and A-FABPs then transfer the ligands to PPARγ upon entering the nucleus to drive adipogenic activities [71]. Unlike FAS, low expression levels of A-FABP are correlated with the progression of human bladder transitional cell carcinoma. When comparing specific types of bladder tumor tissue, A-FABP was mainly detected in cells that were papillary in origin and not invasive urothelial carcinoma [72]. Evidence suggests low-grade bladder tumors have higher levels of A-FABP compared to high-grade bladder tumors [73]. On the other hand, high expression of A-FABP has been observed in tongue squamous cell carcinoma [70]. The differences in tissue types, such as bladder and tongue, may partially account for the discrepancy in the effects of A-FABP expression.

Metabolic changes may occur in nonadipose tissues when they receive fatty acids released by hypertrophic dysfunctional adipose tissue, commonly seen among obese and type II diabetic patients [74]. Nonadipose tissues are not equipped with adequate cellular machinery for excessive amounts of lipid deposits. Therefore, an overload of lipids in these tissues causes a series of organ-specific toxic reactions and results in lipotoxicity, which is lipid-induced metabolic tissue damage and death [75]. Glucuronidation is important for detoxifying the bladder from toxins [76] and may be regulated differentially by fatty acid accumulation. While tissues, such as skeletal muscle and liver, are known to be highly susceptible to lipotoxicity [77], little is known regarding the effects of lipid accumulation in the bladder. Presumably, the functional impairment will occur in most healthy nonadipose tissues; however, this observation may not entirely apply to bladder tissue.

It may be possible that, in bladder tissue, lipid accumulation modifies metabolic functions in a way that strongly upregulates PPARγ and enhances lipid uptake, similar to adipose tissue. Eventually, sufficient amounts of free fatty acids (FFAs) will be present in the bladder due to ectopic fat accumulation, and the bladder may no longer require A-FABP to import additional extracellular FFAs but will heavily utilize FAS for lipid production. FFAs bind PPARγ and other PPAR isoforms and activate transcriptional activity. Other dysregulated metabolic pathways, including those that involve glycolysis [78], can cause a metabolic switch regulated by oncogenes and tumor suppressor genes to favor tumor growth and play a role in bladder carcinogenesis. Together, these observations are consistent with evidence showing lower expression levels of A-FABP and higher expression levels of FAS in more invasive forms of bladder cancer. Increased levels of PPARγ activity may alter the microenvironment in a way that allows for the cells to autonomously synthesize nutrients within the bladder through lipid accumulation and angiogenesis. However, more studies need to be performed to understand the role of PPARγ in bladder cancer.

6. The Impact of Dual-Acting PPAR Agonists

Despite evidence showing PPARγ as the predominant PPAR in urinary bladder epithelium, PPARα has also been found to be expressed in both rabbit and human bladder epithelium. PPARα is activated by a class of synthetic ligands known as fibrates (i.e., fenofibrate) and is predominantly expressed in the liver, heart, brain, skeletal muscle, and kidney. Also, endogenous ligands such as fatty acids can bind PPARα to increase transcriptional activity. Recently, bilirubin was also shown to function as an endogenous PPARα agonist by direct binding [25] and was shown to decrease mRNA expression of PPARγ. Once activated, PPARα regulates genes that encode for mitochondrial and peroxisomal β-oxidation, which reduces dyslipidemia. In addition, activated PPARα functions to hinder hepatic fatty acid synthesis through inhibition of FAS and SREBP1 and therefore lower lipid levels [21, 79, 80]. Dual agonists are a class of drugs that activate both PPARα and PPARγ, thereby combating diabetes mellitus and the metabolic syndrome among patients diagnosed with both conditions [81]. Examples of such dual agonists include ragaglitazar and muraglitazar, which would be of interests for the treatment of obesity and diabetes. However, muraglitazar has been shown to induce gallbladder adenomas in male mice, and ragaglitazar has been demonstrated to induce urinary bladder and renal pelvis tumors in both male and female rats [82].

It is worth noting that certain combinations of PPARα and PPARγ synthetic dual-acting agonists may have a carcinogenic impact on rodents, especially targeting urinary bladder epithelium. In a recent study, Egerod et al. found that rat bladder epithelium expresses both PPARγ and PPARα through a crosstalk link that involves the early growth response-1 (Egr-1) factor [18]. Egr-1 is a transcription factor and has been previously shown to play a role in bladder cancer among different species, including humans [83]. When either PPAR agonist is used alone, there is only slightly increased Egr-1 expression in the rat bladder epithelium [18]. High Egr-1 induction is dependent on the coactivation of PPARα and PPARγ by their respective synthetic ligands fenofibrate and rosiglitazone. Together, fenofibrate and rosiglitazone appear to exert a positive interaction in the bladder epithelium, upregulating high Egr-1 expression. However, this positive interaction is not observed in other tissues, such as the liver, where there are high expression levels of Egr-1 and the absence of carcinogenic effects of dual-acting agonists on rats [18].

It has also been demonstrated that ragaglitazar treatment has a carcinogenic impact on rat bladder epithelium and involves the induction of Egr-1 [82, 84]. Importantly, the fenofibrates that are PPARα agonists have not been shown to induce bladder cancer. PPARα agonists with a different structure, the clofibrates [85], have been shown to weakly enhance BBN-induced bladder carcinogenesis [86]. However, a second report indicated that clofibrates are not carcinogenic [87]. The differences in these studies may be from clofibrate potentially having off-target effects or through possible weak interactions with PPARγ. Furthermore, it is rather a unique characteristic of bladder epithelium to express high levels of both PPARα and PPARγ. While the exact mechanism behind the interactions of PPAR agonists and bladder cancer remains unknown, these studies provide further insight into the relevance of PPAR activation, particularly in bladder cancer development.

7. PP5, a Positive Modulator of PPARγ

PPARγ activity is inhibited by the phosphorylation of serine 112, and, currently, only one phosphatase, protein phosphatase 5 (PP5), has been shown to bind directly to the receptor [26]. PP5 belongs to the PPP-family consisting of serine/threonine protein phosphatases [88, 89]. Evidence has indicated that PP5 activation requires the binding of its tetratricopeptide repeat (TPR) domain to the heat shock protein 90 (Hsp90) chaperone complex [26, 89] (Figure 2). PP5 is a positive modulator of PPARγ in the presence of proadipogenic activity, with PP5 described as a "prolipogenic

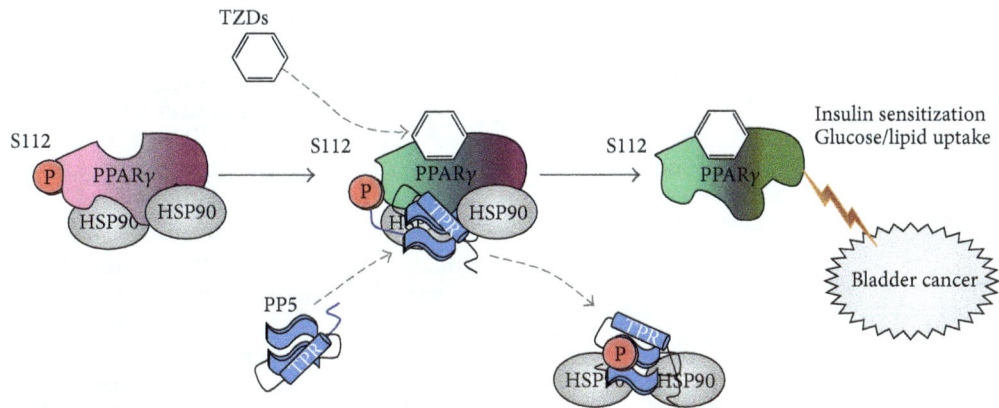

FIGURE 2: Theoretical model of PPARγ and PP5 in bladder cancer. Activation of PPARγ by TZDs recruits PP5 to positively modulate and dephosphorylate Ser-112 (S112). PPARγ is activated once the phosphate group is removed, and a series of PPARγ-mediated activities commence shortly thereafter, including insulin sensitization. PP5 has been shown to mediate PPARγ activity by controlling phosphorylation of S112 in an adipogenic model, and targeting PP5 in the bladder epithelium may potentially affect PPARγ and its carcinogenic effects on the bladder.

phosphatase" [26]. Upon activation by the adipogenic stimulus rosiglitazone, PP5 is recruited to positively modulate the activity of PPARγ by dephosphorylating PPARγ at serine-112 residue [26, 90]. Once dephosphorylated, PPARγ becomes active and regulates genes in metabolic processes, such as adipogenesis. Not only is PP5 a potential target in the treatment of obesity [26], but it may also provide an effective therapeutic intervention for bladder cancer. Other studies have suggested that PP5 plays a role in tumorigenesis. PP5 mRNA levels are remarkably elevated in malignant ascites hepatomas in rats [91]. Also, increased levels of PP5 protein have been observed in human tumor breast tissue and have been linked to the promotion of breast cancer development [92]. It is unknown whether a similar association exists between PP5 and human bladder cancer. The mechanism of PP5 expression and tumorigenesis has yet to be determined, but it may potentially regulate PPARγ in the bladder epithelium similar to adipose, as high levels of PPARγ are also associated with bladder cancer. If PP5 is a positive modulator of PPARγ in the bladder epithelium, then reducing PP5 expression may serve as an alternative therapeutic target to hinder bladder cancer progression. However, these studies are yet to be conducted.

8. Conclusion

Long-term TZD therapy may increase the risk of developing bladder cancer, especially pioglitazone. Rosiglitazone does not appear to have the long-term effects on the bladder. Prolonged and higher PPARγ activity levels are associated with higher incidences of bladder cancer, potentially due to the downstream effects of PPARγ-mediated metabolism. In addition to incidence rates, PPARγ activity is associated with increased bladder cancer cell migration and invasion. Further understanding of the roles of the PPARs and their agonists in the bladder may uncover additional strategies in bladder cancer therapy. Previously, there have not been studies examining the interaction of PP5 with PPARγ in

bladder epithelium and cancer development. It will be of therapeutic importance to determine if the same relationship exists between PP5 and PPARγ in the bladder epithelium as for adipose tissue in the presence of TZD therapy. Bilirubin may offer a therapeutic potential because it activates PPARα and suppresses PPARγ, and fenofibrate has not been associated with bladder cancer. In the future, therapies that target PPARγ, or possibly PP5, may prove to be useful in bladder cancer treatment, particularly among diabetic patients that require long-term health management.

Disclosure

The content is solely the responsibility of the authors and does not necessarily represent the official views of the National Institutes of Health.

Competing Interests

The authors declare that they have no competing interests.

Acknowledgments

This work was supported by the University of Toledo deArce-Memorial Endowment Fund (Terry D. Hinds Jr.). Research reported in this publication was also supported by the National Heart, Lung, and Blood Institute of the National Institutes of Health under Award nos. K01HL125445 (Terry D. Hinds Jr.) and L32MD009154 (Terry D. Hinds Jr.).

References

[1] J. C. Park, D. E. Citrin, P. K. Agarwal, and A. B. Apolo, "Multimodal management of muscle-invasive bladder cancer," Current Problems in Cancer, vol. 38, no. 3, pp. 80–108, 2014.

[2] G. M. Dancik, "An online tool for evaluating diagnostic and prognostic gene expression biomarkers in bladder cancer," BMC Urology, vol. 15, no. 1, article 59, 2015.

[3] Y. Langle, C. Lodillinsky, D. Belgorosky, E. O. Sandes, and A. M. Eiján, "Role of peroxisome proliferator activated receptor-gamma in bacillus calmette-Guérin bladder cancer therapy," *Journal of Urology*, vol. 188, no. 6, pp. 2384–2390, 2012.

[4] American Cancer Society, *Bladder Cancer*, ACS, 2014.

[5] M. C. Hall, S. S. Chang, G. Dalbagni et al., "Guideline for the management of nonmuscle invasive bladder cancer (Stages Ta, T1, and Tis): 2007 update," *Journal of Urology*, vol. 178, no. 6, pp. 2314–2330, 2007.

[6] L. McBeth, M. Grabnar, S. Selman, and T. D. Hinds, "Involvement of the androgen and glucocorticoid receptors in bladder cancer," *International Journal of Endocrinology*, vol. 2015, Article ID 384860, 10 pages, 2015.

[7] H. Chu, M. Wang, and Z. Zhang, "Bladder cancer epidemiology and genetic susceptibility," *Journal of Biomedical Research*, vol. 27, no. 3, pp. 170–178, 2013.

[8] H. Fang, B. Yao, Y. Yan et al., "Diabetes mellitus increases the risk of bladder cancer: an updated meta-analysis of observational studies," *Diabetes Technology and Therapeutics*, vol. 15, no. 11, pp. 914–922, 2013.

[9] Centers for Disease Control and Prevention, *National Diabetes Statistics Report: Estimates of Diabetes and Its Burden in the United States, 2014*, CDC, Atlanta, Ga, USA, 2014.

[10] M. E. Goossens, M. P. Zeegers, M. T. Bazelier, M. L. De Bruin, F. Buntinx, and F. De Vries, "Risk of bladder cancer in patients with diabetes: a retrospective cohort study," *BMJ Open*, vol. 5, no. 6, Article ID e007470, 2015.

[11] A. T. Kharroubi and H. M. Darwish, "Diabetes mellitus: the epidemic of the century," *World Journal of Diabetes*, vol. 6, no. 6, pp. 850–867, 2015.

[12] J. D. Lewis, A. Ferrara, T. Peng et al., "Risk of bladder cancer among diabetic patients treated with pioglitazone: interim report of a longitudinal cohort study," *Diabetes Care*, vol. 34, no. 4, pp. 916–922, 2011.

[13] R. A. Lubet, S. M. Fischer, V. E. Steele, M. M. Juliana, R. Desmond, and C. J. Grubbs, "Rosiglitazone, a PPAR gamma agonist: Potent promoter of hydroxybutyl(butyl)nitrosamine-induced urinary bladder cancers," *International Journal of Cancer*, vol. 123, no. 10, pp. 2254–2259, 2008.

[14] C. Liu, T. Feng, N. Zhu et al., "Identification of a novel selective agonist of PPARgamma with no promotion of adipogenesis and less inhibition of osteoblastogenesis," *Scientific Reports*, vol. 5, article 9530, 2015.

[15] Y. B. Esterson, K. Zhang, S. Koppaka et al., "Insulin sensitizing and anti-inflammatory effects of thiazolidinediones are heightened in obese patients," *Journal of Investigative Medicine*, vol. 61, no. 8, pp. 1152–1160, 2013.

[16] S. Horita, M. Nakamura, N. Satoh, M. Suzuki, and G. Seki, "Thiazolidinediones and edema: recent advances in the pathogenesis of Thiazolidinediones-induced renal sodium retention," *PPAR Research*, vol. 2015, Article ID 646423, 7 pages, 2015.

[17] Y. Guan, Y. Zhang, L. Davis, and M. D. Breyer, "Expression of peroxisome proliferator-activated receptors in urinary tract of rabbits and humans," *American Journal of Physiology—Renal Physiology*, vol. 273, no. 6, pp. F1013–F1022, 1997.

[18] F. L. Egerod, N. Brünner, J. E. Svendsen, and M. B. Oleksiewicz, "PPARα and PPARγ are co-expressed, functional and show positive interactions in the rat urinary bladder urothelium," *Journal of Applied Toxicology*, vol. 30, no. 2, pp. 151–162, 2010.

[19] B. A. Beamer, C. Negri, C.-J. Yen et al., "Chromosomal localization and partial genomic structure of the human peroxisome proliferator activated receptor-gamma (hPPARγ) gene,"

[20] L. Sabatino, A. Fucci, M. Pancione, and V. Colantuoni, "PPARG epigenetic deregulation and its role in colorectal tumorigenesis," *PPAR Research*, vol. 2012, Article ID 687492, 12 pages, 2012.

[21] B. Grygiel-Górniak, "Peroxisome proliferator-activated receptors and their ligands: nutritional and clinical implications—a review," *Nutrition Journal*, vol. 13, no. 1, article 17, 2014.

[22] C. Janani and B. D. Ranjitha Kumari, "PPAR gamma gene—a review," *Diabetes and Metabolic Syndrome: Clinical Research and Reviews*, vol. 9, no. 1, pp. 46–50, 2015.

[23] E. Fuentes, L. Guzmán-Jofre, R. Moore-Carrasco, and I. Palomo, "Role of PPARs in inflammatory processes associated with metabolic syndrome (Review)," *Molecular medicine reports*, vol. 8, no. 6, pp. 1611–1616, 2013.

[24] J. U. Scher and M. H. Pillinger, "15d-PGJ$_2$: the anti-inflammatory prostaglandin?" *Clinical Immunology*, vol. 114, no. 2, pp. 100–109, 2005.

[25] D. E. Stec, K. John, C. J. Trabbic et al., "Bilirubin binding to PPARα inhibits lipid accumulation," *PLoS ONE*, vol. 11, no. 4, Article ID e0153427, 2016.

[26] T. D. Hinds Jr., L. A. Stechschulte, H. A. Cash et al., "Protein phosphatase 5 mediates lipid metabolism through reciprocal control of glucocorticoid receptor and peroxisome proliferator-activated receptor-γ (PPARγ)," *Journal of Biological Chemistry*, vol. 286, no. 50, pp. 42911–42922, 2011.

[27] J. Noble, M. O. Baerlocher, and J. Silverberg, "Management of type 2 diabetes mellitus. Role of thiazolidinediones," *Canadian Family Physician*, vol. 51, pp. 683–687, 2005.

[28] N. D. Shah, V. M. Montori, H. M. Krumholz, K. Tu, G. C. Alexander, and C. A. Jackevicius, "Responding to an FDA warning—geographic variation in the use of rosiglitazone," *New England Journal of Medicine*, vol. 363, no. 22, pp. 2081–2084, 2010.

[29] R. Mamtani, K. Haynes, W. B. Bilker et al., "Association between longer therapy with thiazolidinediones and risk of bladder cancer: a cohort study," *Journal of the National Cancer Institute*, vol. 104, no. 18, pp. 1411–1421, 2012.

[30] J. N. Feige, L. Gelman, L. Michalik, B. Desvergne, and W. Wahli, "From molecular action to physiological outputs: peroxisome proliferator-activated receptors are nuclear receptors at the crossroads of key cellular functions," *Progress in Lipid Research*, vol. 45, no. 2, pp. 120–159, 2006.

[31] S.-S. Choi, J. Park, and J. H. Choi, "Revisiting PPARγ as a target for the treatment of metabolic disorders," *BMB Reports*, vol. 47, no. 11, pp. 599–608, 2014.

[32] F.-Y. Hsiao, P.-H. Hsieh, W.-F. Huang, Y.-W. Tsai, and C.-S. Gau, "Risk of bladder cancer in diabetic patients treated with rosiglitazone or pioglitazone: A Nested Case-control Study," *Drug Safety*, vol. 36, no. 8, pp. 643–649, 2013.

[33] A. M. Gallagher, L. Smeeth, S. Seabroke, H. G. M. Leufkens, and T. P. van Staa, "Risk of death and cardiovascular outcomes with thiazolidinediones: a study with the general practice research database and secondary care data," *PLOS ONE*, vol. 6, no. 12, Article ID e28157, 2011.

[34] H. J. Burstein, G. D. Demetri, E. Mueller, P. Sarraf, B. M. Spiegelman, and E. P. Winer, "Use of the peroxisome proliferator-activated receptor (PPAR) γ ligand troglitazone as treatment for refractory breast cancer: a phase II study," *Breast Cancer Research and Treatment*, vol. 79, no. 3, pp. 391–397, 2003.

Biochemical and Biophysical Research Communications, vol. 233, no. 3, pp. 756–759, 1997.

[35] R. Butler, S. H. Mitchell, D. J. Tindall, and C. Y. F. Young, "Non-apoptotic cell death associated with S-phase arrest of prostate cancer cells via the peroxisome proliferator-activated receptor γ ligand, 15-Deoxy-Δ12,14-prostaglandin J2," *Cell Growth and Differentiation*, vol. 11, no. 1, pp. 49–61, 2000.

[36] K.-I. Inoue, Y. Kawahito, Y. Tsubouchi et al., "Expression of peroxisome proliferator-activated receptor γ in renal cell carcinoma and growth inhibition by its agonists," *Biochemical and Biophysical Research Communications*, vol. 287, no. 3, pp. 727–732, 2001.

[37] S. Kawa, T. Nikaido, H. Unno, N. Usuda, K. Nakayama, and K. Kiyosawa, "Growth inhibition and differentiation of pancreatic cancer cell lines by PPAR ligand troglitazone," *Pancreas*, vol. 24, no. 1, pp. 1–7, 2002.

[38] M.-Y. Li, H. Deng, J.-M. Zhao, D. Dai, and X.-Y. Tan, "Peroxisome proliferator-activated receptor gamma ligands inhibit cell growth and induce apoptosis in human liver cancer BEL-7402 cell," *World Journal of Gastroenterology*, vol. 9, no. 8, pp. 1683–1688, 2003.

[39] T. Shimada, K. Kojima, K. Yoshiura, H. Hiraishi, and A. Terano, "Characteristics of the peroxisome proliferator activated receptor γ (PPARγ) ligand induced apoptosis in colon cancer cells," *Gut*, vol. 50, no. 5, pp. 658–664, 2002.

[40] T.-H. Chang and E. Szabo, "Induction of differentiation and apoptosis by ligands of peroxisome proliferator-activated receptor γ in non-small cell lung cancer," *Cancer Research*, vol. 60, no. 4, pp. 1129–1138, 2000.

[41] A. P. Heaney, M. Fernando, W. H. Yong, and S. Melmed, "Functional PPAR-γ receptor is a novel therapeutic target for ACTH-secreting pituitary adenomas," *Nature Medicine*, vol. 8, no. 11, pp. 1281–1287, 2002.

[42] C. Tseng, "Rosiglitazone reduces breast cancer risk in Taiwanese female patients with type 2 diabetes mellitus," *Oncotarget*, vol. 8, no. 2, pp. 3042–3048, 2017.

[43] C.-H. Tseng, "Rosiglitazone may reduce thyroid cancer risk in patients with type 2 diabetes," *Annals of Medicine*, vol. 45, no. 8, pp. 539–544, 2013.

[44] C.-H. Tseng, "Rosiglitazone may reduce non-melanoma skin cancer risk in Taiwanese," *BMC Cancer*, vol. 15, article 41, 2015.

[45] C.-H. Tseng, "Pioglitazone and bladder cancer: a population-based study of Taiwanese," *Diabetes Care*, vol. 35, no. 2, pp. 278–280, 2012.

[46] C.-H. Tseng, "Pioglitazone does not affect the risk of ovarian cancer: analysis of a nationwide reimbursement database in Taiwan," *Gynecologic Oncology*, vol. 131, no. 1, pp. 135–139, 2013.

[47] C.-H. Tseng, "Pioglitazone and oral cancer risk in patients with type 2 diabetes," *Oral Oncology*, vol. 50, no. 2, pp. 98–103, 2014.

[48] C.-H. Tseng, "Pioglitazone does not affect the risk of kidney cancer in patients with type 2 diabetes," *Metabolism: Clinical and Experimental*, vol. 63, no. 8, pp. 1049–1055, 2014.

[49] C.-H. Tseng, "Pioglitazone and thyroid cancer risk in Taiwanese patients with type 2 diabetes," *Journal of Diabetes*, vol. 6, no. 5, pp. 448–450, 2014.

[50] A. Belfiore, M. Genua, and R. Malaguarnera, "PPAR-γ agonists and their effects on IGF-I receptor signaling: implications for cancer," *PPAR Research*, vol. 2009, Article ID 830501, 18 pages, 2009.

[51] H. Zhao, H. B. Grossman, M. R. Spitz, S. P. Lerner, K. Zhang, and X. Wu, "Plasma levels of insulin-like growth factor-1 and binding protein-3, and their association with bladder cancer risk," *Journal of Urology*, vol. 169, no. 2, pp. 714–717, 2003.

[52] M. Tuccori, K. B. Filion, H. Yin, O. H. Yu, R. W. Platt, and L. Azoulay, "Pioglitazone use and risk of bladder cancer: Population Based Cohort Study," *BMJ*, vol. 352, 2016.

[53] J. D. Lewis, L. A. Habel, C. P. Quesenberry et al., "Pioglitazone use and risk of bladder cancer and other common cancers in persons with diabetes," *The Journal of the American Medical Association*, vol. 314, no. 3, pp. 265–277, 2015.

[54] S. E. Nissen and K. Wolski, "Effect of rosiglitazone on the risk of myocardial infarction and death from cardiovascular causes," *New England Journal of Medicine*, vol. 356, no. 24, pp. 2457–2471, 2007.

[55] C.-H. Tseng, "Rosiglitazone is not associated with an increased risk of bladder cancer," *Cancer Epidemiology*, vol. 37, no. 4, pp. 385–389, 2013.

[56] M. Monami, I. Dicembrini, and E. Mannucci, "Thiazolidinediones and cancer: results of a meta-analysis of randomized clinical trials," *Acta Diabetologica*, vol. 51, no. 1, pp. 91–101, 2014.

[57] C. Bosetti, V. Rosato, D. Buniato, A. Zambon, C. La Vecchia, and G. Corrao, "Cancer risk for patients using thiazolidinediones for type 2 diabetes: a meta-analysis," *Oncologist*, vol. 18, no. 2, pp. 148–156, 2013.

[58] D.-R. Yang, S.-J. Lin, X.-F. Ding et al., "Higher expression of peroxisome proliferator-activated receptor γ or its activation by agonist thiazolidinedione-rosiglitazone promotes bladder cancer cell migration and invasion," *Urology*, vol. 81, no. 5, pp. 1109.e1–1109.e6, 2013.

[59] L. McBeth, A. C. Nwaneri, M. Grabnar, J. Demeter, A. Nestor-Kalinoski, and T. D. Hinds, "Glucocorticoid receptor beta increases migration of human bladder cancer cells," *Oncotarget*, vol. 7, no. 19, pp. 27313–27324, 2016.

[60] E. S. Costanzo, A. K. Sood, and S. K. Lutgendorf, "Biobehavioral influences on cancer progression," *Immunology and Allergy Clinics of North America*, vol. 31, no. 1, pp. 109–132, 2011.

[61] R. R. Langley and I. J. Fidler, "Tumor cell-organ microenvironment interactions in the pathogenesis of cancer metastasis," *Endocrine Reviews*, vol. 28, no. 3, pp. 297–321, 2007.

[62] A. Hoeben, B. Landuyt, M. S. Highley, H. Wildiers, A. T. Van Oosterom, and E. A. De Bruijn, "Vascular endothelial growth factor and angiogenesis," *Pharmacological Reviews*, vol. 56, no. 4, pp. 549–580, 2004.

[63] A. U. Hasan, K. Ohmori, K. Konishi et al., "Eicosapentaenoic acid upregulates VEGF-A through both GPR120 and PPARγ mediated pathways in 3T3-L1 adipocytes," *Molecular and Cellular Endocrinology*, vol. 406, pp. 10–18, 2015.

[64] M. Sankhwar, S. N. Sankhwar, A. Abhishek, and S. Rajender, "Clinical significance of the VEGF level in urinary bladder carcinoma," *Cancer Biomarkers*, vol. 15, no. 4, pp. 349–355, 2015.

[65] F. Roudnicky, C. Poyet, P. Wild et al., "Endocan is upregulated on tumor vessels in invasive bladder cancer where it mediates VEGF-A-induced angiogenesis," *Cancer Research*, vol. 73, no. 3, pp. 1097–1106, 2013.

[66] L. Chang, P. Wu, R. Senthilkumar et al., "Loss of fatty acid synthase suppresses the malignant phenotype of colorectal cancer cells by down-regulating energy metabolism and mTOR signaling pathway," *Journal of Cancer Research and Clinical Oncology*, vol. 142, no. 1, pp. 59–72, 2016.

[67] B. Jiang, E.-H. Li, Y.-Y. Lu et al., "Inhibition of fatty-acid synthase suppresses p-akt and induces apoptosis in bladder cancer," *Urology*, vol. 80, no. 2, pp. 484.e9–484.e15, 2012.

[68] R. M. Kaikaus, N. M. Bass, and R. K. Ockner, "Functions of fatty acid binding proteins," *Experientia*, vol. 46, no. 6, pp. 617–630, 1990.

[69] M. Furuhashi and G. S. Hotamisligil, "Fatty acid-binding proteins: role in metabolic diseases and potential as drug targets," *Nature Reviews Drug Discovery*, vol. 7, no. 6, pp. 489–503, 2008.

[70] D. Lee, K. Wada, Y. Taniguchi et al., "Expression of fatty acid binding protein 4 is involved in the cell growth of oral squamous cell carcinoma," *Oncology Reports*, vol. 31, no. 3, pp. 1116–1120, 2014.

[71] A. Adida and F. Spener, "Adipocyte-type fatty acid-binding protein as inter-compartmental shuttle for peroxisome proliferator activated receptor γ agonists in cultured cell," *Biochimica et Biophysica Acta—Molecular and Cell Biology of Lipids*, vol. 1761, no. 2, pp. 172–181, 2006.

[72] G. Ohlsson, J. M. A. Moreira, P. Gromov, G. Sauter, and J. E. Celis, "Loss of expression of the adipocyte-type fatty acid-binding protein (A-FABP) is associated with progression of human urothelial carcinomas," *Molecular and Cellular Proteomics*, vol. 4, no. 4, pp. 570–581, 2005.

[73] J. E. Celis, M. Østergaard, B. Basse et al., "Loss of adipocyte-type fatty acid binding protein and other protein biomarkers is associated with progression of human bladder transitional cell carcinomas," *Cancer Research*, vol. 56, no. 20, pp. 4782–4790, 1996.

[74] K. Cusi, "The role of adipose tissue and lipotoxicity in the pathogenesis of type 2 diabetes," *Current Diabetes Reports*, vol. 10, no. 4, pp. 306–315, 2010.

[75] C. M. Kusminski, S. Shetty, L. Orci, R. H. Unger, and P. E. Scherer, "Diabetes and apoptosis: lipotoxicity," *Apoptosis*, vol. 14, no. 12, pp. 1484–1495, 2009.

[76] V. L. Sundararaghavan, P. Sindhwani, and T. D. Hinds Jr., "Glucuronidation and UGT isozymes in bladder: new targets for the treatment of uroepithelial carcinomas?" *Oncotarget*, vol. 8, no. 2, pp. 3640–3648, 2016.

[77] T. Suganami, M. Tanaka, and Y. Ogawa, "Adipose tissue inflammation and ectopic lipid accumulation," *Endocrine Journal*, vol. 59, no. 10, pp. 849–857, 2012.

[78] V. R. Conde, P. F. Oliveira, A. R. Nunes et al., "The progression from a lower to a higher invasive stage of bladder cancer is associated with severe alterations in glucose and pyruvate metabolism," *Experimental Cell Research*, vol. 335, no. 1, pp. 91–98, 2015.

[79] Y. Shiomi, T. Yamauchi, M. Iwabu et al., "A novel peroxisome proliferator-activated receptor (PPAR)α agonist and PPARγ antagonist, Z-551, ameliorates high-fat diet-induced obesity and metabolic disorders in mice," *Journal of Biological Chemistry*, vol. 290, no. 23, pp. 14567–14581, 2015.

[80] T. D. Hinds, P. A. Hosick, M. W. Hankins, A. Nestor-Kalinoski, and D. E. Stec, "Mice with hyperbilirubinemia due to Gilbert's Syndrome polymorphism are resistant to hepatic steatosis by decreased serine 73 phosphorylation of PPARα," *American Journal of Physiology—Endocrinology And Metabolism*, 2016.

[81] V. G. Maltarollo, M. Togashi, A. S. Nascimento, and K. M. Honorio, "Structure-based virtual screening and discovery of new PPARδ/γ dual agonist and PPARδ and γ agonists," *PLoS ONE*, vol. 10, no. 3, Article ID e0118790, 2015.

[82] M. B. Oleksiewicz, J. Southgate, L. Iversen, and F. L. Egerod, "Rat urinary bladder carcinogenesis by dual-acting PPARα + γ agonists," *PPAR Research*, vol. 2008, Article ID 103167, 14 pages, 2008.

[83] F. L. Egerod, A. Bartels, N. Fristrup et al., "High frequency of tumor cells with nuclear Egr-1 protein expression in human bladder cancer is associated with disease progression," *BMC Cancer*, vol. 9, article no. 385, 2009.

[84] M. B. Oleksiewicz, I. Thorup, H. S. Nielsen et al., "Generalized cellular hypertrophy is induced by a dual-acting PPAR agonist in rat urinary bladder urothelium in vivo," *Toxicologic Pathology*, vol. 33, no. 5, pp. 552–560, 2005.

[85] L. Giampietro, A. D'Angelo, A. Giancristofaro et al., "Synthesis and structure-activity relationships of fibrate-based analogues inside PPARs," *Bioorganic and Medicinal Chemistry Letters*, vol. 22, no. 24, pp. 7662–7666, 2012.

[86] A. Hagiwara, S. Tamano, T. Ogiso, E. Asakawa, and S. Fukushima, "Promoting effect of the peroxisome proliferator, clofibrate, but not di(2-ethylhexyl)phthalate, on urinary bladder carcinogenesis in F344 rats initiated by N-butyl-N-(4-hydroxybutyl)nitrosamine," *Japanese Journal of Cancer Research*, vol. 81, no. 12, pp. 1232–1238, 1990.

[87] C. E. Torrey, H. G. Wall, J. A. Campbell et al., "Evaluation of the carcinogenic potential of clofibrate in the FVB/Tg.AC mouse after oral administration—Part I," *International Journal of Toxicology*, vol. 24, no. 5, pp. 313–325, 2005.

[88] N. Grankvist, R. E. Honkanen, Å. Sjöholm, and H. Ortsäter, "Genetic disruption of protein phosphatase 5 in mice prevents high-fat diet feeding-induced weight gain," *FEBS Letters*, vol. 587, no. 23, pp. 3869–3874, 2013.

[89] T. D. Hinds Jr. and E. R. Sánchez, "Protein phosphatase 5," *International Journal of Biochemistry and Cell Biology*, vol. 40, no. 11, pp. 2358–2362, 2008.

[90] L. A. Stechschulte, C. Ge, T. D. Hinds, E. R. Sanchez, R. T. Franceschi, and B. Lecka-Czernik, "Protein phosphatase PP5 controls bone mass and the negative effects of rosiglitazone on bone through reciprocal regulation of PPARγ (peroxisome proliferator-activated receptor γ) and RUNX2 (runt-related transcription factor 2)," *Journal of Biological Chemistry*, vol. 291, no. 47, pp. 24475–24486, 2016.

[91] H. Shirato, H. Shima, H. Nakagama et al., "Expression in hepatomas and chromosomal localization of rat protein phosphatase 5 gene," *International Journal of Oncology*, vol. 17, no. 5, pp. 909–912, 2000.

[92] T. Golden, I. V. Aragon, B. Rutland et al., "Elevated levels of Ser/Thr protein phosphatase 5 (PP5) in human breast cancer," *Biochimica et Biophysica Acta (BBA)—Molecular Basis of Disease*, vol. 1782, no. 4, pp. 259–270, 2008.

9

Discovery of Novel Insulin Sensitizers: Promising Approaches and Targets

Yadan Chen,[1] Haiming Ma,[2] Dasheng Zhu,[1] Guowei Zhao,[3] Lili Wang,[4] Xiujuan Fu,[1] and Wei Chen[4]

[1]Department of Pharmacy, The Second Hospital of Jilin University, Changchun 130041, China
[2]Department of Pharmacy, China-Japan Union Hospital of Jilin University, Changchun 130041, China
[3]Department of Pharmacy, Beijing Boai Hospital, China Rehabilitation Research Center, Beijing 100068, China
[4]Beijing Institute of Pharmacology and Toxicology, Beijing 100850, China

Correspondence should be addressed to Xiujuan Fu; fxj462003@163.com and Wei Chen; weichen45@126.com

Academic Editor: Brian N. Finck

Insulin resistance is the undisputed root cause of type 2 diabetes mellitus (T2DM). There is currently an unmet demand for safe and effective insulin sensitizers, owing to the restricted prescription or removal from market of certain approved insulin sensitizers, such as thiazolidinediones (TZDs), because of safety concerns. Effective insulin sensitizers without TZD-like side effects will therefore be invaluable to diabetic patients. The specific focus on peroxisome proliferator-activated receptor γ- (PPARγ-) based agents in the past decades may have impeded the search for novel and safer insulin sensitizers. This review discusses possible directions and promising strategies for future research and development of novel insulin sensitizers and describes the potential targets of these agents. Direct PPARγ agonists, selective PPARγ modulators (sPPARγMs), PPARγ-sparing compounds (including ligands of the mitochondrial target of TZDs), agents that target the downstream effectors of PPARγ, along with agents, such as heat shock protein (HSP) inducers, $5'$-adenosine monophosphate-activated protein kinase (AMPK) activators, 11β-hydroxysteroid dehydrogenase type 1 (11β-HSD1) selective inhibitors, biguanides, and chloroquines, which may be safer than traditional TZDs, have been described. This minireview thus aims to provide fresh perspectives for the development of a new generation of safe insulin sensitizers.

1. Introduction

According to the World Health Organization, the morbidity of diabetes mellitus (DM), which is a global noninfectious epidemic disease, is expected to continue to rise in the coming decades [1]. The surge in type 2 DM (T2DM) that affects more than 90% of diabetic patients can be attributed to the increasing prevalence of insulin resistance (IR) in the general population, which is partially triggered by the widespread occurrence of obesity and metabolic syndrome [2]. IR, which has been considered a root cause of T2DM, is a pathological state in which the target cells in liver, skeletal muscle, and adipose tissue fail to respond properly to insulin, resulting in their inability to efficiently uptake and metabolize glucose [3–5]. A comprehensive review of insulin receptor signaling has been presented previously [4]. IR leads to a loss of response from the peripheral insulin target tissues (mainly the liver, adipose, and muscle tissues) to insulin. Additionally, IR may impair the ability of the pancreatic islets to synthesize and secrete sufficient insulin to address the metabolic needs of the body. The clinical manifestations of IR include hyperinsulinemia, hyperglycemia, hyperlipidemia, increased circulating inflammatory marker levels, and diminished plasma adiponectin levels. Several factors, including defective insulin signal transduction, impaired effectors within insulin-dependent pathways, and enhanced insulin-antagonizing pathways, contribute to the etiology of IR at the cellular level [4]. Thus, it is apparent that T2DM patients urgently require drugs that target the etiology of the disease rather than those that merely ameliorate the symptoms.

Although several mechanism-based drugs, such as dipeptidyl peptidase 4 (DPP-4) inhibitors, and sodium/glucose cotransporter 2 (SGLT2) inhibitors, have been introduced in the

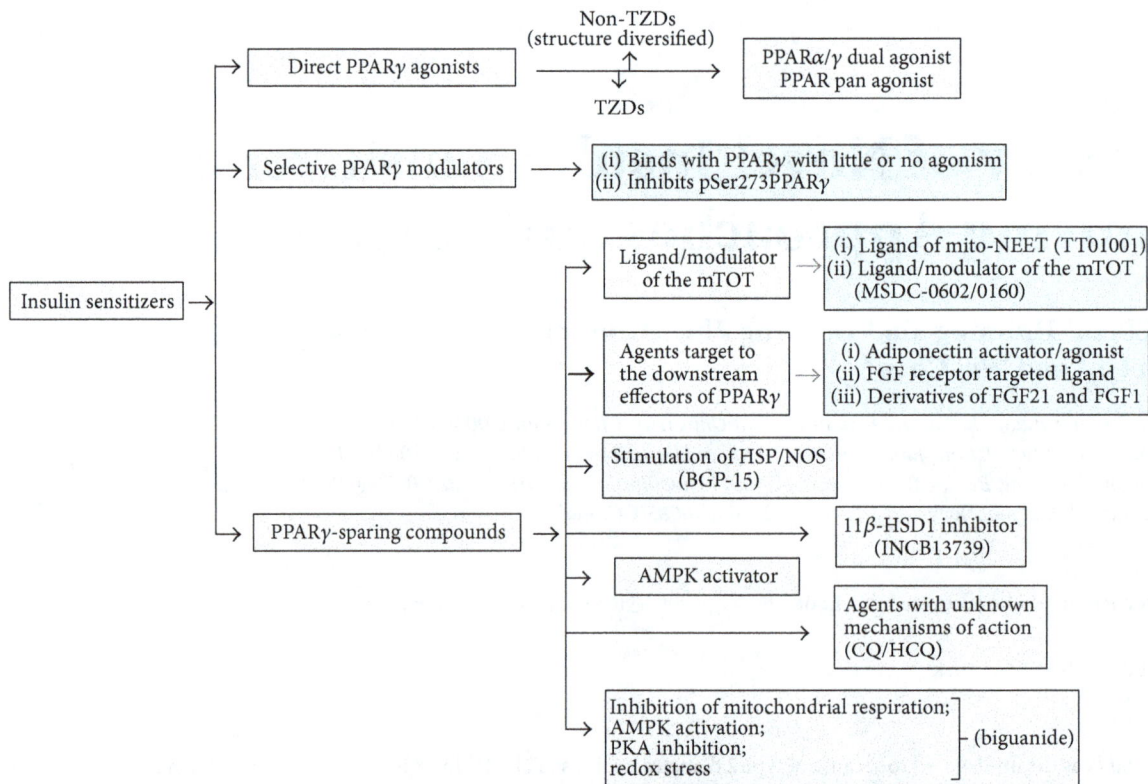

FIGURE 1: *Classification of new-generation insulin sensitizers based on their mechanisms or targets.* AMPK, adenosine monophosphate-activated protein kinase; CQ, chloroquine; FGF, fibroblast growth factor; HCQ, hydroxychloroquine; 11β-HSD1, 11β-hydroxysteroid dehydrogenase type 1; HSP, heat shock protein; mTOT, mitochondrial target of TZDs; mitoNEET, mitochondrial Asn-Glu-Glu-Thr; NOS, nitric oxide synthase; PKA, protein kinase A; PPARγ, peroxisome proliferator-activated receptor γ; TZDs, thiazolidinediones.

market during the past decade for the treatment of T2DM and/or DM-related diseases, none of them specifically target IR except for insulin sensitizers such as thiazolidinediones (TZDs), which are peroxisome proliferator-activated receptor γ (PPARγ) agonists. Insulin sensitizers, which exert positive effects on both insulin target tissues and the pancreas, can potentially reverse the course of the disease and prevent the progression to diabetic complications. Hence, insulin sensitizers would undoubtedly be preferable for T2DM patients, if their side effects, such as fluid retention, weight gain, hemodilution, edema, and congestive heart failure, could be minimized. However, a safe and effective insulin sensitizer remains elusive, as the specific focus on PPARγ-based agents in the past may have partially hampered our efforts towards finding such novel and safer insulin sensitizers. Therefore, this review focuses on recent advances in understanding the pathophysiological mechanisms of IR and describes the PPARγ targets of the classical insulin sensitizers and beyond PPARγ, some newly discovered targets.

2. Classification of New-Generation Insulin Sensitizers

The new-generation insulin sensitizers may be broadly classified as direct PPARγ agonists, selective PPARγ modulators, and PPARγ-sparing compounds (Figure 1). Direct PPARγ

agonists include the pure PPARγ agonists and PPARα/γ dual or PPAR pan agonists. Selective PPARγ modulators are mainly compounds that bind with PPARγ but exhibit little or no agonism and instead inhibit PPARγ phosphorylation at serine 273 in a tissue-selective manner [6]; PPARγ-sparing compounds include those that do not bind with PPARγ but bind with the newly identified mitochondrial targets of TZDs, that is, the mitochondrial outer or inner membrane proteins [7, 8], compounds that target the downstream effectors of PPARγ, such as the adiponectin and fibroblast growth factor 21 (FGF21) signaling pathways, heat shock protein (HSP) inducers, 5′ adenosine monophosphate-activated protein kinase (AMPK) activators, 11β-hydroxysteroid dehydrogenase type 1 (11β-HSD1) inhibitors, and molecules such as biguanides and chloroquines (CQs), whose molecular targets or mechanisms are still not completely understood.

3. Direct PPARγ Agonists

3.1. Pure/Selective PPARγ Agonists. PPARγ is a member of the nuclear hormone receptor (NR) superfamily and belongs to the NR1C subgroup [9]. It is predominantly expressed in the adipose tissue and in low levels in the liver, muscles, and other tissues [6]. TZDs, which are pure PPARγ full agonists, have been widely used to treat T2DM for nearly 20 years and are referred to as the classical "insulin sensitizers," as they act to restore blood glucose to normal levels by increasing the insulin sensitivity of target tissues without the risk of causing hypoglycemia, unlike agents such as secretagogues. The mechanism of action of TZDs involves regulating the expression of a panel of PPARγ downstream target genes associated with glucose and lipid metabolism, adipokines secretion, and inflammatory reactions in target tissues [9, 10]. PPARγ signaling is initiated by the formation of a heterodimer between PPARγ and retinoid X receptor α (RXRα) after the binding of the ligand or agonist to the ligand-binding domain (LBD) of PPARγ and the subsequent dissociation of its corepressors [9, 11]. The PPARγ-RXRα complex then recruits specific coactivators depending on the tissue and cellular environment [6] and regulates gene transcription by binding to specific PPARγ response elements (PPREs) within the promoter region of the target genes (Figure 2). The roles of PPARγ in human and mouse physiology have been reviewed in depth previously [11].

Troglitazone (Rezulin®), the first oral TZD approved in 1997, was discovered before PPARγ was identified as a target of insulin sensitizers. The confirmation of PPARγ as the primary molecular target of TZDs in the mid-1990s spurred the search for novel antidiabetic drugs with stronger PPARγ agonism, although troglitazone was removed from the market in 2001, owing to severe hepatotoxicity [12]. Subsequently, rosiglitazone and pioglitazone, two other pure PPARγ full agonists, were successfully introduced into the market in 1999 for the treatment of T2DM. There was no evidence of hepatotoxicity in clinical trials for either rosiglitazone or pioglitazone [13]. The treatment of T2DM with these drugs was a step toward targeting IR, which is the etiology of the disease, rather than merely promoting insulin release from islet. Therefore, TZDs could potentially rescue the pancreatic islets from the burden of synthesizing and secreting more insulin and consequent functional exhaustion. Although these advantages had resulted in TZDs becoming one of the best-selling drugs in the world for over 10 years, the successive disclosure of adverse events, such as increased cardiovascular risk, fluid retention, bone fractures, hepatotoxicity, and body weight gain, from 2005 onwards posed a severe threat to the clinical prescription of the classical insulin sensitizers [14–16]. Rosiglitazone has been withdrawn by the European Medicines Agency, and its prescription has been restricted by the United States Food and Drug Administration (FDA) [16]. Further, the only available TZD, pioglitazone, carries a black-box warning on the label for potential cardiovascular risks and increased risk of bladder cancer [17]. Thus, the clinical use of first-generation pure PPARγ full agonists has been greatly restricted.

3.2. From Pure PPARγ Agonists to PPARα/γ Dual or PPAR Pan Agonists. In addition to PPARγ, the NR1C subgroup includes two other members, namely, PPARα and PPARβ/δ, which also modulate the expression of a series of target genes that play pleiotropic roles in regulating glucose, lipid, and cholesterol metabolism. These characteristics have made the three PPAR subtypes attractive therapeutic targets for developing novel drugs against T2DM and other metabolic diseases. PPARα agonists (fibrates), which are currently being

marketed as effective hypolipidemic agents that decrease the progression of atherosclerosis, have also been found to improve glucose intolerance in T2DM animals and patients [18, 19]. These findings suggest that the simultaneous activation of both PPARα and PPARγ using a single molecule may combine the advantages of PPARα and PPARγ agonism and avoid some of the disadvantages of pure PPARγ agonists [20]. The development of such potent PPARα/γ dual agonists or PPAR pan agonists as insulin sensitizer candidates was hotly pursued by global pharmaceutical companies from 1998 to 2006, with the expectation of providing a broad spectrum of beneficial metabolic effects [21, 22]. However, the unpredictable side effects, such as carcinogenesis and cardiovascular adverse events, of these newly reported PPARα/γ dual agonists in clinical trials discouraged researchers and almost led to the termination of basic and clinical research on these drugs. Nevertheless, the potential to develop multitargeted PPARα/γ/δ pan agonists as antidiabetic or hypolipidemic drugs is still being actively investigated in some locations [23–26].

4. Selective PPARγ Modulators (sPPARγMs)

As genetic and epidemic studies indicated that the side effects of TZDs were associated with the overactivation of PPARγ, and physiologically appropriate PPARγ activity was beneficial for reducing IR and other T2DM-related risks, partial PPARγ agonists were extensively researched for a short period. Choi et al. reported in 2010 that cyclin-dependent kinase 5-(CDK5-) stimulated phosphorylation at serine 273 of PPARγ (pSer273PPARγ), which led to the dysregulated expression of a set of genes in adipose tissue, especially the epididymal white fat tissue (eWAT), was the critical link between obesity and IR, and pSer273PPARγ inhibition rather than PPARγ agonism was responsible for the insulin-sensitizing and antidiabetic effects of PPARγ agonists [27, 28]. Thus, these distinctive properties of PPARγ suggested the possibility of selectively modulating it such that beneficial therapeutic effects could be attained without the unwanted effects of traditional PPARγ full agonists.

The compounds discovered based on this concept have been variously termed selective PPARγ modulators (sPPARγMs), partial PPARγ agonists, or nonagonist PPARγ ligands in the literature. In this review, we uniformly refer to them as sPPARγMs. Unlike classical PPARγ full agonists, sPPARγMs bind to the LBD of PPARγ in various ways via an activation function 2 motif (AF2) that displays great flexibility in response to diverse ligands, resulting in different receptor conformations and coactivator and/or corepressor recruitment in different tissues [6]. Thus, sPPARγMs selectively regulate the expression of genes that are responsible for insulin sensitization, such as the adiponectin gene, without affecting the transcription of genes related to weight gain, adipogenesis, and fluid retention. Several sPPARγMs, such as UHC1 (modified from SR1664), CMHX008, INT131, balaglitazone, and L312 have been successfully developed by various institutions [29–33] and demonstrated to be potent insulin sensitizers with similar antidiabetic effects as TZDs and better safety profiles, with decreased incidence of TZD-like

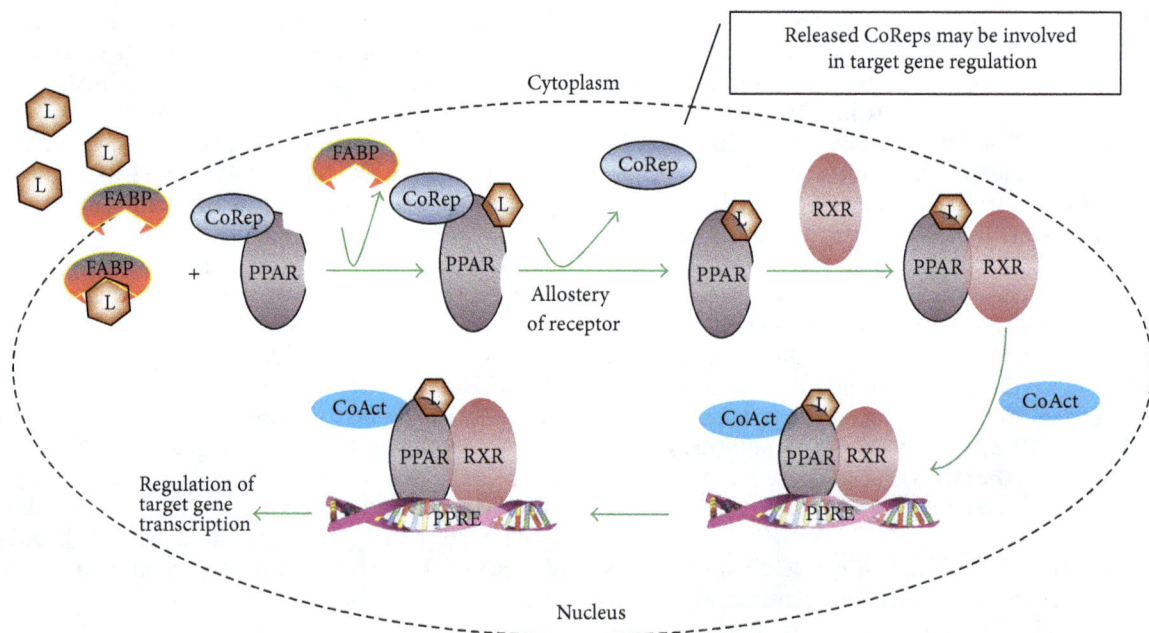

FIGURE 2: *Schematic representation of the mechanism of PPARγ agonist signaling.* L, ligand (including natural ligand and synthetic PPARγ agonist); CoRep, corepressor; CoAct, coactivator; FABP, fatty acid-binding protein; PPAR, peroxisome proliferator-activated receptor; RXR, retinoid X receptor; PPRE, PPARγ response elements.

adverse effects such as heart failure, peripheral edema, and myocardial infarction. These studies suggest that focusing on sPPARγMs presents a great opportunity for developing antidiabetic drugs that offer the desired efficacy of PPARγ agonists without some of their potential adverse effects, although it remains a challenging endeavor. Additionally, it is critical to investigate the different conformations of PPARγ in the presence of distinct ligands, as the ligands interact in different ways with the receptor, recruit different coactivators/corepressors, and exhibit different interactions with the response element, thus triggering the transcription of diverse genes. This may even make it possible to accurately predict the effects of a particular agent.

5. PPARγ-Sparing Compounds

5.1. Ligands/Modulators of the Mitochondrial Targets of TZDs. Several recent studies have proposed that PPARγ could not be completely responsible for the insulin-sensitizing efficacy of the classical TZDs [7, 34, 35]. The identification of a novel binding site for TZDs in the mitochondrial membrane has instead suggested the presence of an alternative, PPARγ-independent mode of action for this class of TZD drugs, which in turn signals the possibility of rationally designing insulin sensitizers that are distinct from PPAR-activating compounds.

5.1.1. MitoNEET (or CDGSH1) Ligands. MitoNEET (mitochondrial Asn-Glu-Glu-Thr), an iron-sulfur- (Fe-S-) containing mitochondrial outer membrane protein that is involved in transferring the Fe-S clusters to the cytosolic aconitase [36],

had been identified by several research groups as a binding target of the insulin sensitizer pioglitazone [37–39]. A potential ligand-binding site, which was identified on the surface of both protomers of the mitoNEET homodimer via blind docking using AutoDock Vina and in vitro fluorescence binding assays, was used as the basis for generating a number of structurally diverse, novel mitoNEET ligands that were structurally distinct from TZDs [39]. Similarly, a mitoNEET ligand, TT01001, which was designed based on the structure of pioglitazone, was reported to show the same potency as pioglitazone in improving hyperglycemia, hyperlipidemia, and glucose intolerance in diabetic (db/db) mice by significantly suppressing the elevated mitochondrial complex activity of skeletal muscles, without activating PPARγ or causing weight gain [40]. MitoNEET has thus been considered a potential target in the treatment of T2DM. Although further studies are required to thoroughly enumerate the physiological role of mitoNEET in regulating the mitochondrial function and its role in DM, current research indicates that alteration of mitochondrial function via mitoNEET may be a valuable insulin-sensitizing strategy.

5.1.2. Mitochondrial Target of TZDs (mTOT) Protein Complex Modulators. As the cross-linking of mitochondrial membranes by TZD probes was observed to occur even in the complete absence of mitoNEET, a study published in 2013 found that mitoNEET was not the primary mitochondrial TZD target [7]. Further studies using radiolabeled TZD probes identified mitochondrial pyruvate carrier 2 (Mpc2 or BRP44), a different protein similar in size to mitoNEET in the inner mitochondrial membrane, as the true binding partner of TZDs. TZDs can rapidly suppress glucose production in perfused livers or isolated hepatocytes and increase glucose uptake in myocytes (within 90 min of TZD treatment) directly by specifically inhibiting Mpc-mediated pyruvate transport into the mitochondria [35, 41]. Mpc, formed by two paralogous subunits, Mpc1 and Mpc2, serves as the channel to facilitate pyruvate transport across the impermeable mitochondrial membrane [8]. Knockdown of Mpc1 or Mpc2 in flies or preincubation with a specific pyruvate transport inhibitor (UK5099) can block the cross-linking of mitochondrial membranes by TZD probes [7]. Importantly, UK5099 can reproduce the effects of TZDs on glucose uptake and hepatic gluconeogenesis from pyruvate [35, 42]. Moreover, mice lacking hepatic MPC2 display impaired hepatic mitochondrial pyruvate metabolism and gluconeogenesis [43]. These data strongly suggest that mild MPC inhibition can be insulin-sensitizing. The newly discovered mTOT should contain at least Mpc1 and Mpc2 as part of a multisubunit complex, along with other unidentified proteins that may vary depending on the cell type [7, 35]. It has also been suggested that mTOT should be viewed as a sensor that signals the coordination multiple parallel pathways in different cells or tissues to increase insulin response and fatty acid oxidation [7, 44, 45].

Subsequently, two new representative mTOT modulators, MSDC-0602 and MSDC-0160, were developed based on this concept by the Metabolic Solutions Development Company in 2013 [45], and phases IIa and IIb trials were completed [46]. Although the PPARγ binding and activating ability of these modulators were much weaker than those of pioglitazone, they displayed equivalent efficacy in managing hyperglycemia in T2DM patients and caused significantly lower fluid retention. Additionally, MSDC-0160 could correct the dysregulated gene expression observed in flies with high-sucrose diet-induced DM [7]. Further, knockdown of the Mpc1 ortholog in flies, which reduced the expression of both Mpc1 and Mpc2, prevented all responses to MSDC-0160 [45]. These data support the hypothesis that the PPARγ binding and activating ability can be uncoupled from the insulin-sensitizing ability. The mitochondrial protein complex, mTOT, thus provides a new target for rationally designing PPARγ-spared insulin sensitizers. However, until the precise molecular target of TZDs is finally identified, utilizing a network pharmacology approach aimed at understanding the comprehensive mechanisms of action of TZDs in improving IR and managing DM appears more reasonable.

5.2. Insulin Sensitizers That Target the Downstream Effectors of PPARγ

5.2.1. Adiponectin Receptor (AdipoR) Activators/Agonists.
Adipokines are pleiotropic molecules that play multiple roles in metabolic and inflammatory responses [47]. In recent years, most research efforts have been focused on studying diabetes associated insulin-sensitizing adipokines, such as adiponectin (also known as Acrp30), vaspin visfatin, metrnl (also known as subfatin), and retinol binding protein 4 (RBP4). [47–50]. Their pathophysiological roles are being actively explored. The adipokine itself or its mimics or

derivatives may become a therapeutic target for diabetes and underlying disturbances.

Adiponectin, an adipokine secreted by adipocytes, was originally identified in 1995 [51] and exists as low-, medium-, and high-molecular weight (LMW, MMW, and HMW) oligomers. While each isoform of adiponectin has distinct biological functions, the HMW oligomer is the most biologically active form with respect to glucose homeostasis and possesses the most potent insulin-sensitizing activity. Research over the past two decades suggests that adiponectin plays an important role in the development of IR [47, 52]. Circulating levels of adiponectin were notably reduced (hypoadiponectinemia) under conditions of obesity, IR, and T2DM, whereas overexpression or administration of adiponectin improved overall insulin action and reversed hyperglycemia in obese mice, independent of plasma insulin levels [52, 53]. Although adiponectin by itself appears to be an effective insulin enhancer, the short half-life (32 min for trimers and 83 min for HMW and MMW proteins [54]) and other limitations have hindered its use as a therapeutic drug. Adiponectin is also considered to play a role in the functioning of other insulin sensitizers, as its levels are reportedly increased by TZD treatment, and the insulin-sensitizing effect of TZDs tends to be impaired in adiponectin-deficient mice [55]. Increased adiponectin levels also promote the PPARγ pathway and form a positive feedback loop that comprehensively addresses the cause of IR and DM.

Adiponectin predominantly binds to the AdipoR1 and AdipoR2 receptors [56], which are abundantly expressed in the skeletal muscle and liver, respectively [57]. These receptors regulate metabolic gene expression and insulin sensitivity in insulin target tissues and play important roles in the development of IR and DM. The reduced expression of AdipoRs in obesity and DM is correlated with a decrease in the effect of adiponectin [52]. Adiponectin exerts its antidiabetic effects by binding to the two AdipoRs and activating the PPARα and AMPK pathways, with APPL1 (adaptor protein, phosphotyrosine interacting with PH domain and leucine zipper 1) as the key adaptor that directly binds to the intracellular domains of AdipoRs via its C-terminal phosphotyrosine binding (PTB) and coiled-coil (CC) domains. This leads to enhanced fatty acid oxidation and decreased hepatic glucose production, which is independent of insulin levels or glucose disposal rate in peripheral tissues [52, 56, 58]. A more comprehensive review of adiponectin signaling has been presented previously [52, 59]. In contrast, the disruption of both AdipoR subtypes has been found to abolish the effects of adiponectin, resulting in elevated lipid accumulation in insulin target issues (mainly the liver and skeletal muscles) and finally leading to IR [56].

Recently, the first orally active AdipoR activator, AdipoRon, which binds to both AdipoRs and ameliorates IR and glucose intolerance in high-fat diet-induced obese mice in an AdipoR-dependent manner, was discovered [60]. AdipoRon has also been shown to reverse the diabetic condition of genetically diabetic db/db mice and prolong their lifespan [61]. Additionally, it exerted cardioprotective effects against postischemic cardiac injury, a common DM-related cardiovascular complication [62]. However, the low affinity of

AdipoR for the currently available small molecule activators is an unresolved challenge. Thus, based on current studies, the AdipoR signaling pathway remains a potential pharmacological target for IR and T2DM, and adiponectin derivatives or orally active small molecules with higher affinity to AdipoR may give rise to novel insulin sensitizers for the treatment of T2DM in the near future.

5.2.2. Fibroblast Growth Factor 21 (FGF21) and Its Derivatives. FGF21, a member of the endocrine FGF subfamily, has been identified as a PPARγ target in the adipose tissue. As a hormone that plays pleiotropic roles in regulating glucose and lipid homeostasis, insulin sensitivity, and cellular oxidative stress, its glucose-lowering effect has been well demonstrated in various diabetic mouse and primate models [63–67]. Recently, FGF1, the prototype of the 22-member FGF family, was found to be transcriptionally regulated by PPARγ in adipose tissue, and the PPRE was identified within the FGF1 gene [65, 68]. FGF1 knockout mice developed severe IR and an aggressive diabetic phenotype when challenged with a high-fat diet [68]. Recombinant FGF1 (rFGF1) administered by injection dose-dependently ameliorated insulin insensitivity and hyperinsulinemia, normalized glucose levels, and increased the hepatic glycogen content in genetically diabetic (ob/ob and db/db) and high-fat diet-induced obese insulin-resistant mice, with no hypoglycemia even at higher doses [69]. Further, there was no resistance to the treatment in ob/ob mice, when the treatment was extended over 1 month. The FGF1-mediated whole-body insulin sensitization was attributed to a simultaneous increase in insulin-dependent glucose uptake in target tissues and suppression of hepatic glucose production.

Studies by Lin et al. [70] revealed that the insulin-sensitizing adipokine, adiponectin, was a downstream effector of FGF21 that coupled the effects of FGF21 in local adipocytes to the liver and skeletal muscles, thus mediating the systemic effects of FGF21 on energy metabolism and insulin sensitivity. Significantly, these benefits were not accompanied by side effects, such as weight gain, fluid retention, and bone loss that are commonly associated with TZDs, the classical insulin sensitizers. Moreover, FGF1 did not stimulate insulin release from the pancreatic islets or possess insulin-mimetic effects but could markedly enhance the glucose-lowering effects of exogenously supplied insulin in streptozotocin-induced type 1 DM (T1DM) mouse models [69], without affecting the blood glucose and insulin levels in chow-fed normoglycemic mice [68]. Similarly, FGF21 increased insulin content and secretion in diabetic islets and protected the pancreatic β cells from apoptosis by activating the extracellular signal-regulated kinase 1/2 (ERK1/2) and Akt signaling pathways [71]. These recent findings collectively indicate that FGF1 and FGF21 possess all the characteristics of a good insulin sensitizer without TZD-like adverse effects.

Other studies have found that FGF1 may be exerting its insulin-sensitizing activity through the FGF1 receptor (FGFR1) in adipose tissue, although it can bind and activate all alternatively spliced forms of the four tyrosine kinase FGF receptors (FGFR1–FGFR4). rFGF1 and rFGF$^{\Delta DNT}$, which are FGF1 ligands generated by removing the first 24 residues from the amino terminus of FGF1, lost their glucose-lowering effect on adipose tissue, specifically in FGFR1 knockout mice [72]. In addition, LY2405319, an engineered FGF21 variant, has recently been found to be effective in alleviating IR in diabetic mice and monkeys [73, 74]. Thus, we can tentatively conclude that FGF receptor-targeted ligands or derivatives of FGF21 and FGF1 are promising insulin sensitizer candidates for fighting T2DM. However, as with all protein-based therapeutics, some major hurdles, such as a short half-life, enzymatic degradation, and low bioavailability, still need to be overcome, and further clinical studies are required to verify whether these candidates can act as effective antidiabetic agents in humans.

5.3. HSP/Nitric Oxide Synthase (NOS) Inducers. BGP-15 [O-(3-piperidino-2-hydroxy-1-propyl)-nicotinic acid], an HSP/chaperone inducer that was originally developed as a chemoprotectant, has been identified as a new type of insulin sensitizer with a novel pharmacological mechanism [75, 76]. BGP-15 has been found to significantly improve insulin sensitivity in both insulin-resistant (ob/ob) mice and diabetic (Goto-Kakizaki [GK]) rats and insulin-resistant patients. Further, BGP-15, which does not activate PPAR, has comparable efficacy to that of rosiglitazone and metformin and produces dose-dependent insulin sensitization in diabetic GK rats and hypercholesterolemic rabbits [76]. A 4-week phase IIb clinical trial involving insulin-resistant, nondiabetic patients demonstrated that BGP-15 can significantly increase whole-body insulin sensitivity and glucose utilization. Moreover, the treatment efficacy was comparable to that associated with 12-13 weeks of rosiglitazone treatment, and BGP-15 was well tolerated with a favorable safety profile. BGP-15 was found to interact directly with heat shock factor 1 (HSF-1) and stabilize the binding of HSF-1 to its DNA response element [77]. Mechanistic studies have shown that BGP-15 functions by inhibiting c-Jun amino-terminal kinase (JNK) phosphorylation and stimulating and upregulating the HSP (HSP90 and HSP72) and NOS (constitutive NOS and neuronal NOS) systems that are decreased or deficient in people suffering from IR or DM [78–82].

The inducible HSP72 is the most abundant of all HSPs, accounting for 1-2% of cellular protein, and is rapidly induced during cellular stress. Intracellular levels of HSP72 and HSP90 have been found to correlate with whole-body glucose utilization. The induced HSPs enhance insulin sensitivity by inhibiting the kinase cascades required for activating IκB kinase (IKK) and c-JNK, the inflammatory signaling protein that plays a vital role in the development of IR, thus preventing the phosphorylation of a key serine residue in insulin receptor substrate 1 (IRS-1) [83]. Subsequently, the insulin-sensitizing effects of BGP-15 are realized through multiple downstream pathways, including those that improve mitochondrial function, protect against hyperglycemia-induced mitochondrial damage, normalize the mitochondrial membrane potential, and prevent mitochondrial depletion and structural alteration [76, 84, 85]. As previous studies have indicated that mitochondrial dysfunction and metabolic overload are possibly the primary causes of IR, BGP-15, which is currently under further development, is a promising drug candidate for improving glycemic control and insulin sensitivity in people with T2DM.

5.4. 11β-HSD1 Inhibitors. 11β-HSD1 oxidoreductase converts the inactive 11-keto forms of GCs (glucocorticoids), such as cortisone, to their active forms, such as cortisol and corticosterone, in metabolically active tissues, including the liver and adipose tissue. Elevated GC levels have been implicated in glucose intolerance, IR, dyslipidemia, and visceral obesity [86, 87]. 11β-HSD1 is upregulated in the adipose tissues of rodents and patients with metabolic syndrome [88, 89]. Animal studies have shown that adipose-specific 11β-HSD1 knockout mice are refractory to diet-induced obesity and show improved glucose tolerance and insulin sensitivity, whereas transgenic mice overexpressing 11β-HSD1 in fat cells have been found to develop glucose intolerance, IR, and dyslipidemia [90, 91]. As inhibition of 11β-HSD1 can decrease the levels of active GCs owing to its specific role in GC interconversion, 11β-HSD1 has been considered an attractive therapeutic target for the treatment of IR, T2DM, and metabolic syndrome [87, 92].

Several structurally diverse and selective 11β-HSD1 inhibitors, such as HIS-388, LG13, and PF-915275, have thus been designed [92, 93]. The antidiabetic activity of these inhibitors has been confirmed to be comparable to that of the classical insulin sensitizer pioglitazone in different insulin-resistant and/or diabetic rodent models [92, 94, 95], where the inhibitors significantly suppressed the levels of plasma and local tissue cortisol, plasma insulin, and fasting or postprandial blood glucose, and improved glucose intolerance and IR. Moreover, some 11β-HSD1 inhibitors have shown the same therapeutic efficacy in human clinical trials as well as in animal studies, with tolerable adverse events and no effects on basal cortisol homeostasis or normal sex hormone levels [96]. However, 11β-HSD1 inhibitors, which are promising insulin sensitizers, are still in the early stages of development, and no drugs of this class have entered phase III clinical trials. Additionally, as 11β-HSD1 is a bidirectional enzyme, which functions as both a reductase (major) and an oxidase (minor), a safer inhibitor that selectively inhibits 11β-HSD1 reductase activity would be preferable [86, 87].

5.5. AMPK Activators/Agonists. AMPK, a phylogenetically conserved serine/threonine kinase, is a master metabolic sensor of cellular energy status that regulates the cellular and whole-body energy balance. It is a heterotrimer consisting of a catalytic α subunit and regulatory β and γ subunits [97]. Several studies have suggested that AMPK is important in regulating insulin signaling, and dysregulation of the AMPK pathway plays critical roles in the development of IR and T2DM [98–100]. AMPK activators have been comprehensively reviewed previously [97]. AMPK activators, such as 5-aminoimidazole-4-carboxamide-1-β-d-ribofuranoside (AICAR), biguanides, and A-769662 (the first direct AMPK activator), have been found to reverse many of the metabolic defects associated with IR, whereas the absence or inhibition of AMPK exacerbates insulin insensitivity in target tissues [97, 101, 102]. These findings have made

AMPK an attractive T2DM drug target during the past two decades. AMPK, which is activated by the phosphorylation of Thr 172 on the activation loop of the catalytic subunit by upstream kinases, stimulates glucose uptake in skeletal muscles and fatty acid oxidation in target tissues and reduces hepatic glucose production and output, partially by inhibiting the mTORC1 (mechanistic target of rapamycin complex 1)/STAT3 (signal transducer and activator of transcription 3)/Notch1 (Notch homolog 1, translocation-associated) signaling pathway [97]. The physiological functions of AMPK have been reviewed in depth previously [97, 103].

As AMPK is involved in numerous pathophysiological processes and implicated in many conditions, such as anemia, inflammation, and tumors, excessive systemic activation of AMPK may undoubtedly cause unwanted side effects, although most of its effects are beneficial. Therefore, in the absence of tissue-selective activation strategies or compounds with isoform specificity, developing a specific AMPK activator into a safer insulin sensitizer is extremely challenging [100]. Thus, despite being a seemingly promising target for drug development, no direct AMPK activators have entered clinical trials as insulin sensitizers yet. However, the effects of some multitarget drugs such as the antidiabetic effects of metformin and TZDs appear to be mediated, at least in part, by the direct or indirect activation of AMPK [104, 105]. Further investigation of AMPK regulation and its role in cellular metabolism may uncover new strategies for efficiently controlling the pharmacological modulation of AMPK using activators.

5.6. Biguanides (Metformin). Metformin is the most representative agent of the biguanide class and the most widely prescribed antidiabetic drug to date, despite its precise mechanism of action being unknown and under active investigation. Studies indicate that metformin decreases IR and improves insulin sensitivity by facilitating the postreceptor transport of insulin and exerting positive effects on insulin receptor expression and tyrosine kinase activity, thus enhancing the insulin-mediated suppression of hepatic glucose production and insulin-stimulated glucose uptake in skeletal muscles and adipose tissues [106, 107]. At the molecular level, inhibition of complex I of the electron transport chain in mitochondria, which was once considered to be a primary target of metformin [108, 109], is believed to enhance cellular glycolysis and AMP production. However, metformin-mediated inhibition of complex I in isolated mitochondria has not been detected directly. Further, some studies, which failed to detect any change in cellular AMP levels, have nevertheless revealed that metformin can activate AMPK efficiently in primary hepatocytes and the liver of mice without affecting the energy state [110]. Moreover, Zhang et al. [111] found that metformin treatment could mimic a state of austere nutrient supply and activate AMPK and inactivate mTORC1 through the AXIN/LKB1-v-ATPase-Ragulator pathway (Figure 3), rather than as a mere consequence of disrupting metabolic processes via the inhibition of oxidative phosphorylation. The inhibition of interstitial fibrosis by metformin may also be attributable to

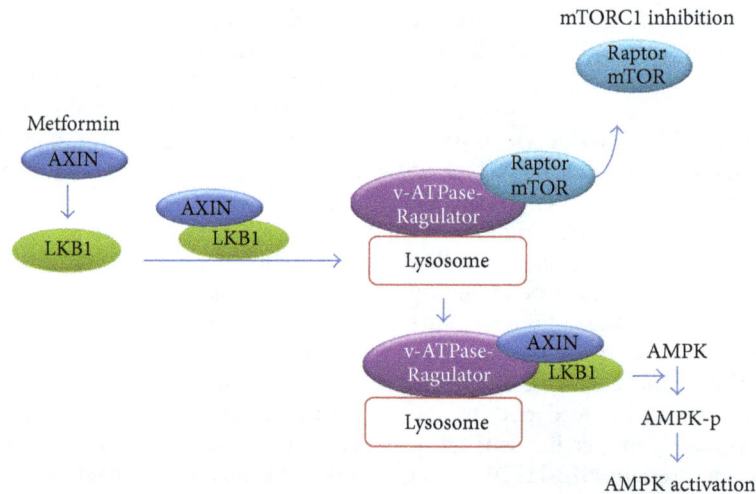

FIGURE 3: *Metformin-mediated activation of 5′ adenosine monophosphate-activated protein kinase (AMPK) through the AXIN/LKB1-v-ATPase-Ragulator pathway.* The lysosomal v-ATPase-Ragulator complex serves as an initiating sensor for switching between AMPK and mechanistic target of rapamycin (mTOR) activation. Metformin can directly act on v-ATPase and promote the translocation of AXIN/LKB1 onto the lysosomal surface to form a complex with v-ATPase-Ragulator, thus leading to AMPK activation and the simultaneous dissociation of Raptor and mTOR, which results in the suppression of mTOR complex 1 (mTORC1) [111].

AMPK activation and transforming growth factor β1 (TGF-β1)/Smad3 signaling suppression, which leads to the suppression of aberrant extracellular matrix (ECM) remodeling in adipose tissues and an increase in systemic insulin sensitivity [112]. As TGF-β1 signaling inhibits the LKB1-AMPK axis and thus facilitates the nuclear translocation of forkhead box protein O1 (FoxO1) and activation of key gluconeogenic genes, such as those of glucose-6-phosphatase (G6P) and phosphoenolpyruvate carboxykinase (PEPCK), suppression of TGF-β1/Smad3 signaling is linked to the suppression of hepatic gluconeogenesis [113].

Although numerous potential mechanisms have been reported for elucidating the metformin-mediated improvement in insulin sensitivity, these mechanisms uniformly indicate that AMPK activation is the central step and differ only with respect to the adaptors between metformin and AMPK activation. Metformin can thus inhibit gluconeogenesis and activate glycolysis by activating hepatic AMPK. In adipose cells, AMPK activation was shown to increase the phosphorylation of the JNK-c-Jun and mTOR-p70S6 kinase pathways and suppress the expression of phosphatase and tension homolog (PTEN), which is a negative regulator of insulin signaling [114]. Metformin also induced glucose transporter type 4 (GLUT4) translocation by increasing the phosphorylation of Cbl and expression of Cbl-associated protein (CAP) signals via AMPK activation [115]. Therefore, AMPK activation, protein kinase A (PKA) inhibition, inhibition of mitochondrial respiration, and redox stress may all play a role in the comprehensive pharmacological effect of metformin against DM. However, unless the exact binding target of metformin is identified, finding a biguanide insulin sensitizer capable of surpassing metformin in efficacy and safety will be challenging.

5.7. Chloroquines (CQs). CQs, which were originally developed as antimalarial drugs, are lately being used to treat autoimmune diseases such as rheumatoid arthritis and lupus erythematosus. Interestingly, several recent studies have demonstrated their beneficial effects against both T1DM and T2DM [116]. Some reports indicate that CQ increases the binding of insulin to its receptor and potentiates insulin-mediated inhibition of hepatic gluconeogenesis [117]. Hydroxychloroquine (HCQ) has been found to significantly increase the insulin sensitivity index (ISI) and show a tendency to reduce IR (as assessed by the homeostatic model assessment for insulin resistance [HOMA-IR]) [118]. However, only a thorough understanding of the mechanisms responsible for these favorable metabolic effects, which currently remain ill-defined, may give rise to an attractive alternative therapeutic option for treating IR and DM. A clinical trial conducted on T2DM patients to investigate the metabolic effects of HCQ on blood glucose, blood pressure, and blood cholesterol was completed in 2015 and aims to contribute to the development of a new therapeutic approach to metabolic syndrome and DM (ClinicalTrials.gov identifier: NCT02026232). Similarly, a "proof-of-concept" randomized double-blinded placebo-controlled trial titled "Rediscovering Hydroxychloroquine as a Novel Insulin Sensitizer" involving insulin-resistant subjects is expected to conclude in 2017 (ClinicalTrials.gov identifier: NCT02124681). This study, which evaluates the insulin-sensitizing effects of HCQ and explores the mechanism by which HCQ affects glucose metabolism and its target organs, may determine whether HCQ can act as a potential therapeutic lead for IR disorders.

6. Conclusion

The critical role played by IR in the pathogenesis of T2DM and the limitations of currently available insulin sensitizers such as TZDs encourage the development of new insulin sensitizers with a higher safety profile. The recent lessons learned from developing powerful PPARγ or PPARα/γ agonists into insulin sensitizers suggest that our efforts towards finding safer insulin sensitizers may be successful only when we go beyond focusing specifically on PPARγ. Moreover, several compounds with completely different modes of action have been identified in recent years. These molecules have shown promising results in early stages of development and represent diverse approaches in the search for a new generation of insulin sensitizers without TZD-like adverse effects. However, several limitations still need to be addressed, and further studies are required before these leads can be successfully developed for the clinical setting. As the identification of a potential drug target and thorough investigation of its pathophysiological functions is a long-term reiterative verification process, whether the drug targets reviewed here would lead to the development of an effective, marketable insulin sensitizer remains to be seen. Therefore, the success of any of the approaches described in this review would represent great progress, and the resulting insulin sensitizer, which would not exhibit TZD-like side effects, will undoubtedly be a valuable antidiabetic agent in the future.

Conflicts of Interest

The authors declare that there are no conflicts of interest regarding the publication of this paper.

Acknowledgments

The research was supported by the National Natural Science Foundation of China (Grant no. 81102308) and the Major Program of the Ministry of Science and Technology of China (Grants nos. 2013ZX09J13301 and 2012ZX09J12109-02C).

References

[1] Global report on diabetes, http://www.who.int/mediacentre/factsheets/fs312/en/.

[2] T. Or, T. Lm, and P. Mr, "Type 2 diabetes mellitus in children and adolescents: a relatively new clinical problem within pediatric practice," *Journal of Medicine and Life*, vol. 9, pp. 235–239, 2016.

[3] H. E. Lebovitz, "Insulin resistance: definition and consequences," *Experimental And Clinical Endocrinology & Diabetes*, vol. 109, supplement 2, pp. S135–S148, 2001.

[4] J. Boucher, A. Kleinridders, and C. Ronald Kahn, "Insulin receptor signaling in normal and insulin-resistant states," *Cold Spring Harbor Perspectives in Biology*, vol. 6, no. 1, Article ID a009191, 2014.

[5] D. D. Sears, G. Hsiao, A. Hsiao et al., "Mechanisms of human insulin resistance and thiazolidinedione-mediated insulin sensitization," *Proceedings of the National Academy of Sciences of the United States of America*, vol. 106, no. 44, pp. 18745–18750, 2009.

[6] L. S. Higgins and A. M. Depaoli, "Selective peroxisome proliferator-activated receptor γ (PPARγ) modulation as a strategy for safer therapeutic PPARγ activation," *The American Journal of Clinical Nutrition*, vol. 91, no. 1, pp. 267S–272S, 2010.

[7] J. R. Colca, W. G. McDonald, G. S. Cavey et al., "Identification of a Mitochondrial Target of Thiazolidinedione Insulin Sensitizers (mTOT)-Relationship to Newly Identified Mitochondrial Pyruvate Carrier Proteins," *PLoS ONE*, vol. 8, no. 5, Article ID e61551, 2013.

[8] K. S. McCommis and B. N. Finck, "Mitochondrial pyruvate transport: a historical perspective and future research directions," *Biochemical Journal*, vol. 466, no. 3, pp. 443–454, 2015.

[9] C. Janani and B. D. Ranjitha Kumari, "PPAR gamma gene—a review," *Diabetes & Metabolic Syndrome*, vol. 9, pp. 46–50, 2015.

[10] J. M. Olefsky, "Treatment of insulin resistance with peroxisome proliferator-activated receptor γ agonists," *Journal of Clinical Investigation*, vol. 106, no. 4, pp. 467–472, 2000.

[11] S. Heikkinen, J. Auwerx, and C. A. Argmann, "PPARγ in human and mouse physiology," *Biochimica et Biophysica Acta: Molecular and Cell Biology of Lipids*, vol. 1771, no. 8, pp. 999–1013, 2007.

[12] H. E. Lebovitz, "Differentiating members of the thiazolidinedione class: a focus on safety," *Diabetes/Metabolism Research and Reviews*, vol. 18, no. 2, pp. S23-S29, 2002.

[13] A. B. King, "A comparison in a clinical setting of the efficacy and side effects of three thiazolidinediones," *Diabetes Care*, vol. 23, no. 4, p. 557, 2000.

[14] P. S. Chaggar, S. M. Shaw, and S. G. Williams, "Review article: thiazolidinediones and heart failure," *Diabetes & Vascular Disease Research*, vol. 6, pp. 146–152, 2009.

[15] A. V. Hernandez, A. Usmani, A. Rajamanickam, and A. Moheet, "Thiazolidinediones and risk of heart failure in patients with or at high risk of type 2 diabetes mellitus: a meta-analysis and meta-regression analysis of placebo-controlled randomized clinical trials," *American Journal of Cardiovascular Drugs*, vol. 11, no. 2, pp. 115–128, 2011.

[16] D. Alemán-González-Duhart, F. Tamay-Cach, S. Álvarez-Almazán, and J. E. Mendieta-Wejebe, "Current advances in the biochemical and physiological aspects of the treatment of type 2 diabetes mellitus with thiazolidinediones," *PPAR Research*, vol. 2016, Article ID 7614270, 2016.

[17] C. H. Tseng, "A review on thiazolidinediones and bladder cancer in human studies," *Journal of Environmental Science and Health. Part C, Environmental Carcinogenesis & Ecotoxicology Reviews*, vol. 32, pp. 1–45, 2014.

[18] S. Haubenwallner, A. D. Essenburg, B. C. Barnett et al., "Hypolipidemic activity of select fibrates correlates to changes in hepatic apolipoprotein C-III expression: a potential physiologic basis for their mode of action," *Journal of Lipid Research*, vol. 36, pp. 2541–2551, 1995.

[19] B. Staels, N. Vu-Dac, V. A. Kosykh et al., "Fibrates downregulate apolipoprotein C-III expression independent of induction of peroxisomal acyl coenzyme A oxidase. A potential mechanism for the hypolipidemic action of fibrates," *Journal of Clinical Investigation*, vol. 95, no. 2, pp. 705–712, 1995.

[20] B. Grygiel-Górniak, "Peroxisome proliferator-activated receptors and their ligands: nutritional and clinical implications—a review," *Nutrition Journal*, vol. 13, article 17, 2014.

[21] N. Zhang, W. Chen, X. Zhou et al., "C333H ameliorated insulin resistance through selectively modulating peroxisome proliferator-activated receptor gamma in brown adipose tissue of db/db mice," *Biological & Pharmaceutical Bulletin*, vol. 36, pp. 980–987, 2013.

[22] C. Fiévet, J.-C. Fruchart, and B. Staels, "PPARα and PPARγ dual agonists for the treatment of type 2 diabetes and the metabolic syndrome," *Current Opinion in Pharmacology*, vol. 6, no. 6, pp. 606–614, 2006.

[23] X.-J. Wang, J. Zhang, S.-Q. Wang, W.-R. Xu, X.-C. Cheng, and R.-L. Wang, "Identification of novel multitargeted PPARα/γ/δ pan agonists by core hopping of rosiglitazone," *Drug Design, Development and Therapy*, vol. 8, pp. 2255–2262, 2014.

[24] A. Tenenbaum and E. Z. Fisman, "Balanced pan-PPAR activator bezafibrate in combination with statin: comprehensive lipids control and diabetes prevention?" *Cardiovascular Diabetology*, vol. 11, article 140, 2012.

[25] W. Chen, S. Fan, X. Xie, N. Xue, X. Jin, and L. Wang, "Novel PPAR pan agonist, ZBH ameliorates hyperlipidemia and insulin resistance in high fat diet induced hyperlipidemic hamster," *PLoS ONE*, vol. 9, no. 4, Article ID e96056, 2014.

[26] M. R. Jain, S. R. Giri, C. Trivedi et al., "Saroglitazar, a novel PPA-Ralpha/gamma agonist with predominant PPARalpha activity, shows lipid-lowering and insulin-sensitizing effects in preclinical models," *Pharmacology Research & Perspectives*, vol. 3, article e00136, 2015.

[27] J. H. Choi, A. S. Banks, J. L. Estall et al., "Anti-diabetic drugs inhibit obesity-linked phosphorylation of PPARγ 3 by Cdk5," *Nature*, vol. 466, no. 7305, pp. 451–456, 2010.

[28] J. H. Choi, A. S. Banks, T. M. Kamenecka et al., "Antidiabetic actions of a non-agonist PPARγ ligand blocking Cdk5-mediated phosphorylation," *Nature*, vol. 477, no. 7365, pp. 477–481, 2011.

[29] S.-S. Choi, E. S. Kim, M. Koh et al., "A novel non-agonist peroxisome proliferator-activated receptor γ (PPARγ) ligand UHC1 blocks PPARγ phosphorylation by cyclin-dependent kinase 5 (CDK5) and improves insulin sensitivity," *Journal of Biological Chemistry*, vol. 289, no. 38, pp. 26618–26629, 2014.

[30] Y. Ming, X. Hu, Y. Song et al., "CMHX008, a novel peroxisome proliferator-activated receptor gamma partial agonist, enhances insulin sensitivity in vitro and in vivo," *PLoS ONE*, vol. 9, no. 7, Article ID e102102, 2014.

[31] R. Agrawal, P. Jain, and S. N. Dikshit, "Balaglitazone: a second generation peroxisome proliferator-activated receptor (PPAR) gamma (γ) agonist," *Mini-Reviews in Medicinal Chemistry*, vol. 12, no. 2, pp. 87–97, 2012.

[32] X. Xie, X. Zhou, W. Chen et al., "L312, a novel PPARγ ligand with potent anti-diabetic activity by selective regulation," *Biochimica et Biophysica Acta—General Subjects*, vol. 1850, no. 1, pp. 62–72, 2015.

[33] D. H. Lee, H. Huang, K. Choi, C. Mantzoros, and Y.-B. Kim, "Selective PPARγ modulator INT131 normalizes insulin signaling defects and improves bone mass in diet-induced obese mice," *American Journal of Physiology—Endocrinology and Metabolism*, vol. 302, no. 5, pp. E552-E560, 2012.

[34] M. Sanz, C. Sánchez-Martín, D. Detaille et al., "Acute mitochondrial actions of glitazones on the liver: a crucial parameter for their antidiabetic properties," *Cellular Physiology and Biochemistry*, vol. 28, no. 5, pp. 899–910, 2011.

[35] A. S. Divakaruni, S. E. Wiley, G. W. Rogers et al., "Thiazolidinediones are acute, specific inhibitors of the mitochondrial pyruvate carrier," *Proceedings of the National Academy of Sciences of the United States of America*, vol. 110, no. 14, pp. 5422–5427, 2013.

[36] G. Tan, D. Liu, F. Pan et al., "His-87 ligand in mitoNEET is crucial for the transfer of iron sulfur clusters from mitochondria to cytosolic aconitase," *Biochemical and Biophysical Research Communications*, vol. 470, no. 1, pp. 226–232, 2016.

[37] J. R. Colca, W. G. McDonald, D. J. Waldon et al., "Mathews, Identification of a novel mitochondrial protein ('mitoNEET') cross-linked specifically by a thiazolidinedione photoprobe,"

American Journal of Physiology. Endocrinology And Metabolism, vol. 286, pp. E252-260, 2004.

[38] M. L. Paddock, S. E. Wiley, H. L. Axelrod et al., "MitoNEET is a uniquely folded 2Fe-2S outer mitochondrial membrane protein stabilized by pioglitazone," *Proceedings of The National Academy of Sciences of The United States of America*, vol. 104, pp. 14342–14347, 2007.

[39] R. M. Bieganski and M. L. Yarmush, "Novel ligands that target the mitochondrial membrane protein mitoNEET," *Journal of Molecular Graphics & Modelling*, vol. 29, no. 7, pp. 965–973, 2011.

[40] T. Takahashi, M. Yamamoto, K. Amikura et al., "A novel Mito-NEET ligand, TT01001, improves diabetes and ameliorates mitochondrial function in db/db mice," *Journal of Pharmacology and Experimental Therapeutics*, vol. 352, no. 2, pp. 338–345, 2015.

[41] P. Raman and R. L. Judd, "Role of glucose and insulin in thiazolidinedione-induced alterations in hepatic gluconeogenesis," *European Journal of Pharmacology*, vol. 409, no. 1, pp. 19–29, 2000.

[42] A. P. Thomas and A. P. Halestrap, "The role of mitochondrial pyruvate transport in the stimulation by glucagon and phenylephrine of gluconeogenesis from L-lactate in isolated rat hepatocytes," *Biochemical Journal*, vol. 198, no. 3, pp. 551–560, 1981.

[43] K. S. McCommis, Z. Chen, X. Fu et al., "Loss of mitochondrial pyruvate carrier 2 in the liver leads to defects in gluconeogenesis and compensation via pyruvate-alanine cycling," *Cell Metabolism*, vol. 22, no. 4, pp. 682–694, 2015.

[44] J. R. Colca, S. P. Tanis, W. G. McDonald, and R. F. Kletzien, "Insulin sensitizers in 2013: new insights for the development of novel therapeutic agents to treat metabolic diseases," *Expert Opinion on Investigational Drugs*, vol. 23, no. 1, pp. 1–7, 2014.

[45] R. C. Shah, D. C. Matthews, R. D. Andrews et al., "An evaluation of MSDC-0160, a prototype mTOT modulating insulin sensitizer, in patients with mild Alzheimer's disease," *Current Alzheimer Research*, vol. 11, no. 6, pp. 564–573, 2014.

[46] J. R. Colca, J. T. Vanderlugt, W. J. Adams et al., "Clinical proof-of-concept study with MSDC-0160, a prototype mTOT-modulating insulin sensitizer," *Clinical Pharmacology and Therapeutics*, vol. 93, no. 4, pp. 352–359, 2013.

[47] V. Andrade-Oliveira, N. O. Câmara, and P. M. Moraes-Vieira, "Adipokines as drug targets in diabetes and underlying disturbances," *Journal of Diabetes Research*, vol. 2015, Article ID 681612, 11 pages, 2015.

[48] R. Dimova and T. Tankova, "The role of vaspin in the development of metabolic and glucose tolerance disorders and atherosclerosis," *BioMed Research International*, vol. 2015, Article ID 823481, 7 pages, 2015.

[49] Z.-Y. Li, J. Song, S.-L. Zheng et al., "Adipocyte Metrnl Antagonizes Insulin Resistance Through PPARγ Signaling," *Diabetes*, vol. 64, no. 12, pp. 4011–4022, 2015.

[50] S. L. Zheng, Z. Y. Li, J. Song, J. M. Liu, and C. Y. Miao, "Metrnl: a secreted protein with new emerging functions," *Acta Pharmacologica Sinica*, vol. 37, pp. 571–579, 2016.

[51] P. E. Scherer, S. Williams, M. Fogliano, G. Baldini, and H. F. Lodish, "A novel serum protein similar to C1q, produced exclusively in adipocytes," *The Journal of Biological Chemistry*, vol. 270, no. 45, pp. 26746–26749, 1995.

[52] H. Ruan and L. Q. Dong, "Adiponectin signaling and function in insulin target tissues," *Journal of Molecular Cell Biology*, vol. 8, no. 2, pp. 101–109, 2016.

[53] T. Yamauchi, J. Kamon, H. Waki et al., "Globular adiponectin protected ob/ob mice from diabetes and ApoE-deficient mice from atherosclerosis," *Journal of Biological Chemistry*, vol. 278, no. 4, pp. 2461–2468, 2003.

[54] N. Halberg, T. D. Schraw, Z. V. Wang et al., "Systemic fate of the adipocyte-derived factor adiponectin," *Diabetes*, vol. 58, no. 9, pp. 1961–1970, 2009.

[55] A. R. Nawrocki, M. W. Rajala, E. Tomas et al., "Mice lacking adiponectin show decreased hepatic insulin sensitivity and reduced responsiveness to peroxisome proliferator-activated receptor γ agonists," *The Journal of Biological Chemistry*, vol. 281, no. 5, pp. 2654–2660, 2006.

[56] T. Yamauchi, Y. Nio, T. Maki et al., "Targeted disruption of AdipoR1 and AdipoR2 causes abrogation of adiponectin binding and metabolic actions," *Nature Medicine*, vol. 13, no. 3, pp. 332–339, 2007.

[57] T. Yamauchi, J. Kamon, Y. Ito et al., "Cloning of adiponectin receptors that mediate antidiabetic metabolic effects," *Nature*, vol. 423, no. 6941, pp. 762–769, 2003.

[58] A. H. Berg, T. P. Combs, X. Du, M. Brownlee, and P. E. Scherer, "The adipocyte-secreted protein Acrp30 enhances hepatic insulin action," *Nature Medicine*, vol. 7, no. 8, pp. 947–953, 2001.

[59] M. Iwabu, T. Yamauchi, M. Okada-Iwabu, and T. Kadowaki, "Adiponectin receptor-targeted therapy for lifestyle-related diseases," *Clinical Calcium*, vol. 26, pp. 413–418, 2016.

[60] M. Okada-Iwabu, T. Yamauchi, M. Iwabu et al., "A small-molecule AdipoR agonist for type 2 diabetes and short life in obesity," *Nature*, vol. 503, no. 7477, pp. 493–499, 2013.

[61] M. Okada-Iwabu, M. Iwabu, K. Ueki, T. Yamauchi, and T. Kadowaki, "Perspective of small-molecule adipoR agonist for type 2 diabetes and short life in obesity," *Diabetes & Metabolism Journal*, vol. 39, pp. 363–372, 2015.

[62] Y. Zhang, J. Zhao, R. Li et al., "AdipoRon, the first orally active adiponectin receptor activator, attenuates postischemic myocardial apoptosis through both AMPK-mediated and AMPK-independent signalings," *American Journal of Physiology—Endocrinology and Metabolism*, vol. 309, no. 3, pp. E275-E282, 2015.

[63] J. A. Seo and N. H. Kim, "Fibroblast growth factor 21: a novel metabolic regulator," *Diabetes & Metabolism Journal*, vol. 36, pp. 26–28, 2012.

[64] I. Dostalova, D. Haluzikova, and M. Haluzik, "Fibroblast growth factor 21: a novel metabolic regulator with potential therapeutic properties in obesity/type 2 diabetes mellitus," *Physiological Research*, vol. 58, pp. 1–7, 2009.

[65] P. A. Dutchak, T. Katafuchi, A. L. Bookout et al., "Fibroblast growth factor-21 regulates PPARγ activity and the antidiabetic actions of thiazolidinediones," *Cell*, vol. 148, no. 3, pp. 556–567, 2012.

[66] M. M. Véniant, G. Sivits, J. Helmering et al., "Pharmacologic effects of FGF21 are independent of the 'browning' of white adipose tissue," *Cell Metabolism*, vol. 21, no. 5, pp. 731–738, 2015.

[67] M. A. Gomez-Samano, M. Grajales-Gomez, J. M. Zuarth-Vazquez et al., "Fibroblast growth factor 21 and its novel association with oxidative stress," *Redox Biology*, vol. 11, pp. 335–341, 2017.

[68] J. W. Jonker, J. M. Suh, A. R. Atkins et al., "A PPARγ-FGF1 axis is required for adaptive adipose remodelling and metabolic homeostasis," *Nature*, vol. 485, no. 7398, pp. 391–394, 2012.

[69] J. M. Suh, J. W. Jonker, M. Ahmadian et al., "Endocrinization of FGF1 produces a neomorphic and potent insulin sensitizer," *Nature*, vol. 513, no. 7518, pp. 436–439, 2014.

[70] Z. Lin, H. Tian, K. S. L. Lam et al., "Adiponectin mediates the metabolic effects of FGF21 on glucose homeostasis and insulin sensitivity in mice," *Cell Metabolism*, vol. 17, no. 5, pp. 779–789, 2013.

[71] X. Y. Chen, G. M. Li, Q. Dong, and H. Peng, "miR-577 inhibits pancreatic β-cell function and survival by targeting fibroblast growth factor 21 (FGF-21) in pediatric diabetes," *Genetics and Molecular Research*, vol. 14, no. 4, pp. 15462–15470, 2015.

[72] H. Ohta and N. Itoh, "Fgf signaling in adipocytes as a target for metabolic diseases," *Molecular Metabolism*, vol. 2, no. 1, pp. 3-4, 2013.

[73] A. C. Adams, C. A. Halstead, B. C. Hansen et al., "LY2405319, an engineered FGF21 variant, improves the metabolic status of diabetic monkeys," *PLoS ONE*, vol. 8, no. 6, Article ID e65763, 2013.

[74] A. Kharitonenkov, J. M. Beals, R. Micanovic et al., "Rational design of a fibroblast growth factor 21-based clinical candidate, LY2405319," *PLoS ONE*, vol. 8, no. 3, Article ID e58575, 2013.

[75] B. Literáti-Nagy, E. Kulcsár, Z. Literáti-Nagy et al., "Improvement of insulin sensitivity by a novel drug, BGP-15, in insulin-resistant patients: a proof of concept randomized double-blind clinical trial," *Hormone And Metabolic Research*, vol. 41, no. 5, pp. 374–380, 2009.

[76] B. Literáti-Nagy, K. Tory, B. Peitl et al., "Improvement of insulin sensitivity by a novel drug candidate, BGP-15, in different animal studies," *Metabolic Syndrome and Related Disorders*, vol. 12, no. 2, pp. 125–131, 2014.

[77] I. Gombos, T. Crul, S. Piotto et al., "Membrane-lipid therapy in operation: the HSP co-inducer BGP-15 activates stress signal transduction pathways by remodeling plasma membrane rafts," *PLoS ONE*, vol. 6, no. 12, Article ID e28818, 2011.

[78] I. Kurucz, Á. Morva, A. Vaag et al., "Decreased expression of heat shock protein 72 in skeletal muscle of patients with type 2 diabetes correlates with insulin resistance," *Diabetes*, vol. 51, no. 4, pp. 1102–1109, 2002.

[79] C. R. Bruce, A. L. Carey, J. A. Hawley, and M. A. Febbraio, "Intramuscular heat shock protein 72 and heme oxygenase-1 mRNA are reduced in patients with type 2 diabetes: Evidence that insulin resistance is associated with a disturbed antioxidant defense mechanism," *Diabetes*, vol. 52, no. 9, pp. 2338–2345, 2003.

[80] C. Sóti, E. Nagy, Z. Giricz, L. Vígh, P. Csermely, and P. Ferdinandy, "Heat shock proteins as emerging therapeutic targets," *British Journal of Pharmacology*, vol. 146, no. 6, pp. 769–780, 2005.

[81] R. R. Shankar, Y. Wu, H.-Q. Shen, J.-S. Zhu, and A. D. Baron, "Mice with gene disruption of both endothelial and neuronal nitric oxide synthase exhibit insulin resistance," *Diabetes*, vol. 49, no. 5, pp. 684–687, 2000.

[82] S. R. Kashyap, L. J. Roman, J. Lamont et al., "Insulin resistance is associated with impaired nitric oxide synthase activity in skeletal muscle of type 2 diabetic subjects," *Journal of Clinical Endocrinology and Metabolism*, vol. 90, no. 2, pp. 1100–1105, 2005.

[83] J. Chung, A.-K. Nguyen, D. C. Henstridge et al., "HSP72 protects against obesity-induced insulin resistance," *Proceedings of the National Academy of Sciences of the United States of America*, vol. 105, no. 5, pp. 1739–1744, 2008.

[84] D. C. Henstridge, C. R. Bruce, B. G. Drew et al., "Activating HSP72 in rodent skeletal muscle increases mitochondrial number and oxidative capacity and decreases insulin resistance," *Diabetes*, vol. 63, no. 6, pp. 1881–1894, 2014.

[85] K. Sumegi, K. Fekete, C. Antus et al., "BGP-15 protects against oxidative stress- or lipopolysaccharide-induced mitochondrial destabilization and reduces mitochondrial production of reactive oxygen species," *PloS One*, vol. 12, article e0169372, 2017.

[86] M. Wang, "Inhibitors of 11β-hydroxysteroid dehydrogenase type 1 in antidiabetic therapy," in *Handbook of Experimental Pharmacology*, pp. 127–146, 2011.

[87] R. Ge, Y. Huang, G. Liang, and X. Li, "11β-Hydroxysteroid dehydrogenase type 1 inhibitors as promising therapeutic drugs for diabetes: status and development," *Current Medicinal Chemistry*, vol. 17, no. 5, pp. 412–422, 2010.

[88] W. Chen, L. L. Wang, H. Y. Liu, L. Long, and S. Li, "Peroxisome proliferator-activated receptor delta-agonist, GW501516, ameliorates insulin resistance, improves dyslipidaemia in monosodium L-glutamate metabolic syndrome mice," *Basic & Clinical Pharmacology & Toxicology*, vol. 103, pp. 240–246, 2008.

[89] P. Anagnostis, N. Katsiki, F. Adamidou et al., "11beta-Hydroxysteroid dehydrogenase type 1 inhibitors: novel agents for the treatment of metabolic syndrome and obesity-related disorders?" *Metabolism: Clinical and Experimental*, vol. 62, no. 1, pp. 21–33, 2013.

[90] H. Masuzaki, H. Yamamoto, C. J. Kenyon et al., "Transgenic amplification of glucocorticoid action in adipose tissue causes high blood pressure in mice," *The Journal of Clinical Investigation*, vol. 112, no. 1, pp. 83–90, 2003.

[91] E. E. Kershaw, N. M. Morton, H. Dhillon, L. Ramage, J. R. Seckl, and J. S. Flier, "Adipocyte-specific glucocorticoid inactivation protects against diet-induced obesity," *Diabetes*, vol. 54, no. 4, pp. 1023–1031, 2005.

[92] S. Okazaki, T. Takahashi, T. Iwamura et al., "HIS-388, a novel orally active and long-acting 11β-hydroxysteroid dehydrogenase type 1 inhibitor, ameliorates insulin sensitivity and glucose intolerance in diet-induced obesity and nongenetic type 2 diabetic murine models," *Journal of Pharmacology and Experimental Therapeutics*, vol. 351, no. 1, pp. 181–189, 2014.

[93] L. Zhao, Y. Pan, K. Peng et al., "Inhibition of 11β-HsD1 by LG13 improves glucose metabolism in type 2 diabetic mice," *Journal of Molecular Endocrinology*, vol. 55, no. 2, pp. 119–131, 2015.

[94] A. Joharapurkar, N. Dhanesha, G. Shah, R. Kharul, and M. Jain, "11β-Hydroxysteroid dehydrogenase type 1: potential therapeutic target for metabolic syndrome," *Pharmacological Reports*, vol. 64, no. 5, pp. 1055–1065, 2012.

[95] S. Y. Byun, Y. J. Shin, K. Y. Nam, S. P. Hong, and S. K. Ahn, "A novel highly potent and selective 11β-hydroxysteroid dehydrogenase type 1 inhibitor, UI-1499," *Life Sciences*, vol. 120, pp. 1–7, 2015.

[96] J. Rosenstock, S. Banarer, V. A. Fonseca et al., "The 11-β-hydroxysteroid dehydrogenase type 1 inhibitor INCB13739 improves hyperglycemia in patients with type 2 diabetes inadequately controlled by metformin monotherapy," *Diabetes Care*, vol. 33, no. 7, pp. 1516–1522, 2010.

[97] K. A. Coughlan, R. J. Valentine, N. B. Ruderman, and A. K. Saha, "AMPK activation: a therapeutic target for type 2 diabetes?" *Diabetes, Metabolic Syndrome and Obesity: Targets and Therapy*, vol. 7, pp. 241–253, 2014.

[98] S. Fogarty and D. G. Hardie, "Development of protein kinase activators: AMPK as a target in metabolic disorders and cancer," *Biochimica et Biophysica Acta*, vol. 1804, no. 3, pp. 581–591, 2010.

[99] K. A. Weikel, N. B. Ruderman, and J. M. Cacicedo, "Unraveling the actions of AMP-activated protein kinase in metabolic diseases: systemic to molecular insights," *Metabolism: Clinical and Experimental*, vol. 65, no. 5, pp. 634–645, 2016.

[100] J. Kim, G. Yang, Y. Kim, J. Kim, and J. Ha, "AMPK activators: mechanisms of action and physiological activities," *Experimental & Molecular Medicine*, vol. 48, p. e224, 2016.

[101] H. Li, J. Lee, C. He, M.-H. Zou, and Z. Xie, "Suppression of the mTORC1/STAT3/Notch1 pathway by activated AMPK prevents hepatic insulin resistance induced by excess amino acids," *American Journal of Physiology—Endocrinology and Metabolism*, vol. 306, no. 2, pp. E197-E209, 2014.

[102] D. G. Hardie, "AMP-activated protein kinase: a key regulator of energy balance with many roles in human disease," *Journal of Internal Medicine*, vol. 276, no. 6, pp. 543–559, 2014.

[103] N. B. Ruderman, D. Carling, M. Prentki, and J. M. Cacicedo, "AMPK, insulin resistance, and the metabolic syndrome," *The Journal of Clinical Investigation*, vol. 123, no. 7, pp. 2764–2772, 2013.

[104] L. G. D. Fryer, A. Parbu-Patel, and D. Carling, "The anti-diabetic drugs rosiglitazone and metformin stimulate AMP-activated protein kinase through distinct signaling pathways," *The Journal of Biological Chemistry*, vol. 277, no. 28, pp. 25226–25232, 2002.

[105] I. Osman and L. Segar, "Pioglitazone, a PPARγ agonist, attenuates PDGF-induced vascular smooth muscle cell proliferation through AMPK-dependent and AMPK-independent inhibition of mTOR/p70S6K and ERK signaling," *Biochemical Pharmacology*, vol. 101, pp. 54–70, 2016.

[106] K. Mahmood, M. Naeem, and N. A. Rahimnajjad, "Metformin: the hidden chronicles of a magic drug," *European Journal of Internal Medicine*, vol. 24, no. 1, pp. 20–26, 2013.

[107] X. Yang, Z. Xu, C. Zhang, Z. Cai, and J. Zhang, "Metformin, beyond an insulin sensitizer, targeting heart and pancreatic beta cells," *Biochimica et Biophysica Acta*, vol. 16, pp. 30243–30245, 2016.

[108] S. Andrzejewski, S. P. Gravel, M. Pollak, and J. St-Pierre, "Metformin directly acts on mitochondria to alter cellular bioenergetics," *Cancer & Metabolism*, vol. 2, p. 12, 2014.

[109] A. Luengo, L. B. Sullivan, and M. G. V. Heiden, "Understanding the complex-I-ty of metformin action: Limiting mitochondrial respiration to improve cancer therapy," *BMC Biology*, vol. 12, no. 1, article 82, 2014.

[110] L. He and F. E. Wondisford, "Metformin action: concentrations matter," *Cell Metabolism*, vol. 21, no. 2, pp. 159–162, 2015.

[111] C. S. Zhang, M. Li, T. Ma et al., "Metformin activates ampk through the lysosomal pathway," *Cell Metabolism*, vol. 24, pp. 521-522, 2016.

[112] T. Luo, A. Nocon, J. Fry et al., "AMPK activation by metformin suppresses abnormal extracellular matrix remodeling in adipose tissue and ameliorates insulin resistance in obesity," *Diabetes*, vol. 65, no. 8, pp. 2295–2310, 2016.

[113] H. Yadav, S. Devalaraja, S. T. Chung, and S. G. Rane, "TGF-β1/Smad3 Pathway Targets PP2A-AMPK-FoxO1 Signaling to Regulate Hepatic Gluconeogenesis," *Journal of Biological Chemistry*, vol. 292, no. 8, pp. 3420–3432, 2017.

[114] S. K. Lee, J. O. Lee, J. H. Kim et al., "Metformin sensitizes insulin signaling through AMPK-mediated pten down-regulation in preadipocyte 3T3-L1 cells," *Journal of Cellular Biochemistry*, vol. 112, no. 5, pp. 1259–1267, 2011.

[115] J. O. Lee, S. K. Lee, J. H. Kim et al., "Metformin regulates glucose transporter 4 (GLUT4) translocation through AMP-activated protein kinase (AMPK)-mediated Cbl/CAP signaling in 3T3-L1 preadipocyte cells," *Journal of Biological Chemistry*, vol. 287, no. 53, pp. 44121–44129, 2012.

[116] M. P. Hage, M. R. Al-Badri, and S. T. Azar, "A favorable effect of hydroxychloroquine on glucose and lipid metabolism beyond its anti-inflammatory role," *Therapeutic Advances in Endocrinology and Metabolism*, vol. 5, no. 4, pp. 77–85, 2014.

[117] A. P. Bevan, J. R. Christensen, J. Tikerpae, and G. D. Smith, "Chloroquine augments the binding of insulin to its receptor," *Biochemical Journal*, vol. 311, no. 3, pp. 787–795, 1995.

[118] E. Mercer, L. Rekedal, R. Garg, B. Lu, E. M. Massarotti, and D. H. Solomon, "Hydroxychloroquine improves insulin sensitivity in obese non-diabetic individuals," *Arthritis Research & Therapy*, vol. 14, article R135, 2012.

10

The Hepatoprotection by Oleanolic Acid Preconditioning: Focusing on PPARα Activation

Wenwen Wang,[1] Kan Chen ⓘ,[1] Yujing Xia ⓘ,[1] Wenhui Mo,[2] Fan Wang,[3] Weiqi Dai,[4,5] and Peiqin Niu ⓘ[1,6]

[1]*Department of Gastroenterology, Shanghai Tenth People's Hospital, Tongji University School of Medicine, Shanghai 200072, China*
[2]*Department of Gastroenterology, Minhang Hospital, Fudan University, Shanghai 201100, China*
[3]*Department of Oncology, Shanghai General Hospital, Shanghai Jiaotong University School of Medicine, Shanghai 200080, China*
[4]*Department of Gastroenterology, Zhongshan Hospital, Fudan University, Shanghai 200032, China*
[5]*Shanghai Institute of Liver Diseases, Zhongshan Hospital, Fudan University, Shanghai 200032, China*
[6]*Shanghai Tenth People's Hospital Chongming Branch, Tongji University School of Medicine, Shanghai 202157, China*

Correspondence should be addressed to Peiqin Niu; niuniu1657@126.com

Academic Editor: Swasti Tiwari

Objective. Previous studies have characterized the hepatoprotective and anti-inflammatory properties of oleanolic acid (OA). This study aimed to investigate the molecular mechanisms of OA hepatoprotection in concanavalin A- (ConA-) induced acute liver injury. *Materials and Methods*. ConA (20 mg/kg) was intravenously injected to induce acute liver injury in Balb/C mice. OA pretreatment (20, 40, and 80 mg/kg) was administered subcutaneously once daily for 3 consecutive days prior to treatment with ConA; 2, 8, and 24 h after ConA injection, the levels of serum liver enzymes and the histopathology of major factors and inflammatory cytokines were determined. *Results*. OA reduced the release of serum liver enzymes and inflammatory factors and prevented ConA mediated damage to the liver. OA elevated the expression levels of peroxisome proliferator-activated receptor alpha (PPARα) and decreased the phosphorylation of c-Jun NH2-terminal kinase (JNK). *Conclusion*. OA exhibits anti-inflammatory properties during ConA-induced acute liver injury by attenuating apoptosis and autophagy through activation of PPARα and downregulation of JNK signaling.

1. Introduction

The liver is a metabolic and immunological organ that performs a variety of functions, including deoxidation, glycogen storage, and secretory protein synthesis. The onset of liver injury may occur in response to various factors like excessive alcohol use, infections, chemical drugs, and autoimmune disorders [1]. Concanavalin A (ConA) is a mitogenic plant lectin extracted from *Canavalia brasiliensis* [2] that has been used to model liver injury *in vivo*. ConA-induced liver injury is a well-established model to explore the pathogenesis of liver injury [3–5], as it is characterized by elevated liver enzymes and inflammatory cytokines, such as TNF-α, IL-1β, IL-4, and IL-6, leading to the activation of T cells, sinusoidal endothelial cells (SECs), and Kupffer cells (KCs) [3, 6–9].

Furthermore, animal studies have shown that apoptosis and autophagy are associated with ConA-induced liver injury in a c-Jun NH2-terminal kinase- (JNK-) dependent manner [10–13]. Oleanonic acid (3β-hydroxyolean-12-en-28-oic acid, OA) is a pentacyclic terpenoid found in the form of free acids and triterpenoid saponin glycosides in plants [14, 15]. Previous studies have demonstrated that OA and its derivatives possess anticancer, antidiabetic, anti-HIV, antioxidant, and anti-inflammatory [16–20] properties. However, OA's most well characterized properties are hepatoprotective, and it alleviates acute chemical-induced liver injury and chronic liver fibrosis and cirrhosis [21, 22]. OA has even been used as an over-the-counter drug to treat liver disorders in China [15]. Though the exact mechanistic targets modulated by OA during liver injury are unknown, several groups have suggested that ERK, JNK, PI3K/Akt, and Nrf2 may be involved [23–27].

Peroxisome proliferator-activated receptors (PPARs) are a group of nuclear receptors which function as transcription factors and regulate gene expression by binding their heterodimeric partner retinoid X receptors at specific PPAR-response elements [28]. PPARs used to be predominantly associated with lipid metabolism, but follow-up studies have suggested that PPARs participate in the regulation of inflammation and immunity [29, 30]. PPARα, abundantly expressed in hepatocytes, the heart, muscle tissues, adipose tissues, and the kidney, is one of three identified isoforms of PPARs (α, β/δ, and γ). Studies have confirmed that PPARα is a transcriptional activator of lipid metabolism and also a suppressor of acute phase immunity in both humans and rodents [31]. PPARα is also associated with alterations in the development of both B and T lymphocytes [30, 32].

This study aimed to investigate the role of OA in ConA-induced liver injury and the underlying signaling pathways associated with its hepatoprotective properties. Based on the mechanisms of hepatoprotection of OA during liver injury induced by other small molecules like phalloidin [33], CCl4 [34], and acetaminophen [25], we hypothesized that OA attenuated ConA-induced liver injury in a PPARα- and JNK-dependent manner.

2. Materials and Methods

2.1. Chemicals and Reagents. ConA and OA were obtained from Sigma-Aldrich (St. Louis, MO, USA). The alanine aminotransferase (ALT) and the aspartate aminotransferase (AST) microplate test kits were obtained from the Nanjing Jiancheng Bioengineering Institute (Jiancheng Biotech, China). The enzyme-linked immunosorbent assay (ELISA) kits were acquired from eBioscience (San Diego, CA, USA). The RNA polymerase chain reaction (PCR) kit was purchased from Takara Biotechnology (Dalian, China). The antibodies for PPARα, JNK, p-JNK, TRAF2, Bax, Bcl-2, LC3, Beclin 1, and caspase-3 were provided by Proteintech (Chicago, IL, USA). The IL-1β, IL-6, and TNF-α antibodies were from Abcam (Cambridge, MA, USA). The TdT-mediated dUTP nick end labeling (TUNEL) apoptosis assay kit was from Roche (Roche Ltd, Basel, Switzerland).

2.2. Animals. Male Balb/c mice, 6–8 weeks old, weighing 23 ± 2 g, were supplied by Shanghai SLAC Laboratory Animal Co. Ltd. (Shanghai, China). The mice were housed in plastic cages at a temperature of 24°C with a 12 h light-dark cycle and were provided with food and water ad libitum. All our animal experiments conformed to the National Institutes of Health Guidelines and were approved by the Animal Care and Use Committee of Shanghai Tongji University. No animals died or became severely ill prior to reaching our experimental endpoints.

2.3. Experimental Design. OA was prepared as an injectable suspension with olive oil and was administered once daily subcutaneously for 3 consecutive days with doses of either 20, 40, or 80 mg/kg prior to ConA injection. ConA was dissolved in saline to a concentration of 2.5 mg/mL and injected at a dose of 20 mg/kg [35, 36] in the caudal vein to induce acute liver injury.

The mice were randomly divided into seven groups:

(1) Normal control group ($n = 6$): mice were given saline.

(2) Oil control group ($n = 6$): mice were given an equal volume of olive oil.

(3) OA group ($n = 6$): mice were given 40 mg/kg OA suspension.

(4) ConA group ($n = 18$): mice were injected with 20 mg/kg ConA via caudal vein.

(5) ConA + OA 20 mg/kg group ($n = 18$): mice were given 20 mg/kg OA for 3 days before ConA injection.

(6) ConA + OA 40 mg/kg group ($n = 18$): mice were given 40 mg/kg OA for 3 days before ConA injection.

(7) ConA + OA 80 mg/kg group ($n = 18$): mice were given 80 mg/kg OA for 3 days before ConA injection.

2.4. Biochemical Analysis. Blood samples were collected by retroorbital bleeding, and the collected blood was centrifuged at 3000 r/min for 10 min at 4°C to obtain sera. The activities of serum alanine aminotransferase (ALT) and aspartate aminotransferase (AST) were determined using commercial assay kits. The levels of IL-1β, IL-6, and TNF-α were determined using ELISA kits, per manufacturer's instructions.

2.5. Histopathology and Quantification of Liver Injury. Liver tissues were removed from a portion of the left lobe, fixed in 4% paraformaldehyde, embedded in paraffin, sliced to 5-micron thick sections, and stained with hematoxylin and eosin (H&E). Inflammation and tissue damage were assessed using a light microscope. 5 fields (200x magnification) were evaluated from 4 to 6 individual animals per group by an experienced pathologist. Liver sections were blind to observer. The percentages of necrotic area were used for statistical analysis [37]. Based on the severity and distribution of the necrosis, the overall grade of necrotic lesion was evaluated by a scoring system from 0 to 4: 0: none; 1: mild; 2: moderate; 3: marked; 4: severe to diffuse.

2.6. Immunohistochemistry. Liver tissues were prepared as paraffin-embedded sections, dewaxed in xylene, and dehydrated in ethanol. Antigen retrieval was achieved using citrate buffer and incubation at 95°C water for 20 min. To block the activity of endogenous peroxidases, the sections were incubated with 3% hydrogen peroxide for 10 min at 37°C. Nonspecific binding was blocked with 5% bovine serum albumin for 30 min. Liver sections were then incubated overnight at 4°C with the following primary antibodies and dilutions: IL-1β (1 : 100), IL-6 (1 : 100), TNF-α (1 : 100), PPARα (1 : 50), phospho-JNK (1 : 100), LC3 (1 : 50), Beclin 1 (1 : 50), Bcl-2 (1 : 100), and Bax (1 : 100). The slices were then washed three times and incubated with secondary antibodies. A diaminobenzidine kit was used to measure antibody binding under a light microscope. The ratios of stained and total area were calculated using Image-Pro Plus software (version 6.0).

2.7. TUNEL Staining. The prepared paraffin sections were dewaxed in xylene for 5–10 min twice and dehydrated with ethanol. Proteinase K without DNase was added at a concentration of 20 micrograms/mL for 15–30 min. TUNEL reaction buffer was added to the slices after washing according to the manufacturer's protocols, and the sections were observed under a light microscope to determine the number of apoptotic cells.

2.8. Quantification of mRNA by Reverse Transcription PCR (RT-PCR). Total RNA in liver tissues was reverse-transcribed into cDNA using the reverse transcription kit (TaKaRa Biotechnology, China) and the resulting cDNA was used for real-time PCR analysis using SYBR Premix EX Taq (TaKaRa Biotechnology, China) with a 7900HT fast real-time PCR system (Applied Biosystems, CA, USA). Oligonucleotide primer sequences are listed in Table 1. The relative expression levels were calculated using the $2^{-\Delta\Delta Ct}$ method and normalized to β-actin.

2.9. Western Blot Analysis. Total protein was extracted using radio immunoprecipitation assay lysis buffer with protease inhibitors (PI) with phenylmethane-sulfonyl fluoride from liver tissues and stored at −80°C. Protein concentrations were determined using a BCA protein assay kit according to the manufacturer's instructions (Kaiji, China). Equivalent amounts of total protein (120 microgram) were separated in 7.5%–12.5% SDS-polyacrylamide gels and then transferred to polyvinylidene fluoride membranes. Nonspecific binding was blocked with phosphate-buffered saline (PBS) containing 0.1% Tween 20 (PBST) and 5% nonfat milk (dissolved with PBS) for 1 h, and the membranes were incubated overnight at 4°C with the following primary antibodies and dilutions: β-actin (1:1000) LC3 (1:1000), Beclin 1 (1:500), Bcl-2 (1:1000), Bax (1:500), caspase-3 (1:500), JNK (1:1000), phospho-JNK (1:500), and TRAF2 (1:1000). Membranes were washed with PBST three times and incubated with horseradish peroxidase-conjugated anti-rabbit or anti-mouse secondary antibodies (1:2000) for 1 h at room temperature. Finally, membranes were washed three times and scanned with the Odyssey two-color infrared laser imaging system.

2.10. Statistical Analysis. All data are expressed as means ± standard error. The differences between groups were analyzed using one-way analysis of variance. A P value < 0.05 was considered as statistically significant. Statistical analyses were performed using Graphpad Prism Software (version 6.0, San Diego, CA, USA).

3. Results

3.1. Oleanolic Acid (OA) Is Safe and Tolerable in Mice. To determine the safety and tolerability of OA, 18 mice were given equal volumes of either saline, olive oil, or OA (40 mg/kg) suspension for 3 days and then sacrificed to examine signs of liver dysfunction. There were no significant differences in the expression levels of liver enzymes and inflammatory cytokines between the three groups (Figures 1(a) and 1(b)). Liver biopsies showed no pathological and morphological

changes in response to OA (Figure 1(c)). Thus, OA appears to be safe and tolerable in these mice.

3.2. OA Alleviates Liver Injury Induced by ConA. We found that, after ConA injection, SECs, KCs, and CD4$^+$ Th cells were activated, resulting in elevated levels of cytokines and edema and necrosis in hepatocytes [6, 7]. The levels of ALT and AST were also increased in response to ConA (Figure 2(a)). The most significant increases occurred at 8 h, and OA markedly alleviated the activities of these transaminases. The reduction in ConA-dependent changes was most prominent in the intermediately dosed mice (40 mg/kg). As shown in Figure 2(b), furthermore, liver tissue in oil group showed well preserved hepatic architecture with intact liver lobules. 8 hours after ConA administration, ConA group showed diffuse necrosis, congestion, and partially severe inflammation, and the integrality of hepatic lobules was destroyed. In OA pretreatment group, narrowed necrotic area, slight congestion, and milder lymphocytic accumulation were seen compared to treatment with ConA alone. The patterns of liver tissue of these five groups in 2 h and 24 h were similar to the 2 h. Again, the intermediately dosed mice (40 mg/kg) showed the least amount of necrosis. Table 2 showed the pathological score of liver injury 8 h after ConA administration. These results suggest that pretreatment with OA can attenuate ConA-induced liver injury in mice.

3.3. OA Pretreatment Reduces the Production of TNF-α, IL-1β, and IL-6 in ConA-Induced Liver Injury. Expectedly, the expression levels of inflammatory cytokines were all elevated after ConA injection. The mRNA and protein expression levels of TNF-α and IL-6 peaked at 2 h and then declined at 8 and 24 h, while the levels of IL-1β peaked at 8 h. Pretreatment with OA markedly decreased cytokines expression levels compared to ConA treated mice, and the medium dose (40 mg/kg) had the most potent effect on attenuating inflammation (Figures 3(a) and 3(b)). Furthermore, western blotting and TNF-α, IL-1β, and IL-6 immunohistochemistry analysis also confirmed that OA significantly reduced the production of TNF-α, IL-1β, and IL-6 on protein level (Figures 3(c) and 3(d)).

3.4. OA Reduces Autophagy and Apoptosis in ConA-Induced Liver Injury. We assessed the activation of apoptosis and autophagy by measuring the expression levels of caspase-3, caspase-9, Bcl-2, Bax, Beclin 1, and LC3. Previous studies have identified that caspase-3, caspase-9, Bcl-2, and Bax played important roles in regulating apoptosis, and Beclin 1 and LC3 are known mediators of autophagy. The expression levels of Bcl-2, an antiapoptotic marker, were downregulated in response to ConA, and OA pretreatment abrogated this effect. Bax, caspase-3, caspase-9, Beclin 1, and LC3 were all highly expressed in mice given ConA, and these levels were reduced in response to OA pretreatment (Figures 4(a) and 4(b)). Immunohistochemistry analysis and TUNEL staining confirmed these results (Figures 4(c) and 4(d)). These findings suggest that OA regulates autophagy and apoptosis and protects hepatocytes from pathological damage induced by ConA.

TABLE 1: Oligonucleotide primer sequences used for qRT-PCR.

Gene	Forward (5'-3')	Reverse (3'-5')
β-Actin	GGCTGTATTCCCCTCCATCG	CCAGTTGGTAACAATGCCATGT
IL-1β	CGATCGCGCAGGGGCTGGGCGG	AGGAACTGACGGTACTGATGGA
IL-6	CTGCAAGAGACTTCCATCCAG	AGTGGTATAGACAGGTCTGTTGG
TNF-α	CAGGCGGTGCCTATGTCTC	CGATCACCCCGAAGTTCAGTAG
PPARα	AACATCGAGTGTCGAATATGTGG	CCGAATAGTTCGCCGAAAGAA
Caspase-3	ATGGAGAACAACAAAACCTCAGT	TTGCTCCCATGTATGGTCTTTAC
Caspase-9	TCCTGGTACATCGAGACCTTG	AAGTCCCTTTCGCAGAAACAG
Bcl-2	GCTACCGTCGTCGTGACTTCGC	CCCCACCGAACTCAAAGAAGG
Bax	AGACAGGGGCCTTTTTGCTAC	AATTCGCCGGAGACACTCG
Beclin 1	ATGGAGGGGTCTAAGGCGTC	TGGGCTGTGGTAAGTAATGGA
LC3	GACCGCTGTAAGGAGGTGC	AGAAGCCGAAGGTTTCTTGGG
TRAF2	AGAGAGTAGTTCGGCCTTTCC	AGAGAGTAGTTCGGCCTTTCC

TABLE 2: Pathological score for liver injury of 8 h.

	0	1	2	3	4	Mean
Oil	6	0	0	0	0	0.00
ConA	0	0	0	4	2	3.33*
OA (20 mg/kg)	0	3	2	1	0	1.67#
OA (40 mg/kg)	1	4	1	0	0	1.00+
OA (80 mg/kg)	0	5	1	0	0	1.17^

Notes. $n = 6$; *$P < 0.05$ for oil versus ConA; #$P < 0.05$ for ConA + OA (20 mg/kg) versus ConA; +$P < 0.05$ for ConA + OA (40 mg/kg) versus ConA; ^$P < 0.05$ for ConA + OA (80 mg/kg) versus ConA.

3.5. OA Inhibits ConA-Induced Liver Injury via Activation of PPARα and Suppression of JNK Signaling. Previous studies have suggested that attenuation of JNK signaling could effectively alleviate ConA-induced liver injury and that PPARα participates in the regulation of inflammation and immunity. Therefore, we hypothesized that PPARα and JNK signaling are involved in the hepatoprotective effects of OA.

We found that PPARα protein and mRNA levels were significantly reduced in ConA treated mice, and pretreatment with OA abrogated this effect. The protein and mRNA levels of TRAF2 and the phosphorylation of JNK were markedly increased in the ConA group, and OA reduced the expression levels of TRAF2 and the activation of JNK (Figures 5(a)–5(c)). Our findings support the premise that OA has the ability to attenuate ConA-induced liver injury and that activation of PPARα and suppression of JNK signaling may be one of the underlying mechanisms (Figure 6).

4. Discussion

OA is a pentacyclic triterpenoid found in a variety of medicinal herbs [14]. Due to its hepatoprotective properties, OA has been developed in China as a an oral remedy for the treatment of acute and chronic liver disorders [15]. Liu et al. [38] have shown that the hepatoprotective effects of OA are not evident until 24 h after exposure but are retained for at least 72 h. However, the underlying mechanisms of OA hepatoprotection during liver injury remain unknown.

Numerous animal studies have illustrated that OA protects against liver injury induced by small molecules like phalloidin, CCl4, and acetaminophen, by reducing serum transaminase levels and preventing necrosis [33, 34, 38]. To further investigate the pathways modulated by OA, we established a model of ConA-induced liver injury and verified the hepatoprotective effects of OA. In our study, ConA elevated serum aminotransferase levels, suggesting that ConA could damage hepatocytes and induce pathological lesions in mouse livers. Expectedly, OA attenuated the effects of ConA and alleviated ConA mediated liver injury and inflammation.

Wang et al. [8] have previously studied the mechanisms of ConA-triggered immune responses in mice. ConA was shown to bind the mannose gland on the surface of SECs, facilitating its binding to KCs. CD4+ Th cells can then identify the ConA-modified major histocompatibility complex presented by KCs and become activated, mediating the release of cytokines like TNF-α. SECs and KCs also secrete IL-1 and IL-6, which suggests that both KCs and SECs mediate liver injury along with CD4+ Th cells. Our study demonstrates that pretreatment with OA mitigates the inflammatory response mediated by ConA, as it reduced the levels of proinflammatory cytokines.

It has been shown that OA exerts its protective effects by binding and activating the PPAR nuclear receptor, PPARα [39], which participates in the regulation of inflammation and immunity. Genetic ablation of PPARα can promote NF-KB and c-jun activation in T lymphocytes, leading to increased

(a)

(b)

(c)

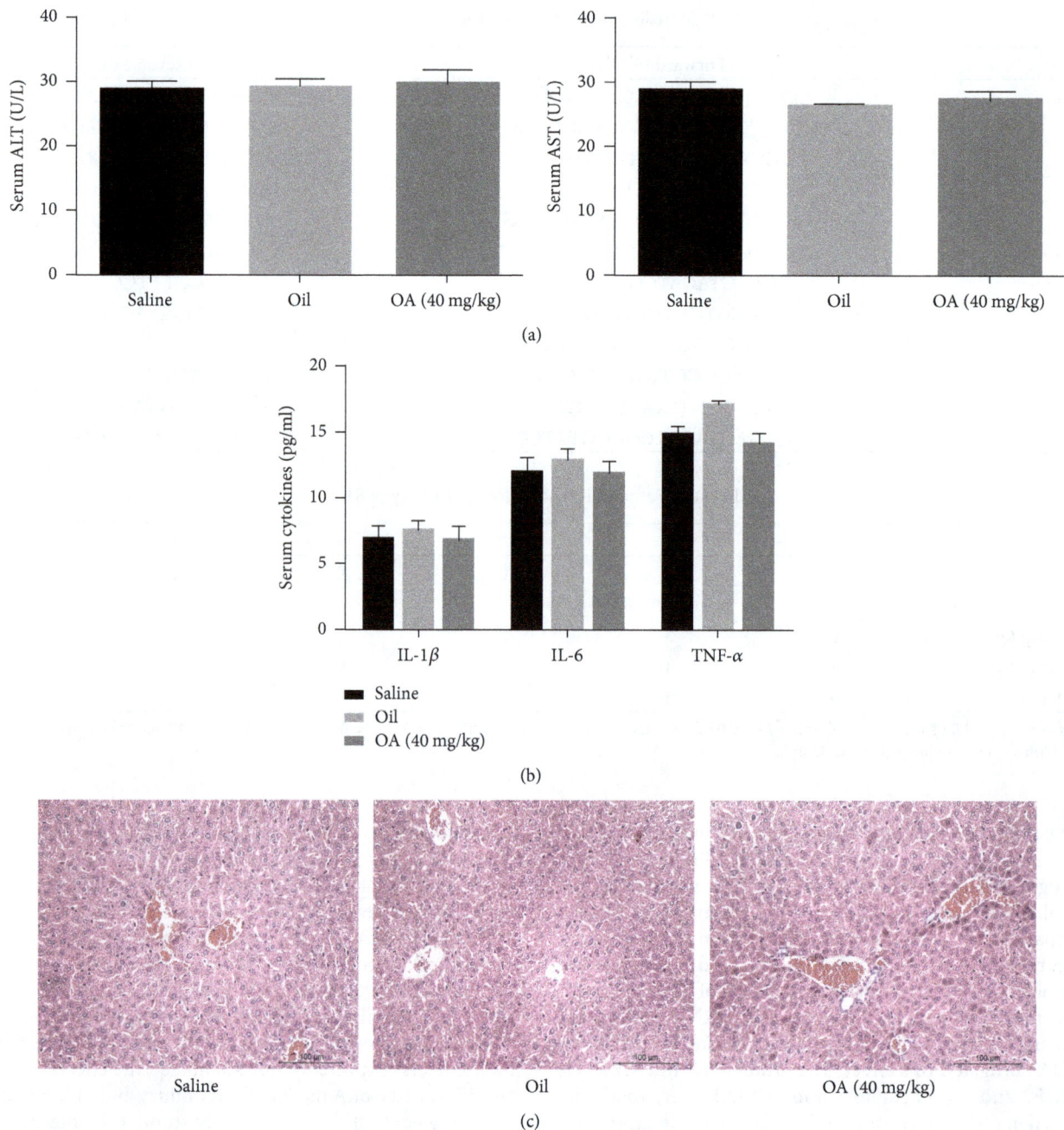

FIGURE 1: *OA is safe and tolerable in mice. Notes.* (a, b) The levels of serum ALT and AST (a) and of IL-1β, IL-6, and TNF-α (b) are expressed as means ± standard error ($n = 6$, $P > 0.05$). (c) Representative hematoxylin and eosin (H&E) stained sections of livers from saline, olive oil, and OA treated mice (200x magnification).

production of IFN-γ and TNF, and lower expression levels of 2 Th2 cytokines [32]. We therefore hypothesized that OA can promote the expression of PPARα. We found that ConA could, in fact, reduce both PPARα mRNA and protein expression levels, an affect that was abrogated by pretreatment with OA.

TNF-α and IL-1β are known activators of JNK signaling [40–42]. TNFR2 binds TRAF2 directly, inducing TRAF2 degradation and activating JNK, which modulates gene transcription [43]. OA has been shown to inhibit the

phosphorylation of JNK, attenuating B cell dysfunction and mitochondrial apoptosis [33, 44]. To discern the contribution of JNK signaling to OA's ability to alleviate ConA-induced liver injury, we assessed the phosphorylation of JNK and the expression levels of Bcl-2, Bax, Beclin 1, LC3B, caspase-3, and caspase-9 in liver tissue. When phosphorylated, JNK translocates from the cytoplasm to the nucleus, mediating the phosphorylation and activation of transcription factor c-Jun and upregulating expression of proapoptotic Bcl2-associated gene Bax and downregulating the expression of Bcl-2, thereby

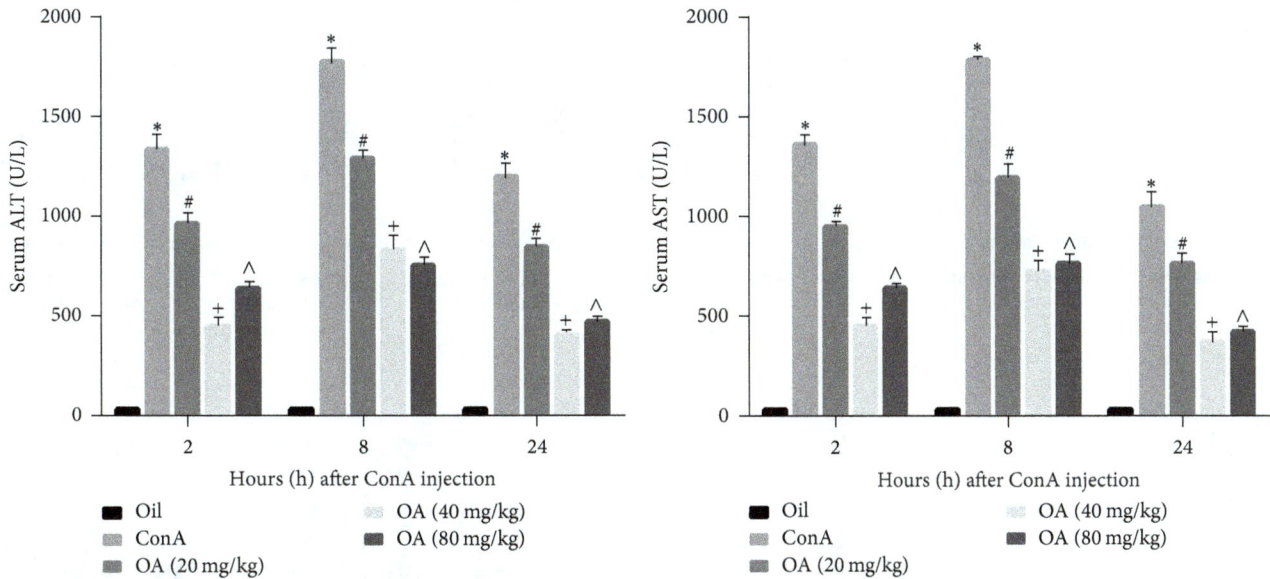

(a)

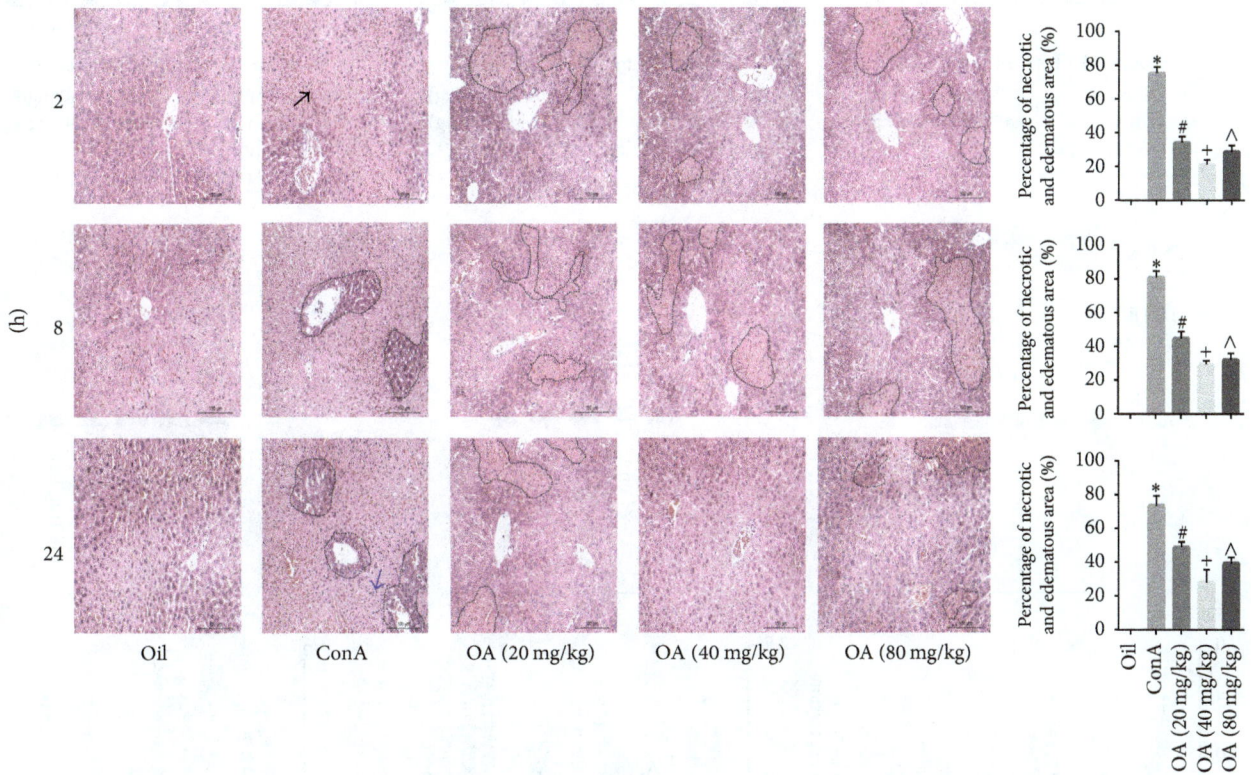

(b)

FIGURE 2: *Pathological liver injury induced by ConA is attenuated by OA*. *Notes*. (a) Serum aminotransferase activities were determined at 2, 8, and 24 h after intravenous injection of 20 mg/kg ConA. Olive oil injected animals were used as a control. (b) Representative hematoxylin and eosin (H&E) staining of livers. Scale bar: 200 microns. Necrotic area was outlined with dotted line, black arrows indicate representative areas of injury, and blue arrows indicate leukocyte adhesion to vascular endothelium. The percentage of necrotic and edematous areas on the basis of H&E liver sections was analyzed with Image-Pro Plus 6.0 (original magnification, ×200). Data were presented as means ± standard error ($n = 6$; $^*P < 0.05$ for oil versus ConA; $^\#P < 0.05$ for ConA + OA (20 mg/kg) versus ConA; $^+P < 0.05$ for ConA + OA (40 mg/kg) versus ConA; $^\wedge P < 0.05$ for ConA + OA (80 mg/kg) versus ConA).

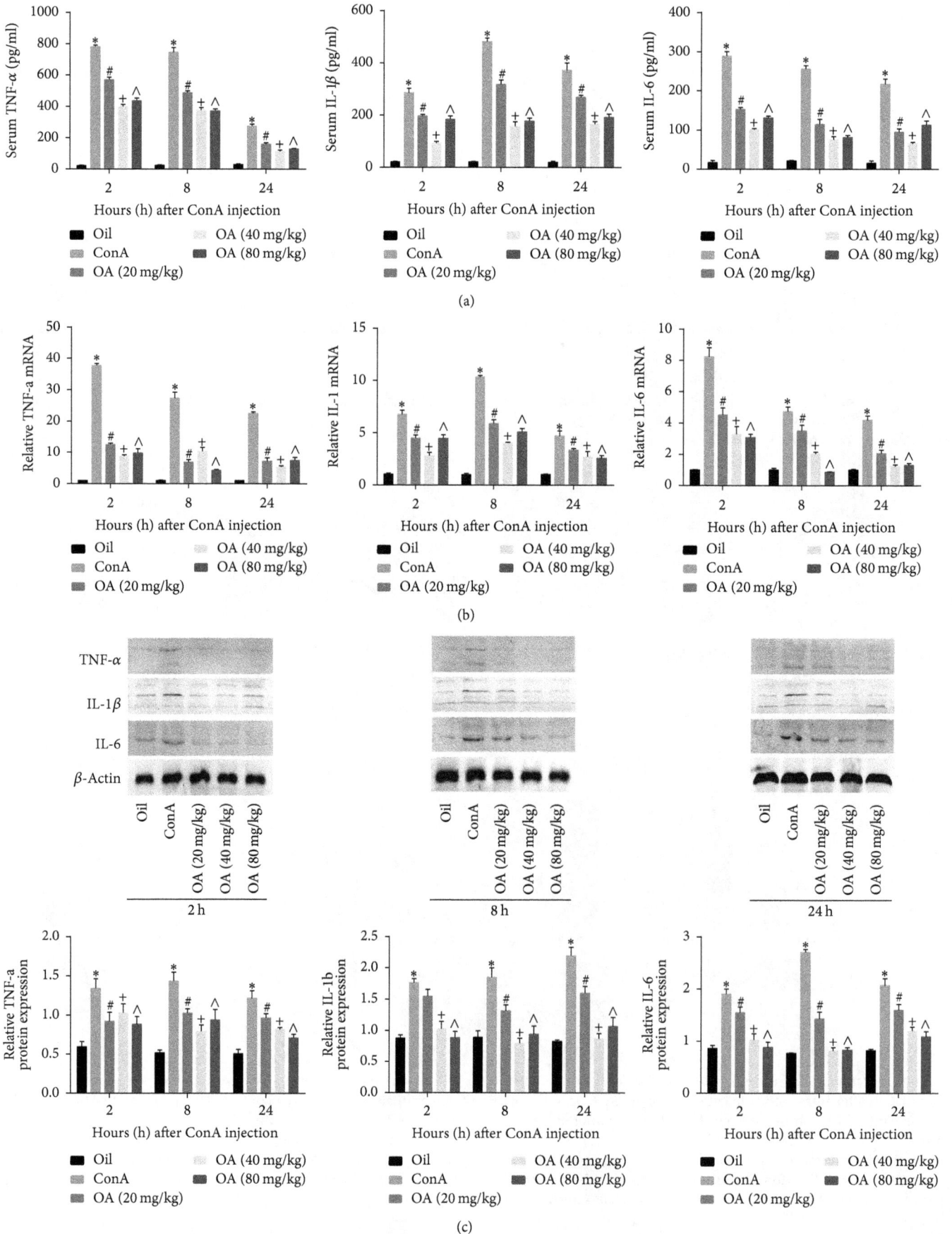

(a)

(b)

(c)

FIGURE 3: Continued.

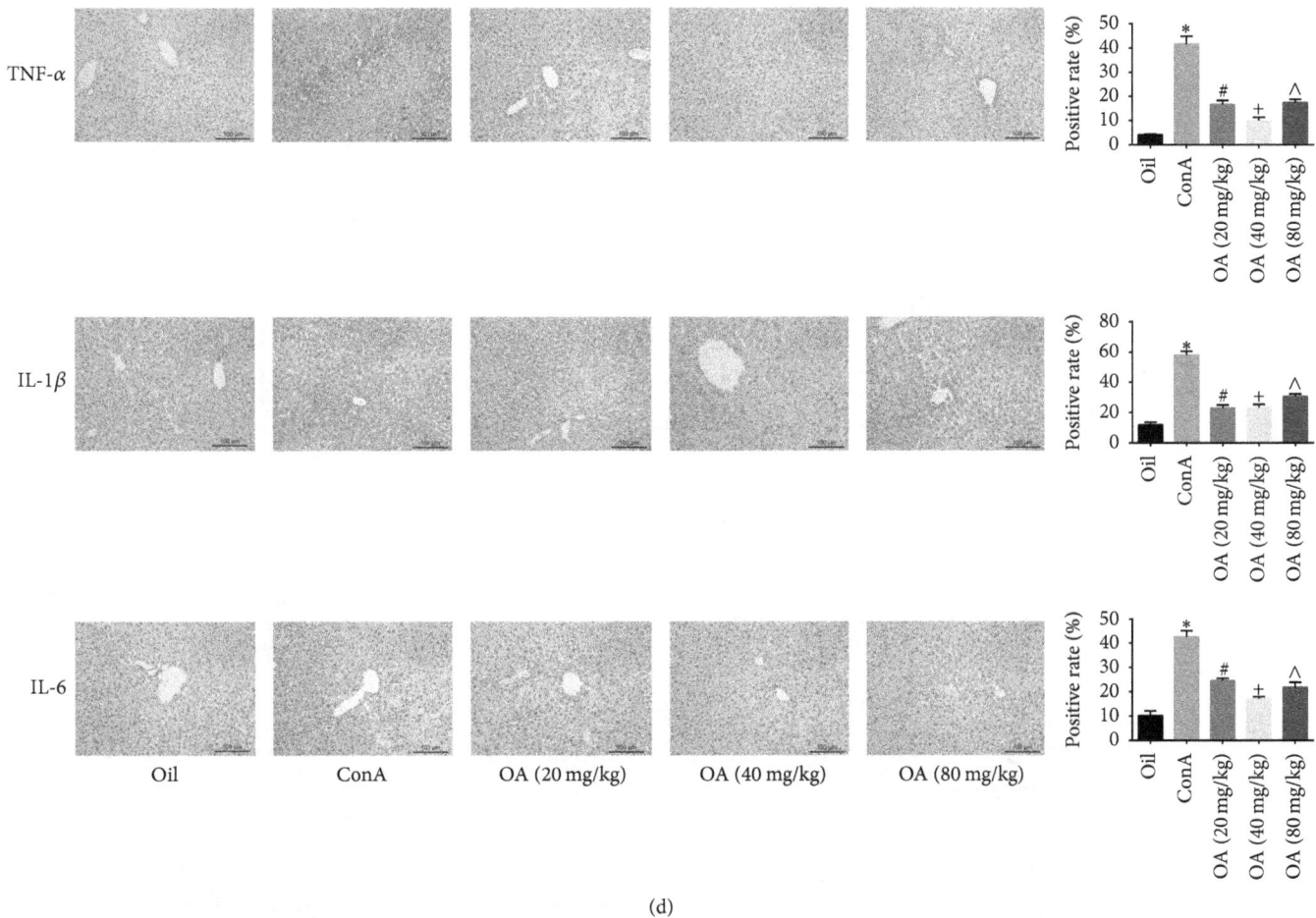

(d)

FIGURE 3: *OA attenuates the production of inflammatory cytokines in ConA-induced liver injury. Notes.* (a, b) The relative plasma (a) and mRNA (b) TNF-α, IL-1β, and IL-6 levels at 2, 8, and 24 h after ConA injection and pretreatment with low (20 mg/kg), intermediate (40 mg/kg), and high (80 mg/kg) doses of OA. (c) Protein levels of TNF-α, IL-1β, and IL-6 were evaluated by western blotting and the gray values were calculated. (d) Immunohistochemistry staining (200x magnification) of TNF-α, IL-1β, and IL-6 in liver tissues after 8 h of treatment with ConA. The ratio of brown area to total area was analyzed with Image-Pro Plus 6.0 ($n = 6$; $^*P < 0.05$ for oil versus ConA; $^#P < 0.05$ for ConA + OA (20 mg/kg) versus ConA; $^+P < 0.05$ for ConA + OA (40 mg/kg) versus ConA; $^\wedge P < 0.05$ for ConA + OA (80 mg/kg) versus ConA).

promoting apoptosis through caspase-9 and caspase-3 [45]. We found that phosphorylation of JNK and the expression of Bax, caspase-3, and caspase-9 were elevated in response to ConA, while the expression of Bcl-2 was reduced, effects that was reversed by OA. We therefore infer that OA attenuates apoptosis via inhibition of JNK in hepatocytes. Furthermore, JNK has been shown to promote the transcription of Beclin 1 [46]. Beclin 1, the first identified mammalian autophagy protein [47], has been reported to interact with the antiapoptotic protein Bcl-2 as well as other Bcl family members via its BH3 (Bcl-2 homology 3) domain, leading to inhibition of Beclin 1 activity and autophagy [48–50]. As an autophagic effector protein, LC3 (microtubule-associated protein 1 light chain 3) levels can modulate autophagic flux and can be used as a marker of autophagic activation [51–53]. OA pretreatment abrogated the increased expression levels of Beclin 1 and LC3 mediated by ConA, suggesting that OA alleviates liver injury by also inhibiting autophagy.

In conclusion, OA exhibits hepatoprotective effects via activation of PPARα and inhibition of apoptosis and autophagy through inhibition of JNK signaling.

Conflicts of Interest

The authors report no conflicts of interest regarding the publication of this paper.

Acknowledgments

The authors express their gratitude to all the members of Central Laboratory of the Shanghai Tenth People's Hospital of Tongji University. Particularly thanks are due to the assistance of Professor Xiangyue Yu from Clinical Pathology Diagnosis Center of Shanghai Tenth People's Hospital. This work was supported by the National Natural Science Foundation of China (Grant nos. 81670472 and 81500466).

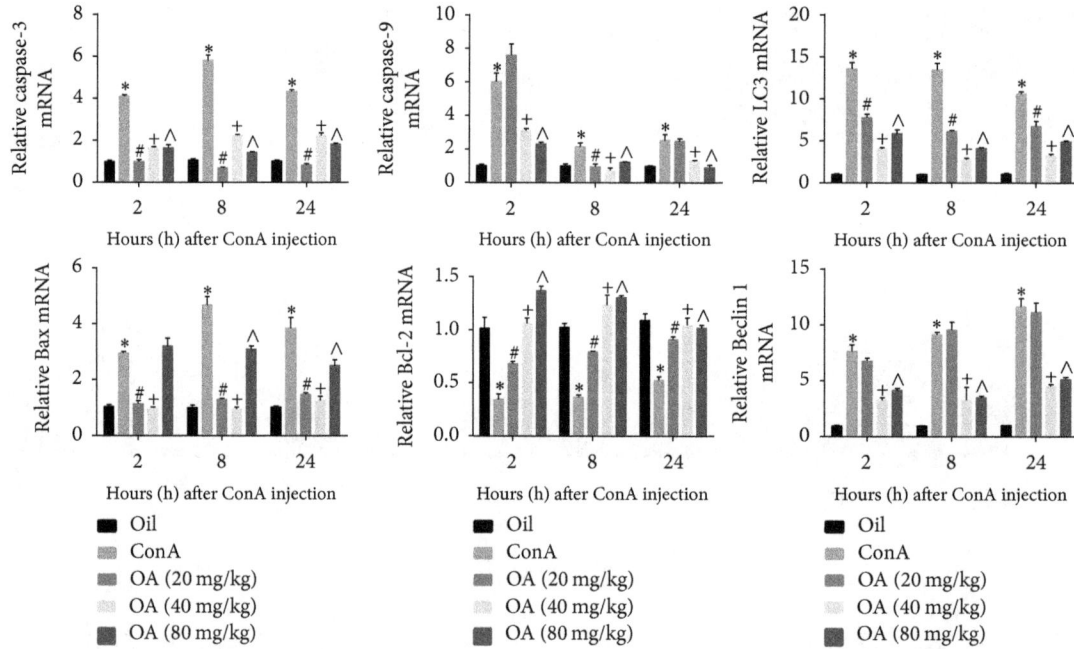

(a)

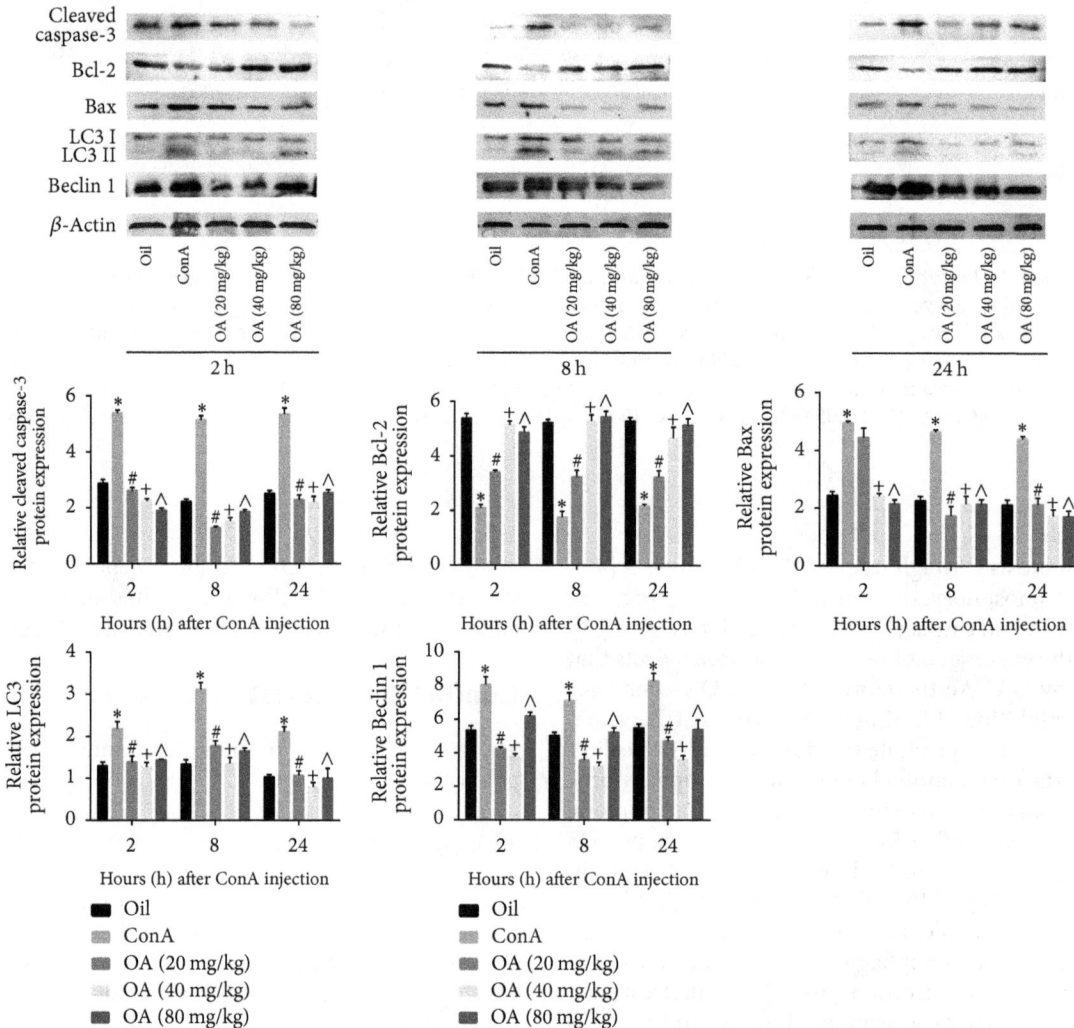

(b)

FIGURE 4: Continued.

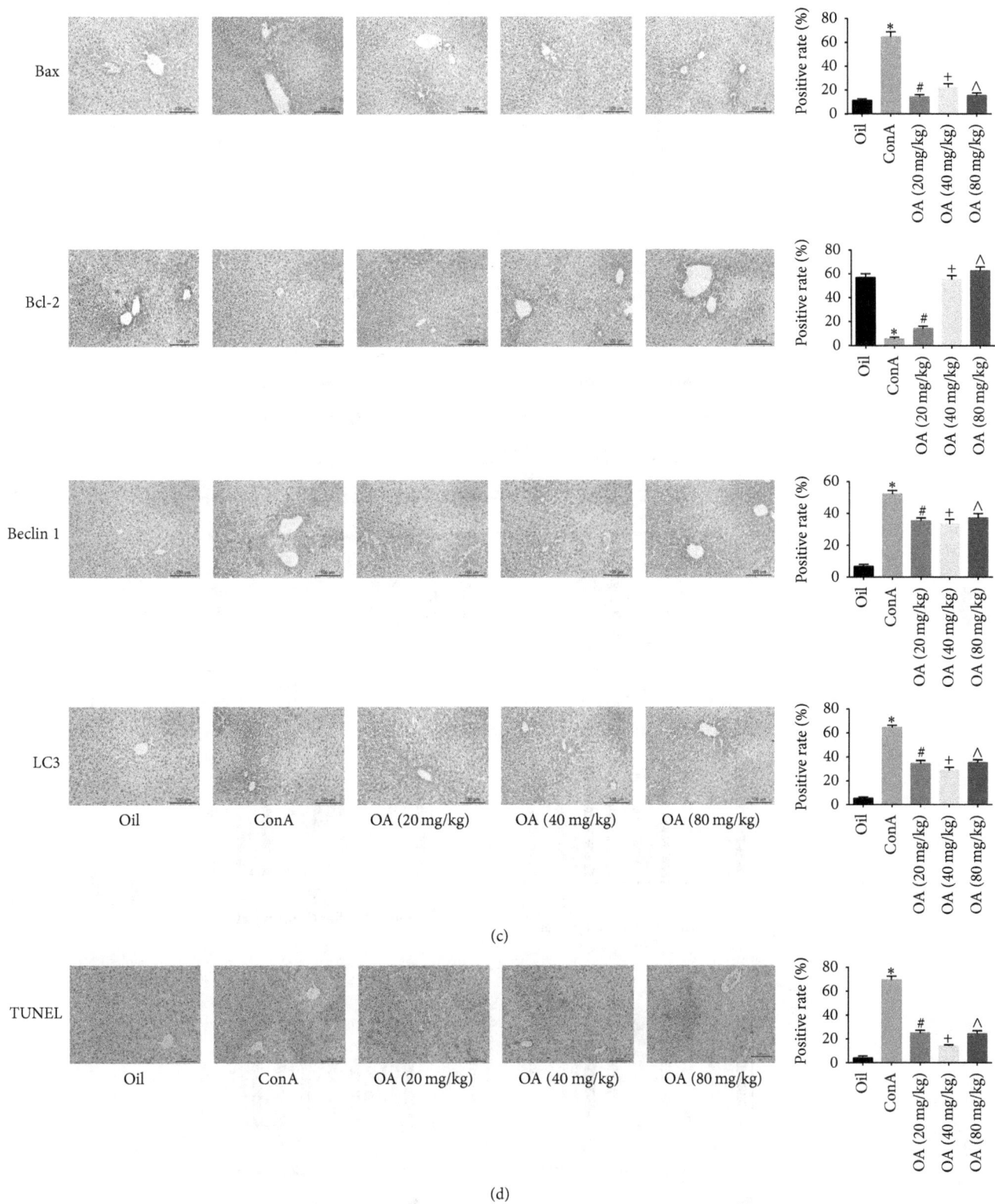

FIGURE 4: *OA regulates autophagy and apoptosis in ConA-induced liver injury. Notes.* (a) mRNA levels of caspase-3, caspase-9, Bcl-2, Bax, LC3, and Beclin 1 were determined using real-time PCR. (b) Protein expression of caspase-3, Bcl-2, Bax, Beclin 1, and LC3 was evaluated by western blot. (c) Representative immunohistochemistry images (200x magnification) show the expression levels of Bax, Bcl-2, Beclin 1, and LC3 at 8 h of exposure to ConA. (d) TUNEL staining (200x magnification) of liver tissue at 8 h represents apoptotic cells ($n = 6$; $^*P < 0.05$ for oil versus ConA; $^\#P < 0.05$ for ConA + OA (20 mg/kg) versus ConA; $^+P < 0.05$ for ConA + OA (40 mg/kg) versus ConA; $^\wedge P < 0.05$ for ConA + OA (80 mg/kg) versus ConA).

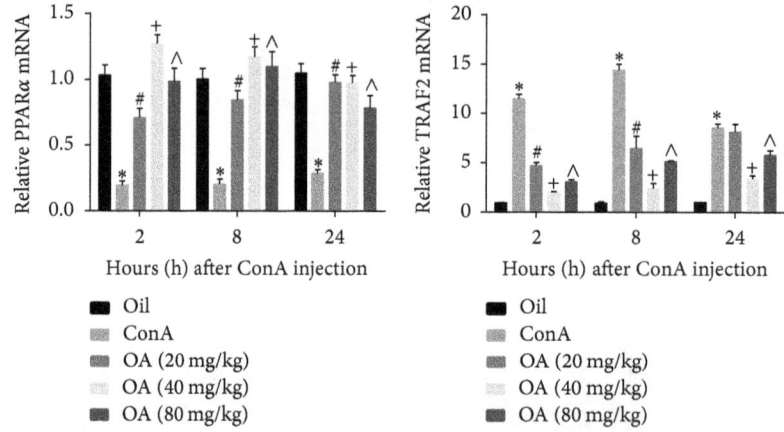

(a)

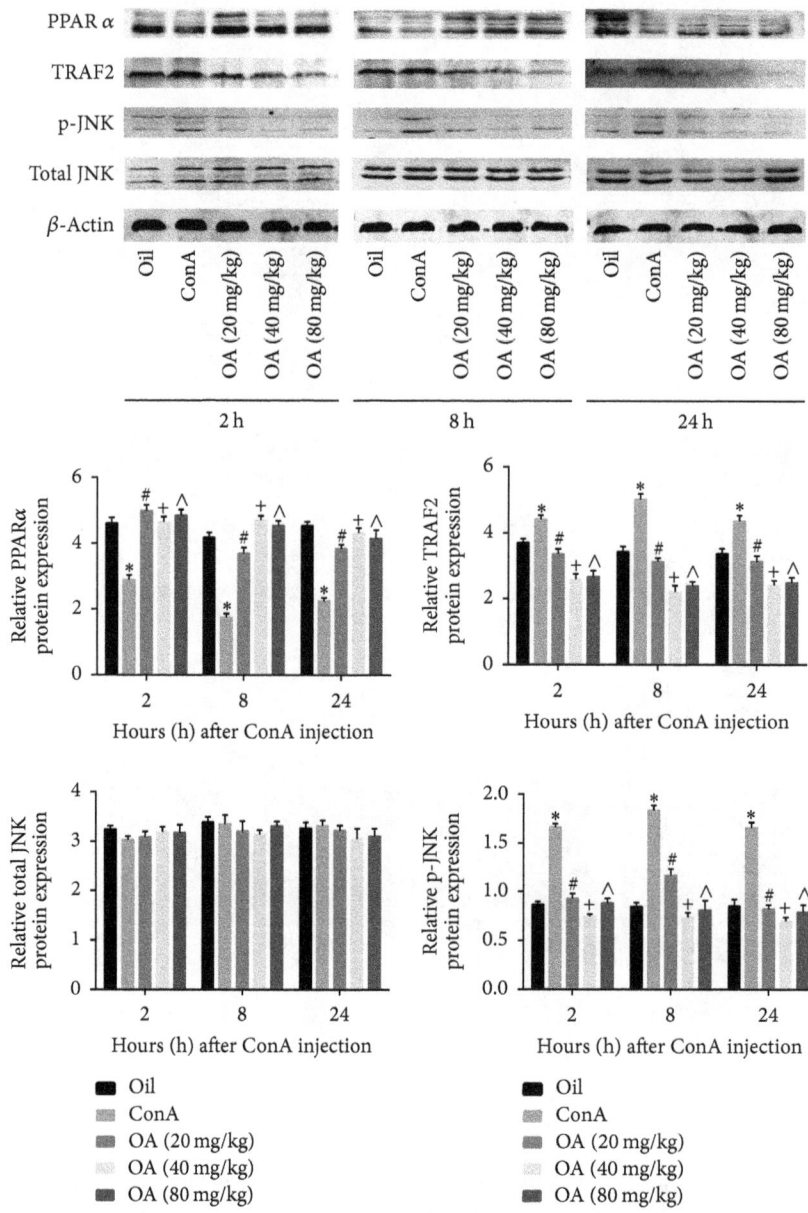

(b)

FIGURE 5: Continued.

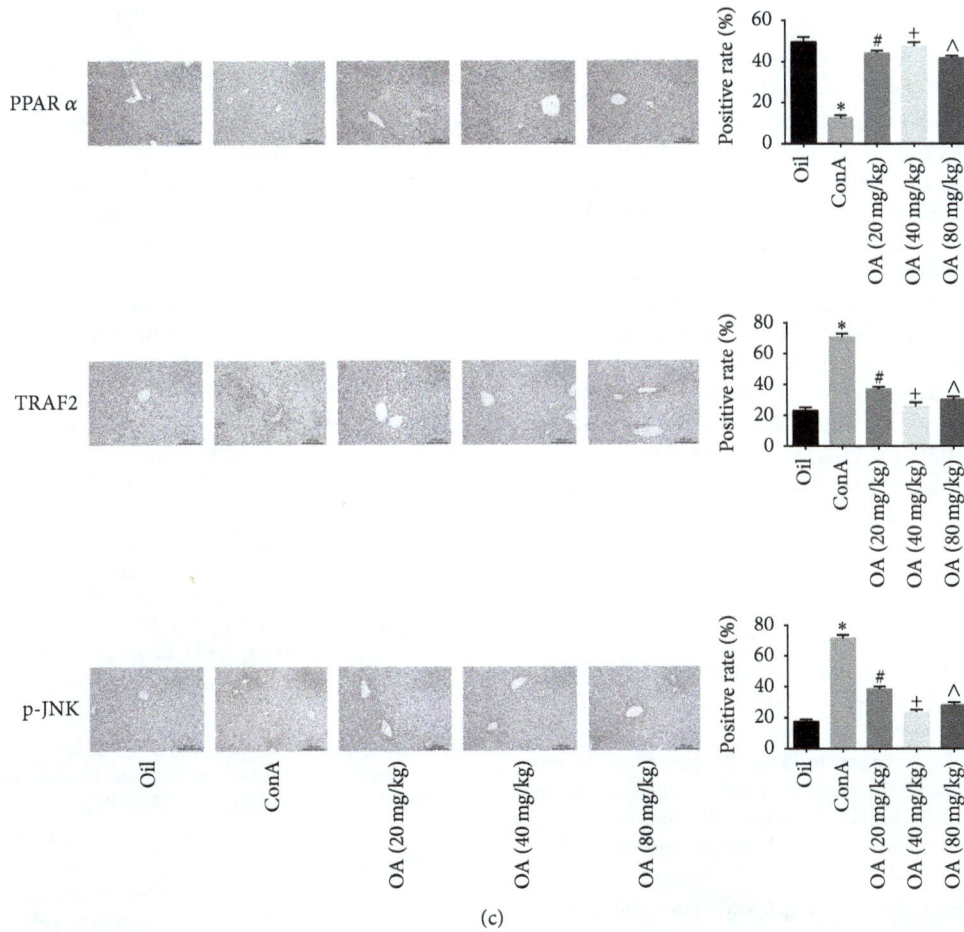

(c)

FIGURE 5: *OA regulates PPARα and JNK signaling in ConA-induced liver injury. Notes.* (a) mRNA expression levels of PPARα and TRAF2 were measured with real-time PCR. (b) Protein expression levels of PPARα, TRAF2, total JNK, and phospho-JNK were determined using western blot. (c) Representative immunohistochemistry images (200x magnification) were used to evaluate the expression levels of PPARα, TRAF2, and phospho-JNK after 8 h of exposure to ConA ($n = 6$; [*]$P < 0.05$ for oil versus ConA; [#]$P < 0.05$ for ConA + OA (20 mg/kg) versus ConA; [+]$P < 0.05$ for ConA + OA (40 mg/kg) versus ConA; [^]$P < 0.05$ for ConA + OA (80 mg/kg) versus ConA).

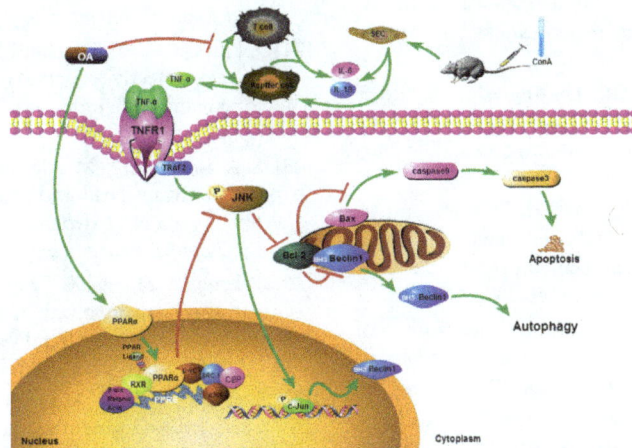

FIGURE 6: *A schematic representation of the pathways modulated by OA in response to ConA.* In our ConA-induced liver injury model, OA activates PPARα leading to decreased expression of cytokines, including TNF-α, IL-1β, and IL-6. OA also attenuates JNK signaling activated by TNF-α. Furthermore, OA suppresses the phosphorylation of JNK. Activated JNK inhibits Bcl-2 activity, thus promoting the activation of caspase-9 induced by Bax expression and the activation of Beclin 1. OA exhibits hepatoprotective effects via attenuating apoptosis and autophagy through regulating JNK signaling and activating PPARα.

Supplementary Materials

To support our viewpoint that oleanolic acid is purely acting as a PPARα ligand in this case, real-time PCR and western blot were used to evaluate the expression level of CPT1A and ACOX1, which were both target genes of PPARα. As is shown in Supplemental Figure, the mRNA and protein expression of CPT1A and ACOX1 were both reduced in ConA group, and these levels were significantly upregulated in response to OA pretreatment. Our findings further indicated that OA exhibited liver protection by acting as a PPARα ligand. OA is related to CPT1A and ACOX1 in ConA-induced liver injury. Notes: (A) mRNA expression levels of CPT1A and ACOX1 were measured with real-time PCR; (B) protein expression levels of CPT1A and ACOX1 were determined using western blot ($n = 6$; $^*P < 0.05$ for oil versus ConA; $^\#P < 0.05$ for ConA + OA (20 mg/kg) versus ConA; $^+P < 0.05$ for ConA + OA (40 mg/kg) versus ConA; $^\wedge P < 0.05$ for ConA + OA (80 mg/kg) versus ConA). *(Supplementary Materials)*

References

[1] M. Ghabril, N. Chalasani, and E. Bjornsson, "Drug-induced liver injury: a clinical update," *Current Opinion in Gastroenterology*, vol. 26, pp. 222–226, 2010.

[2] P. A. Soares, C. O. Nascimento, T. S. Porto, M. T. Correia, A. L. Porto, and M. G. Carneiro-da-Cunha, "Purification of a lectin from Canavalia ensiformis using PEG–citrate aqueous two-phase system," *J Chromatogr B Analyt Technol Biomed Life Sci*, vol. 879, pp. 457–460, 2011.

[3] G. Sass, S. Heinlein, A. Agli, R. Bang, J. Schümann, and G. Tiegs, "Cytokine expression in three mouse models of experimental hepatitis," *Cytokine*, vol. 19, no. 3, pp. 115–120, 2002.

[4] S. Li, Y. Xia, K. Chen et al., "Epigallocatechin-3-gallate attenuates apoptosis and autophagy in concanavalin a-induced hepatitis by inhibiting BNIP3," *Drug Design, Development and Therapy*, vol. 10, pp. 631–647, 2016.

[5] S. Xu, L. Wu, Q. Zhang et al., "Pretreatment with propylene glycol alginate sodium sulfate ameliorated concanavalin A-induced liver injury by regulating the PI3K/Akt pathway in mice," *Life Sciences*, vol. 185, pp. 103–113, 2017.

[6] M. L. Miller, Y. Sun, and Y. X. Fu, "Cutting edge: B and T lymphocyte attenuator signaling on NKT cells inhibits cytokine release and tissue injury in early immune responses," *The Journal of Immunology*, vol. 183, pp. 32–36, 2009.

[7] F. Gantner, M. Leist, S. Küsters, K. Vogt, H.-D. Volk, and G. Tiegs, "T cell stimulus-induced crosstalk between lymphocytes and liver macrophages results in augmented cytokine release," *Experimental Cell Research*, vol. 229, no. 1, pp. 137–146, 1996.

[8] H.-X. Wang, M. Liu, S.-Y. Weng et al., "Immune mechanisms of Concanavalin a model of autoimmune hepatitis," *World Journal of Gastroenterology*, vol. 18, no. 2, pp. 119–125, 2012.

[9] F. Heymann, K. Hamesch, R. Weiskirchen, and F. Tacke, "The concanavalin A model of acute hepatitis in mice," *Laboratory Animal*, vol. 49, pp. 12–20, 2015.

[10] E. Guo, R. Li, J. Yang et al., "FK866 attenuates acute hepatic failure through c-jun-N-terminal kinase (JNK)-dependent autophagy," *Scientific Reports*, vol. 7, no. 1, article no. 2206, 2017.

[11] K. Chen, J. Li, S. Li et al., "15d-PGJ2 alleviates ConA-induced acute liver injury in mice by up-regulating HO-1 and reducing

[12] hepatic cell autophagy," *Biomedicine & Pharmacotherapy*, vol. 80, pp. 183–192, 2016.

[12] J. Li et al., "Protective effects of astaxanthin on ConA-induced autoimmune hepatitis by the JNK/p-JNK pathway-mediated inhibition of autophagy and apoptosis," *PLoS One*, vol. 10, Article ID e0120440, 2015.

[13] H. M. Ni, X. Chen, W. X. Ding, M. Schuchmann, and X. M. Yin, "Differential roles of JNK in ConA/GalN and ConA-induced liver injury in mice," *The American Journal of Pathology*, vol. 173, pp. 962–972, 2008.

[14] N. Sultana and A. Ata, "Oleanolic acid and related derivatives as medicinally important compounds," *Journal of Enzyme Inhibition and Medicinal Chemistry*, vol. 23, pp. 739–756, 2008.

[15] J. Pollier and A. Goossens, "Oleanolic acid," *Phytochemistry*, vol. 77, pp. 10–15, 2012.

[16] A. Petronelli, G. Pannitteri, and U. Testa, "Triterpenoids as new promising anticancer drugs," *Anticancer Drugs*, vol. 20, pp. 880–892, 2009.

[17] X. Wang, R. Liu, W. Zhang et al., "Oleanolic acid improves hepatic insulin resistance via antioxidant, hypolipidemic and anti-inflammatory effects," *Molecular and Cellular Endocrinology*, vol. 376, no. 1-2, pp. 70–80, 2013.

[18] P. Dzubak, M. Hajduch, D. Vydra et al., "Pharmacological activities of natural triterpenoids and their therapeutic implications," *Natural Product Reports*, vol. 23, no. 3, pp. 394–411, 2006.

[19] Z. Ovesna, K. Kozics, and D. Slamenova, "Protective effects of ursolic acid and oleanolic acid in leukemic cells," *Mutation Research*, vol. 600, pp. 131–137, 2006.

[20] L. I. Somova, F. O. Shode, P. Ramnanan, and A. Nadar, "Antihypertensive, antiatherosclerotic and antioxidant activity of triterpenoids isolated from *Olea europaea*, subspecies *africana* leaves," *Journal of Ethnopharmacology*, vol. 84, no. 2-3, pp. 299–305, 2003.

[21] J. Liu, "Oleanolic acid and ursolic acid: research perspectives," *Journal of Ethnopharmacology*, vol. 100, no. 1-2, pp. 92–94, 2005.

[22] J. Liu, "Pharmacology of oleanolic acid and ursolic acid," *Journal of Ethnopharmacology*, vol. 49, no. 2, pp. 57–68, 1995.

[23] C. D. Klaassen and S. A. Reisman, "Nrf2 the rescue: effects of the antioxidative/electrophilic response on the liver," *Toxicology and Applied Pharmacology*, vol. 244, pp. 57–65, 2010.

[24] J. Liu, Q. Wu, Y. F. Lu, and J. Pi, "New insights into generalized hepatoprotective effects of oleanolic acid: key roles of metallothionein and Nrf2 induction," *Biochemical Pharmacology*, vol. 76, pp. 922–928, 2008.

[25] S. A. Reisman, L. M. Aleksunes, and C. D. Klaassen, "Oleanolic acid activates Nrf2 and protects from acetaminophen hepatotoxicity via Nrf2-dependent and Nrf2-independent processes," *Biochemical Pharmacology*, vol. 77, no. 7, pp. 1273–1282, 2009.

[26] J. Feng, P. Zhang, X. Chen, and G. He, "PI3K and ERK/Nrf2 pathways are involved in oleanolic acid-induced heme oxygenase-1 expression in rat vascular smooth muscle cells," *Journal of Cellular Biochemistry*, vol. 112, pp. 1524–1531, 2011.

[27] X. Wang, X.-L. Ye, R. Liu et al., "Antioxidant activities of oleanolic acid in vitro: possible role of Nrf2 and MAP kinases," *Chemico-Biological Interactions*, vol. 184, no. 3, pp. 328–337, 2010.

[28] J. D. Tugwood, I. Issemann, R. G. Anderson, K. R. Bundell, W. L. McPheat, and S. Green, "The mouse peroxisome proliferator activated receptor recognizes a response element in the 5' flanking sequence of the rat acyl CoA oxidase gene," *EMBO Journal*, vol. 11, no. 2, pp. 433–439, 1992.

[29] Q. Yang, Y. Xie, A. M. Eriksson, B. D. Nelson, and J. W. DePierre, "Further evidence for the involvement of inhibition of cell proliferation and development in thymic and splenic atrophy induced by the peroxisome proliferator perfluoroctanoic acid in mice," *Biochemical Pharmacology*, vol. 62, no. 8, pp. 1133–1140, 2001.

[30] Q. Yang and F. J. Gonzalez, "Peroxisome proliferator-activated receptor alpha regulates B lymphocyte development via an indirect pathway in mice," *Biochemical Pharmacology*, vol. 68, pp. 2143–2150, 2004.

[31] S. Kersten and R. Stienstra, "The role and regulation of the peroxisome proliferator activated receptor alpha in human liver," *Biochimie*, vol. 136, pp. 75–84, 2017.

[32] S. E. Dunn, S. S. Ousman, R. A. Sobel et al., "Peroxisome proliferator–activated receptor (PPAR)α expression in T cells mediates gender differences in development of T cell–mediated autoimmunity," *The Journal of Experimental Medicine*, vol. 204, no. 2, pp. 321–330, 2007.

[33] Y. F. Lu, J. Liu, K. C. Wu, and C. D. Klaassen, "Protection against phalloidin-induced liver injury by oleanolic acid involves Nrf2 activation and suppression of Oatp1b2," *Toxicology Letters*, vol. 232, pp. 326–332, 2015.

[34] Z. Yu, W. Sun, W. Peng, R. Yu, G. Li, and T. Jiang, "Pharmacokinetics in Vitro and in Vivo of Two Novel Prodrugs of Oleanolic Acid in Rats and Its Hepatoprotective Effects against Liver Injury Induced by CCl4," *Molecular Pharmaceutics*, vol. 13, no. 5, pp. 1699–1710, 2016.

[35] C. Wang, Y. Xia, Y. Zheng et al., "Protective effects of N-acetyl-cysteine in concanavalin a-induced hepatitis in mice," *Mediators of Inflammation*, vol. 2015, Article ID 189785, 17 pages, 2015.

[36] Y. Wang, L. Zhou, Y. Li et al., "The Effects of Berberine on Concanavalin A-Induced Autoimmune Hepatitis (AIH) in Mice and the Adenosine 5'-Monophosphate (AMP)-Activated Protein Kinase (AMPK) Pathway," *Medical Science Monitor*, vol. 23, pp. 6150–6161, 2017.

[37] B. Bhushan, C. Walesky, M. Manley et al., "Pro-regenerative signaling after acetaminophen-induced acute liver injury in mice identified using a novel incremental dose model," *The American Journal of Pathology*, vol. 184, no. 11, pp. 3013–3025, 2014.

[38] J. Liu, Y. Liu, C. Madhu, and C. D. Klaassen, "Protective effects of oleanolic acid on acetaminophen-induced hepatotoxicity in mice," *Journal of Pharmacology and Experimental Therapeutics*, vol. 266, pp. 1607–1613, 1993.

[39] S. W. Lim, S. P. Hong, S. W. Jeong et al., "Simultaneous effect of ursolic acid and oleanolic acid on epidermal permeability barrier function and epidermal keratinocyte differentiation via peroxisome proliferator-activated receptor-α," *The Journal of Dermatology*, vol. 34, no. 9, pp. 625–634, 2007.

[40] T. Liu, Y. Xia, J. Li et al., "Shikonin Attenuates Concanavalin A-Induced Acute Liver Injury in Mice via Inhibition of the JNK Pathway," *Mediators of Inflammation*, vol. 2016, Article ID 2748367, 14 pages, 2016.

[41] J. Li, K. Chen, S. Li et al., "Pretreatment with Fucoidan from Fucus vesiculosus Protected against ConA-Induced Acute Liver Injury by Inhibiting Both Intrinsic and Extrinsic Apoptosis," *PLoS ONE*, vol. 11, no. 4, Article ID e0152570, 2016.

[42] C. R. Weston and R. J. Davis, "The JNK signal transduction pathway," *Current Opinion in Cell Biology*, vol. 19, pp. 142–149, 2007.

[43] L. Cabal-Hierro, N. Artime, J. Iglesias et al., "A TRAF2 binding independent region of TNFR2 is responsible for TRAF2 depletion and enhancement of cytotoxicity driven by TNFR1," *Oncotarget*, vol. 5, no. 1, pp. 224–236, 2014.

[44] X. Wang et al., "Protective effect of oleanolic acid against beta cell dysfunction and mitochondrial apoptosis: crucial role of ERK-NRF2 signaling pathway," *Journal of Biological Regulators & Homeostatic Agents*, vol. 27, pp. 55–67, 2013.

[45] J. P. Renton, N. Xu, J. J. Clark, and M. R. Hansen, "Interaction of neurotrophin signaling with Bcl-2 localized to the mitochondria and endoplasmic reticulum on spiral ganglion neuron survival and neurite growth," *Journal of Neuroscience Research*, vol. 88, pp. 2239–2251, 2010.

[46] Y. Y. Zhou, Y. Li, W. Q. Jiang, and L. F. Zhou, "MAPK/JNK signalling: a potential autophagy regulation pathway," *Bioscience Reports*, vol. 35, 2015.

[47] A. Oberstein, P. D. Jeffrey, and Y. Shi, "Crystal structure of the Bcl-XL-Beclin 1 peptide complex: Beclin 1 is a novel BH3-only protein," *The Journal of Biological Chemistry*, vol. 282, Article ID M700492200, pp. 13123–13132, 2007.

[48] S. Pattingre, A. Tassa, X. Qu et al., "Bcl-2 antiapoptotic proteins inhibit Beclin 1-dependent autophagy," *Cell*, vol. 122, no. 6, pp. 927–939, 2005.

[49] K. Chen, J. Li, S. Li et al., "15-Deoxy-$\Delta^{12,14}$-prostaglandin J_2 alleviates hepatic ischemia-reperfusion injury in mice via inducing antioxidant response and inhibiting apoptosis and autophagy," *Acta Pharmacologica Sinica*, vol. 38, no. 5, pp. 672–687, 2017.

[50] J. Feng, Q. Zhang, W. Mo et al., "Salidroside pretreatment attenuates apoptosis and autophagy during hepatic ischemia–reperfusion injury by inhibiting the mitogen-activated protein kinase pathway in mice," *Drug Design, Development and Therapy*, vol. 11, pp. 1989–2006, 2017.

[51] P. Jiang and N. Mizushima, "LC3- and p62-based biochemical methods for the analysis of autophagy progression in mammalian cells," in *Methods*, pp. 13–18, 2015.

[52] J. Li, K. Chen, S. Li et al., "Protective effect of fucoidan from fucus vesiculosus on liver fibrosis via the TGF-β1/Smad pathway-mediated inhibition of extracellular matrix and autophagy," *Drug Design, Development and Therapy*, vol. 10, pp. 619–630, 2016.

[53] T. Liu, Q. Zhang, W. Mo et al., "The protective effects of shikonin on hepatic ischemia/reperfusion injury are mediated by the activation of the PI3K/Akt pathway," *Scientific Reports*, vol. 7, Article ID 44785, 2017.

11

Signaling Mechanisms of Selective PPARγ Modulators in Alzheimer's Disease

Manoj Govindarajulu,[1] Priyanka D. Pinky ⓘ,[1] Jenna Bloemer ⓘ,[1] Nila Ghanei,[1]
Vishnu Suppiramaniam ⓘ,[1,2] and Rajesh Amin ⓘ[1,2]

[1]Department of Drug Discovery and Development, Harrison School of Pharmacy, Auburn University, Auburn, AL, USA
[2]Center for Neuroscience, Auburn University, Auburn, AL, USA

Correspondence should be addressed to Rajesh Amin; rha0003@auburn.edu

Academic Editor: Paul D. Drew

Alzheimer's disease (AD) is a chronic neurodegenerative disease characterized by abnormal protein accumulation, synaptic dysfunction, and cognitive impairment. The continuous increase in the incidence of AD with the aged population and mortality rate indicates the urgent need for establishing novel molecular targets for therapeutic potential. Peroxisome proliferator-activated receptor gamma (PPARγ) agonists such as rosiglitazone and pioglitazone reduce amyloid and tau pathologies, inhibit neuroinflammation, and improve memory impairments in several rodent models and in humans with mild-to-moderate AD. However, these agonists display poor blood brain barrier permeability resulting in inadequate bioavailability in the brain and thus requiring high dosing with chronic time frames. Furthermore, these dosing levels are associated with several adverse effects including increased incidence of weight gain, liver abnormalities, and heart failure. Therefore, there is a need for identifying novel compounds which target PPARγ more selectively in the brain and could provide therapeutic benefits without a high incidence of adverse effects. This review focuses on how PPARγ agonists influence various pathologies in AD with emphasis on development of novel selective PPARγ modulators.

1. Introduction

Alzheimer's disease (AD) is the sixth leading cause of mortality in the United States. In 2018, an estimated 5.7 million Americans of all ages are living with Alzheimer's dementia and this is projected to increase to 14 million by 2050 [1]. However, there are limited options to prevent the progression of the disease. Moreover, the continuous increase in mortality rates due to AD reinforces the critical need for identifying novel molecular targets with therapeutic potential. For example, the failure of several recent potential therapies in clinical trials for improving cognitive deficits in AD by reducing amyloid beta (Aβ) levels, suggests a need to explore alternative approaches for AD treatment that are not focused upon altering Aβ levels.

Pathological correlations between type 2 diabetes mellitus (DM) and AD provide direct links for the development of cognitive deficits in both diseases and suggest potential application of antidiabetic drugs for AD [2, 3]. Type 2 DM is a disorder of altered glucose regulation and is associated with cognitive decline [4]. Although there are direct links between AD and DM in the manifestation of cognitive impairment, there is an understanding that impaired insulin signaling directly alters memory in AD. Insulin signaling in the brain has a significant role in modulating neuroendocrine and neurotrophic functions including synaptic plasticity [5, 6]. Therefore, extensive investigation of these correlations between the two diseases will potentiate the identification of novel therapeutic targets for the treatment of AD.

Peroxisome proliferator-activated receptors (PPARs), a subfamily of nuclear receptors, play a crucial role in regulating insulin sensitivity and may serve as potential therapeutic targets for AD. Recently, pharmacological activation by a class of PPAR subtype, PPARγ agonists thiazolidinediones (TZDs), has been found to improve learning and memory in transgenic AD animal models [7, 8]. Furthermore, meta-analysis studies indicate that pioglitazone treatment may offer therapeutic benefits in patients with early or mild-to-moderate AD [9]. Further analysis of these studies showed a significant reduction in amyloid beta and tau pathology measured in cerebral blood flow samples from AD patients. The anti-inflammatory properties and improved glucose metabolism by TZDs have helped explain how it improves cognition in AD patients and transgenic animal models of DM and AD [10, 11]. However, the molecular signaling mechanisms mediated by central PPARγ activation resulting in improved cognition in AD have not been extensively investigated. Furthermore, the use of these drugs for cognitive deficits in diabetes and AD is limited due to their poor bioavailability in the brain and off-target effects [12, 13]. Therefore, there is a critical need to develop PPARγ targeted agents that display improved tolerability. To understand the significance of these chemical and pharmacological standpoints, the molecular structure and how PPARγ modulates different cellular targets need to be more thoroughly evaluated.

Recently, the focus of PPARγ has intensified, as new ligands and novel biological roles have emerged for the receptor activity, particularly for its therapeutic potential in neurodegenerative disorders, such as AD. The present review discusses the beneficial role of PPARγ ligands on the pathologies of AD and the therapeutic potential of selective PPARγ modulators as future therapy for AD.

2. Overview of PPARs

2.1. Isoforms and Expression.
The PPARs are part of a subfamily of nuclear receptors that regulate several important cellular processes by activating or repressing transcription via their ligand binding domain (LBD) and DNA-binding domains (DBD) [14]. The initial PPAR (PPARα) was cloned as a nuclear receptor from a mouse-liver genetic (cDNA) library that was activated by several endogenous and xenobiotic compounds known as peroxisome proliferators. PPARs are named for their property of increasing both the number and activity of liver peroxisomes after administering high dose of these substances for a chronic time frame in rodents. Additionally, marked liver abnormalities progressing to liver carcinomas were noted, indicating that these substances at high doses strongly induce peroxisome proliferation [15].

The PPARs are mainly divided into PPARα, PPARβ/δ, and PPARγ. All the PPARs consist of distinct functional domains including an N-terminal transactivation domain (AF1), a highly conserved DBD, and a C-terminal ligand binding domain (LBD) that contains a ligand transactivation function (AF2). Each subtype displays distinct effects on the body; for example, PPARα regulates whole body energy homeostasis by reducing lipid levels, regulating glucose homeostasis, and reducing insulin resistance [16]. PPAR β/δ regulates lipid metabolism and myelination in the brain while PPARγ regulates lipid and glucose homeostasis, mitochondrial biogenesis, and inflammation [17].

The PPARγ receptor is unique in that despite being expressed from the same gene, it has different promoters and 5'-exons. Hence, it consists of three isoforms, namely,

PPARγ-1, PPARγ-2, and PPARγ-3. PPARγ-1 and PPARγ-3 are similar, while PPARγ-2 differs in the ligand-independent region at the N-terminus. PPARγ-2 has an extra 30 amino acid residues in the amino end, which provides a potent transcriptional activity compared to PPARγ-1 [18]. PPARγ-1 is expressed in almost all cells while PPARγ-2 is restricted in the adipose tissue [19]. In the CNS (central nervous system), all the three subtypes of PPARs are expressed, with PPAR β/δ being the most abundant subtype [20, 21]. PPARα is involved in acetylcholine metabolism, excitatory neurotransmission, and oxidative stress defense [22]. PPARβ/δ is ubiquitously expressed in all cell types including immature oligodendrocytes and promotes differentiation and myelination in the CNS [23, 24], while PPARγ is expressed predominantly in microglia and astrocytes and regulates inflammation in the CNS [25].

2.2. PPAR Signaling.
PPARs regulate the expression of various genes through a complex set of mechanisms. The homo PPAR forms a heterodimer with another class of nuclear receptors, retinoid X receptors (RXR). During unstimulated conditions, the heterodimer complex is associated with corepressors (NCoR and SMRT), which suppress gene transcription [26]. Ligand binding to the hydrophobic pocket of the PPAR receptor induces conformational changes in the LBD structure, thereby resulting in its activation. Changes in the conformation on ligand binding lead to release of corepressors NCoR/SMRT or Not1, which generally prevents gene transcription, respectively. Release of corepressor with full agonist results in the stabilization of the LBD, resulting in binding of coactivators CBP/P300, p160/SRC-1, and vitamin D receptor interacting protein (DRIP) or thyroid hormone receptor associated protein (TRAP) complexes resulting in the activation of the PPAR molecule. Once activated, the PPAR/retinoid X receptor heterodimer stimulates peroxisome proliferator response elements (PPRE) in the promoter region of target genes. This scaffold recruits histone acetyl transferases and the gene transcription machinery (RNA polymerase complex), which together initiate chromatin relaxation to permit transcription of target genes [27] as depicted in Figure 1. Coactivator PGC-1α gene expression is particularly important in mediating cognition and has shown protective effects against AD. In addition, it regulates mitochondrial biogenesis, oxidative metabolism, fatty acid oxidation, and gluconeogenesis via PPARs; these effects on mitochondria, in turn, can improve brain function [28].

Apart from the above-mentioned action of PPARs involving gene transcription in the nucleus, nongenomic actions associated with the cytoplasmic PPARs have been observed. Nongenomic regulation of PPARγ is mediated by interaction with cytosolic second messengers, including kinases and phosphatases [29]. For instance, in response to mitogen stimulation, the MAP/ERK kinase, MAPK kinase (MEK)-1, binds directly to the AF2 domain of PPARγ, leading to the sequestration of PPARγ in the cytoplasm. Selective inhibition of this MEK1/PPAR interaction has been proposed to offer novel pharmacological treatments of various cancers, metabolic disorders, and inflammation [30]. Recent studies indicate that posttranslational control of PPARs occurs through

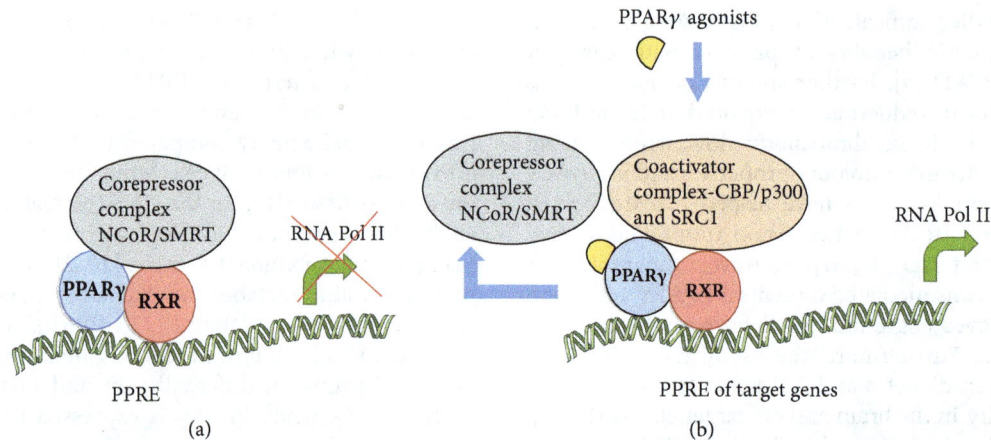

FIGURE 1: Mechanism of action of PPARγ agonists. (a) During unstimulated conditions, the heterodimer is associated with corepressors which suppress gene transcription. (b) Binding of PPARγ agonist induces release of corepressor complex, while binding to coactivator complex, thereby stimulating the response elements of target genes. This scaffold recruits histone acetyl transferase and RNA polymerase leading to transcription of target genes.

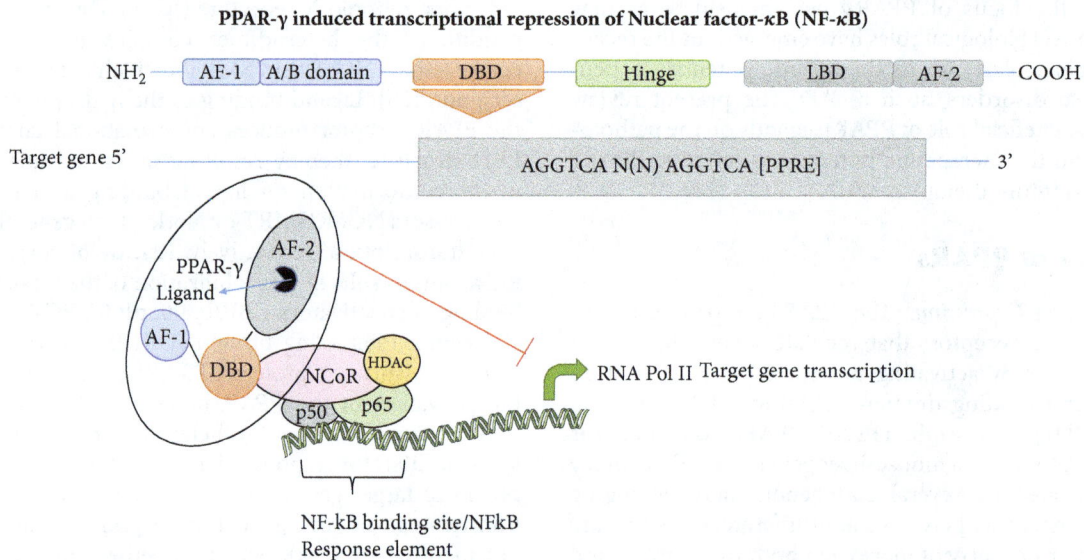

FIGURE 2: PPARγ mediated transrepression of NF-κB through SUMOylation modification. Binding of PPARγ ligand to the AF-2 domain at Lys-365 position is important in regulation of inflammatory gene expression through transrepression. Additionally, recruitment of NCoR with inhibition of NCoR proteosomal degradation occurs.

phosphorylation, SUMOylation, ubiquitination, and nitration [31]. The phosphorylation of PPARγ occurs at several sites via different kinases including MAPKs. An N-terminal serine phosphorylation (Ser82 in PPARγ-1 and Ser112 in PPARγ-2), mediated by MAPKs, reduces the transcriptional activity of PPARγ-1 and PPARγ-2 (in cells activated by serum) [32, 33]. Phosphorylation as a mechanism of action of PPARγ agonists has been recently suggested linking its role to obesity, inflammation, and insulin resistance [34]. For instance, rosiglitazone was found to inhibit phosphorylation of PPARγ at Ser273 by cyclin-dependent kinase 5 (CDK5) in adipose tissue. This leads to transcription of insulin-response genes (such as adiponectin and adipsin) thereby mediating antidiabetic effects. As CDK5 is activated by inflammatory

mediators, targeting CDK5/PPARγ regulation may offer new avenues in treating various disorders where inflammation is a key component. SUMOylation is a posttranslational modification that regulates the stability, nuclear/cytosolic ratio, and activity of several transcription factors. Of importance is the transcriptional repression of inflammatory genes such as inducible nitric oxide synthase (iNOS) and TNF-α, which are regulated by NF-kB pathway. Additionally, SUMOylation also induces recruitment of PPAR corepressors, such as NCoR as depicted in Figure 2.

The LBD of PPARγ consisting of the transcriptional AF2 motif associated with helix 12 mediates most of the pharmacological actions of PPARγ agonists [47]. The importance of AF2 motif in regulating PPARγ targeted genes has been extensively studied, thereby allowing us to understand the mechanism of ligand-induced transcriptional activation by PPARγ [48, 49]. AF2 helix is in an equilibrium state between closed (active) and open (inactive) conformations in the absence of the ligand [50]. However, binding to a full agonist leads to AF2 helix getting locked in closed (active) state, thereby allowing recruitment of coactivators for transcriptional activation [51]. Hence, developing novel PPARγ ligands that stabilize the AF2 helix in distinct states between closed and open conformations would offer therapeutic advantage which is discussed in subsequent sections.

Several studies have reported that the locking of AF2 helix in its closed conformation is responsible for the antidiabetic effects as well as several side effects noted with PPARγ agonists like TZDs [52–54]. Hence, developing novel PPARγ ligands that stabilize the AF2 helix in distinct states between the closed and open conformations will selectively recruit coactivators for newer therapeutic benefits with reduced side effects [55–57].

Recently, several natural and synthetic PPARγ agonists have been developed to treat various disorders, out of which the selective PPARγ modulators (SPPARγMs) have attracted considerable attention because of their ability to selectively target PPARγ activity states, thereby offering therapeutic efficacy with minimal side effects [58–61]. Currently, no SPPARγMs have been successfully used in clinical practice, and mechanistically it remains unclear how to achieve selective PPARγ activation. The subsequent sections discuss the role of PPARγ in modulating the pathologies of AD followed by SPPARγMs under development for treating AD.

3. Overview of AD

Pathological changes related to AD occur many years before clinical symptoms are present. The traditional theory for the development of AD has been the amyloid beta cascade hypothesis, which postulates that pathogenic amyloid beta is the primary cause for development of AD and leads to the hyperphosphorylation of tau protein. However, it is becoming increasingly clear that a multitude of pathological mechanisms are likely at play to promote development of clinical AD [62]. Therefore, therapeutics with multiple mechanisms of action against AD pathology may be desirable in treatment of the disorder. Some early pathological processes which are increasingly recognized to contribute to AD include neuroinflammation [63], mitochondrial dysfunction [64], and dysregulated insulin signaling [65]. Amyloid beta accumulation occurs prior to clinical symptoms and persists throughout the course of the disease. Occurrence of memory dysfunction later in the disease is correlated with the severity of synaptic deficits and severity of tau pathology [66]. Therefore, an ideal AD drug may target multiple facets of the disease including inflammatory and metabolic components occurring early in disease, along with reducing pathogenic amyloid beta, hyperphosphorylated tau, and synaptic dysfunction later in the disease. In fact, PPARγ signaling exerts several potential beneficial mechanisms in early, as well as in late, AD, as it reduces inflammation, improves metabolic processes, and

may directly reduce levels of pathogenic amyloid beta and hyperphosphorylated tau. The hallmarks of AD relating to its pathologies are illustrated in Figure 3.

4. PPARγ in Alzheimer's Disease

4.1. Genetic Alterations Relating PPARγ to AD. Genome-wide association studies (GWAS) indicate a strong association between late onset Alzheimer's disease (LOAD) and over twenty genomic loci [67, 68]. One of the strongest genetic risk factors of LOAD is ApoE, and the presence of the ApoE4 allele is associated with an increased accumulation of Aβ. Several studies have shown increased ApoE-mRNA levels in LOAD brains and that cis-genetic variability contributes to differential ApoE gene expression [69–71]. Furthermore, chromosome 19q13.32, a gene rich region consisting of TOMM40, ApoE, and APOC1 genes, is implicated in several phenotypes including AD. This region exhibits a complex regulation and is enriched in potential PPARγ binding sites. PPARγ agonists decreased the levels of the TOMM40, ApoE, and APOC1-mRNAs, with the greatest effect on ApoE-mRNA through transcriptional regulation [72]. Furthermore, a study done by Barrera et al. investigated the effect of PPARγ knockdown on expression of twenty-four late onset AD-associated genes and demonstrated that PPARγ regulates the expression of seven LOAD-associated genes. Upregulation of six genes (ABCA7, ApoE, CASS4, CELF1, PTK2B, and ZCWPW1) and downregulation of one gene (*DSG2*) were noted and indicate that PPARγ agonists may represent an attractive class of drugs for preventing or delaying the onset of late onset AD [73].

4.2. PPARγ in Early Stages of AD

4.2.1. PPARγ and Amyloid Beta. AD is pathologically characterized by deposition of extracellular fibrillar amyloid derived from proteolytic cleavage of amyloid precursor protein (APP) and formation of senile plaques. An imbalance between Aβ production and its clearance leads to Aβ accumulation, which further leads to tau hyperphosphorylation and neurodegeneration [74]. PPARγ agonists have also been observed to reduce Aβ levels either by reducing the Aβ production or enhancing its clearance. Several studies have demonstrated the role of PPARγ agonists in decreasing Aβ accumulation. For instance, pioglitazone-treated APP transgenic mice showed reduced transcription and expression of β-secretase enzyme that processes APP to generate Aβ [75]. However, other studies have shown that APP processing and Aβ production are not affected by pioglitazone suggesting that decrease in Aβ levels by PPARγ agonists may be due to Aβ clearance [76].

Aβ clearance in the brain is mediated by enzymatic and nonenzymatic pathways. Some of the key enzymes include insulin-degrading enzyme (IDE), neprilysin (NEP), and matrix metalloproteinase (MMP)-9. The nonenzymatic pathway includes (1) drainage through perivascular basement membranes, (2) phagocytosis by microglia or astrocytes, and (3) clearance mediated by receptors such as low-density lipoprotein receptor-related protein 1 (LRP1) and

Preclinical AD

Prodromal AD

Alzheimer's Disease Progression

MCI due to AD (7-10 yrs)

Mild AD (2-5 yrs)

Moderate AD (2-5 yrs)

Severe AD (3-6 yrs)

Medial temporal lobe
No clinical symptoms but have underlying AD pathology

Medial temporal lobe-
Entorhinal cortex and hippocampus
Short term memory loss and attention deficit

Lateral temporal and parietal lobes-
Longer time to accomplish normal daily tasks, compromised judgement and confusion, mood and personality changes

Frontal lobes-
Shortened attention span, difficulty with language and organizing thoughts, loss of impulse control, anxiety and perceptual motor problems

Occipital lobes-
Visual problems, weight loss, lack of bowel and bladder control, difficulty swallowing and repeated infections

Oxidative stress, Energy dysregulation Mitochondrial dysfunction

Amyloid-Beta plaques Neurofibrillary tangles Neuroinflammation

Neurotransmitter dysfunction Impaired synaptic plasticity

Neurodegeneration Neuronal death

DISEASE MODIFYING DRUGS
Early treatment with novel therapeutics leads to delay in progression of disease. Ideal time to start therapy

CURRENT TREATMENT
MAJORITY OF FAILURES
Treatment unlikely to provide therapeutic effects or alter the disease progression as neurodegeneration and neuronal death has occurred

Delay the onset of AD by decreasing Aβ production and prevent tangle formation

Delay the onset of cognitive impairment by decreasing accumulated Aβ and decrease neurodegeneration by anti-Tau or neuroprotective drugs

Delay the onset or progression of AD by preventing neuronal loss, enhance the function of remaining neurons and neurotransmitter repletion

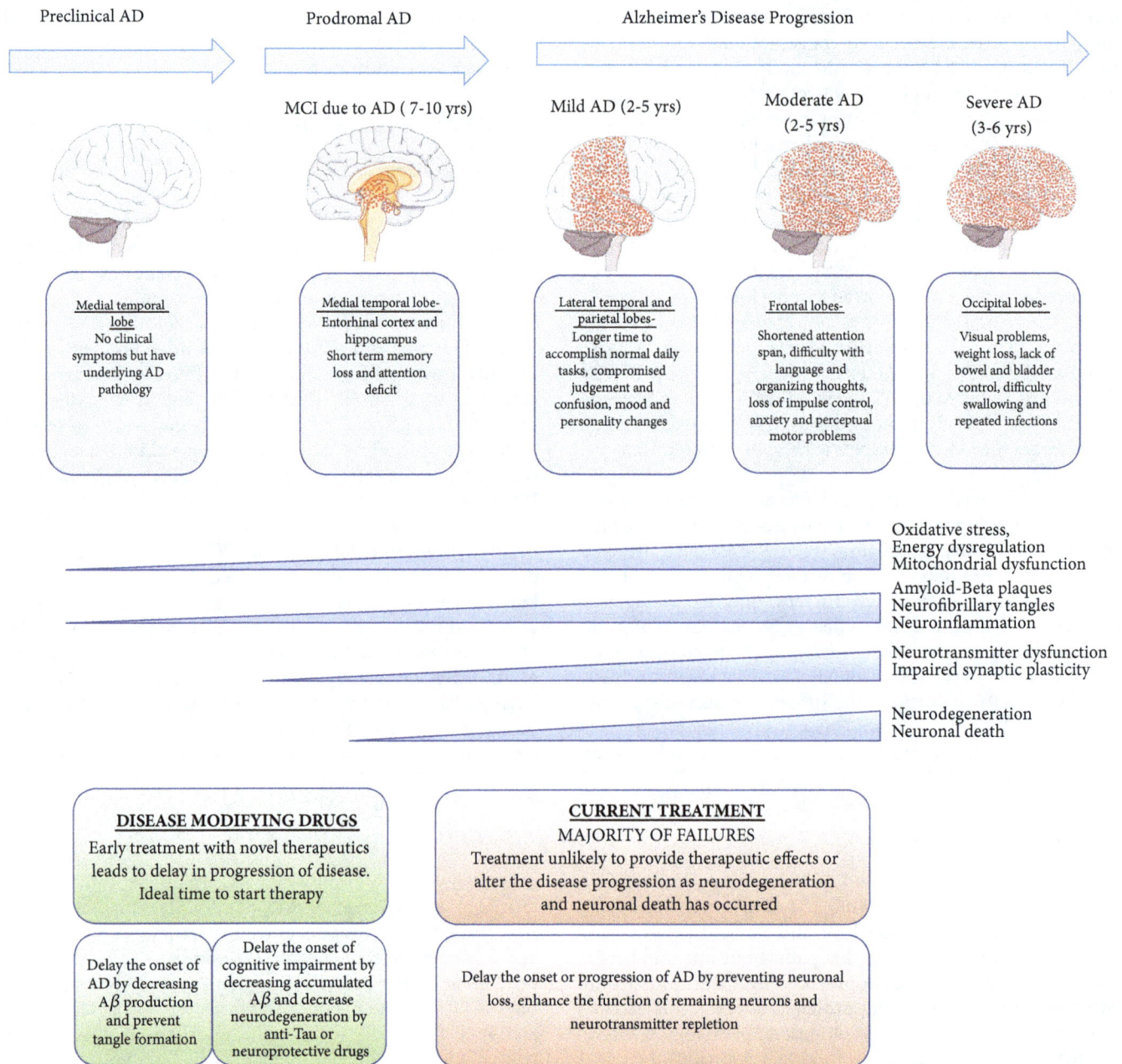

FIGURE 3: Description of progressive clinical stages and pathologies associated with Alzheimer's disease (AD) for relevance in developing therapeutic strategies for mitigating progression of AD.

P-glycoprotein localized predominantly on the abluminal side of the cerebral endothelium [77, 78].

LRP1 is important in mediating endocytosis of various proteins such as ApoE and Aβ.

Low-density lipoprotein (LDL) receptor-related protein 1 (LRP1) is a transmembrane receptor involved in the endocytosis of more than 40 structurally different ligands, including ApoE, and Aβ peptide [79, 80]. Levels of LRP1 are found to be decreased in AD patients indicating its role in mediating Aβ metabolism. PPARγ transcriptionally regulates LRP1 gene due to the presence of PPRE on the LRP1 promoter region [81]. A study by Rondon-Ortiz et al.

reported that rosiglitazone transcriptionally activated LRP1 gene in a concentration dependent manner in HepG2 cells [82]. Similarly, rosiglitazone upregulated LRP1 expression at both the mRNA and protein levels, via PPARγ activation [83]. *In vivo* studies utilizing AD models need to be performed to validate the role of PPARγ agonists and LRP1 in AD.

Apolipoprotein E (ApoE) is a lipoprotein expressed predominantly in the brain and is known to enhance Aβ degradation and phagocytosis in the microglia and astrocytes [74]. PPARγ agonists (rosiglitazone and pioglitazone) have also been shown to induce Aβ degradation by increasing apolipoprotein E (ApoE) concentrations in the brain

[76]. ApoE can increase the concentration of Aβ degrading enzyme neprilysin and insulin in astrocytes and microglia facilitating Aβ degradation [84]. In a recent study utilizing APP/Presenilin-1 mouse model [85], activation of PPARγ enhances the microglial uptake of Aβ resulting in reduced cortical and hippocampal Aβ level. This effect is mediated by scavenger receptor CD36, which is a well-known player of phagocytosis. This finding can be further confirmed by observance of reduced microglial response to fibrillar Aβ response in CD36 null mice [86]. Additionally, pioglitazone treatment on APP/PS1 mice increased the levels of ATP-binding cassette transporter (ABCA1) and ApoE, thereby decreasing the levels of Aβ by 50%. In addition, the expression and processing levels of APP and of Aβ-degrading enzymes were not altered, suggesting that the changes seen in amyloid deposition were a result of Aβ catabolism [87]. Similar results were obtained with rosiglitazone treatment in a J20 mouse model [88] and with the APP/PS1 mice [89]. These studies suggest that TZDs enhance amyloid clearance in cell lines of microglia and astrocytes treated with Aβ and these effects are related to the activation of the ApoE pathway. Interestingly, rosiglitazone improved cognition in mild-to-moderate AD patients that did not carry ApoE4 allele. In contrast, no improvements were noted in cognitive test in ApoE4 positive patients, indicating that the amyloid clearance pathway dependent on TZDs also depends on the expression of functional ApoE4 [36]. The compelling results from animal models of Alzheimer's disease underline the beneficial effects of PPARγ agonists on attenuating Aβ pathologies for future therapies.

4.2.2. PPARγ and Neuroinflammation. Several failures in AD clinical trials have encouraged researchers to look at treatment in the presymptomatic phase, where inflammation plays a vital role in the progression of neurodegeneration. One of the many potential beneficial effects of PPARγ is its ability to downregulate inflammatory gene expression in immune cells [90, 91]. For example, PPARγ activation has been shown to modulate the microglial response to amyloid deposition in such a way that it increases Aβ phagocytosis and decreases cytokine release [85]. The inflammatory hypothesis of AD involves activation of glial cells (microglia and astrocytes) by Aβ, which produces proinflammatory substances as a driving factor for neurodegeneration. Interestingly, a large meta-analysis reported that use of nonsteroidal anti-inflammatory drugs (NSAIDs), many of which have been shown to directly activate PPARγ, is associated with a reduced risk of developing AD [92]. NSAID medications have provided key evidence that AD progression or initiation is related to neuroinflammation and that PPARγ may mediate beneficial properties of NSAIDs in relation to AD. Commonly used NSAIDs including ibuprofen, indomethacin, and sulindac have been demonstrated to activate PPARγ [93]. Under physiological conditions, the expression of PPARγ in the brain is relatively less. However, its expression as measured by mRNA levels is elevated in AD patients, suggesting that PPAR may play a crucial role in modulating the pathology of AD [94]. Collectively, these findings led to the concept that PPARγ could be an important target for mitigating

brain inflammation in AD. More specifically, the activation of PPARγ suppressed various transcription factors involved in inflammation such as nuclear factor-kB (NF-kB), Stat-1, and transcription factors activator protein-1 [95] which are important proinflammatory genes as illustrated in Figure 4.

Additionally, PPARγ also downregulates cyclooxygenase-2 (COX-2), metalloproteinase-9 (MMP-9), inducible nitric oxide synthase (iNOS), proinflammatory cytokines, chemokines, and interleukins [96–98]. Thus, a reduction in PPARγ activation may contribute to chronic inflammation, and pharmacological treatment with PPARγ agonists may diminish expression of inflammatory genes. Several PPARγ ligands, both natural (15d-PGJ2, docosahexaenoic acid) and synthetic (NSAIDs and TZDs), were shown to inhibit the expression of interleukin-6 (IL-6), TNFα, and cyclooxygenase-2 (COX-2) from monocytic and microglial cell cultures stimulated with Aβ [99]. Similarly, the anti-inflammatory effects of PPARγ agonists like rosiglitazone and pioglitazone were noted in several AD mouse models [100, 101]. For example, the treatment with pioglitazone reduced astrocytes and microglial activation in the cortex and hippocampus of the A/T mouse that expresses high levels of Aβ and TGF-β1 [87]. At the same time, injection of rosiglitazone into the brain of Wistar rats, previously treated with Aβ oligomers, prevented the increase of inflammatory cytokines levels resulting in an improvement in cognitive decline and prevention of microglia activation [102]. Interestingly, similar effects were also observed in the AD transgenic mouse models J20 and APP/PS1 with oral administration of rosiglitazone [88]. Targeting microglia and astrocyte polarization may serve as therapeutic option. Cyclin-dependent kinase 5 (CDK5) is involved in activation of microglia and astrocytes and may serve as a potential therapeutic target for PPARγ agonist therapy. This possibility is supported in a report where pioglitazone treatment, in conditional CDK5 knockout mice, displayed significant reduction in the activation of microglia and astrocytes and neuronal loss resulting in improved survival rates [103]. Mechanistically, CDK5 is a protein kinase, whose dysregulation contributes to synaptic loss and tau hyperphosphorylation in the AT8 epitope (present in the AD brain) after stimulation of Aβ fibrils [104, 105]. Together, these findings suggest that an anti-inflammatory property by TZDs involves regulating microglia and astrocytes inflammation and may involve CDK5.

Recently, PPARγ has been implicated in macrophage polarization from M1, the classically activated phenotype, to M2, the alternatively activated phenotype, in several neurodegenerative diseases. M1 microglia have proinflammatory and neurotoxic properties through secretion of proinflammatory cytokines (interleukin IL-1α, IL-1β, TNF, and NO) [106, 107]. Alternatively, activated M2 microglia exhibit an anti-inflammatory phenotype and neurotrophic effect and degrade toxic aggregates due to anti-inflammatory interleukin production [106, 107]. The importance of PPARγ in regulating the M1/M2 phenotypic switch has been confirmed by Amine Bouhlel et al., who demonstrated that activation of PPARγ potentiates the polarization of circulating monocytes to macrophages of the M2 phenotype [108]. Subsequent studies reported that an active PPARγ pathway is a prominent

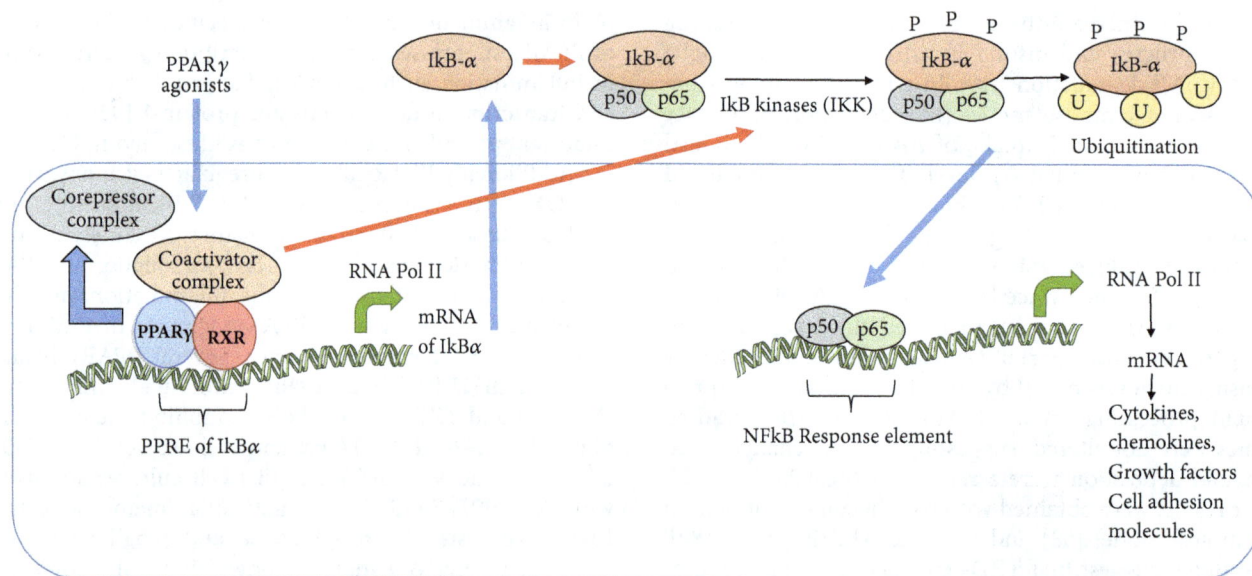

FIGURE 4: PPARγ agonist mediated transrepression of NF-kB signaling. Activation of PPARγ occurs upon binding of PPARγ agonists through association of heterodimer with coactivator complex to form a transcriptional complex. This complex binds to the PPARγ response element (PPRE) of IkBα gene, thereby inducing the expression of IkBα. An additional transrepressive mechanism involves inhibition of IKKα/β, an upstream kinase of IkBα. Consequently, degradation of IkBα and subsequent nuclear-translocation and activation of NF-kB (p50/p65) fail to occur, resulting in inhibition of inflammatory gene expression.

feature of alternatively activated (M2) macrophages and that M2-type responses are compromised in the absence of PPARγ expression. PPARγ expression is important for the full expression of certain genes characteristic of M2 macrophages, especially the gene encoding arginase-I, a direct PPAR target [109].

The small molecule SNU-BP was recently observed to inhibit inflammatory cytokine production and iNOS activity in LPS-stimulated microglia by PPARγ activation [110]. In addition, SNU-BP also increased IL-4 and arginase-1 expression, which are considered as M2 microglial phenotype markers; thus SNU-BP further evaluation of in vivo testing will help decipher a novel mechanism for this compound for mitigating early AD. Conversely, 12-month-old APP/PS1 mice treated with pioglitazone showed a significant reduction of the immunofluorescence intensity of microglial activator marker M1 in the surrounding area of amyloid deposits and elevated expression of M2 markers. Reduction in the levels of GFAP-immuno-reactive astrocytes surrounding amyloid plaques and internalized Aβ peptides in astrocytes of pioglitazone-treated animals were noted. Together, these findings suggest that TZDs treatment not only reduced the inflammatory response by microglia and astrocytes but also facilitated the removal of Aβ deposits presumably through enhancing the phagocytic activity of these cells.

Interestingly, some of the anti-inflammatory effects of PPARγ agonists appear to be independent of PPARγ activity. For instance, the rank order potency of drugs that activate PPARγ is often inconsistent with the anti-inflammatory efficacy, and expression of PPARγ does not correlate with the observed anti-inflammatory effects. Moreover, part of the anti-inflammatory effects of TZDs is unaffected in PPARγ

knockout models, and secretion of both IL-6 and TNF-α is inhibited equally in both wild type and PPARγ deficient macrophages [111]. Together, these data indicate that some anti-inflammatory effects of TZDs may be due to PPARγ independent effects, thus suggesting that there exists a significant gap in understanding the mechanisms to explain how TZDs and PPARs confer their anti-inflammatory properties for AD and thus warrant further investigation.

4.2.3. PPARγ and Mitochondrial Function. Apoptosis, programmed cell death, is thought to be intimately involved in AD pathogenesis. Aβ localized to the mitochondrial membrane can initiate the intrinsic apoptotic pathway causing neuronal cell death [112]. Dysregulated metabolism results from altered mitochondrial trafficking and enhanced mitochondrial degradation, which can lead to alteration in tau and microtubular instability [113]. Increasing evidence suggests that PPAR ligands are involved in mitochondrial regulation in adipose tissue [114, 115] and other organs [116, 117] indicating a potential benefit against mitochondrial dysregulation in AD. PPAR-γ coactivator 1 alpha (PGC1-α) is highly expressed in the brain and acts as a critical transcriptional coactivator for mitochondrial biogenesis and cellular energy metabolism. Decreased hippocampal PGC1-α has been observed in postmortem analysis of AD patients [118]. Decreased PGC1-α expression has been reported to result in reduced mitochondrial density in various brain areas, including midbrain, cortex, and cerebellum accompanied with reduced ATP levels [119]. Both PPARα and PPARγ agonists prevent mitochondrial size reduction by enhancing PGC1-α expression in cultured hippocampal neurons [120]. In the APP23 mouse model of AD, PGC1-α gene delivery improves spatial and recognition memory along with reduction in Aβ level through a decrease in BACE1 activity [121]. However, excess PGC1-α can also exert deleterious effects via mitochondrial proliferation and produce toxicity in the heart [122], muscles [123], and brain, leading to cognitive impairment [124, 125]. Therefore, an ideal therapeutic approach would be to increase the PGC1-α level via an indirect mechanism, i.e., through PPAR ligands. Studies on N2A cells showed that treatment with rosiglitazone increased mitochondrial mass and function through the activation of PGC1-α mediated by the PKA/CREB/AMPK pathway [126]. In another study, chronic treatment with pioglitazone attenuated oxidative damage, restored mitochondrial respiratory activity, and enhanced mitochondrial biogenesis in Wistar rats injected with Aβ [127]. Taken together it can be stated that further research for novel therapeutic development of PPAR compounds will explore how these ligands will enhance mitochondrial function.

4.2.4. PPARγ, Insulin Signaling, and Brain Insulin Resistance.

Insulin signaling is known to play a crucial role in the process of memory formation as insulin receptors are densely located in key areas of the brain, namely, olfactory bulb, hypothalamus, hippocampus, cerebral cortex, striatum, and cerebellum [128–131]. Insulin is essential to maintain normal neuronal homeostasis and survival, thus promoting learning and memory specially in the hippocampus [132]. For instance, brain specific insulin receptor knockout animal model showed increased tau hyperphosphorylation with altered Akt and GSK3β expression [133]. Additionally, diet induced insulin resistance in AD mice displayed increased Aβ peptide and advanced plaque formation [134]. These studies indicate that insulin resistance serves as an underlying mechanism for the development of Aβ production in the brain and associated sporadic memory impairment [135, 136].

Postmortem studies in AD patients have shown significantly reduced levels of insulin as well as insulin like growth factor (IGF-1 and IGF2) and insulin receptor substrate-1 (IRS-1) in the brain [137]. Abnormal insulin signaling leads to impaired neuronal oxidative metabolism [138]. The increase in oxidative stress and mitochondrial dysfunction can lead to aberrant posttranslational modification of APP and accumulation of Aβ in neurons [139]. Because of these shared features between AD and diabetes, AD has also been referred to as type III diabetes mellitus, leading to a growing interest in using insulin sensitizing agents as a potential therapy for AD [100, 140]. Rosiglitazone, a PPARγ agonist, improved neuronal insulin resistance in high fat diet rat model by increasing the phosphorylation of AKT/PKB at Ser473. Additionally, high fat diet induced brain mitochondrial dysfunction and oxidative stress were attenuated by rosiglitazone [141].

The Wnt signaling pathway is important in mediating several functions in the central nervous system, including neuroprotection and synaptic plasticity, and deregulated Wnt signaling has been shown to be associated with AD [142]. Dysfunctional Wnt signaling is associated with Aβ deposition, tau hyperphosphorylation, and cognitive impairment as reviewed by Tapia-Rojas et al. [143]. In view of the energy dysregulation associated with AD, Wnt signaling has been shown to act as a central integrator of metabolic signals from peripheral organs to the brain, thereby promoting adequate glucose utilization in the neurons [144]. Furthermore, dysfunctional glucose utilization is also associated with several neurological disorders, indicating that Wnt signaling is important in AD pathogenesis [145, 146]. These findings suggest that pharmacological activation of Wnt pathway would be a feasible therapeutic approach for the treatment of AD.

4.3. PPARγ in Later Stages of AD

4.3.1. PPARγ and Tau. Tau proteins are microtubule associated proteins that under normal physiological conditions interact with tubulin for microtubule assembly by mediating microtubule stabilization [147]. However, under pathological conditions such as AD, tau proteins undergo hyperphosphorylation resulting in neurotoxicity. Homeostasis maintained between kinase-mediated phosphorylation and protein phosphatases-mediated dephosphorylation is important in regulating the phosphorylation state of tau protein [148]. Various important kinases regulate tau phosphorylation, including cyclin-dependent kinases (CDK2 and CDK5), GSK-3β, mitogen-activated protein kinase (MAPK), extracellular signal-regulated protein kinase 1/2 (ERK1/2), c-Jun N-terminal kinase (JNK), Akt, protein kinase a (PKA), and calcium-calmodulin protein kinase 2 (CaMKII). Contrarily, PP1, PP2A, PP2B, and PP2C are important phosphatases that contribute to dephosphorylation of tau. Recent studies have shown that PPARs can also exert an effect on tau pathology. In vitro cellular studies using troglitazone and pioglitazone revealed reduced hyperphosphorylation of tau at Ser202, Ser396, and Ser404 in a tau transfected cell model involving GSK3β [149]. In the 3xTg-AD mouse model, treatment with pioglitazone resulted in significantly reduced tau phosphorylated-positive neurons in the hippocampus and improved cognitive deficits [150]. These studies also revealed that treatment with pioglitazone reduced tau phosphorylation at Ser202, Ser396, Ser404, Ser422, and Thr231 in cerebral cortex and CA1 area of hippocampus. Although these findings suggest that PPARγ stimulation can reduce tau hyperphosphorylation, further mechanistic studies are needed to determine the signaling mechanism by which PPARγ offers neuroprotection against tau hyperphosphorylation. Interestingly, the pan-PPAR agonist bezafibrate was shown to reduce tau phosphorylation in a P301 mice model by reducing iNOS and cyclooxygenase-2 in microglia [151]. Although role of PPARγ in Aβ mediated pathogenesis is exhaustively studied, its role in tauopathy needs to be explored for potential mechanism for reducing the hyperphosphorylation in-depth. A great variation can be noticed in the existing literature which is likely due to variation in the animal model studied and the time point of study.

4.3.2. PPARγ and Synaptic Plasticity. Moderate to severe stages of AD are characterized by synaptic failure which leads to cognitive decline and memory dysfunction. Synaptic function is dependent on specialized structures on neuronal processes called dendritic spines, and the loss of dendritic spines directly correlates with the loss of synaptic function. One of the key mediators for increasing dendritic density and synaptic plasticity is neurotrophins, including brain-derived neurotrophic factor (BDNF) [152]. Several studies have reported beneficial effects of PPARγ agonists in improving synaptic plasticity. Rosiglitazone has been shown to prevent dendritic spine loss and improve synaptic function in hippocampal neurons treated with Aβ oligomers [126]. Decreased expression of BDNF mRNA and protein levels were noted in hippocampi of db/db mice which were restored with rosiglitazone treatment. Furthermore, PPARγ has been shown to transcriptionally regulate BDNF expression as demonstrated from promoter activity assays wherein ligand activation of PPARγ induced the BDNF promoter in a log dose-dependent manner [153]. Similarly, Aβ injected rats treated with pioglitazone had reduced caspase-3 activation and increased BDNF levels, which was correlated with improved synaptic plasticity [127]. These observations suggest that PPARγ agonists prevent the impairment of synaptic plasticity by increasing BDNF expression and dendrite spine density.

Numerous studies have reported that kinases, such as CDK5, are also vital in the regulation of synaptic plasticity [154]. For example, a recent study showed that pioglitazone, via a proteasome-dependent manner, decreased the expression levels of p35 resulting in reduced CDK5 activity in neurons [154]. Moreover, blockage of CDK5 by pioglitazone prevented long-term potentiation (LTP) defects at CA3-CA1 synapses in APP/PS1 mice [155]. Alternatively, rosiglitazone was reported to induce an increase in the expression of neurotrophic factor-α1 (NF-α1), a neuroprotective protein, which increases prosurvival protein BCL 2 expression and provides neuroprotection in hippocampus [156]. Neurotrophins, such as nerve growth factor (NGF), can also induce PPARγ activation via the tyrosine kinase (TrkA) dependent signaling pathway and promote cell survival and differentiation [157]. PGC-1α gene therapy also increases NGF and exerts neuroprotective effects in AD mouse models [158]. These observations describe the significance of TZDs towards mitigating AD via improving mitochondrial function and synapse plasticity and reducing memory loss. Overall, PPARγ activation can simultaneously promote mitochondrial functions, improve metabolic and energy regulation, modulate neuroinflammation, stimulate axonal growth and myelination, and clear toxic Aβ from the brain [159].

5. PPARγ Agonists

5.1. Conventional PPARγ Agonists: Drawbacks and Limitations. Rosiglitazone and pioglitazone have been recognized as potential treatments for the AD through their insulin sensitizing and anti-inflammatory effects [160]. Several clinical studies have tested the efficacy of TZDs treatments in AD [161]. However, some clinical trials utilizing pioglitazone have failed to show therapeutic benefit [162, 163]. A meta-analysis study showed insufficient evidence to support use of rosiglitazone in amnestic mild cognitive impairment and AD patients. Interestingly, pioglitazone showed efficacy especially

in patients with comorbid diabetes mellitus [164]. However, another meta-analysis indicated that there is no statistically significant benefit with PPAR agonists in mild-to-moderate AD patients [165]. However, as previously stated, full agonists of PPARγ mediated closed conformation of the AF2 helix is responsible for many TZDs side effects [52–54]. Some of the most common adverse effects noted with conventional PPAR agonists include edema and heart enlargement [35, 166]. Discovery and development of specific novel PPARγ ligands with improved therapeutic profiles provide a molecular framework for future developments of pharmacological PPARγ agonists with advantages over current TZDs drugs. Review of several clinical trials utilizing PPARγ agonists in the treatment of AD has been summarized in Table 1, with references and highlights of the study.

5.2. New Direction for PPARγ Agonists: Development of Selective PPARγ Modulators (SPPARγMs). Selective PPARγ modulators (SPPARγMs) have attracted considerable attention because of their ability to selectively target PPARγ activity states. Several investigators have characterized and identified promising SPPARγMs that serve as partial agonists for PPARγ in cell based transcriptional activity and adipogenic assays [167, 168]. SPPARγMs specifically bind to the LBD of PPARγ via an activation function 2 motif (AF2). This offers greater flexibility in response to diverse ligands, resulting in different receptor conformations and coactivator and/or corepressor recruitment in different tissues [169]. Several SPPARγMs in preclinical studies have demonstrated strong insulin sensitizing activity in diet induced obese C57/BL6 mice with attenuated adverse effects on adiposity, weight gain, and cardiac related complications compared to potent full PPARγ agonists [170]. To further explain, the mechanism by which SPPARγMs uniquely interact with the receptor results in diminished conformational stability of the receptor when compared to traditional TZDs. Co-crystallography studies of the PPARγ LBD complexed with full PPARγ agonist rosiglitazone demonstrated strong hydrogen bonding with the Tyr473 site in helix 12 of the human PPARγ LBD. In contrast, rational drug design utilizing molecular modeling and crystallography structure analysis performed on the PPARγ LBD with SPPARγMs revealed that these compounds have the inability to form hydrogen bonding with Tyr473 due to the bonding distance with the carboxylic acid moiety [171, 172]. Findings from NMR studies have indicated that SPPARγMs induce a less stable confirmation than full PPARγ agonists (Figure 5) [173]. In addition, the Tyr473 site, within the helix 12 transcriptional activation function 2 domain, is involved in activation of the transcriptional coactivator binding pocket of the LBD [174]. Alteration of this site leads to the potential inability to directly stabilize this region and may serve as the physical basis for the differential receptor coactivator interaction, altered transcriptional activity, and reduced deleterious effects upon the heart and body associated with current full PPARγ agonists. Traditional PPARγ agonists, which display strong interaction with Tyr473, displace the inhibitory cofactors NCoR/SMRT and recruit P300/CBP, which confirms the most stable confirmation of the ligand binding pocket. These

TABLE 1: Clinical trials of PPARγ agonists.

Title	Treatment	# Of subjects	Methods	Inclusion criteria	Major outcome(s)	Results of major outcome(s)	Reference
Efficacy of rosiglitazone in a genetically defined population with mild-to-moderate AD	Rosi 2mg, Rosi 4mg, Rosi 8mg, or placebo daily for 24 weeks	511	RCT	Probable AD, MMSE score of 16-26	ADAS-Cog and CIBIC+	No significant difference; exploratory analyses suggested that ApoE4 non-carriers exhibited cognitive improvement with 8mg dose of Rosi	[35]
Rosiglitazone monotherapy in mild-to-moderate AD: results from a randomized, double-blind, placebo-controlled phase III study.	Rosi XR 2mg, Rosi XR 8 mg, donepezil 10mg, or placebo daily for 24 weeks	693	RCT	Probable AD, MMSE score of 10-23	ADAS-Cog and CIBIC+	No significant difference for Rosi group vs. placebo; no interaction between treatment and ApoE status	[36]
Rosiglitazone does not improve cognition or global function when used as adjunctive therapy to AChE inhibitors in mild-to-moderate AD: two phase 3 studies.	Rosi XR 2mg, Rosi XR 8 mg, or placebo daily for 48 weeks in addition to an AChEI	2,822	RCT	Mild-moderate probable AD, MMSE score of 10-26	ADAS-Cog and CDR-SB	No significant difference; no interaction between treatment and ApoE status	[37]
Efficacy of PPAR-γ agonist pioglitazone in mild AD	Pio 15-30 mg daily or no treatment for 6 months	42	randomized, open-label	Mild AD, Clinical Dementia Rating score of 0.5 or 1	MMSE, ADAS-Cog	Significant improvement in MMSE and ADAS-cog from baseline in pio treated subjects	[38]
Biomarker Qualification for Risk of MCI Due to AD and Safety and Efficacy Evaluation of Pioglitazone in Delaying Its Onset (TOMMORROW)	Pio 0.8mg SR daily or placebo for up to 5 years	3,494	RCT	Cognitively normal patients	Time to diagnosis of MCI due to AD for subjects in the high-risk stratum	Trial discontinued due to inadequate treatment effect; full results not yet published	[39]
Telmisartan vs. Perindopril in Hypertensive Mild-Moderate AD Patients (SARTAN-AD)	Telmi 40mg, Telmi 80mg, perindopril 2mg, perindopril 4mg, or perindopril 8mg daily for 12 months	goal of 240	Randomized, open label	Probable AD or possible AD dementia due to concomitant cerebrovascular disease, MMSE 16-27	Ventricular enlargement, cognitive function based on ADAS-cog and cognitive battery	Trial is ongoing	[40]
Effects of telmisartan on the level of Aβ1-42, interleukin-1β, TNFα and cognition in hypertensive patients with AD	Telmi 40-80mg or amlodipine 5-10 mg daily for 6 months	48	Randomized	Probable AD and essential hypertension	ADAS-Cog and MMSE	Significant improvement in MMSE and ADAS-cog in Telmi treated subjects compared to amlodipine treated subjects	[41]
Phase 2a Feasibility Study of T3D-959 in Subjects with Mild to Moderate AD	T3D-959* 3mg, 10mg, 30mg, or 90mg once daily for 2 weeks	36	Randomized, open-label	Mild-to-moderate AD, MMSE score of 14 -26	FDG-PET Imaging, ADAS-Cog	Trends towards improvement in ADAS-Cog	[42]

Clinical trials of PPARγ agonists. AChEI: acetylcholinesterase inhibitor; AD: Alzheimer's disease; ADAS-Cog: Alzheimer's disease assessment scale cognitive subscale; ApoE: apolipoprotein E; CDR-SB: clinical dementia rating scale sum of boxes; CIBIC+: clinician's interview-based impression of change with caregiver input; FDG-PET: fluorodeoxyglucose-positron emission tomography; MMSE: mini mental status exam; PPAR-γ: peroxisome proliferator activated receptor gamma; Pio: pioglitazone; Rosi: rosiglitazone; Telmi: telmisartan; *T3D-959 is a dual PPARδ/γ agonist.

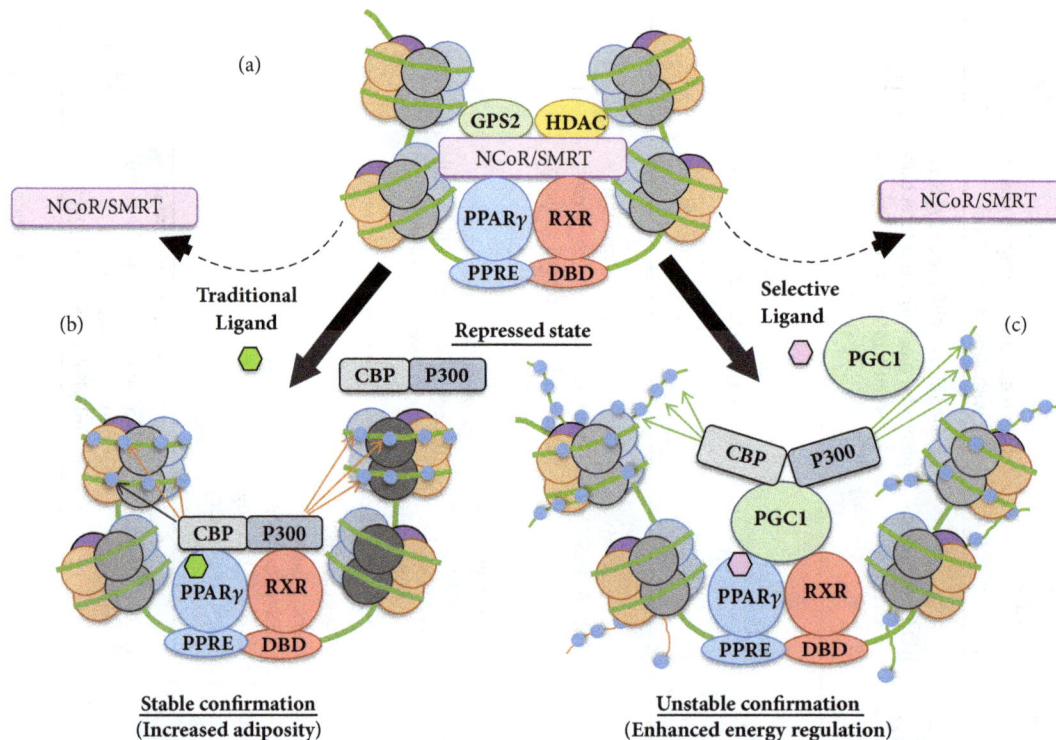

FIGURE 5: PPARγ receptor (a) is in the repressed state due to the transcriptional cofactor inhibitors NCoR/SMRT binding with PPARγ and preventing the transcription of target genes. When traditional (full agonist, (b)) or selective agonist (c) changes the confirmation of the PPARγ receptor and corepressors NCoR/SMRT come off. Traditional agonists (full agonist) such as rosiglitazone or pioglitazone promote a stable confirmation of the PPARγ-RXR confirmation with coactivators CBP/P300. However, selective agonists can induce an unstable confirmation of the PPARγ complex and allow alternative interactions with nontraditional coactivators, potentially PGC-1α, thus inducing alternative gene expression.

cofactors serve as histone acetylators and thus conform the receptor to the adipogenic gene in a stable confirmation. SPPARγMs that lack interaction with Tyr473 induce less stable confirmation and thus allow predictions for alternative cofactor associations with the receptor including PGC-1α. The potential of SPPARγMs in AD is just beginning and will likely lead to development of therapeutic targets for mitigating AD. Tyr473 in the AF2 region of the LBD has been shown to be a critical site of interaction between the full agonists and the PPARγ receptor. Studies on mutant PPARγ-LBD, where Tyr473 is replaced with alanine, revealed that interaction with Tyr473 is necessary for full agonist activity [175]. To this, various SPPARγMs such as SPPARγM2, GW0072, INT131, and PA082 have been observed not to interact with Tyr473 residue. Recently, Bruning and coworkers demonstrated that several SPPARγMs (BVT13, nTZDpa, MRL-20, MRL-24, SR145, and SR147) cause activation of PPARγ by interaction and stabilization of the β-sheet and H3 rather than AF2 helix of the LBD, which acts as a novel coactivator interaction site [176]. It suggests that the structurally diverse SPPARγMs, due to their distinct physical interaction with the receptor, uniquely bind to the receptor, resulting in diminished conformational stability compared with full agonists. Figure 5 illustrates the conformational changes in PPARγ/RXR receptor induced by the binding of full agonists or SPPARγMs, leading to coregulator heterodimer dissociation/recruitment, which forms the molecular basis for selective gene regulation that triggers specific metabolic effects. Studies with several SPPARγMs have mainly focused on four families of coregulators: NCoR and silencing mediator for retinoid and thyroid hormone receptors (SMRT), the p300 and CREB binding protein (CBP) family, the PPARγ coactivator 1 (PGC-1) family, and the p160 family, which are composed of three related coactivators (SRC1/NCoA1, GRIP1/TIF2/SRC2, and pCIP/RAC3/ACTR/AIB1/TRAM1/SRC3). Corepressors NCoR and Not1 and SMRT are known to downregulate full PPARγ agonist-mediated transcriptional activity and inhibit adipogenesis [177]. Several SPPARγMs that induce selective PPARγ or lack displacement of corepressors have been observed to display partial or antagonistic effects on adipogenesis and yet maintained insulin sensitization. For example, telmisartan and halofenate, which act as a SPPARγMs, induce reduced dissociation of corepressors and thus are partially adipogenic, while GW0072 (PPARγ repressor) does not dissociate corepressors resulting in preventing adipogenesis. However, they all are effective insulin sensitizers. Alternatively, FK614 causes NCoR dissociation equal to that of rosiglitazone and is a full agonist in adipogenesis assay, but shows several characteristics of SPPARγM in vivo [173]. Since the corepressor dissociation studies with SPPARγMs are limited and given that SPPARγMs display diverse activity in adipogenesis assay, their effects on AD needs to be further

TABLE 2

Ligand	Classification	Model	Amyloid	Other pathologies	references
NP00111 and NP01138 (Novel TZDs)	PPARγ agonist	cerebral cortex of embryonic day 18 rats	Decreased Aβ	Prevented activation of microglia and suppressed inflammatory markers. Restricted cortical or hippocampal neuronal cell death	[43]
Pirinixic acid derivate MH84	Dual gamma-secretase/PPARγ modulator	Thy-1 AβPP$_{SL}$ mice	reduced cerebral levels of Aβ40	NA	[44]
INT131	SPPARMs- non-thiazolidinedione compound	Rat primary hippocampal neurons	Improved neuronal survival against Aβ	increased dendritic branching, improved mitochondrial functions	[45]
T3D-959	Dual PPAR-δ/PPARγ agonist	streptozotocin-induced AD mouse model	reduced Aβ	Reduced levels of oxidative stress, normalized expression of phospho-tau and choline acetyltransferase.	[42]
		Intracerebral streptozotocin (i.c. STZ) model	-NA-	Improved Brain Insulin/IGF Signaling and reduced neuroinflammation	[46]

PPARγ agonists in various models of AD and its effects on various pathologies. Amyloid beta (Aβ), peroxisome proliferator-activated receptor gamma (PPAR-γ), thiazolidinediones (TZDs), streptozotocin (STZ).

explored with respect to corepressor interaction and its role in PPARγ-mediated insulin sensitization. Coactivators CBP/p300, TIF2 and SRC-3 seem to favor fat accumulation [178], and therefore their recruitment may not be desirable, while the physiological role of other coactivators, such as SRC1 and PGC-1α, is more associated with energy regulation. Thus, the specific recruitment of TIF2 over SRC1 may be a reason for lipid accumulation observed following rosiglitazone treatment in diabetic patients [179]. Interestingly, MBX-102, a SPPARγM, promotes higher recruitment of CBP, TIF2, SRC1, and PGC-1α when compared to a full agonist [173]. Other SPPARγMs including FMOC-leucine, PA-082, GW0072, and FK614 favor the recruitment of PGC-1α over that of SRC-1, TIF2, or p300 when compared with rosiglitazone [60, 180]. The role of PGC-1α is important for PPARγ activity as it acts as a docking surface for integrating the actions of transcription factors and cofactors for regulation of mitochondrial biogenesis and oxidative capacity [181]. Also, it has been shown that rosiglitazone upregulates the constitutively low expression of PGC-1α in white adipose tissue [182]. In the aged brain, PGC-1α regulates the expression of sirtuin 3, which is a factor related to the aging process [183]. It has been observed that brains from patients with neurodegenerative diseases display low levels of PGC-1α which leads to mitochondrial dysfunction and oxidative stress [184]. PGC-1α regulates mitochondrial density in neurons and PGC-1α–knockout mice showed an increased sensitivity to the degeneration of dopaminergic and glutamatergic neurons in the brain [185]. Moreover, alternative studies have demonstrated that the reduction of mitochondrial gene expression in PGC-1α–knockout mice leads to neuronal dysfunction [186]. Given that PGC-1α plays a crucial role in neuronal function and regulates mitochondrial function, PGC-1α could ameliorate mitochondrial

dysfunction and improve cognitive function in AD [118, 187]. Therefore, SPPARγMs favoring the recruitment of PGC-1α may lead to the discovery of new drug therapy for AD. Some of the newer PPARγ agonists in several disease models are listed in Table 2, with references and highlights of the study.

6. Conclusions and Future Directions

Following the utilization of PPARγ agonists for type 2 diabetes mellitus in improving insulin sensitivity, the pleiotropic effects of PPARγ in neurodegenerative diseases like AD have been increasingly investigated in recent years. Extensive research undertaken to improve the efficacy and/or safety of first-generation PPARγ agonists (the TZDs) has led to a greater understanding of the complexity of PPAR regulation, specifically the importance of coactivator and corepressor proteins. Developing novel agonists that exploit cofactor biology to derive better agents and reduce the unwanted deleterious effects is currently in process. Recent efforts to demonstrate differential cofactor recruitment and to develop better preclinical efficacy/safety profiles of SPPARγMs compared to conventional PPARγ agonists are underway. Future directions in PPAR research are likely to focus on optimizing the PPAR subtype interaction profile, maximizing inhibition of PPARγ phosphorylation, and screening against off-target activity.

Disclosure

There was no involvement of anyone other than the authors who (1) has an interest in the outcome of the work, (2) is affiliated to an organization with such an interest, or (3) was employed or paid by a funder, in the commissioning, conception, planning, design, conduct, or analysis of the work, the preparation or editing of the manuscript, or the decision to publish.

Conflicts of Interest

The authors declare that there are no conflicts of interest regarding the publication of this paper.

Acknowledgments

The current study was supported by funding to Drs. Amin and Suppiramaniam, NIHR15AG048643.

References

[1] Alzheimer's Association, "2018 Alzheimers disease facts and figures," *Alzheimer's & Dementia*, vol. 14, no. 3, pp. 367–429, 2018, http://linkinghub.elsevier.com/retrieve/pii/S1552526018300414.

[2] B. Chami, A. J. Steel, S. M. De La Monte, and G. T. Sutherland, "The rise and fall of insulin signaling in Alzheimer's disease," *Metabolic Brain Disease*, vol. 31, no. 3, pp. 497–515, 2016, http://www.ncbi.nlm.nih.gov/pubmed/26883429.

[3] S. M. de la Monte, M. Tong, N. Lester-Coll, M. Plater Jr, and J. R. Wands, "Therapeutic rescue of neurodegeneration in experimental type 3 diabetes: Relevance to Alzheimer's disease," *Journal of Alzheimer's Disease*, vol. 10, no. 1, pp. 89–109, 2006, http://www.ncbi.nlm.nih.gov/pubmed/16988486.

[4] A. Ott, R. P. Stolk, F. van Harskamp, H. A. P. Pols, A. Hofman, and M. M. B. Breteler, "Diabetes mellitus and the risk of dementia: the Rotterdam Study," *Neurology*, vol. 53, no. 9, pp. 1937–1942, 1999, http://www.ncbi.nlm.nih.gov/pubmed/10599761.

[5] E. Recio-Pinto, F. F. Lang, and D. N. Ishii, "Insulin and insulin-like growth factor II permit nerve growth factor binding and the neurite formation response in cultured human neuroblastoma cells," *Proceedings of the National Acadamy of Sciences of the United States of America*, vol. 81, no. 8, pp. 2562–2566, 1984, http://www.ncbi.nlm.nih.gov/pubmed/6326132.

[6] H. Sancheti, G. Akopian, F. Yin et al., "Age-dependent modulation of synaptic plasticity and insulin mimetic effect of lipoic acid on a mouse model of alzheimer's disease," *PLoS ONE*, vol. 8, no. 7, p. e69830, 2013, http://www.ncbi.nlm.nih.gov/pubmed/23875003.

[7] W. A. Pedersen, P. J. McMillan, J. J. Kulstad, J. B. Leverenz, S. Craft, and G. R. Haynatzki, "Rosiglitazone attenuates learning and memory deficits in Tg2576 Alzheimer mice," *Experimental Neurology*, vol. 199, no. 2, pp. 265–273, 2006, http://www.ncbi.nlm.nih.gov/pubmed/16515786.

[8] L. Escribano, A.-M. Simón, E. Gimeno et al., "Rosiglitazone rescues memory impairment in Alzheimer's transgenic mice: mechanisms involving a reduced amyloid and tau pathology," *Neuropsychopharmacology*, vol. 35, no. 7, pp. 1593–1604, 2010, http://www.ncbi.nlm.nih.gov/pubmed/20336061.

[9] H. Cheng, Y. Shang, L. Jiang et al., "The peroxisome proliferators activated receptor-gamma agonists as therapeutics for the treatment of Alzheimer's disease and mild-to-moderate Alzheimer's disease: a meta-analysis," *International Journal of Neuroscience*, vol. 126, no. 4, pp. 299–307, 2015, http://www.tandfonline.com/doi/full/10.3109/00207454.2015.1015722.

[10] F. Masciopinto, N. Di Pietro, C. Corona et al., "Effects of long-term treatment with pioglitazone on cognition and glucose metabolism of PS1-KI, 3xTg-AD and wild-type mice," *Cell Death & Disease*, vol. 3, no. 12, pp. e448–e448, 2012, http://www.ncbi.nlm.nih.gov/pubmed/23254291.

[11] L.-Y. Jiang, S.-S. Tang, X.-Y. Wang et al., "PPARγ agonist pioglitazone reverses memory impairment and biochemical changes in a mouse model of type 2 diabetes mellitus," *CNS Neuroscience & Therapeutics*, vol. 18, no. 8, pp. 659–666, 2012, http://www.ncbi.nlm.nih.gov/pubmed/22620268.

[12] G. Landreth, Q. Jiang, S. Mandrekar, and M. Heneka, "PPARγ agonists as therapeutics for the treatment of Alzheimer's disease," *Neurotherapeutics*, vol. 5, no. 3, pp. 481–489, 2008, http://www.ncbi.nlm.nih.gov/pubmed/18625459.

[13] A. Kermani and A. Garg, "Thiazolidinedione-Associated Congestive Heart Failure and Pulmonary Edema," *Mayo Clinic Proceedings*, vol. 78, no. 9, pp. 1088–1091, 2003, http://www.ncbi.nlm.nih.gov/pubmed/12962163.

[14] L. Nagy and J. W. R. Schwabe, "Mechanism of the nuclear receptor molecular switch," *Trends in Biochemical Sciences*, vol. 29, no. 6, pp. 317–324, 2004, http://www.ncbi.nlm.nih.gov/pubmed/15276186.

[15] J. C. Corton, S. P. Anderson, and A. Stauber, "Central role of peroxisome proliferator–activated receptors in the actions of peroxisome proliferators," *Annual Review of Pharmacology and Toxicology*, vol. 40, no. 1, pp. 491–518, 2000, http://www.ncbi.nlm.nih.gov/pubmed/10836145.

[16] S. Neschen, K. Morino, J. Dong et al., "n-3 Fatty acids preserve insulin sensitivity in vivo in a peroxisome proliferator-activated receptor-alpha–Dependent manner," *Diabetes*, vol. 56, no. 4, pp. 1034–1041, 2007, http://www.ncbi.nlm.nih.gov/pubmed/17251275.

[17] R. C. Scarpulla, R. B. Vega, and D. P. Kelly, "Transcriptional integration of mitochondrial biogenesis," *Trends in Endocrinology & Metabolism*, vol. 23, no. 9, pp. 459–466, 2012, http://www.ncbi.nlm.nih.gov/pubmed/22817841.

[18] Y. Zhu, C. Qi, J. R. Korenberg et al., "Structural organization of mouse peroxisome proliferator-activated receptor gamma (mPPAR gamma) gene: alternative promoter use and different splicing yield two mPPAR gamma isoforms," *Proceedings of the National Acadamy of Sciences of the United States of America*, vol. 92, no. 17, pp. 7921–7925, 1995, http://www.ncbi.nlm.nih.gov/pubmed/7644514.

[19] G. Medina-Gomez, S. L. Gray, L. Yetukuri et al., "PPAR gamma 2 prevents lipotoxicity by controlling adipose tissue expandability and peripheral lipid metabolism," *PLoS Genetics*, vol. 3, no. 4, p. e64, 2007, http://dx.plos.org/10.1371/journal.pgen.0030064.

[20] M. T. Heneka and G. E. Landreth, "PPARs in the brain," *Biochimica et Biophysica Acta (BBA)—Molecular and Cell Biology of Lipids*, vol. 1771, no. 8, pp. 1031–1045, 2007, http://www.ncbi.nlm.nih.gov/pubmed/17569578.

[21] S. Moreno, S. Farioli-Vecchioli, and M. P. Cerù, "Immunolocalization of peroxisome proliferator-activated receptors and retinoid X receptors in the adult rat CNS," *Neuroscience*, vol. 123, no. 1, pp. 131–145, 2004, http://www.ncbi.nlm.nih.gov/pubmed/14667448.

[22] K. Murakami, K. Tobe, T. Ide et al., "A novel insulin sensitizer acts as a coligand for peroxisome proliferator-activated receptor-α (PPAR-α) and PPAR-γ. Effect of PPAR-α activation on abnormal lipid metabolism in liver of Zucker fatty rats," *Diabetes*, vol. 47, no. 12, pp. 1841–1847, 1998, http://www.ncbi.nlm.nih.gov/pubmed/9836514.

[23] I. Saluja, J. G. Granneman, and R. P. Skoff, "PPAR delta agonists stimulate oligodendrocyte differentiation in tissue culture,"

Glia, vol. 33, no. 3, pp. 191–204, 2001, http://www.ncbi.nlm.nih.gov/pubmed/11241737.

[24] P. E. Polak, S. Kalinin, C. Dello Russo et al., "Protective effects of a peroxisome proliferator-activated receptor-β/δ agonist in experimental autoimmune encephalomyelitis," *Journal of Neuroimmunology*, vol. 168, no. 1-2, pp. 65–75, 2005, http://www.ncbi.nlm.nih.gov/pubmed/16098614.

[25] P. D. Storer, J. Xu, J. Chavis, and P. D. Drew, "Peroxisome proliferator-activated receptor-gamma agonists inhibit the activation of microglia and astrocytes: implications for multiple sclerosis," *Journal of Neuroimmunology*, vol. 161, no. 1-2, pp. 113–122, 2005, http://www.ncbi.nlm.nih.gov/pubmed/15748950.

[26] B. Desvergne and W. Wahli, "Peroxisome Proliferator-Activated Receptors: Nuclear Control of Metabolism," *Endocrine Reviews*, vol. 20, no. 5, pp. 649–688, 1999, http://www.ncbi.nlm.nih.gov/pubmed/10529898.

[27] J.-D. Lin, C. Handschin, and B. M. Spiegelman, "Metabolic control through the PGC-1 family of transcription coactivators," *Cell Metabolism*, vol. 1, no. 6, pp. 361–370, 2005, https://www.sciencedirect.com/science/article/pii/S1550413105001427.

[28] M. P. Mattson, "Energy intake and exercise as determinants of brain health and vulnerability to injury and disease," *Cell Metabolism*, vol. 16, no. 6, pp. 706–722, 2012, http://www.ncbi.nlm.nih.gov/pubmed/23168220.

[29] D. Li, K. Chen, N. Sinha et al., "The effects of PPAR-γ ligand pioglitazone on platelet aggregation and arterial thrombus formation," *Cardiovascular Research*, vol. 65, no. 4, pp. 907–912, 2005, https://academic.oup.com/cardiovascres/article-lookup/doi/10.1016/j.cardiores.2004.11.027.

[30] E. Burgermeister and R. Seger, "MAPK kinases as nucleocytoplasmic shuttles for PPARγ," *Cell Cycle*, vol. 6, no. 13, pp. 1539–1548, 2007, http://www.ncbi.nlm.nih.gov/pubmed/17611413.

[31] M. Luconi, G. Cantini, and M. Serio, "Peroxisome proliferator-activated receptor gamma (PPARγ): is the genomic activity the only answer?" *Steroids*, vol. 75, no. 8-9, pp. 585–594, 2010, http://www.ncbi.nlm.nih.gov/pubmed/19900469.

[32] H. S. Camp and S. R. Tafuri, "Regulation of Peroxisome Proliferator-activated Receptor γ Activity by Mitogen-activated Protein Kinase," *The Journal of Biological Chemistry*, vol. 272, no. 16, pp. 10811–10816, 1997, http://www.ncbi.nlm.nih.gov/pubmed/9099735.

[33] E. Hu, J. B. Kim, P. Sarraf, and B. M. Spiegelman, "Inhibition of adipogenesis through MAP kinase-mediated phosphorylation of PPARγ," *Science*, vol. 274, no. 5295, pp. 2100–2103, 1996, http://www.ncbi.nlm.nih.gov/pubmed/8953045.

[34] J. H. Choi, A. S. Banks, J. L. Estall et al., "Anti-diabetic drugs inhibit obesity-linked phosphorylation of PPARγ 3 by Cdk5," *Nature*, vol. 466, no. 7305, pp. 451–456, 2010, http://www.ncbi.nlm.nih.gov/pubmed/20651683.

[35] M. E. Risner, A. M. Saunders, J. F. B. Altman et al., "Efficacy of rosiglitazone in a genetically defined population with mild-to-moderate Alzheimer's disease," *The Pharmacogenomics Journal*, vol. 6, no. 4, pp. 246–254, 2006, http://www.ncbi.nlm.nih.gov/pubmed/16446752.

[36] M. Gold, C. Alderton, M. Zvartau-Hind et al., "Rosiglitazone monotherapy in mild-to-moderate alzheimer's disease: results from a randomized, double-blind, placebo-controlled phase III study," *Dementia and Geriatric Cognitive Disorders*, vol. 30, no. 2, pp. 131–146, 2010, http://www.ncbi.nlm.nih.gov/pubmed/20733306.

[37] C. Harrington, S. Sawchak, C. Chiang et al., "Rosiglitazone Does Not Improve Cognition or Global Function when Used as Adjunctive Therapy to AChE Inhibitors in Mild-to-Moderate Alzheimers Disease: Two Phase 3 Studies," *Current Alzheimer Research*, vol. 8, no. 5, pp. 592–606, 2011, http://www.ncbi.nlm.nih.gov/pubmed/21592048.

[38] T. Sato, H. Hanyu, K. Hirao, H. Kanetaka, H. Sakurai, and T. Iwamoto, "Efficacy of PPAR-γ agonist pioglitazone in mild Alzheimer disease," *Neurobiology of Aging*, vol. 32, no. 9, pp. 1626–1633, 2011, http://www.ncbi.nlm.nih.gov/pubmed/19923038.

[39] Biomarker Qualification for Risk of Mild Cognitive Impairment (MCI) Due to Alzheimer's Disease (AD) and Safety and Efficacy Evaluation of Pioglitazone in Delaying Its Onset - Tabular View, https://clinicaltrials.gov/ct2/show/record/NCT01931566?view=record.

[40] Telmisartan vs. Perindopril in Hypertensive Mild-Moderate Alzheimer's Disease Patients - Tabular View - ClinicalTrials.gov, https://clinicaltrials.gov/ct2/show/record/NCT02085265.

[41] W. Li, J. Zhang, F. Lu, M. Ma, J. Wang, and A. Suo, "Effects of telmisartan on the level of Aβ1-42, interleukin-1β, tumor necrosis factor α and cognition in hypertensive patients with Alzheimer's disease," *Zhonghua Yi Xue Za Zhi*, vol. 92, no. 39, pp. 2743–2746, 2012, http://www.ncbi.nlm.nih.gov/pubmed/23290159.

[42] M. Tong, C. Deochand, J. Didsbury, and S. M. de la Monte, "T3D-959: A Multi-Faceted Disease Remedial Drug Candidate for the Treatment of Alzheimer's Disease," *Journal of Alzheimer's Disease*, vol. 51, no. 1, pp. 123–138, 2016, http://www.ncbi.nlm.nih.gov/pubmed/26836193.

[43] R. Luna-Medina, M. Cortes-Canteli, M. Alonso, A. Santos, A. Martínez, and A. Perez-Castillo, "Regulation of inflammatory response in neural cells in vitro by thiadiazolidinones derivatives through peroxisome proliferator-activated receptor gamma activation," *The Journal of Biological Chemistry*, vol. 280, no. 22, pp. 21453–21462, 2005, http://www.ncbi.nlm.nih.gov/pubmed/15817469.

[44] M. Pohland, M. Pellowska, H. Asseburg et al., "MH84 improves mitochondrial dysfunction in a mouse model of early Alzheimer's disease," *Alzheimer's Research & Therapy*, vol. 10, no. 1, p. 18, 2018, http://www.ncbi.nlm.nih.gov/pubmed/29433569.

[45] J. A. Godoy, J. M. Zolezzi, and N. C. Inestrosa, "INT131 increases dendritic arborization and protects against Aβ toxicity by inducing mitochondrial changes in hippocampal neurons," *Biochemical and Biophysical Research Communications*, vol. 490, no. 3, pp. 955–962, 2017, http://www.ncbi.nlm.nih.gov/pubmed/28655613.

[46] S. M. de la Monte, M. Tong, I. Schiano, and J. Didsbury, "Improved Brain Insulin/IGF Signaling and Reduced Neuroinflammation with T3D-959 in an Experimental Model of Sporadic Alzheimer's Disease," *Journal of Alzheimer's Disease*, vol. 55, no. 2, pp. 849–864, 2016, http://www.ncbi.nlm.nih.gov/pubmed/27802237.

[47] D. Moras and H. Gronemeyer, "The nuclear receptor ligand-binding domain: structure and function," *Current Opinion in Cell Biology*, vol. 10, no. 3, pp. 384–391, 1998, http://www.ncbi.nlm.nih.gov/pubmed/9640540.

[48] B. A. Johnson, E. M. Wilson, Y. Li, D. E. Moller, R. G. Smith, and G. Zhou, "Ligand-induced stabilization of PPARγ monitored by NMR spectroscopy: implications for nuclear receptor activation," *Journal of Molecular Biology*, vol. 298, no. 2, pp. 187–194, 2000, http://www.ncbi.nlm.nih.gov/pubmed/10764590.

[49] T. S. Hughes, M. J. Chalmers, S. Novick et al., "Ligand and receptor dynamics contribute to the mechanism of graded PPARγ agonism," *Structure*, vol. 20, no. 1, pp. 139–150, 2012, http://www.ncbi.nlm.nih.gov/pubmed/22244763.

[50] R. T. Nolte, G. B. Wisely, S. Westin et al., "Ligand binding and co-activator assembly of the peroxisome proliferator-activated receptor-γ," *Nature*, vol. 395, no. 6698, pp. 137–143, 1998, http://www.ncbi.nlm.nih.gov/pubmed/9744270.

[51] R. T. Gampe, V. G. Montana, M. H. Lambert et al., "Asymmetry in the PPARγ/RXRα crystal structure reveals the molecular basis of heterodimerization among nuclear receptors," *Molecular Cell*, vol. 5, no. 3, pp. 545–555, 2000, http://www.ncbi.nlm.nih.gov/pubmed/10882139.

[52] U. Grether, W. Klaus, B. Kuhn, H. P. Maerki, P. Mohr, and M. B. Wright, "New insights on the mechanism of PPAR-targeted drugs," *ChemMedChem*, vol. 5, no. 12, pp. 1973–1976, 2010, http://doi.wiley.com/10.1002/cmdc.201000446.

[53] L. Guasch, E. Sala, C. Valls et al., "Structural insights for the design of new PPARgamma partial agonists with high binding affinity and low transactivation activity," *Journal of Computer-Aided Molecular Design*, vol. 25, no. 8, pp. 717–728, 2011, http://www.ncbi.nlm.nih.gov/pubmed/21691811.

[54] T. S. Hughes, P. K. Giri, I. M. de Vera et al., "An alternate binding site for PPARγ ligands," *Nature Communications*, vol. 5, no. 1, 2014, http://www.nature.com/articles/ncomms4571.

[55] M. B. Wright, M. Bortolini, M. Tadayyon, and M. Bopst, "Minireview: challenges and opportunities in development of PPAR agonists," *Molecular Endocrinology*, vol. 28, no. 11, pp. 1756–1768, 2014, http://www.ncbi.nlm.nih.gov/pubmed/25148456.

[56] S. Garcia-Vallvé, L. Guasch, S. Tomas-Hernández et al., "Peroxisome Proliferator-Activated Receptor γ (PPARγ) and Ligand Choreography: Newcomers Take the Stage," *Journal of Medicinal Chemistry*, vol. 58, no. 14, pp. 5381–5394, 2015, http://pubs.acs.org/doi/10.1021/jm501155f.

[57] M. Ahmadian, J. M. Suh, N. Hah et al., "PPARγ signaling and metabolism: the good, the bad and the future," *Nature Medicine*, vol. 99, no. 5, pp. 557–566, 2013, http://www.ncbi.nlm.nih.gov/pubmed/23652116.

[58] C. Pirat, A. Farce, N. Lebègue et al., "Targeting Peroxisome Proliferator-Activated Receptors (PPARs): Development of Modulators," *Journal of Medicinal Chemistry*, vol. 55, no. 9, pp. 4027–4061, 2012, http://www.ncbi.nlm.nih.gov/pubmed/22260081.

[59] G. Pochetti, C. Godio, N. Mitro et al., "Insights into the mechanism of partial agonism: crystal structures of the peroxisome proliferator-activated receptor γ ligand-binding domain in the complex with two enantiomeric ligands," *The Journal of Biological Chemistry*, vol. 282, no. 23, pp. 17314–17324, 2007, http://www.ncbi.nlm.nih.gov/pubmed/17403688.

[60] F. Zhang, B. E. Lavan, and F. M. Gregoire, "Selective Modulators of PPAR-γ Activity: Molecular Aspects Related to Obesity and Side-Effects," *PPAR Research*, Article ID 32696, pp. 1–7, 2007, http://www.ncbi.nlm.nih.gov/pubmed/17389769.

[61] W. Zheng, X. Feng, L. Qiu et al., "Identification of the antibiotic ionomycin as an unexpected peroxisome proliferator-activated receptor γ (PPARγ) ligand with a unique binding mode and effective glucose-lowering activity in a mouse model of diabetes," *Diabetologia*, vol. 56, no. 2, pp. 401–411, 2013, http://www.ncbi.nlm.nih.gov/pubmed/23178929.

[62] A. Kumar, A. Singh, and Ekavali, "A review on Alzheimer's disease pathophysiology and its management: an update," *Pharmacological Reports*, vol. 67, no. 2, pp. 195–203, 2015, http://www.ncbi.nlm.nih.gov/pubmed/25712639.

[63] M. R. Bronzuoli, A. Iacomino, L. Steardo, and C. Scuderi, "Targeting neuroinflammation in Alzheimer's disease," *Journal of Inflammation Research*, vol. 9, pp. 199–208, 2016, http://www.ncbi.nlm.nih.gov/pubmed/27843334.

[64] I. G. Onyango, J. Dennis, and S. M. Khan, "Mitochondrial dysfunction in Alzheimer's disease and the rationale for bioenergetics based therapies," *Aging and Disease (A&D)*, vol. 7, no. 2, pp. 201–214, 2016, http://www.ncbi.nlm.nih.gov/pubmed/27114851.

[65] S. T. Ferreira, J. R. Clarke, T. R. Bomfim, and F. G. de Felice, "Inflammation, defective insulin signaling, and neuronal dysfunction in Alzheimer's disease," *Alzheimer's & Dementia*, vol. 10, no. 1, pp. S76–S83, 2014, http://www.ncbi.nlm.nih.gov/pubmed/24529528.

[66] M. Sheng, B. L. Sabatini, and T. C. Südhof, "Synapses and Alzheimer's disease," *Cold Spring Harbor Perspectives in Biology*, vol. 4, no. 5, 2012, http://www.ncbi.nlm.nih.gov/pubmed/22491782.

[67] J-C. Lambert, C. A. Ibrahim-Verbaas, D. Harold, A. C. Naj, R. Sims, C. Bellenguez et al., "Meta-analysis of 74,046 individuals identifies 11 new susceptibility loci for Alzheimer's disease," *Nature Genetics*, vol. 45, no. 12, pp. 1452–1458, 2013, http://www.ncbi.nlm.nih.gov/pubmed/24162737.

[68] L. Bertram, M. B. McQueen, K. Mullin, D. Blacker, and R. E. Tanzi, "Systematic meta-analyses of Alzheimer disease genetic association studies: the AlzGene database," *Nature Genetics*, vol. 39, no. 1, pp. 17–23, 2007, http://www.ncbi.nlm.nih.gov/pubmed/17192785.

[69] A. Payton, P. Sindrewicz, V. Pessoa et al., "A TOMM40 poly-T variant modulates gene expression and is associated with vocabulary ability and decline in nonpathologic aging," *Neurobiology of Aging*, vol. 39, pp. 217.e1–217.e7, 2016, http://www.ncbi.nlm.nih.gov/pubmed/26742953.

[70] W. K. Gottschalk and M. Mihovilovic, "The Role of Upregulated APOE in Alzheimer's Disease Etiology," *Journal of Alzheimer's Disease & Parkinsonism*, vol. 6, no. 1, 2016, http://www.ncbi.nlm.nih.gov/pubmed/27104063.

[71] C. Linnertz, L. Anderson, W. Gottschalk et al., "The cis-regulatory effect of an Alzheimer's disease-associated poly-T locus on expression of TOMM40 and apolipoprotein E genes," *Alzheimer's & Dementia*, vol. 10, no. 5, pp. 541–551, 2014, http://www.ncbi.nlm.nih.gov/pubmed/24439168.

[72] S. Subramanian, W. K. Gottschalk, S. Y. Kim, A. D. Roses, and O. Chiba-Falek, "The effects of PPARγ on the regulation of the TOMM40-APOE-C1 genes cluster," *Biochimica et Biophysica Acta (BBA) - Molecular Basis of Disease*, vol. 1863, no. 3, pp. 810–816, 2017, https://www.sciencedirect.com/science/article/pii/S092544391730008X.

[73] J. Barrera, S. Subramanian, O. Chiba-Falek, and J. Fuh, "Probing the role of PPARγ in the regulation of late-onset Alzheimer's disease-associated genes," *PLoS ONE*, vol. 13, no. 5, p. e0196943, 2018, http://dx.plos.org/10.1371/journal.pone.0196943.

[74] S. H. Barage and K. D. Sonawane, "Amyloid cascade hypothesis: pathogenesis and therapeutic strategies in Alzheimer's disease," *Neuropeptides*, vol. 52, pp. 1–18, 2015, http://www.ncbi.nlm.nih.gov/pubmed/26149638.

[75] M. T. Heneka, M. Sastre, L. Dumitrescu-Ozimek et al., "Acute treatment with the PPARγ agonist pioglitazone and ibuprofen reduces glial inflammation and Aβ1-42 levels in APPV717I

transgenic mice," *Brain*, vol. 128, no. 6, pp. 1442–1453, 2005, http://www.ncbi.nlm.nih.gov/pubmed/15817521.

[76] S. Mandrekar-Colucci, J. C. Karlo, and G. E. Landreth, "Mechanisms underlying the rapid peroxisome proliferator-activated receptor-γ-mediated amyloid clearance and reversal of cognitive deficits in a murine model of Alzheimer's disease," *The Journal of Neuroscience*, vol. 32, no. 30, pp. 10117–10128, 2012, http://www.ncbi.nlm.nih.gov/pubmed/22836247.

[77] M. Shibata, S. Yamada, S. R. Kumar et al., "Clearance of Alzheimer's amyloid-β1-40 peptide from brain by LDL receptor-related protein-1 at the blood-brain barrier," *The Journal of Clinical Investigation*, vol. 106, no. 12, pp. 1489–1499, 2000, http://www.ncbi.nlm.nih.gov/pubmed/11120756.

[78] R. Deane, Z. Wu, A. Sagare et al., "LRP/amyloid β-peptide interaction mediates differential brain efflux of Aβ isoforms," *Neuron*, vol. 43, no. 3, pp. 333–344, 2004, http://www.ncbi.nlm.nih.gov/pubmed/15294142.

[79] A. P. Lillis, L. B. Van Duyn, J. E. Murphy-Ullrich, and D. K. Strickland, "LDL receptor-related protein 1: Unique tissue-specific functions revealed by selective gene knockout studies," *Physiological Reviews*, vol. 88, no. 3, pp. 887–918, 2008, http://www.ncbi.nlm.nih.gov/pubmed/18626063.

[80] A. Ramanathan, A. R. Nelson, A. P. Sagare, and B. V. Zlokovic, "Impaired vascular-mediated clearance of brain amyloid beta in Alzheimer's disease: the role, regulation and restoration of LRP1," *Frontiers in Aging Neuroscience*, vol. 7, 2015, http://www.ncbi.nlm.nih.gov/pubmed/26236233.

[81] A. Gauthier, G. Vassiliou, F. Benoist, and R. McPherson, "Adipocyte Low Density Lipoprotein Receptor-related Protein Gene Expression and Function Is Regulated by Peroxisome Proliferator-activated Receptor γ," *The Journal of Biological Chemistry*, vol. 278, no. 14, pp. 11945–11953, 2003, http://www.ncbi.nlm.nih.gov/pubmed/12551936.

[82] A. N. Rondón-Ortiz, C. L. Lino Cardenas, J. Martínez-Málaga et al., "High Concentrations of Rosiglitazone Reduce mRNA and Protein Levels of LRP1 in HepG2 Cells," *Frontiers in Pharmacology*, vol. 8, p. 772, 2017, http://www.ncbi.nlm.nih.gov/pubmed/29201005.

[83] J. H. Moon, H. J. Kim, H. M. Kim et al., "Upregulation of hepatic LRP1 by rosiglitazone: a possible novel mechanism of the beneficial effect of thiazolidinediones on atherogenic dyslipidemia," *Molecular Endocrinology*, vol. 49, no. 3, pp. 165–174, 2012, http://www.ncbi.nlm.nih.gov/pubmed/22889684.

[84] Q. Jiang, C. Y. D. Lee, S. Mandrekar et al., "ApoE promotes the proteolytic degradation of Aβ," *Neuron*, vol. 58, no. 5, pp. 681–693, 2008, http://www.ncbi.nlm.nih.gov/pubmed/18549781.

[85] M. Yamanaka, T. Ishikawa, A. Griep, D. Axt, M. P. Kummer, and M. T. Heneka, "PPARγ/RXRA-induced and CD36-mediated microglial amyloid-β phagocytosis results in cognitive improvement in amyloid precursor protein/presenilin 1 mice," *The Journal of Neuroscience*, vol. 32, no. 48, pp. 17321–17331, 2012, http://www.ncbi.nlm.nih.gov/pubmed/23197723.

[86] L. A. Medeiros, T. Khan, J. B. El Khoury et al., "Fibrillar Amyloid Protein Present in Atheroma Activates CD36 Signal Transduction," *The Journal of Biological Chemistry*, vol. 279, no. 11, pp. 10643–10648, 2004.

[87] P. F. Chapman, G. L. White, M. W. Jones et al., "Impaired synaptic plasticity and learning in aged amyloid precursor protein transgenic mice," *Nature Neuroscience*, vol. 2, no. 3, pp. 271–276, 1999, http://www.ncbi.nlm.nih.gov/pubmed/10195221.

[88] K. Hsiao, P. Chapman, S. Nilsen et al., "Correlative memory deficits, Aβ elevation, and amyloid plaques in transgenic mice," *Science*, vol. 274, no. 5284, pp. 99–102, 1996, http://www.ncbi.nlm.nih.gov/pubmed/8810256.

[89] K. Johnson-Wood, M. Lee, R. Motter et al., "Amyloid precursor protein processing and A 42 deposition in a transgenic mouse model of Alzheimer disease," *Proceedings of the National Acadamy of Sciences of the United States of America*, vol. 94, no. 4, pp. 1550–1555, 1997, http://www.ncbi.nlm.nih.gov/pubmed/9037091.

[90] C. Jiang, A. T. Ting, and B. Seed, "PPAR-γ agonists inhibit production of monocyte inflammatory cytokines," *Nature*, vol. 391, no. 6662, pp. 82–86, 1998, http://www.ncbi.nlm.nih.gov/pubmed/9422509.

[91] M. Ricote, J. Huang, L. Fajas et al., "Expression of the peroxisome proliferator-activated receptor γ (PPARγ) in human atherosclerosis and regulation in macrophages by colony stimulating factors and oxidized low density lipoprotein," *Proceedings of the National Acadamy of Sciences of the United States of America*, vol. 95, no. 13, pp. 7614–7619, 1998, http://www.ncbi.nlm.nih.gov/pubmed/9636198.

[92] C. Zhang, Y. Wang, D. Wang, J. Zhang, and F. Zhang, "NSAID Exposure and Risk of Alzheimer's Disease: An Updated Meta-Analysis From Cohort Studies," *Frontiers in Aging Neuroscience*, vol. 10, p. 83, 2018.

[93] A. C. Puhl, F. A. Milton, A. Cvoro et al., "Mechanisms of Peroxisome Proliferator Activated Receptor γ Regulation by Non-steroidal Anti-inflammatory Drugs," *Nuclear Receptor Signaling*, vol. 13, no. 1, 2018, http://www.ncbi.nlm.nih.gov/pubmed/26445566.

[94] Y. Kitamura, S. Shimohama, H. Koike et al., "Increased Expression of Cyclooxygenases and Peroxisome Proliferator-Activated Receptor-γ in Alzheimer's Disease Brains," *Biochemical and Biophysical Research Communications*, vol. 254, no. 3, pp. 582–586, 1999, http://www.ncbi.nlm.nih.gov/pubmed/9920782.

[95] M. Ricote, A. C. Li, T. M. Willson, C. J. Kelly, and C. K. Glass, "The peroxisome proliferator-activated receptor-γ is a negative regulator of macrophage activation," *Nature*, vol. 391, no. 6662, pp. 79–82, 1998.

[96] R. Kapadia, J.-H. Yi, and R. Vemuganti, "Mechanisms of anti-inflammatory and neuroprotective actions of PPAR-gamma agonists," *Frontiers in Bioscience*, vol. 13, no. 5, pp. 1813–1826, 2008, http://www.ncbi.nlm.nih.gov/pubmed/17981670.

[97] M. T. Heneka, T. Klockgether, and D. L. Feinstein, "Peroxisome proliferator-activated receptor-gamma ligands reduce neuronal inducible nitric oxide synthase expression and cell death in vivo," *The Journal of Neuroscience*, vol. 20, no. 18, pp. 6862–6867, 2000, http://www.ncbi.nlm.nih.gov/pubmed/10995830.

[98] S. Lenglet, F. Montecucco, and F. Mach, "Role of Matrix Metalloproteinases in Animal Models of Ischemic Stroke," *Current Vascular Pharmacology*, vol. 13, no. 2, pp. 161–166, 2015, https://www.ingentaconnect.com/content/ben/cvp/2015/00000013/00000002/art00005.

[99] C. K. Combs, D. E. Johnson, J. C. Karlo, S. B. Cannady, and G. E. Landreth, "Inflammatory Mechanisms in Alzheimer's Disease: Inhibition of β-Amyloid-Stimulated Proinflammatory Responses and Neurotoxicity by PPARγ Agonists," *The Journal of Neuroscience*, vol. 20, no. 2, pp. 558–567, 2000, http://www.ncbi.nlm.nih.gov/pubmed/10632585.

[100] N. Nicolakakis, T. Aboulkassim, B. Ongali et al., "Complete rescue of cerebrovascular function in aged Alzheimer's disease transgenic mice by antioxidants and pioglitazone, a peroxisome proliferator-activated receptor γ agonist," *The Journal of Neuroscience*, vol. 28, no. 37, pp. 9287–9296, 2008, http://www.ncbi.nlm.nih.gov/pubmed/18784309.

[101] E. M. Toledo and N. C. Inestrosa, "Activation of Wnt signaling by lithium and rosiglitazone reduced spatial memory impairment and neurodegeneration in brains of an APPswe/PSEN1ΔE9 mouse model of Alzheimer's disease," *Molecular Psychiatry*, vol. 15, no. 3, pp. 272–285, 2010, http://www.ncbi.nlm.nih.gov/pubmed/19621015.

[102] M. E. Calhoun, P. Burgermeister, A. L. Phinney et al., "Neuronal overexpression of mutant amyloid precursor protein results in prominent deposition of cerebrovascular amyloid," *Proceedings of the National Acadamy of Sciences of the United States of America*, vol. 96, no. 24, pp. 14088–14093, 1999, http://www.ncbi.nlm.nih.gov/pubmed/10570203.

[103] E. Utreras, R. Hamada, M. Prochazkova et al., "Suppression of neuroinflammation in forebrain-specific Cdk5 conditional knockout mice by PPARγ agonist improves neuronal loss and early lethality," *Journal of Neuroinflammation*, vol. 11, no. 1, p. 28, 2014, http://www.ncbi.nlm.nih.gov/pubmed/24495352.

[104] J. P. Lopes, C. R. Oliveira, and P. Agostinho, "Neurodegeneration in an Aβ-induced model of Alzheimer's disease: The role of Cdk5," *Aging Cell*, vol. 9, no. 1, pp. 64–77, 2010, http://www.ncbi.nlm.nih.gov/pubmed/19895631.

[105] F. Roselli, P. Livrea, and O. F. X. Almeida, "CDK5 is essential for soluble amyloid β-induced degradation of GKAP and remodeling of the synaptic actin cytoskeleton," *PLoS ONE*, vol. 6, no. 7, Article ID e23097, 2011, http://dx.plos.org/10.1371/journal.pone.0023097.

[106] A. Michelucci, T. Heurtaux, L. Grandbarbe, E. Morga, and P. Heuschling, "Characterization of the microglial phenotype under specific pro-inflammatory and anti-inflammatory conditions: effects of oligomeric and fibrillar amyloid-β," *Journal of Neuroimmunology*, vol. 210, no. 1-2, pp. 3–12, 2009, http://www.ncbi.nlm.nih.gov/pubmed/19269040.

[107] J. Y. Choi, J. Y. Kim, J. Y. Kim, J. Park, W. T. Lee, and J. E. Lee, "M2 Phenotype Microglia-derived Cytokine Stimulates Proliferation and Neuronal Differentiation of Endogenous Stem Cells in Ischemic Brain," *Experimental Neurobiology*, vol. 26, no. 1, p. 33, 2017, http://www.ncbi.nlm.nih.gov/pubmed/28243165.

[108] M. A. Bouhlel, B. Derudas, E. Rigamonti et al., "PPARγ activation primes human monocytes into alternative m2 macrophages with anti-inflammatory properties," *Cell Metabolism*, vol. 6, no. 2, pp. 137–143, 2007, http://www.ncbi.nlm.nih.gov/pubmed/17681149.

[109] J. I. Odegaard, R. R. Ricardo-Gonzalez, M. H. Goforth et al., "Macrophage-specific PPARγ controls alternative activation and improves insulin resistance," *Nature*, vol. 447, no. 7148, pp. 1116–1120, 2007, http://www.ncbi.nlm.nih.gov/pubmed/17515919.

[110] G. J. Song, Y. Nam, M. Jo et al., "A novel small-molecule agonist of PPAR-γ potentiates an anti-inflammatory M2 glial phenotype," *Neuropharmacology*, vol. 109, pp. 159–169, 2016, http://www.ncbi.nlm.nih.gov/pubmed/27288982.

[111] A. Chawla, Y. Barak, L. Nagy, D. Liao, P. Tontonoz, and R. M. Evans, "PPAR-γ dependent and independent effects on macrophage-gene expression in lipid metabolism and inflammation," *Nature Medicine*, vol. 7, no. 1, pp. 48–52, 2001, http://www.ncbi.nlm.nih.gov/pubmed/11135615.

[112] M. Obulesu and M. J. Lakshmi, "Apoptosis in Alzheimer's disease: an understanding of the physiology, pathology and therapeutic avenues," *Neurochemical Research*, vol. 39, no. 12, pp. 2301–2312, 2014, http://www.ncbi.nlm.nih.gov/pubmed/25322820.

[113] R. Castellani, K. Hirai, G. Aliev et al., "Role of mitochondrial dysfunction in Alzheimer's disease," *Journal of Neuroscience Research*, vol. 70, no. 3, pp. 357–360, 2002, http://www.ncbi.nlm.nih.gov/pubmed/12391597.

[114] I. Bogacka, H. Xie, G. A. Bray, and S. R. Smith, "Pioglitazone induces mitochondrial biogenesis in human subcutaneous adipose tissue in vivo," *Diabetes*, vol. 54, no. 5, pp. 1392–1399, 2005, http://www.ncbi.nlm.nih.gov/pubmed/15855325.

[115] L. Qiang, L. Wang, N. Kon et al., "Brown remodeling of white adipose tissue by SirT1-dependent deacetylation of Pparγ," *Cell*, vol. 150, no. 3, pp. 620–632, 2012, http://www.ncbi.nlm.nih.gov/pubmed/22863012.

[116] G. Haemmerle, T. Moustafa, G. Woelkart et al., "ATGL-mediated fat catabolism regulates cardiac mitochondrial function via PPAR-α and PGC-1," *Nature Medicine*, vol. 17, no. 9, pp. 1076–1085, 2011, http://www.ncbi.nlm.nih.gov/pubmed/21857651.

[117] D. M. Muoio and T. R. Koves, "Skeletal muscle adaptation to fatty acid depends on coordinated actions of the PPARs and PGC1α: implications for metabolic disease," *Applied Physiology, Nutrition, and Metabolism*, vol. 32, no. 5, pp. 874–883, 2007, http://www.ncbi.nlm.nih.gov/pubmed/18059612.

[118] W. Qin, V. Haroutunian, P. Katsel et al., "PGC-1α expression decreases in the Alzheimer disease brain as a function of dementia," *JAMA Neurology*, vol. 66, no. 3, pp. 352–361, 2009, http://www.ncbi.nlm.nih.gov/pubmed/19273754.

[119] P. Wareski, A. Vaarmann, V. Choubey et al., "PGC-1α and PGC-1β regulate mitochondrial density in neurons," *The Journal of Biological Chemistry*, vol. 284, no. 32, pp. 21379–21385, 2009, http://www.ncbi.nlm.nih.gov/pubmed/19542216.

[120] J. M. Zolezzi, C. Silva-Alvarez, D. Ordenes et al., "Peroxisome Proliferator-Activated Receptor (PPAR) γ and PPARα Agonists Modulate Mitochondrial Fusion-Fission Dynamics: Relevance to Reactive Oxygen Species (ROS)-Related Neurodegenerative Disorders?" *PLoS ONE*, vol. 8, no. 5, Article ID e64019, 2013, http://dx.plos.org/10.1371/journal.pone.0064019.

[121] L. Katsouri, Y. M. Lim, K. Blondrath et al., "PPARγ-coactivator-1α gene transfer reduces neuronal loss and amyloid-β generation by reducing β-secretase in an Alzheimer's disease model," *Proceedings of the National Acadamy of Sciences of the United States of America*, vol. 113, no. 43, pp. 12292–12297, 2016, http://www.ncbi.nlm.nih.gov/pubmed/27791018.

[122] L. K. Russell, C. M. Mansfield, J. J. Lehman et al., "Cardiac-Specific Induction of the Transcriptional Coactivator Peroxisome Proliferator-Activated Receptor γ Coactivator-1α Promotes Mitochondrial Biogenesis and Reversible Cardiomyopathy in a Developmental Stage-Dependent Manner," *Circulation Research*, vol. 94, no. 4, pp. 525–533, 2004, http://www.ncbi.nlm.nih.gov/pubmed/14726475.

[123] S. Miura, E. Tomitsuka, Y. Kamei et al., "Overexpression of Peroxisome Proliferator-Activated Receptor γ Co-Activator-1α Leads to Muscle Atrophy with Depletion of ATP," *The American Journal of Pathology*, vol. 169, no. 4, pp. 1129–1139, 2006, http://www.ncbi.nlm.nih.gov/pubmed/17003473.

[124] J. Clark, J. M. Silvaggi, T. Kiselak et al., "Pgc-1α overexpression downregulates Pitx3 and increases susceptibility to MPTP toxicity associated with decreased Bdnf," *PLoS ONE*,

vol. 7, no. 11, Article ID e48925, 2012, http://dx.plos.org/10.1371/journal.pone.0048925.

[125] C. Ciron, S. Lengacher, J. Dusonchet, P. Aebischer, and B. L. Schneider, "Sustained expression of PGC-1α in the rat nigrostriatal system selectively impairs dopaminergic function," *Human Molecular Genetics*, vol. 21, no. 8, pp. 1861–1876, 2012, http://www.ncbi.nlm.nih.gov/pubmed/22246294.

[126] M.-C. Chiang, Y.-C. Cheng, H.-M. Chen, Y.-J. Liang, and C.-H. Yen, "Rosiglitazone promotes neurite outgrowth and mitochondrial function in N2A cells via PPARgamma pathway," *Mitochondrion*, vol. 14, no. 1, pp. 7–17, 2014, http://www.ncbi.nlm.nih.gov/pubmed/24370585.

[127] A. Prakash and A. Kumar, "Role of nuclear receptor on regulation of BDNF and neuroinflammation in hippocampus of β-amyloid animal model of Alzheimer's disease," *Neurotoxicity Research*, vol. 25, no. 4, pp. 335–347, 2014, http://www.ncbi.nlm.nih.gov/pubmed/24277156.

[128] J. L. Marks, D. Porte, W. L. Stahl, and D. G. Baskin, "Localization of insulin receptor mRNA in rat brain by in situ hybridization," *Endocrinology*, vol. 127, no. 6, pp. 3234–3236, 1990, http://www.ncbi.nlm.nih.gov/pubmed/2249648.

[129] J. W. Unger and M. Betz, "Insulin receptors and signal transduction proteins in the hypothalamo-hypophyseal system: a review on morphological findings and functional implications," *Histology Histopathology Journal*, vol. 13, no. 4, pp. 1215–1224, 1998, http://www.ncbi.nlm.nih.gov/pubmed/9810512.

[130] G. A. Werther, A. Hogg, B. J. Oldfield et al., "Localization and characterization of insulin receptors in rat brain and pituitary gland using in vitro autoradiography and computerized densitometry," *Endocrinology*, vol. 121, no. 4, pp. 1562–1570, 1987, http://www.ncbi.nlm.nih.gov/pubmed/3653038.

[131] W. Zhao, H. Chen, H. Xu et al., "Brain insulin receptors and spatial memory. Correlated changes in gene expression, tyrosine phosphorylation, and signaling molecules in the hippocampus of water maze trained rats," *The Journal of Biological Chemistry*, vol. 274, no. 49, pp. 34893–34902, 1999, http://www.ncbi.nlm.nih.gov/pubmed/10574963.

[132] J. Bloemer, S. Bhattacharya, R. Amin, and V. Suppiramaniam, "Impaired insulin signaling and mechanisms of memory loss," *Progress in Molecular Biology and Translational Science*, vol. 121, pp. 413–449, 2014, http://www.ncbi.nlm.nih.gov/pubmed/24373245.

[133] M. Schubert, D. Gautam, D. Surjo et al., "The role for neuronal insulin resistance in neurodegenerative diseases," *Proceedings of the National Academy of Sciences of the United States of America*, vol. 101, no. 9, pp. 3100–3105, 2004, http://www.ncbi.nlm.nih.gov/pubmed/14981233.

[134] L. Ho, W. Qin, P. N. Pompl, Z. Xiang, J. Wang et al., "Diet-induced insulin resistance promotes amyloidosis in a transgenic mouse model of Alzheimer's disease," *The FASEB Journal*, vol. 18, no. 7, pp. 902–904, 2004, http://www.ncbi.nlm.nih.gov/pubmed/15033922.

[135] A. R. Pathan, A. B. Gaikwad, B. Viswanad, and P. Ramarao, "Rosiglitazone attenuates the cognitive deficits induced by high fat diet feeding in rats," *European Journal of Pharmacology*, vol. 589, no. 1-3, pp. 176–179, 2008, http://www.ncbi.nlm.nih.gov/pubmed/18602098.

[136] X.-L. Li, S. Aou, Y. Oomura, N. Hori, K. Fukunaga, and T. Hori, "Impairment of long-term potentiation and spatial memory in leptin receptor-deficient rodents," *Neuroscience*, vol. 113, no. 3, pp. 607–615, 2002, http://www.ncbi.nlm.nih.gov/pubmed/12150780.

[137] E. Steen, B. M. Terry, E. J. Rivera et al., "Impaired insulin and insulin-like growth factor expression and signaling mechanisms in Alzheimer's disease–Is this type 3 diabetes?" *Journal of Alzheimer's Disease*, vol. 7, no. 1, pp. 63–80, 2005, http://www.ncbi.nlm.nih.gov/pubmed/15750215.

[138] S. Hoyer and H. Lannert, "Inhibition of the Neuronal Insulin Receptor Causes Alzheimer-like Disturbances in Oxidative/Energy Brain Metabolism and in Behavior in Adult Rats," *Annals of the New York Academy of Sciences*, vol. 893, no. 1, pp. 301–303, 1999, http://www.ncbi.nlm.nih.gov/pubmed/10672254.

[139] G.-J. Chen, J. Xu, S. A. Lahousse, N. L. Caggiano, and S. M. De la Monte, "Transient hypoxia causes Alzheimer-type molecular and biochemical abnormalities in cortical neurons: Potential strategies for neuroprotection," *Journal of Alzheimer's Disease*, vol. 5, no. 3, pp. 209–228, 2003, http://www.ncbi.nlm.nih.gov/pubmed/12897406.

[140] P. L. Mcclean, V. Parthsarathy, E. Faivre, and C. Holscher, "The diabetes drug liraglutide prevents degenerative processes in a mouse model of Alzheimer's disease," *The Journal of Neuroscience*, vol. 31, no. 17, pp. 6587–6594, 2011, http://www.ncbi.nlm.nih.gov/pubmed/21525299.

[141] N. Pipatpiboon, W. Pratchayasakul, N. Chattipakorn, and S. C. Chattipakorn, "PPARγ agonist improves neuronal insulin receptor function in hippocampus and brain mitochondria function in rats with insulin resistance induced by long term high-fat diets," *Endocrinology*, vol. 153, no. 1, pp. 329–338, 2012, http://www.ncbi.nlm.nih.gov/pubmed/22109891.

[142] N. C. Inestrosa and L. Varela-Nallar, "Wnt signaling in the nervous system and in Alzheimer's disease," *Journal of Molecular Cell Biology*, vol. 6, no. 1, pp. 64–74, 2014, http://www.ncbi.nlm.nih.gov/pubmed/24549157.

[143] C. Tapia-Rojas and N. Inestrosa, "Loss of canonical Wnt signaling is involved in the pathogenesis of Alzheimer's disease," *Neural Regeneration Research*, vol. 13, no. 10, p. 1705, 2018, http://www.ncbi.nlm.nih.gov/pubmed/30136680.

[144] P. Cisternas, P. Salazar, C. Silva-Álvarez, L. F. Barros, and N. C. Inestrosa, "Activation of Wnt Signaling in Cortical Neurons Enhances Glucose Utilization through Glycolysis," *The Journal of Biological Chemistry*, vol. 291, no. 50, pp. 25950–25964, 2016, http://www.ncbi.nlm.nih.gov/pubmed/27703002.

[145] E. A. Winkler, Y. Nishida, A. P. Sagare et al., "GLUT1 reductions exacerbate Alzheimer's disease vasculo-neuronal dysfunction and degeneration," *Nature Neuroscience*, vol. 18, no. 4, pp. 521–530, 2015, http://www.ncbi.nlm.nih.gov/pubmed/25730668.

[146] Z. Chen and C. Zhong, "Decoding Alzheimer's disease from perturbed cerebral glucose metabolism: Implications for diagnostic and therapeutic strategies," *Progress in Neurobiology*, vol. 108, pp. 21–43, 2013, http://www.ncbi.nlm.nih.gov/pubmed/23850509.

[147] D. W. Cleveland, S. Y. Hwo, and M. W. Kirschner, "Physical and chemical properties of purified tau factor and the role of tau in microtubule assembly," *Journal of Molecular Biology*, vol. 116, no. 2, pp. 227–247, 1977, http://www.ncbi.nlm.nih.gov/pubmed/146092.

[148] A. Mietelska-Porowska, U. Wasik, M. Goras, A. Filipek, and G. Niewiadomska, "Tau protein modifications and interactions: their role in function and dysfunction," *International Journal of Molecular Sciences*, vol. 15, no. 3, pp. 4671–4713, 2014, http://www.mdpi.com/1422-0067/15/3/4671.

[149] C. d'abramo, R. Ricciarelli, M. A. Pronzato, and P. Davies, "Troglitazone, a peroxisome proliferator-activated receptor-gamma agonist, decreases tau phosphorylation in CHOtau4R cells," *Journal of Neurochemistry*, vol. 98, no. 4, pp. 1068–1077, 2006, http://doi.wiley.com/10.1111/j.1471-4159.2006.03931.x.

[150] B. L. Adler, M. Yarchoan, H. M. Hwang et al., "Neuroprotective effects of the amylin analogue pramlintide on Alzheimer's disease pathogenesis and cognition," *Neurobiology of Aging*, vol. 35, no. 4, pp. 793–801, 2014, http://www.ncbi.nlm.nih.gov/pubmed/24239383.

[151] M. Dumont, C. Stack, C. Elipenahli et al., "Bezafibrate administration improves behavioral deficits and tau pathology in P301S mice," *Human Molecular Genetics*, vol. 21, no. 23, Article ID dds355, pp. 5091–5105, 2012.

[152] T. Falkenberg, A. K. Mohammed, B. Henriksson, H. Persson, B. Winblad, and N. Lindefors, "Increased expression of brain-derived neurotrophic factor mRNA in rat hippocampus is associated with improved spatial memory and enriched environment," *Neuroscience Letters*, vol. 138, no. 1, pp. 153–156, 1992, http://www.ncbi.nlm.nih.gov/pubmed/1407655.

[153] T. Kariharan, G. Nanayakkara, K. Parameshwaran et al., "Central activation of PPAR-gamma ameliorates diabetes induced cognitive dysfunction and improves BDNF expression," *Neurobiology of Aging*, vol. 36, no. 3, pp. 1451–1461, 2015, https://www.sciencedirect.com/science/article/pii/S0197458014006344?via%3Dihub.

[154] F. Plattner, M. Angelo, and K. P. Giese, "The roles of cyclin-dependent kinase 5 and glycogen synthase kinase 3 in tau hyperphosphorylation," *The Journal of Biological Chemistry*, vol. 281, no. 35, pp. 25457–25465, 2006, http://www.ncbi.nlm.nih.gov/pubmed/16803897.

[155] J. Chen, S. Li, W. Sun, J. Li, and J. Padmanabhan, "Antidiabetes drug pioglitazone ameliorates synaptic defects in AD transgenic mice by inhibiting cyclin-dependent kinase5 activity," *PLoS ONE*, vol. 10, no. 4, Article ID e0123864, 2015, http://dx.plos.org/10.1371/journal.pone.0123864.

[156] E. Thouennon, Y. Cheng, V. Falahatian, N. X. Cawley, and Y. P. Loh, "Rosiglitazone-activated PPARγ induces neurotrophic factor-α1 transcription contributing to neuroprotection," *Journal of Neurochemistry*, vol. 134, no. 3, pp. 463–470, 2015, http://www.ncbi.nlm.nih.gov/pubmed/25940785.

[157] K. M. Fuenzalida, M. C. Aguilera, D. G. Piderit et al., "Peroxisome Proliferator-activated Receptor γ Is a Novel Target of the Nerve Growth Factor Signaling Pathway in PC12 Cells," *The Journal of Biological Chemistry*, vol. 280, no. 10, pp. 9604–9609, 2005, http://www.jbc.org/cgi/doi/10.1074/jbc.M409447200.

[158] L. Aloe, M. L. Rocco, P. Bianchi, and L. Manni, "Nerve growth factor: from the early discoveries to the potential clinical use," *Journal of Translational Medicine*, vol. 10, no. 1, p. 239, 2012, http://www.ncbi.nlm.nih.gov/pubmed/23190582.

[159] J. M. Zolezzi, M. J. Santos, S. Bastías-Candia, C. Pinto, J. A. Godoy, and N. C. Inestrosa, "PPARs in the central nervous system: roles in neurodegeneration and neuroinflammation," *Biological Reviews*, vol. 92, no. 4, pp. 2046–2069, 2017, http://doi.wiley.com/10.1111/brv.12320.

[160] B. W. Miller, K. C. Willett, and A. R. Desilets, "Rosiglitazone and Pioglitazone for the Treatment of Alzheimer's Disease," *Annals of Pharmacotherapy*, vol. 45, no. 11, pp. 1416–1424, 2011, http://journals.sagepub.com/doi/10.1345/aph.1Q238.

[161] M. T. Heneka, A. Fink, and G. Doblhammer, "Effect of pioglitazone medication on the incidence of dementia," *Annals of Neurology*, vol. 78, no. 2, pp. 284–294, 2015, http://www.ncbi.nlm.nih.gov/pubmed/25974006.

[162] D. S. Geldmacher, T. Fritsch, M. J. McClendon, and G. Landreth, "A randomized pilot clinical trial of the safety of pioglitazone in treatment of patients with alzheimer disease," *JAMA Neurology*, vol. 68, no. 1, pp. 45–50, 2011, http://www.ncbi.nlm.nih.gov/pubmed/20837824.

[163] Takeda and Zinfandel Pharmaceuticals Discontinue TOMMORROW Trial Following Planned Futility Analysis, https://www.takeda.com/newsroom/newsreleases/2018/takeda-tommorrow-trial/.

[164] J. Liu, L. Wang, and J. Jia, "Peroxisome Proliferator-Activated Receptor-Gamma Agonists for Alzheimer's Disease and Amnestic Mild Cognitive Impairment: A Systematic Review and Meta-Analysis," *Drugs & Aging*, vol. 32, no. 1, pp. 57–65, 2015, http://www.ncbi.nlm.nih.gov/pubmed/25504005.

[165] H. Cheng, Y. Shang, and L. Jiang, "The peroxisome proliferators activated receptor-gamma agonists as therapeutics for the treatment of Alzheimer's disease and mild-to-moderate Alzheimer's disease: a meta-analysis," *International Journal of Neuroscience*, vol. 126, no. 4, pp. 299–307, 2015, http://www.ncbi.nlm.nih.gov/pubmed/26001206.

[166] B. W. Miller, K. C. Willett, and A. R. Desilets, "Rosiglitazone and Pioglitazone for the Treatment of Alzheimer's Disease," *Annals of Pharmacotherapy*, vol. 45, no. 11, pp. 1416–1424, 2011, http://www.ncbi.nlm.nih.gov/pubmed/22028424.

[167] S. Gathiaka, G. Nanayakkara, T. Boncher et al., "Design, development and evaluation of novel dual PPARδ/PPARγ agonists," *Bioorganic & Medicinal Chemistry Letters*, vol. 23, no. 3, pp. 873–879, 2013, http://www.ncbi.nlm.nih.gov/pubmed/23273519.

[168] K. Liu, L. Xu, J. P. Berger et al., "Discovery of a Novel Series of Peroxisome Proliferator-Activated Receptor α/γ Dual Agonists for the Treatment of Type 2 Diabetes and Dyslipidemia," *Journal of Medicinal Chemistry*, vol. 48, no. 7, pp. 2262–2265, 2005, http://www.ncbi.nlm.nih.gov/pubmed/15801817.

[169] L. S. Higgins and A. M. Depaoli, "Selective peroxisome proliferator-activated receptor γ (PPARγ) modulation as a strategy for safer therapeutic PPARγ activation," *American Journal of Clinical Nutrition*, vol. 91, no. 1, pp. 267S–272S, 2010, https://academic.oup.com/ajcn/article/91/1/267S/4597134.

[170] M. Laplante, H. Sell, K. L. MacNaul, D. Richard, J. P. Berger, and Y. Deshaies, "PPAR-gamma activation mediates adipose depot-specific effects on gene expression and lipoprotein lipase activity: mechanisms for modulation of postprandial lipemia and differential adipose accretion," *Diabetes*, vol. 52, no. 2, pp. 291–299, 2003, http://www.ncbi.nlm.nih.gov/pubmed/12540599.

[171] J. L. Oberfield, J. L. Collins, C. P. Holmes et al., "A peroxisome proliferator-activated receptor gamma ligand inhibits adipocyte differentiation," *Proceedings of the National Acadamy of Sciences of the United States of America*, vol. 96, no. 11, pp. 6102–6106, 1999, http://www.ncbi.nlm.nih.gov/pubmed/10339548.

[172] E. Burgermeister, A. Schnoebelen, A. Flament et al., "A novel partial agonist of peroxisome proliferator-activated receptor-γ (PPARγ) recruits PPARγ-coactivator-1α, prevents triglyceride accumulation, and potentiates insulin signaling in vitro," *Molecular Endocrinology*, vol. 20, no. 4, pp. 809–830, 2006, http://www.ncbi.nlm.nih.gov/pubmed/16373399.

[173] J. P. Berger, A. E. Petro, K. L. Macnaul et al., "Distinct properties and advantages of a novel peroxisome proliferator-activated protein γ selective modulator," *Molecular Endocrinology*, vol. 17, no. 4, pp. 662–676, 2003, http://www.ncbi.nlm.nih.gov/pubmed/12554792.

[174] S.-H. Sheu, T. Kaya, D. J. Waxman, and S. Vajda, "Exploring the binding site structure of the PPARγ ligand-binding domain by computational solvent mapping," *Biochemistry*, vol. 44, no. 4, pp. 1193–1209, 2005, http://www.ncbi.nlm.nih.gov/pubmed/15667213.

[175] L. L. Atkinson, M. A. Fischer, and G. D. Lopaschuk, "Leptin activates cardiac fatty acid oxidation independent of changes in the AMP-activated protein kinase-acetyl-CoA carboxylase-malonyl-CoA axis," *The Journal of Biological Chemistry*, vol. 277, no. 33, pp. 29424–29430, 2002, http://www.ncbi.nlm.nih.gov/pubmed/12058043.

[176] J. B. Bruning, M. J. Chalmers, S. Prasad et al., "Partial agonists activate PPARγ using a helix 12 independent mechanism," *Structure*, vol. 15, no. 10, pp. 1258–1271, 2007, http://www.ncbi.nlm.nih.gov/pubmed/17937915.

[177] I. A. Voutsadakis, "Peroxisome proliferator activated receptor-γ and the ubiquitin-proteasome system in colorectal cancer," *World Journal of Gastrointestinal Oncology*, vol. 2, no. 5, pp. 235–241, 2010, http://www.ncbi.nlm.nih.gov/pubmed/21160623.

[178] N. Viswakarma, Y. Jia, L. Bai et al., "Coactivators in PPAR-Regulated Gene Expression," *PPAR Research*, Article ID 250126, pp. 1–21, 2010, http://www.ncbi.nlm.nih.gov/pubmed/20814439.

[179] S. M. Watkins, P. R. Reifsnyder, H. Pan, J. B. German, and E. H. Leiter, "Lipid metabolome-wide effects of the PPARγ agonist rosiglitazone," *Journal of Lipid Research*, vol. 43, no. 11, pp. 1809–1817, 2002, http://www.ncbi.nlm.nih.gov/pubmed/12401879.

[180] M. Einstein, T. E. Akiyama, G. A. Castriota et al., "The differential interactions of peroxisome proliferator-activated receptor γ ligands with Tyr473 is a physical basis for their unique biological activities," *Molecular Pharmacology*, vol. 73, no. 1, pp. 62–74, 2008, http://www.ncbi.nlm.nih.gov/pubmed/17940191.

[181] L. Cui, H. Jeong, F. Borovecki, C. N. Parkhurst, N. Tanese, and D. Krainc, "Transcriptional repression of PGC-1α by mutant huntingtin leads to mitochondrial dysfunction and neurodegeneration," *Cell*, vol. 127, no. 1, pp. 59–69, 2006, http://www.ncbi.nlm.nih.gov/pubmed/17018277.

[182] M. H. Karimfar, K. Haghani, A. Babakhani, and S. Bakhtiyari, "Rosiglitazone, but Not Epigallocatechin-3-Gallate, Attenuates the Decrease in PGC-1α Protein Levels in Palmitate-Induced Insulin-Resistant C2C12 Cells," *Lipids*, vol. 50, no. 6, pp. 521–528, 2015, http://www.ncbi.nlm.nih.gov/pubmed/25893813.

[183] X. Kong, R. Wang, Y. Xue et al., "Sirtuin 3, a new target of PGC-1α, plays an important role in the suppression of ROS and mitochondrial biogenesis," *PLoS ONE*, vol. 5, no. 7, Article ID e11707, 2010, http://dx.plos.org/10.1371/journal.pone.0011707.

[184] X. Zhang, X. Ren, Q. Zhang et al., "PGC-1α/ERRα-Sirt3 pathway regulates DAergic neuronal death by directly deacetylating SOD2 and ATP synthase β," *Antioxidants & Redox Signaling*, vol. 24, no. 6, pp. 312–328, 2016, http://www.ncbi.nlm.nih.gov/pubmed/26421366.

[185] H. Jiang, S. Kang, S. Zhang et al., "Adult Conditional Knockout of PGC-1α Leads to Loss of Dopamine Neurons," *eNeuro*, vol. 3, no. 4, 2016, http://www.ncbi.nlm.nih.gov/pubmed/27622213.

[186] J. Lin, P.-H. Wu, P. T. Tarr et al., "Defects in adaptive energy metabolism with CNS-linked hyperactivity in PGC-1α null mice," *Cell*, vol. 119, no. 1, pp. 121–135, 2004, http://www.ncbi.nlm.nih.gov/pubmed/15454086.

[187] G. Sweeney and J. Song, "The association between PGC-1α and Alzheimer's disease," *Anatomy & Cell Biology*, vol. 49, no. 1, pp. 1–6, 2016, http://www.ncbi.nlm.nih.gov/pubmed/27051562.

12

High Glucose Induces Autophagy through PPARγ-Dependent Pathway in Human Nucleus Pulposus Cells

Chang Jiang,[1] Shuhao Liu ⓘ,[1] Yuanwu Cao ⓘ,[1] and Hongping Shan[2]

[1]*Department of Orthopaedics, Zhongshan Hospital, Fudan University, Shanghai, China*
[2]*Department of Nephrology, Pudong Medical Center, Fudan University, Shanghai, China*

Correspondence should be addressed to Yuanwu Cao; cywzjcyw@163.com

Academic Editor: Lingyan Xu

Diabetes mellitus is a multiorgan disorder affecting many types of connective tissues, including bone and cartilage. High glucose could accelerate the autophagy in nucleus pulposus (NP) cells. In our present study, we investigated whether peroxisome proliferator-activated receptor γ (PPAR-γ) pathway is involved into autophagy regulation in NP cells under high glucose condition. After NP cells were treated with different high glucose concentrations for 72 hours, the rate of autophagy increased. Moreover, the levels of PPARγ, Beclin-1, and LC3II were significantly increased and p62 was significantly decreased compared to control group. Then, NP cells were treated with high glucose plus PPARγ agonist or PPARγ antagonist, respectively. The rate of autophagy and the levels of Beclin-1 and LC3II increased, but p62 decreased when PPARγ agonist was used. On the contrary, the rate of autophagy and the levels of Beclin-1 and LC3II decreased, while p62 increased when PPARγ antagonist was added. These results suggested that autophagy induced by high glucose in NP cells was through PPARγ-dependent pathway.

1. Introduction

Low back pain is highly prevalent and accounts for low life quality, and it is widely accepted that back pain has relationship with lumbar disc degeneration (LDD). Although the strength of the association is still controversial [1, 2], deterioration of intervertebral disc (IVD) could lead ultimately to the development of symptomatic degenerative disorders such as disc herniation, spinal stenosis, and degenerative spondylolisthesis.

Many evidences showed that diabetes mellitus (DM) is important in the aetiology of LDD. It was reported that there is a higher incidence of degenerative disc diseases in patients with DM than in the non-DM population [3] and patients with DM had poorer surgical outcomes versus non-DM patients [4].

The decrease in the number of viable nucleus pulposus (NP) cells in diabetes was thought to be one of the initial triggers of disc degeneration. In vitro studies, high glucose has been proved to accelerate autophagy [5], apoptosis [6], and senescence [7] in adult rat NP cells in a dose- and time-dependent manner. Both apoptosis and senescence of IVD

cells can lead to the decrease of viable cells. The role of autophagy is relatively complex. Initially, autophagy can promote cell survival and avert apoptosis during stress responses by turning over the intracellular organelles and molecules through the lysosomal pathway. However, when autophagy is prolonged, proteins and organelles essential for basic homeostasis and cell survival are degraded, which can lead to cell death. But the mechanism of autophagy in NP cell under high glucose is still unclear.

Peroxisome proliferator-activated receptors (PPAR) are a kind of ligand-activated transcription factors that regulate vital genes in cell differentiation and various metabolic processes. The family of PPARs in mammals comprises three isoforms: PPARα, PPARβ/δ, and PPARγ [8]. Activation of PPARα induces lipid metabolism and regulates energy homeostasis, whereas the activation of PPARβ/δ enhances fatty acid metabolism. On the other hand, activation of PPARγ leads to an improvement of insulin resistance, followed by glucose metabolism.

PPARγ is expressed in white and brown adipose tissue, the large intestine, and spleen. A plethora of evidence implicates that PPARγ plays a central role in numerous diseases, including obesity, diabetes, and atherosclerosis [9–11]. But up to now, PPARγ has never been reported in the NP cells and in intervertebral disc degeneration in previous literature.

Giving the role of PPARγ in glucose metabolism and the role of high glucose in intervertebral disc degeneration, we supposed that the high glucose condition induces autophagy via PPARγ-dependent pathway in our present study.

2. Methods

2.1. Cell Preparation. An intervertebral disc (L45) was harvested from a forty-four-year-old female patient who accepted transforaminal lumbar interbody fusion operation because of lumbar disc herniation. The disc degeneration was grade III according to Pfirrmann classification. The disc was dissected carefully under a microscope to obtain only the NP tissues under aseptic condition. Then, the harvested NP tissues were cut as small as possible(<1 mm3), digested with 0.25% type II collagenase for 4 h, and filtered with a sieve of 70 microns. After being washed with phosphate-buffered saline (PBS) twice, the NP cells were cultured in a culture flask with DMEM low-glucose medium supplemented with 10% fetal bovine serum (FBS) and 1% penicillin-streptomycin (Gibco BRL) at 37°C in a humidified atmosphere (95% air, 5% CO2). Medium was changed two or three days later. When the cells reached 80%–90% confluence, they were split once (passage 1) and grown to 80%–90% confluence again. The cells after 3 passages were used for subsequent experiments.

2.2. Cell Culture. The cells after 3 passages were cultured in DMEM containing 5.6 mM (normal control), 0.1 or 0.2 M glucose, supplemented with 10% fetal bovine serum, and 1% penicillin-streptomycin (Gibco BRL) and maintained at 5% CO2 on poly-L-lysine coated plates. For pharmacologic intervention of glucose-induced cell change, cells at 0.2 M glucose medium were switched to 0.2 M glucose medium with 25 uM/L T0070907 or rosiglitazone (Selleck Chemicals, Shanghai, China), respectively.

2.3. Western Blot. NP cells were harvested for protein quantification by using RIPA (Beyotime, Shanghai, China) with 1% phenylmethanesulfonyl fluoride (PMSF). Protein concentrations were assayed by a BCA kit (Piece, Biotechnology, MA, USA). Protein sample was electrophoresed on 12% polyacrylamide gel in the presence of SDS-PAGE and transferred onto a polyvinylidene difluoride membrane (millipor). Blots were blocked for 1 h at room temperature with 5% nonfat dry milk in TBST buffer. Afterward, the membranes were incubated with the primary antibodies against LC3II/I (CST, 1:1000); Beclin1 (CST, 1:1000); PPARγ (Proteinteck, 1:500); p62 (CST, 1:10000); and GAPDH (Abcam, 1:10000) overnight at 4°C and HRP-conjugated secondary antibodies (CST, 1:2000) at room temperature. The bands were visualized by using ECL substrate (ThermoFisher) and analyzed by ImageJ software. The protein expression was normalized to control GAPDH levels.

2.4. Real-Time PCR. After being washed with PBS, total RNA was extracted from NP cells by using TriZol reagents (Invitrogen, California, USA) by following the manufacturer's protocol and its absorbance at 260/280 nm was detected to evaluate the RNA quality. The absorbance of 1.8–2.0 was considered to be good. cDNA was synthesized using SuperScript™ RT reagent kit with gDNA Eraser (Takara, Shiga, Japan) from 1 ug RNA. For PCR amplification, 10 ul of reaction volume included 5 ul of 2Power SYBR Green PCR Master Mix (ABI, Waltham, Massachusetts, USA), 0.25 ul each primer, 1 ug cDNA, and 3.5 ul sterile distilled water. The cycle threshold (Ct) values were collected and normalized to the housekeeping gene GAPDH. The $2^{-\Delta\Delta CT}$ method was used to calculate the relative mRNA levels of each target gene. The primers for PPARγ were 5′-TACTGTCGGTTTCAGAAATGCC-3′ (forward) and 5′-GTCAGCGGACTCTGGATTCAG-3′ (backward).

2.5. Fluorescence Microscopy. NP cells were cultured and grown to 80% confluence in 24-well plate. Appropriate amount of virus fluid containing packaged pL-CMV-TO-GFP-HLC3B (constructed by ourselves) was added to the medium. NP cells were incubated for 6 h at 37°C. The medium containing virus was replaced with DMEM supplemented with 10% fetal bovine serum (FBS) and 1% penicillin-streptomycin (Gibco BRL) and the NP cells were incubated for another 30 h at 37°C. Then, these transfected NP cells were treated as described in the section of cell culture. At last, autophagy in NP cells was observed and evaluated by fluorescence microscope. Autophagy rates were calculated by the number of autophagy cells over total ones under 10x lens.

2.6. Statistics. All experiments were repeated at least three times. The data were presented as means ± SD (standard deviation). SPSS 21.0 was used for all statistical analyses of the data. Comparison of data was performed using the one-way ANOVA test. Differences were considered statistically significant at $p < 0.05$.

3. Results

3.1. High Glucose-Induced Autophagy in NP Cells. The NP cells were divided into three groups as control group, 0.1 M high glucose group, and 0.2 M high glucose group according to glucose concentration(5.6 mM, 0.1 M, and 0.2 M). To evaluate the role of high glucose on autophagy in NP cells, we next not only display the autophagy cells using GFP-LC3B tracer technique but also examine and compare the LC3, Beclin-1, and p62 expression in the NP cells in all three groups by western blot. Beclin-1 and microtubule-associated protein-1 light chain 3 (LC3) are required for autophagosome formation and maturation, one of the important steps for autophagy. p62 protein called the autophagy-specific substrate can be degraded together with LC3-II. The impaired autophagy is accompanied by accumulation of p62. GFP-LC3B would form spots when autophagy occurs. And the more spots, the more autophagy. By using GFP-LC3B tracer technique, the rate of autophagy in NP cells was 6.67 ± 0.86%, 8.15 ± 0.85%, and

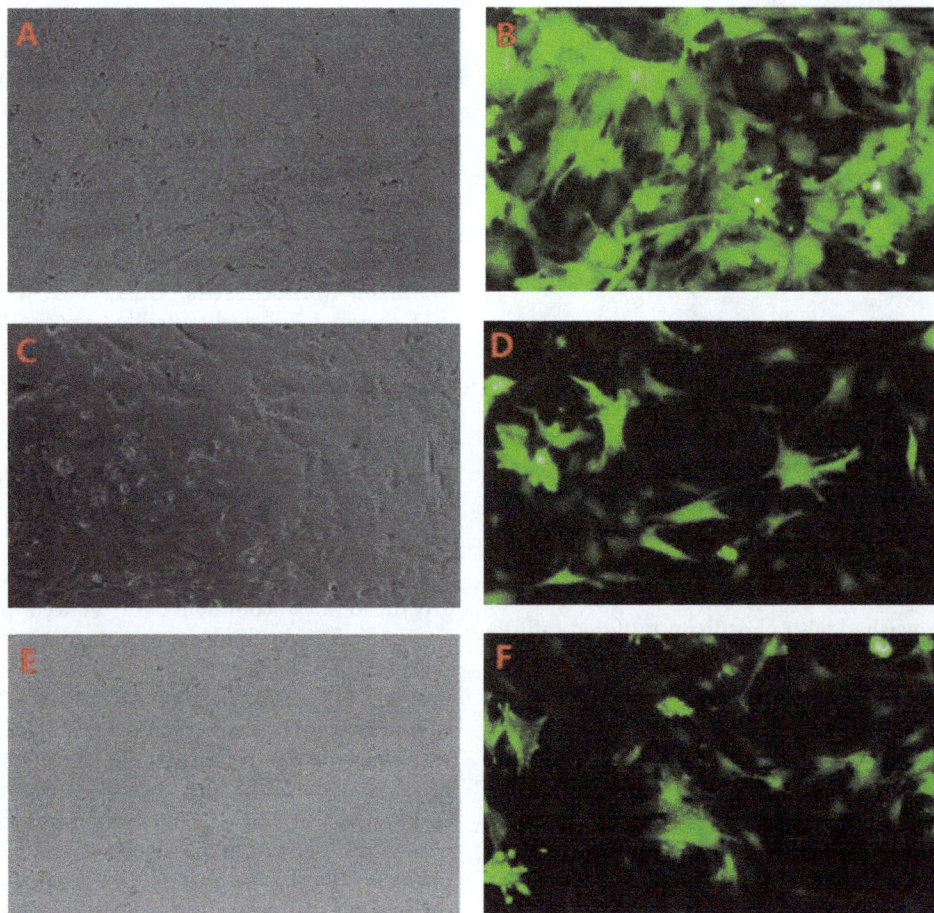

FIGURE 1: GFP-LC3B tracer technique showed that autophagy was induced in NP cells treated with high glucose condition ((A, C, E) light microscope; (B, D, F) fluorescence microscope. (A) and (B) represent glucose concentration as 5.6 mM; (C) and (D) as 0.1 M; (E) and (F) as 0.2 M, resp.).

10.57 ± 1.21% in control group, 0.1 M glucose group, and 0.2 M glucose, respectively (Figure 1). The rate of autophagy increased with the increase of glucose concentration. And the western blot analysis showed an increased expression of Beclin-1 and LC3-II and a decreased expression of p62 in the NP cells treated with high glucose concentrations when compared with the control group (Figure 2). The ratio of LC3-II/LC3-I expression increased under high glucose conditions, too. Moreover, it was also shown that the expression of Beclin-1, LC3-II, and p62 was changed almost in a glucose concentration-dependent manner.

3.2. PPARγ Was Expressed in NP Cells and Upregulated by High Glucose. Although PPARγ has been confirmed to be expressed in many tissues, it has never been studied in NP cells. In order to evaluate whether NP cells also express the PPARγ and the role of high glucose on PPARγ expression, Real-Time PCR and western blot were used. By PCR and western blot examination, the presence of PPARγ was detected at both RNA and protein levels in NP cells. When compared with the control group, it showed that the expression of PPARγ increased in the NP cells treated with high

glucose and the increase of PPARγ content was almost paralleled with the elevation of glucose concentration (Figure 3).

3.3. PPARγ Activation Induced Autophagy in NP Cells. Considering that high glucose not only induced autophagy but also upregulated the expression of PPARγ in NP cells, it was supposed by us that the PPARγ should have a relationship with autophagy in NP cells under high glucose. To better understand this relationship, PPARγ agonist and antagonist were added to the 0.2 M high glucose medium. Then the LC3, Beclin-1, and p62 expressions in the NP cells were examined and compared by western blot again. The western blot analysis showed an increased expression of Beclin-1 and LC3-II and a decrease expression of p62 in the NP cells treated with PPARγ agonist when compared with the 0.2 M high glucose condition (Figure 4). On the contrary, the expression of Beclin-1 and LC3-II decreased and the expression of p62 increased in the NP cells when treated with PPARγ antagonist (Figure 5).

Similarly, the autophagy in NP cells was also traced by using GFP-LC3B technique, when the agonist or antagonist was added (Figure 6). It showed that the autophagy in NP

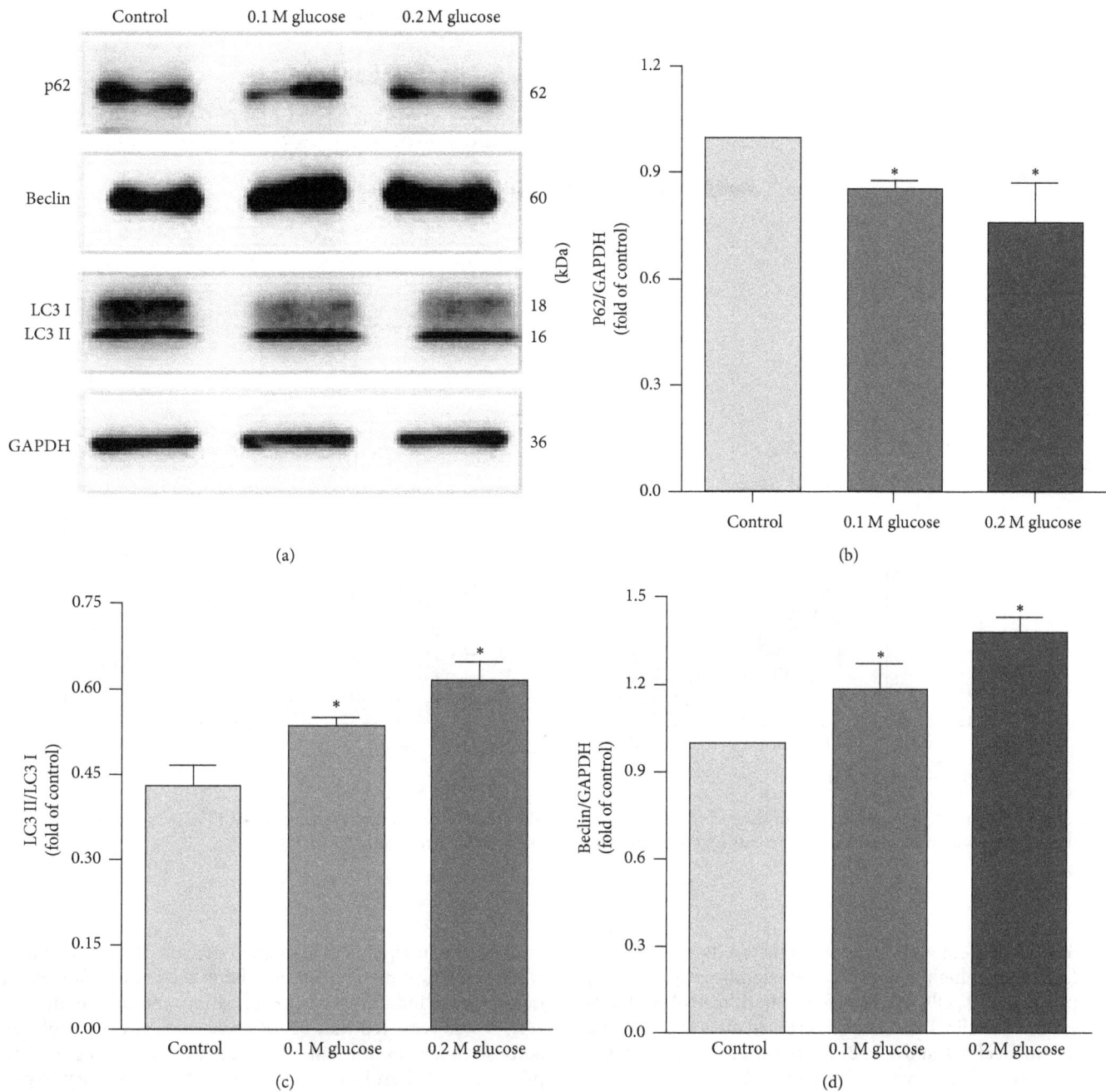

(a)

(b)

(c)

(d)

FIGURE 2: Western blot showed an increased expression of Beclin-1 and LC3-II and a decreased expression of p62 in the NP cells treated with high glucose. * represents a significant difference from the control group ($p < .05$).

cells increased and the rate of autophagy was 15.08 ± 1.77% when the agonist was added. While the rate of autophagy decreased to 7.38±0.75% when the antagonist was added, and it was almost the same as that in the control group (Figure 7).

4. Discussion

Glucose is an important fuel of nearly all organisms. It was used to be thought to lead to the elucidation of the electron transport chain and oxidative phosphorylation and complete the aerobic glucose metabolism for ATP generation through a common set of metabolic pathways. But now, it is known that glucose can be metabolized in multiple pathways providing not only an energy supply, but also participant in many important metabolites, such as cell growth and function. In recent years, high glucose has been proved to regulate autophagy in many cells, such as podocytes, renal tubular epithelial cells, and NP cells [5, 12, 13].

(a)

(b)

(c)

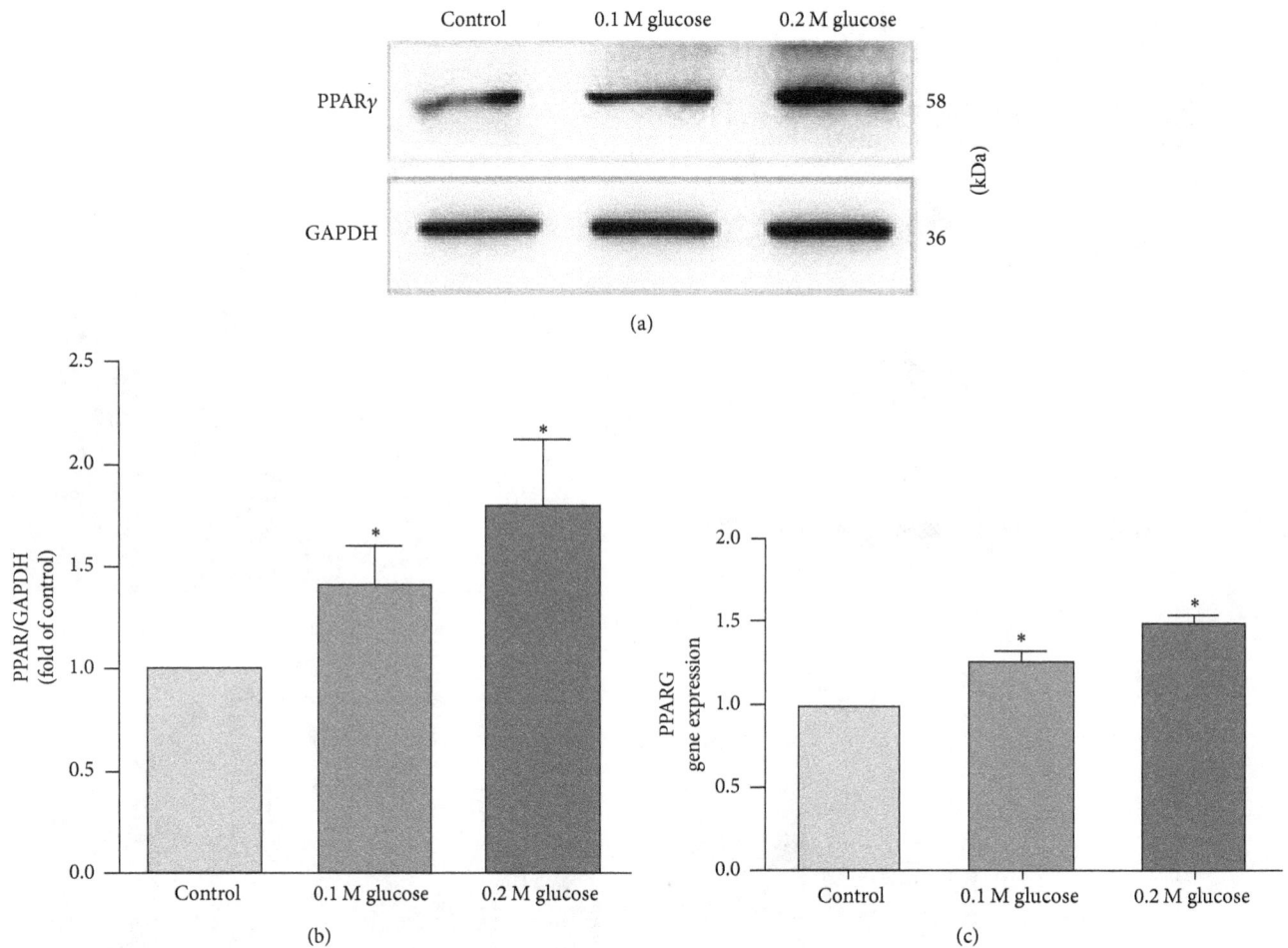

FIGURE 3: Real-Time PCR and western blot showed that PPARγ expressed in the NP cells and the expression of PPARγ increased when NP cells were treated with high glucose. ∗ represents a significant difference from the control group ($p < .05$).

To be consistent with those previous results, our findings emphasize that high glucose could significantly enhance autophagy in NP cells. We have found both mRNA and protein levels of Beclin-1 and LC3B increased after high glucose treatment. Beclin-1 and LC3B are required for autophagosome formation and maturation, which is one of the most important steps of autophagy. We have also found that p62 protein decreased under high glucose. p62 is an autophagy-specific substrate, which can be degraded together with LC3-II. The accumulation of p62 indicated impaired autophagy. These findings indicated that the autophagy in NP cells activated by high glucose treatment and the autophagic flux was efficient. GFP-LC3B tracer technique also provided similar outcomes. When autophagy occurs, GFP-LC3B forms spots in cytoplasm. The more spots represents the higher level of autophagy. Our results showed that NP cells under 0.1 M and 0.2 M glucose resulted in more green spots than control, which revealed that glucose can certainly activate the autophagy in NP cells. However, the pathway of autophagy in NP cells under the high glucose condition is unclear.

PPARγ is a nuclear hormone receptor that comprises an agonist-dependent activation domain, DNA binding domain, and agonist-independent activation domain. It is one of pathways in glucose metabolism involving the control of energy homeostasis, inflammation, proliferation, and differentiation [14]. It was reported that PPARγ was expressed not only in adipose tissue [15, 16], but also in breast, colon, lung, ovary, prostate, and thyroid [17]. However, whether PPARγ is expressed in human NP and how it can affect NP cells are unclear.

Here, it was the first time to identify that human NP cells also presented expression of PPARγ by Real-Time PCR and western blot. Moreover, the expression of PPARγ was found to be upregulated under high glucose treatment and the increase of PPARγ was almost in direct proportion of the glucose concentration. Interestingly, the change pattern of PPARγ in NP cells in our study varied with Schwann cells reported by Kim et al. [18]. The result in his study showed that chronic high glucose conditions retained normal PPAR levels in Schwann cells. The differences between Kim and us might be attributed to the differences in cell types, glucose concentration, and time of treatment.

There is no final conclusion about whether PPARγ could activate or inactivate autophagy [19]. In our present study,

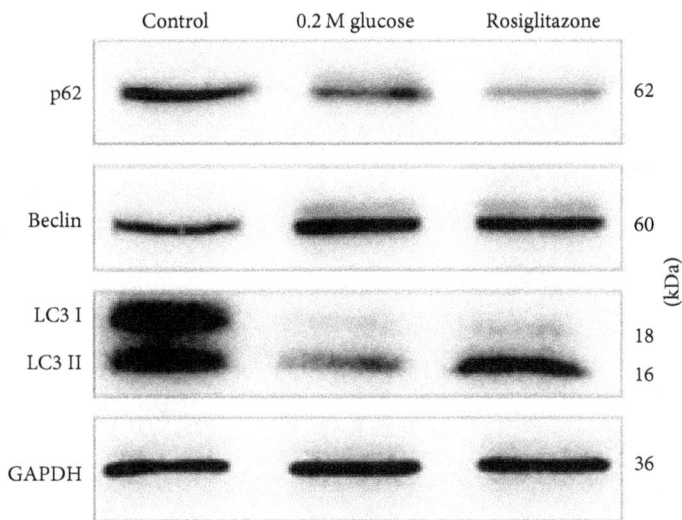

(a)

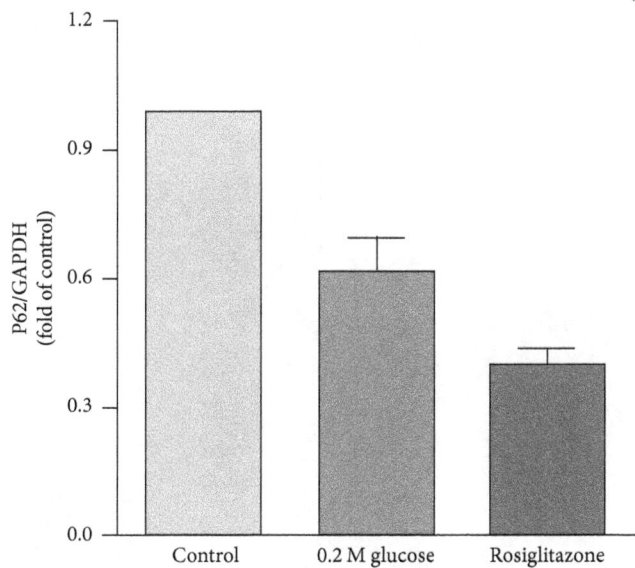

(b)

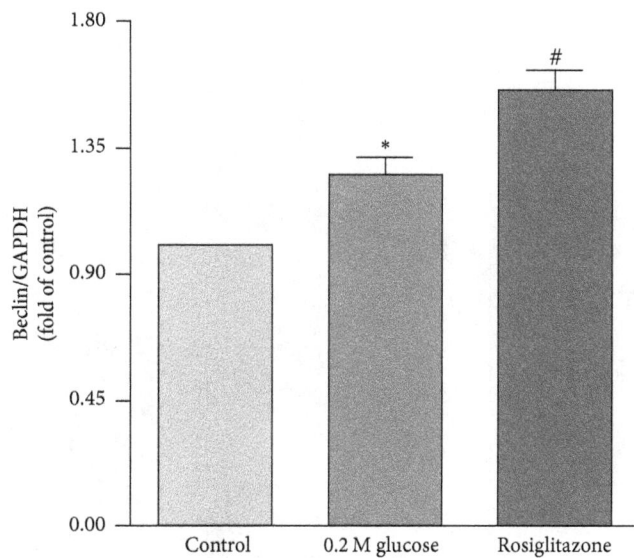

(c)

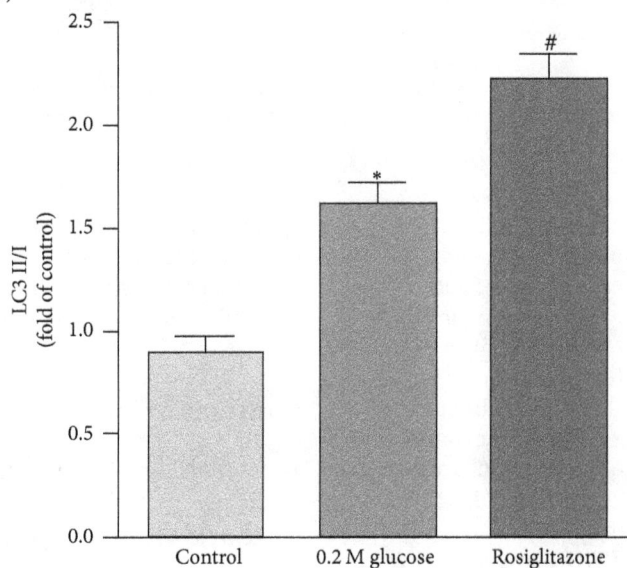

(d)

FIGURE 4: Western blot analysis showed an increased expression of Beclin-1 and LC3-II and a decreased expression of p62 in the NP cells treated with PPARγ agonist. # represents a significant difference from 0.2 M high glucose condition ($p < .05$).

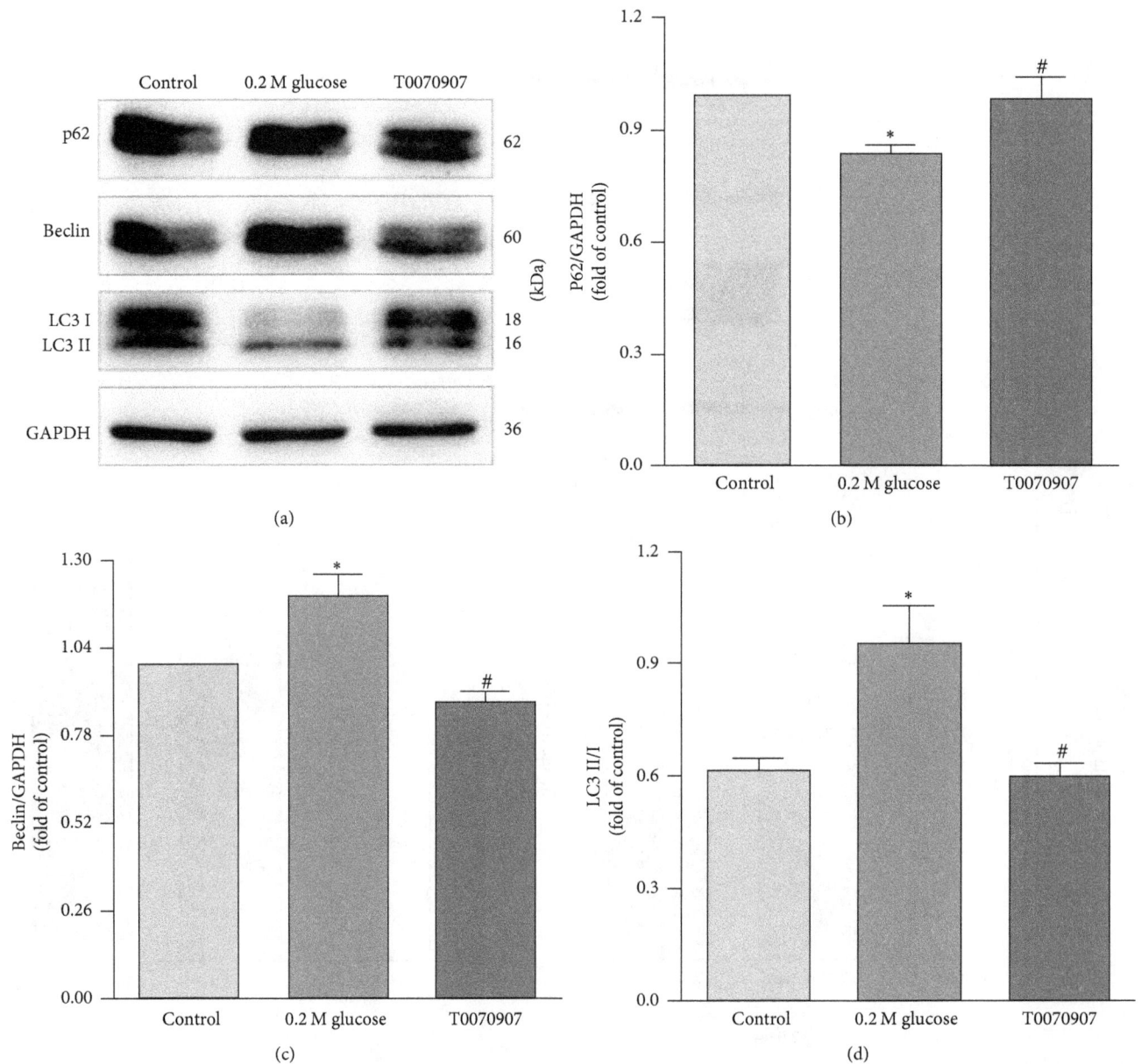

(a)

(b)

(c)

(d)

FIGURE 5: Western blot showed that the expression of Beclin-1 and LC3-II decreased and p62 increased in the NP cells when treated with PPARγ antagonist. # represents a significant difference from 0.2 M high glucose condition ($p < .05$).

PPARγ was also found to have a relationship with autophagy in NP cells under high glucose condition and the increase of PPARγ content was associated with the degree of autophagy. But whether the increase of PPARγ is the upstream or the concomitant phenomenon of autophagy by high glucose needs be further studied. To better understand the relationship between PPARγ and autophagy under high glucose condition in NP cells, the PPARγ agonist and antagonist were added to DMEM with 0.2 M glucose. Our results revealed that PPARγ agonist increased the autophagy in NP cells and the antagonist (T0070907) was opposite. According to these findings, we determined that PPARγ was the upstream of autophagy and PPARγ activation could further induce autophagy in NP cells under high glucose condition.

In summary, high glucose treatment could upregulate PPARγ, which further activated autophagy in NP cells. Further observations are needed to uncover the specific signaling molecules on the PPARγ-related autophagy induced by high glucose in NP.

Conflicts of Interest

The authors declare that they have no conflicts of interest.

Authors' Contributions

Chang Jiang and Shuhao Liu contributed equally to this work as co-first authors.

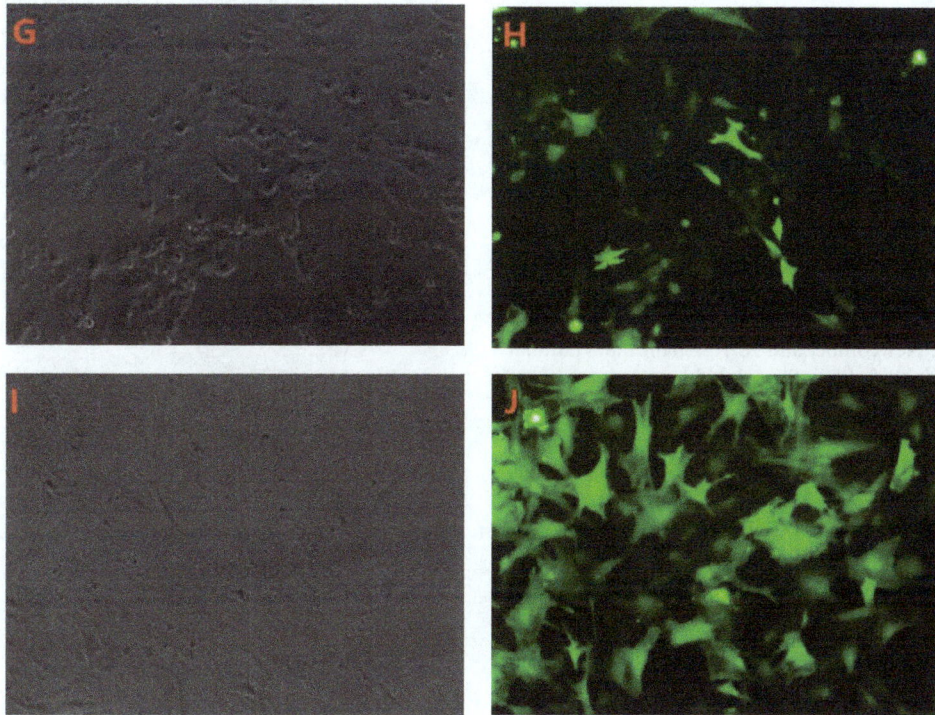

FIGURE 6: It showed that the autophagy in NP cells increased when the agonist was added to the high glucose medium, while it decreased when the antagonist was added ((G, I) light microscope; (H, J) fluorescence microscope. (G) and (H) represent as 0.2 M high glucose + agonist; (I) and (J) as 0.2 M high glucose + antagonist, resp.).

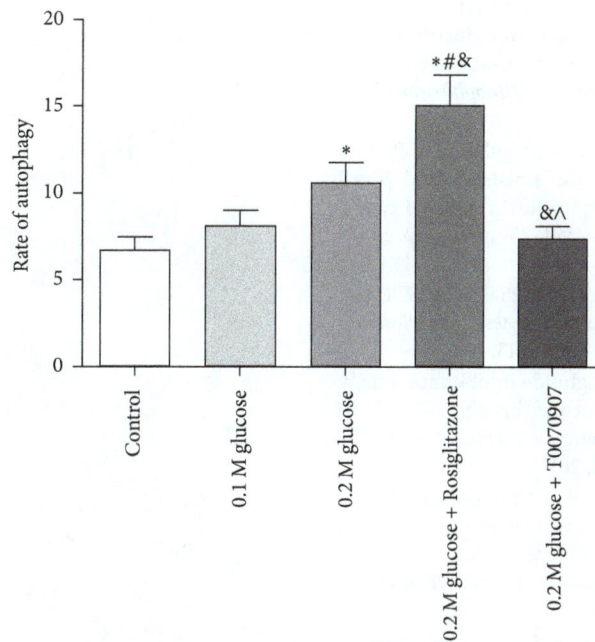

FIGURE 7: The rate of autophagy under different medium conditions was shown and the PPARγ activation could induce autophagy significantly. * represents a significant difference from the control group; # represents a significant difference from the 0.1 M glucose condition; & represents a significant difference from 0.2 M glucose condition; and ∧ represents a significant difference from 0.2 M high glucose condition plus agonist ($p < .05$).

References

[1] A. Endean, K. T. Palmer, and D. Coggon, "Potential of magnetic resonance imaging findings to refine case definition for mechanical low back pain in epidemiological studies: A systematic review," *The Spine Journal*, vol. 36, no. 2, pp. 160–169, 2011.

[2] A. J. MacGregor, T. Andrew, P. N. Sambrook et al., "Structural, psychological, and genetic influences on low back and neck pain: a study of adult female twins," *Arthritis Care & Research*, vol. 51, no. 2, pp. 160–167, 2004.

[3] N. Sakellaridis, "The influence of diabetes mellitus on lumbar intervertebral disk herniation," *World Neurosurgery*, vol. 66, no. 2, pp. 152–154, 2006.

[4] R. J. Mobbs, R. L. Newcombe, and K. N. Chandran, "Lumbar discectomy and the diabetic patient: Incidence and outcome," *Journal of Clinical Neuroscience*, vol. 8, no. 1, pp. 10–13, 2001.

[5] C.-G. Kong, J.-B. Park, M. S. Kim, and E.-Y. Park, "High glucose accelerates autophagy in adult rat intervertebral disc cells," *Asian Spine Journal*, vol. 8, no. 5, pp. 543–548, 2014.

[6] H.-Y. Won, J.-B. Park, E.-Y. Park, and K. D. Riew, "Effect of hyperglycemia on apoptosis of notochordal cells and intervertebral disc degeneration in diabetic rats," *Journal of Neurosurgery: Spine*, vol. 11, no. 6, pp. 741–748, 2009.

[7] J.-G. Kong, J.-B. Park, D. Lee, and E.-Y. Park, "Effect of high glucose on stress-induced senescence of nucleus pulposus cells of adult rats," *Asian Spine Journal*, vol. 9, no. 2, pp. 155–161, 2015.

[8] P. Balakumar and G. Jagadeesh, "PPAR ligands and cardiovascular disorders: friend or foe," *Curr Mol Pharmacol*, vol. 5, no. 2, pp. 219–223, 2012.

[9] E. Y. Hsia, M. L. Goodson, J. X. Zou, M. L. Privalsky, and H.-W. Chen, "Nuclear receptor coregulators as a new paradigm for therapeutic targeting," *Advanced Drug Delivery Reviews*, vol. 62, no. 13, pp. 1227–1237, 2010.

[10] D. Kim, K.-K. Park, S. K. Lee, S.-E. Lee, and J.-K. Hwang, "Cornus kousa F.Buerger ex Miquel increases glucose uptake through activation of peroxisome proliferator-activated receptor γ and insulin sensitization," *Journal of Ethnopharmacology*, vol. 133, no. 2, pp. 803–809, 2011.

[11] A. K. Sharma, S. Bharti, S. Goyal et al., "Upregulation of PPARγ by Aegle marmelos ameliorates insulin resistance and β-cell dysfunction in high fat diet fed-streptozotocin induced type 2 diabetic rats," *Phytotherapy Research*, vol. 25, no. 10, pp. 1457–1465, 2011.

[12] T. Ma, J. Zhu, X. Chen, D. Zha, P. C. Singhal, and G. Ding, "High glucose induces autophagy in podocytes," *Experimental Cell Research*, vol. 319, no. 6, pp. 779–789, 2013.

[13] X. Zhao, G. Liu, H. Shen et al., "Liraglutide inhibits autophagy and apoptosis induced by high glucose through GLP-1R in renal tubular epithelial cells," *International Journal of Molecular Medicine*, vol. 35, no. 3, pp. 684–692, 2015.

[14] T. Imai, R. Takakuwa, S. Marchand et al., "Peroxisome proliferator-activated receptor γ is required in mature white and brown adipocytes for their survival in the mouse," *Proceedings of the National Acadamy of Sciences of the United States of America*, vol. 101, no. 13, pp. 4543–4547, 2004.

[15] B. M. Spiegelman, "PPAR-γ: adipogenic regulator and thiazolidinedione receptor," *Diabetes*, vol. 47, no. 4, pp. 507–514, 1998.

[16] P. Tontonoz, E. Hu, and B. M. Spiegelman, "Stimulation of adipogenesis in fibroblasts by PPARγ2, a lipid-activated transcription factor," *Cell*, vol. 79, no. 7, pp. 1147–1156, 1994.

[17] K. G. Lambe and J. D. Tugwood, "A Human peroxisome-proliferator-activated receptor-gamma is activated by inducers of adipogenesis, including thiazolidinedione drugs," *European Journal of Biochemistry*, vol. 239, no. 1, pp. 1–7, 1996.

[18] E. S. Kim, F. Isoda, I. Kurland, and C. V. Mobbs, "Glucose-induced metabolic memory in Schwann cells: Prevention by PPAR agonists," *Endocrinology*, vol. 154, no. 9, pp. 3054–3066, 2013.

[19] J. Yao, K. Zheng, and X. Zhang, "Rosiglitazone exerts neuroprotective effects via the suppression of neuronal autophagy and apoptosis in the cortex following traumatic brain injury," *Molecular Medicine Reports*, vol. 12, no. 5, pp. 6591–6597, 2015.

13

Mediating Roles of PPARs in the Effects of Environmental Chemicals on Sex Steroids

Qiansheng Huang[1,2] and Qionghua Chen[3]

[1]*Key Lab of Urban Environment and Health, Institute of Urban Environment, Chinese Academy of Sciences, Xiamen 361021, China*
[2]*Center for Excellence in Regional Atmospheric Environment, Institute of Urban Environment, Chinese Academy of Sciences, Xiamen 361021, China*
[3]*The First Affiliated Hospital of Xiamen University, Xiamen 361003, China*

Correspondence should be addressed to Qiansheng Huang; qshuang@iue.ac.cn

Academic Editor: Christopher Lau

Peroxisome proliferator-activated receptors (PPARs) are ligand-activated nuclear receptors that are widely involved in various physiological functions. They are widely expressed through the reproductive system. Their roles in the metabolism and function of sex steroids and thus the etiology of reproductive disorders receive great concern. Various kinds of exogenous chemicals, especially environmental pollutants, exert their adverse impact on the reproductive system through disturbing the PPAR signaling pathway. Chemicals could bind to PPARs and modulate the transcription of downstream genes containing PPRE (peroxisome proliferator response element). This will lead to altered expression of genes related to metabolism of sex steroids and thus the abnormal physiological function of sex steroids. In this review, various kinds of environmental ligands are summarized and discussed. Their interactions with three types of PPARs are classified by various data from transcript profiles, PPRE reporter in cell line, in silico docking, and gene silencing. The review will contribute to the understanding of the roles of PPARs in the reproductive toxicology of environmental chemicals.

1. Introduction

Peroxisome proliferator-activated receptors (PPARs) are ligand-activated nuclear receptors which are widely involved in various physiological and pathological processes [1]. The family contains three subtypes (PPARα, PPARβ/δ, and PPARγ) with various ligand specificity, tissue distribution, and biological function. PPARs are detectable in various compartments of the reproductive system, including hypothalamus, pituitary, testis, ovary, uterus, and adrenal and mammary gland. PPARs are widely involved in reproductive function, such as ovarian function, gestation, and communication between mother and fetus [2–4]. Sex steroids, also named as gonadal steroids, are defined as steroid hormones that interact with receptors of androgen, estrogen, and progesterone in vertebrates [5]. Sex steroids are produced by gonads (ovaries or testes) and adrenal glands. Further conversion could occur in other tissues such as livers and fats. PPARs are critical for the metabolism and physiological function of sex hormones [2, 6].

Large amounts of pollutants have been released into the environmental media as a consequence of rapid industrialization and urbanization. Exposure to pollutants has been reported to be a big risk for reproductive health [7]. The mechanism through which pollutants elicit adverse effects is still not fully understood. However, it is widely accepted that pollutants could adversely affect the reproductive function through disturbing the metabolism and function of sex steroids [8]. Pollutants could bind to PPARs and then modulate the PPAR signaling pathways involved in the reproductive function. Hydrophobic interactions are the primary driving force for the binding between pollutants and PPARs. Most of the amino acid residues are hydrophobic around the binding pocket which located inside the protein structure of PPARs [9]. The sequences of amino acids which form the pocket are conserved across species. Results from reporter cell lines also show that environmental ligands (BPA derivatives, phthalates, and PFAAs) share similar affinity for PPARγ of zebrafish and human [10].

In this review, the interactions between PPARs and sex steroids are presented. Various kinds of PPAR ligands, especially environmental chemicals, are summarized. The pathways through which exogenous chemicals exert their impact on the metabolism and function of sex steroids via PPARs are depicted.

2. Interaction between PPARs and Sex Steroids

Androgens and estrogens are the primary types of sex steroids. Exogenous testosterone significantly inhibited the expression of PPARγ in primary hepatocytes isolated from brown trout [11]. 17β-Estradiol could regulate the expression of PPARγ in human peripheral blood eosinophils [12]. Additionally, precursors of sex steroids also interact with PPARs. For example, dehydroepiandrosterone (DHEA) induced elevated expression of both PPARα and PPARβ/δ in the muscle of mice [13]. Conversely, PPARs have an important impact on sex steroids. Single nucleotide polymorphism (SNP) of PPARs significantly affected the level of sex steroids and was linked to hormone related diseases. For example, the SNP of PPARγ at P12A (Pro12Ala, rs1801282) was linked to a gynecological disease: polycystic ovary syndrome (PCOS) as PCOS patients with CG genotype showed lower free testosterone and other hormones than that of GG genotype [14]. Peroxisome proliferators (PPs) are a group of chemicals which function through PPARs. PPs could impair the function of endocrine tissues by regulating the expression of phase I and phase II steroid metabolism enzymes [15], including P450 enzymes and 17β-hydroxysteroid dehydrogenase IV [16]. Apart from their impact on metabolism, PPs could also disturb the physiological function of sex steroids. They have been reported to mimic or interfere with the action of sex steroids and then induce reproductive disorders [17]. In addition, receptors of sex steroids were also reported to interplay with PPARs. For example, estrogen receptor alpha (ERα) binds to the PPRE sequence of PPARγ and represses its transactivation in MCF-7 cells [18]. Bidirectional interplay occurs between PPARγ and ER [19].

Sources of PPs contain endogenous and exogenous chemicals. Endogenous essential fatty acids (FAs) and their derivative eicosanoids are able to activate the PPAR signaling pathway [20]. 17β-Estradiol could suppress the expression of PPARα regulating genes [21]. In addition to these endogenous chemicals, chemicals from environmental media, drugs, and other external sources are also reported to disturb the PPAR signaling pathway and then affect metabolism and function of sex steroids.

3. Environmental Chemicals as Exogenous Ligands

A lot of environmental chemicals act as exogenous ligands to PPARs. These chemicals are widely detectable in the human body and have received widespread public health attention [52]. PPARs have been regarded as a bridge to link the environmental chemicals and their health impact [53]. Chemicals which could modulate the PPAR signaling pathway and affect the sex steroids are classified and listed as follows. They are also shown in Table 1.

3.1. Phthalates. Phthalates were widely reported as reproductive toxicants. Fetal exposure to environmentally relevant di(2-ethylhexyl) phthalate (DEHP) decreased serum levels of steroid hormones in adult male mice and antagonism of PPARγ diminished the toxic effect [22]. In our study, PPARγ was thought to transduce the toxicity of DEHP at 0.2–2 μM in both primary cultured endometrial cells and endometrial adenocarcinoma cell line (ishikawa) [23]. We also obtained consistent results in a marine fish model where the expressions of PPARγ and aromatase were both enhanced after fish embryo exposure to DEHP at 0.1–1 mg/L [24]. In vivo, DEHP is metabolized to mono(2-ethylhexyl) phthalate (MEHP) which could activate both PPARα and PPARγ and then suppress the transcription of aromatase and estradiol production in the ovary. These have been verified both in rat ovarian granulosa cell models [26] and in the ovary of rat models [25]. Direct exposure to MEHP at the dose of 50 μM also inhibited the expression of aromatase by activating PPARα or PPARγ in rat granulosa cells [27]. Due to the adverse health outcome of commonly used compounds, phthalate-alternative compounds have been emerging. Some of these chemicals also showed various affinities to PPARs and different influences on reproductive function according to docking studies [30, 54–56]. For example, diisononyl phthalate (DINP) showed DEHP-like affinity to PPARα. Di(2-ethylhexyl) terephthalate (DEHT) has the paraisomer structure of DEHP and shows a very weak affinity to PPARα.

3.2. Perfluoroalkyl Acids. Perfluoroalkyl acids (PFAAs), characteristic of fully fluorinated carbon chains, are widely used in consumer goods and industrial products. Concerns have arisen regarding human exposure and adverse outcome, especially due to extremely long biologic retention time [57]. Treatments with perfluorononanoic acid (PFNA), perfluorooctanoic acid (PFOA), perfluorodecanoic acid (PFDA), perfluoroundecanoic acid (PFUnDA), and perfluorooctane sulfonate (PFOS) all dose-dependently activated PPARα using a PPRE reporter system [31, 33]. PFOS and PFOA are top two members in toxicological studies. Our study showed that the effects of PFOS (1–16 mg/L) were different on the expression of these three types of PPARs in the larvae of *O. melastigma* [37]. PFOA (5 mg/kg) exposure affected the expression of PPARs in a tissue dependent manner in fetal and postnatal CD-1 mice [34]. Both PFOS and PFOA can induce PPARs-mediated transcriptional activity determined by PPRE reporter assay [31, 33, 35, 36, 38, 39]. This led to alterations in immune response and other physiological processes [58]. However, the mediating roles of PPARs are not consistently recognized. Several studies confirm that PFOA can exert its toxicity independently of PPARα [59, 60]. It is worth mentioning that four weeks' PFOA treatment (5 mg/kg) increased the expression of enzymes catalyzing the biosynthesis of steroid hormone and enhanced serum levels of progesterone in PPARα knockout female mice [61]. Apart

TABLE 1: Various kinds of environmental activators of PPARs and their impact on sex steroids.

Chemicals	PPARs subtype	Methods	Effects on sex steroids	Experimental model	References
DEHP	α, γ	Docking, transcript profiles, antagonism	Enhanced expression of aromatase, altered levels of estradiol	Rat, endometrial cells, fish	[22–25]
MEHP	α, β/δ, γ	Antagonism, transcript profiles	Decreased expression of aromatase and estradiol production	Rat ovarian granulosa cells, rat model, human liposarcoma cells, 3T3-L1 cells	[25–29]
DEHT	α	Docking	No significant impact	Rat model	[30]
PFNA	α, β/δ, γ	Transcript profiles, PPRE reporter	Elevated expression of CYP4A	Zebrafish, monkey kidney CV-1 cell line	[31, 32]
PFOA	α, γ	PPRE reporter, transcript profiles, antagonism, gene silencing	/	Monkey kidney CV-1 cell line, mice	[31, 33–36]
PFOS	α, γ	PPRE reporter, transcript profiles, antagonism, gene silencing	/	Monkey kidney CV-1 cell line, O. melastigma, mice	[31, 33, 35–39]
PFDA	α	PPRE reporter	/	Monkey kidney CV-1 cell line	[31]
PFUnDA	α	PPRE reporter	/	monkey kidney CV-1 cell line	[31]
TBBPA	γ	PPRE reporter	Increased apelin expression and secretion	Epithelial ovarian cancer cell line (OVCAR-3)	[40, 41]
TCBPA	γ	PPRE reporter	Increased apelin expression and secretion	OVCAR-3	[40, 41]
BPA	a, β/δ, γ	Transcript profiles, PPRE reporter, docking	Decreased expression of aromatase and estradiol production	Human ovarian granulosa cell, mouse embryo fibroblasts, OVCAR-3	[41–46]
PCB77	a, β/δ, γ	Docking, antagonism	/	Cell model, mice model	[47]
PCB18	a, β/δ, γ	Docking, antagonism	/	Cell model, mice model	[7, 47]
PCB126	α	Transcript profiles	Altered the secretion of estradiol	Rat model, mice model	[48]
DDT	γ	Transcript profiles	Enhanced expression of CYP4A	Human mesenchymal stem cells	[49]
2,4-D	γ	Transcript profiles, gene silencing	Decreased cholesterol levels	Mice leydig cells, mice model	[6]
TBT	a, β/δ, γ	PPRE reporter	Inhibition of gonad development	Juvenile salmon, cell model	[50, 51]
EE2	γ	Transcript profiles	/	Brown trout	[11]

"/" indicated data is not available as we known; The experimental methods to support the interaction between chemicals and PPARs are depicted as follows. *Antagonism*: PPARs was antagonized by specific antagonist. Then, the effects elicited by chemicals were re-assessed. If the effects were diminished or enhanced, the mediating roles of PPARs could be confirmed; *Transcript profiles*: Transcript profiles of PPARs were modulated by chemicals treatment; *Docking*: Computing methods to predict the structural binding between chemicals and PPARs; *PPRE reporter*: Reporter system was constructed by transfecting the luciferase reporting plasmid containing PPRE sequence into the cells. Then, the cells were treated with chemicals to determine whether chemicals functioned through activating PPARs; *Gene silencing*: The expression of PPARs was inhibited by RNAi or gene knockout. Then, the effects elicited by chemicals were re-assessed. If the effects were diminished or enhanced, the mediating roles of PPARs could be confirmed; *Abbreviation*: di-(2-ethylhexyl) phthalate, DEHP; mono-(2-ethylhexyl) phthalate, MEHP; di(2-ethylhexyl) terephthalate, DEHT; perfluorododecanoic acid, PFDoA; perfluorononanoic acid, PFNA; perfluorooctanoic acid, PFOA; perfluorodecanoic acid, PFDA; perfluoroundecanoic acid, PFUnDA; perfluorooctane sulfonate, PFOS; BPA diglycidyl ether, BADGE; tetrabromobisphenol A, TBBPA; tetrachlorobisphenol A, TCBPA; bisphenol A, BPA; polychlorinated biphenyls, PCB; dichlorodiphenyltrichloroethane, DDT; 2,3,7,8-tetrachlorodibenzo-p-dioxin, TCDD; 2,4-dichlorophenoxyacetic acid, 2,4-D; organotin, TBT; ethinylestradiol, EE2.

from the toxicological studies, a lot of epidemiological studies also revealed the effects of PFOA on reproduction. Positive or negative association was reported by publications from C8 science panel [62–64]. Different members of PFAAs show various impacts on PPAR signaling due to their various chain lengths and functional groups [65, 66]. Thus, toxicities of other family members are being studied. For example, perfluorododecanoic acid (PFDoA) administration (3 mg/kg) led to reduced serum levels of 17β-estradiol in prepubertal female rats; however, the roles of PPARs have not been verified yet [67].

3.3. Bisphenol A (BPA) and Its Derivatives.
BPA is widely used in plastic bottles, paper, and other daily commodities. Due to structural similarity with 17β-estradiol, the estrogenic activity of BPA via ER activation was widely studied. In addition to ERs, BPA also show an affinity to human PPARγ as confirmed by data from docking and PPRE reporter studies [9, 42, 43]. The affinity was ranked as ERRγ > ERα > PPARγ. BPA exposure (0–100 μM) led to reduced expression of aromatase and decreased level of E2 secretion in human ovarian granulosa cells, which also happened after overexpression of the PPARγ [44]. By contrast, the same level range of BPA showed no significant effect on the expression of both PPARγ and aromatase in human endometrial stromal fibroblast cells [68]. To be noted, low dose effects were observed in the toxicology of BPA. A low dose was considered to be a dose below the range typically used in toxicological studies of chemicals [69]. Biphasic U- or inverted U-shaped dose-response curves have been observed when evaluating the effects of BPA on reproduction and other health outcomes. Competitive binding to PPARs and other receptors between BPA and sex hormone might contribute to this low dose effect [70]. Derivatives of BPA could also interfere with PPARs. Brominated or chlorinated derivatives of BPA display their adverse impact through PPARs. Both tetrabromobisphenol A (TBBPA) and tetrachlorobisphenol A (TCBPA) show binding affinity to PPARγ as indicated by reporter cell lines [40, 71]. Of further note, TBBPA (0.01–10 μM) can also induce the expression of aromatase and thus enhance estrogen synthesis independently of PPARγ in human choriocarcinoma JEG-3 cells [72, 73].

3.4. Dioxin-Like Chemicals.
Dioxin and its structure-like chemicals are widely accepted as the ligands to aryl hydrocarbon receptor (AHR). They also interplay with PPARs as confirmed by in silico docking experiments [47]. An in vivo study using male rat model revealed that polychlorinated biphenyls 126 (PCB126) exposure at the dose of 5 μmol/kg inhibited the mRNA expression of PPARα and its downstream genes acyl-CoA oxidase (Acox1) and hydroxy-3-methylglutaryl-CoA synthase 2 (Hmgcs2) in liver [48]. In our study using both cells and mice models, PCB126 exposure at human relevant levels induces the expression of HSD17B7 and enhances the secretion of estradiol in endometrium [7]. Molecular evidence confirmed the existence of two PPRE sites at the promoter of cytochrome P4501A1 (CYP1A1). Thus, direct activation of CYP1A1 by PPARα without AHR might be a new pathway to link PCBs and PPARs [74, 75].

However, strong evidence is still needed to confirm the link.

3.5. Pesticides.
A lot of pesticides show disrupting effects on metabolism and function of sex steroids, such as deltamethrin [76], linuron [77], and methomyl [78]. The mediating function of PPARs is being studied in the toxicity of pesticides. For example, a large in vitro reporter gene assay screening study with 200 pesticides showed that PPARs did not have a major role in the toxicity of pesticides. Various kinds of pesticides were examined including 29 organochlorines, 11 diphenyl ethers, 56 organophosphorus pesticides, 12 pyrethroids, 22 carbamates, 11 acid amides, 7 triazines, 8 ureas, and 44 others. Results showed that only three (diclofop-methyl, pyrethrins, and imazalil) could activate PPARα and none of them could activate PPARγ. The agonist roles of these three pesticides were further confirmed in mice [79]. In a study that has raised wide ecotoxicological concern, the mRNA level of PPARγ was induced by DDT at the doses of 100 pM-10 μM in human mesenchymal stem cells [49]. To be noted, direct evidence is still expected on the effects of pesticides on sex steroids through PPAR signaling.

3.6. Other Pollutants.
Organotin compounds are ubiquitously present in environment media. The compounds have been reported to alter endocrine functions in juvenile salmon and human choriocarcinoma cell lines [50, 80]. Tributyltin (TBT) could activate all three types of RXR (retinoid X receptor): PPARα, PPARβ/δ, and PPARγ heterodimers by PPRE luciferase experiment [51]. 2,4-Dichlorophenoxyacetic acid (2,4-D) is a possible endocrine disruptor. Treatment with 2,4-D decreased the level of testosterone in mice serum and testis through inhibiting the expression of 3-hydroxy-3-methylglutaryl coenzyme A synthase 1 and reductase, which led to decreased cholesterol levels. PPARα exerted a critical role as its silencing diminished these toxic effects [6].

3.7. Pollutant Mixtures.
In addition to individual pollutants, chemical mixtures also display reproductive toxicity through PPARs. Combined exposure to 2,3,7,8-tetrachlorodibenzo-p-dioxin (TCDD) and DEHP led to decreased estradiol synthesis in human granulosa cell line—KGN. Direct activation of AHR and transactivation of PPARs are indispensable parts in this molecular response pathway [81]. Chemical mixtures extracted from natural water could also disturb the function of steroid hormones where PPARs act as key regulators [82, 83]. In our study, cotreatment with DEHP and PCBs promoted the expression of PPARγ but not the other PPAR types in mice liver [84].

4. Conclusion and Perspectives

PPARs, especially the subtype of α and γ, have important roles in mediating the toxicological outcomes caused by environmental ligands. Various kinds of environmental pollutants show impacts on the metabolism and function of sex steroids through disturbing the PPARs signaling pathways. The interactions between PPARs and environmental chemicals have been revealed through various approaches including molecular docking, PPRE reporter, transcript profiles, and gene silencing which are performed in silico, in vitro, and in vivo. Future studies that should be carried out include (1) structural biological studies on crystal structures of pollutants bound to PPARs and (2) further evaluation of the crosstalk between PPARs and other classical nuclear receptors, such as ER and AHR. These studies will help reveal the roles of PPARs in the toxicology of environmental pollutants on sex steroids.

Conflicts of Interest

The authors declare that there are no conflicts of interest regarding the publication of this article.

Acknowledgments

This work was supported by the National Natural Science Foundation of China (21477123 and 81571418).

References

[1] B. Gross, M. Pawlak, P. Lefebvre, and B. Staels, "PPARs in obesity-induced T2DM, dyslipidaemia and NAFLD," *Nature Reviews Endocrinology*, vol. 13, no. 1, pp. 36–49, 2017.

[2] M. Vitti, G. Di Emidio, M. Di Carlo et al., "Peroxisome proliferator-activated receptors in female reproduction and fertility," *PPAR Research*, vol. 2016, Article ID 4612306, 12 pages, 2016.

[3] J. Yang, L. Chen, X. Zhang et al., "PPARs and female reproduction: evidence from genetically manipulated mice," *PPAR Research*, vol. 2008, Article ID 723243, 8 pages, 2008.

[4] P. Froment, F. Gizard, D. Defever, B. Staels, J. Dupont, and P. Monget, "Peroxisome proliferator-activated receptors in reproductive tissues: from gametogenesis to parturition," *Journal of Endocrinology*, vol. 189, no. 2, pp. 199–209, 2006.

[5] G. Guerriero, "Vertebrate sex steroid receptors: Evolution, ligands, and neurodistribution," *Annals of the New York Academy of Sciences*, vol. 1163, pp. 154–168, 2009.

[6] Y. Harada, N. Tanaka, M. Ichikawa et al., "PPARα-dependent cholesterol/testosterone disruption in Leydig cells mediates 2,4-dichlorophenoxyacetic acid-induced testicular toxicity in mice," *Archives of Toxicology*, vol. 90, no. 12, pp. 3061–3071, 2016.

[7] Q. Huang, Y. Chen, Q. Chen et al., "Dioxin-like rather than non-dioxin-like PCBs promote the development of endometriosis through stimulation of endocrine-inflammation interactions," *Archives of Toxicology*, vol. 91, no. 4, pp. 1915–1924, 2017.

[8] Z. R. Craig, W. Wang, and J. A. Flaws, "Endocrine-disrupting chemicals in ovarian function: Effects on steroidogenesis, metabolism and nuclear receptor signaling," *Reproduction*, vol. 142, no. 5, pp. 633–646, 2011.

[9] L. Li, Q. Wang, Y. Zhang, Y. Niu, X. Yao, and H. Liu, "The molecular mechanism of bisphenol A (BPA) as an endocrine disruptor by interacting with nuclear receptors: Insights from molecular dynamics (MD) simulations," *PLoS ONE*, vol. 10, no. 3, Article ID e0120330, 2015.

[10] M. Grimaldi, A. Boulahtouf, V. Delfosse, E. Thouennon, W. Bourguet, and P. Balaguer, "Reporter Cell Lines to Evaluate The Selectivity of Chemicals for Human and Zebrafish Estrogen and Peroxysome Proliferator Activated γ Receptors," *Frontiers in Neuroscience*, vol. 9, Article ID 00212, 212 pages, 2015.

[11] C. Lopes, T. V. Madureira, N. Ferreira, I. Pinheiro, L. F. C. Castro, and E. Rocha, "Peroxisome proliferator-activated receptor gamma (PPARγ) in brown trout: Interference of estrogenic and androgenic inputs in primary hepatocytes," *Environmental Toxicology and Pharmacology*, vol. 46, pp. 328–336, 2016.

[12] S. Ueki, M. Oguma, A. Usami et al., "Regulation of peroxisome proliferator-activated receptor-γ expression in human eosinophils by estradiol," *International Archives of Allergy and Immunology*, vol. 149, Supplement 1, pp. 51–56, 2009.

[13] N. Horii, K. Sato, N. Mesaki, and M. Iemitsu, "DHEA Administration Activates Transcription of Muscular Lipid Metabolic Enzymes via PPARα and PPARδ in Obese Rats," *Hormone and Metabolic Research*, vol. 48, no. 3, pp. 207–212, 2016.

[14] M. Yilmaz et al., "Pro12Ala polymorphism of the peroxisome proliferator-activated receptor-gamma gene in women with polycystic ovary syndrome," *Gynecological Endocrinology*, vol. 22, no. 6, pp. 336–342, 2006.

[15] L.-Q. Fan, L. You, H. Brown-Borg, S. Brown, R. J. Edwards, and J. C. Corton, "Regulation of phase I and phase II steroid metabolism enzymes by PPARα activators," *Toxicology*, vol. 204, no. 2-3, pp. 109–121, 2004.

[16] L.-Q. Fan, R. C. Cattley, and J. C. Corton, "Tissue-specific induction of 17β-hydroxysteroid dehydrogenase type IV by peroxisome proliferator chemicals is dependent on the peroxisome proliferator-activated receptor α," *Journal of Endocrinology*, vol. 158, no. 2, pp. 237–246, 1998.

[17] S. De Coster and N. van Larebeke, "Endocrine-disrupting chemicals: associated disorders and mechanisms of action," *Journal of Environmental and Public Health*, vol. 2012, Article ID 713696, 52 pages, 2012.

[18] D. Bonofiglio, S. Gabriele, S. Aquila et al., "Estrogen receptor α binds to peroxisome proliferator-activated receptor response element and negatively interferes with peroxisome proliferator-activated receptor γ signaling in breast cancer cells," *Clinical Cancer Research*, vol. 11, no. 17, pp. 6139–6147, 2005.

[19] X. Wang and M. W. Kilgore, "Signal cross-talk between estrogen receptor alpha and beta and the peroxisome proliferator-activated receptor gammal in MDA-MB-231 and MCF-7 breast cancer cells," *Molecular and Cellular Endocrinology*, vol. 194, no. 1-2, pp. 123–133, 2002.

[20] F. Echeverría, M. Ortiz, R. Valenzuela, and L. A. Videla, "Long-chain polyunsaturated fatty acids regulation of PPARs, signaling: Relationship to tissue development and aging," *Prostaglandins Leukotrienes and Essential Fatty Acids*, vol. 114, pp. 28–34, 2016.

[21] M. Yoon, "PPARα in obesity: sex difference and estrogen involvement," *PPAR Research*, vol. 2010, Article ID 584296, 16 pages, 2010.

[22] S. Lee, D. B. Martinez-Arguelles, E. Campioli, and V. Papadopoulos, "Fetal exposure to low levels of the plasticizer DEHP predisposes the adult male adrenal gland to endocrine disruption," *Endocrinology*, vol. 158, no. 2, pp. 304–318, 2017.

[23] Q. S. Huang et al., "The inflammation response to DEHP through PPAR gamma in endometrial cells," *International Journal of Environmental Research and Public Health*, vol. 13, no. 3, p. 13, 2016.

[24] T. Ye, M. Kang, Q. Huang et al., "Accumulation of Di(2-ethylhexyl) Phthalate Causes Endocrine-Disruptive Effects in Marine Medaka (Oryzias melastigma) Embryos," *Environmental Toxicology*, vol. 31, no. 1, pp. 116–127, 2016.

[25] C. Xu, J.-A. Chen, Z. Qiu et al., "Ovotoxicity and PPAR-mediated aromatase downregulation in female Sprague-Dawley

rats following combined oral exposure to benzo[a]pyrene and di-(2-ethylhexyl) phthalate," *Toxicology Letters*, vol. 199, no. 3, pp. 323–332, 2010.

[26] T. Lovekamp-Swan, A. M. Jetten, and B. J. Davis, "Dual activation of PPARα and PPARγ by mono-(2-ethylhexyl) phthalate in rat ovarian granulosa cells," *Molecular and Cellular Endocrinology*, vol. 201, no. 1-2, pp. 133–141, 2003.

[27] T. Lovekamp-Swan and B. J. Davis, "Mechanisms of phthalate ester toxicity in the female reproductive system," *Environmental Health Perspectives*, vol. 111, no. 2, pp. 139–145, 2003.

[28] E. Campioli, A. Batarseh, J. Li, and V. Papadopoulos, "The endocrine disruptor mono-(2-ethylhexyl) phthalate affects the differentiation of human liposarcoma cells (SW 872)," *PLoS ONE*, vol. 6, no. 12, Article ID e28750, 2011.

[29] J. N. Feige, L. Gelman, D. Rossi et al., "The endocrine disruptor monoethyl-hexyl-phthalate is a selective peroxisome proliferator-activated receptor γ modulator that promotes adipogenesis," *Journal of Biological Chemistry*, vol. 282, no. 26, pp. 19152–19166, 2007.

[30] M. A. Babich, "Review of Exposure And Toxicity Data for Phthalate Substitutes," Tech. Rep., 2010, http://www.cpsc.gov/PageFiles/126546/phthalsub.pdf.

[31] H. Ishibashi, H. Iwata, E.-Y. Kim et al., "Contamination and effects of perfluorochemicals in baikal seal (Pusa sibirica). 2. Molecular characterization, expression level, and transcriptional activation of peroxisome proliferator-activated receptor α," *Environmental Science and Technology*, vol. 42, no. 7, pp. 2302–2308, 2008.

[32] W. Zhang, Y. Zhang, H. Zhang, J. Wang, R. Cui, and J. Dai, "Sex differences in transcriptional expression of FABPs in zebrafish liver after chronic perfluorononanoic acid exposure," *Environmental Science and Technology*, vol. 46, no. 9, pp. 5175–5182, 2012.

[33] H. Ishibashi, E.-Y. Kim, and H. Iwata, "Transactivation potencies of the Baikal seal (Pusa sibirica) peroxisome proliferator-activated receptor α by perfluoroalkyl carboxylates and sulfonates: Estimation of PFOA induction equivalency factors," *Environmental Science and Technology*, vol. 45, no. 7, pp. 3123–3130, 2011.

[34] B. D. Abbott, C. R. Wood, A. M. Watkins, K. Tatum-Gibbs, K. P. Das, and C. Lau, "Effects of perfluorooctanoic acid (PFOA) on expression of peroxisome proliferator-activated receptors (PPAR) and nuclear receptor-regulated genes in fetal and postnatal CD-1 mouse tissues," *Reproductive Toxicology*, vol. 33, no. 4, pp. 491–505, 2012.

[35] W. Xia, Y.-J. Wan, X. Wang et al., "Sensitive bioassay for detection of PPARα potentially hazardous ligands with gold nanoparticle probe," *Journal of Hazardous Materials*, vol. 192, no. 3, pp. 1148–1154, 2011.

[36] J. P. Vanden Heuvel, J. T. Thompson, S. R. Frame, and P. J. Gillies, "Differential activation of nuclear receptors by perfluorinated fatty acid analogs and natural fatty acids: A comparison of human, mouse, and rat peroxisome proliferator-activated receptor-α, -β, and -γ, liver X receptor-β, and retinoid X receptor-α," *Toxicological Sciences*, vol. 92, no. 2, pp. 476–489, 2006.

[37] C. Fang, X. Wu, Q. Huang et al., "PFOS elicits transcriptional responses of the ER, AHR and PPAR pathways in Oryzias melastigma in a stage-specific manner," *Aquatic Toxicology*, vol. 106-107, pp. 9–19, 2012.

[38] M. L. Takacs and B. D. Abbott, "Activation of mouse and human peroxisome proliferator-activated receptors (α, β/δ, γ) by perfluorooctanoic acid and perfluorooctane sulfonate," *Toxicological Sciences*, vol. 95, no. 1, pp. 108–117, 2007.

[39] J. M. Shipley, C. H. Hurst, S. S. Tanaka et al., "trans-activation of PPARα and induction of PPARα target genes by perfluorooctane-based chemicals," *Toxicological Sciences*, vol. 80, no. 1, pp. 151–160, 2004.

[40] A. Riu, M. Grimaldi, A. le Maire et al., "Peroxisome proliferator-activated receptor γ is a target for halogenated analogs of bisphenol A," *Environmental Health Perspectives*, vol. 119, no. 9, pp. 1227–1232, 2011.

[41] M. Hoffmann, E. Fiedor, and A. Ptak, "Bisphenol A and its derivatives tetrabromobisphenol A and tetrachlorobisphenol A induce apelin expression and secretion in ovarian cancer cells through a peroxisome proliferator-activated receptor gamma-dependent mechanism," *Toxicology Letters*, vol. 269, pp. 15–22, 2017.

[42] G. Biasiotto, I. Zanella, A. Masserdotti et al., "Municipal wastewater affects adipose deposition in male mice and increases 3T3-L1 cell differentiation," *Toxicology and Applied Pharmacology*, vol. 297, pp. 32–40, 2016.

[43] D. Montes-Grajales and J. Olivero-Verbel, "Computer-aided identification of novel protein targets of bisphenol A," *Toxicology Letters*, vol. 222, no. 3, pp. 312–320, 2013.

[44] J. Kwintkiewicz, Y. Nishi, T. Yanase, and L. C. Giudice, "Peroxisome proliferator-activated receptor-γ mediates bisphenol A inhibition of FSH-stimulated IGF-1, aromatase, and estradiol in human granulosa cells," *Environmental Health Perspectives*, vol. 118, no. 3, pp. 400–406, 2010.

[45] C. H. Hurst and D. J. Waxman, "Activation of PPARα and PPARγ by environmental phthalate monoesters," *Toxicological Sciences*, vol. 74, no. 2, pp. 297–308, 2003.

[46] E. Grasselli, K. Cortese, A. Voci et al., "Direct effects of Bisphenol A on lipid homeostasis in rat hepatoma cells," *Chemosphere*, vol. 91, no. 8, pp. 1123–1129, 2013.

[47] I. A. Sheikh, A. A. Khweek, and M. A. Beg, "Peroxisome proliferator-activated receptors as potential targets for carcinogenic activity of polychlorinated biphenyls: A computational perspective," *Anticancer Research*, vol. 36, no. 11, pp. 6117–6124, 2016.

[48] G. S. Gadupudi, W. D. Klaren, A. K. Olivier, A. J. Klingelhutz, and L. W. Robertson, "PCB126-induced disruption in gluconeogenesis and fatty acid oxidation precedes fatty liver in male rats," *Toxicological Sciences*, vol. 149, no. 1, pp. 98–110, 2016.

[49] A. L. Strong, Z. Shi, M. J. Strong et al., "Effects of the endocrine-disrupting chemical DDT on self-renewal and differentiation of human Mesenchymal stem cells," *Environmental Health Perspectives*, vol. 123, no. 1, pp. 42–48, 2015.

[50] N. Pavlikova, T. M. Kortner, and A. Arukwe, "Modulation of acute steroidogenesis, peroxisome proliferator-activated receptors and CYP3A/PXR in salmon interrenal tissues by tributyltin and the second messenger activator, forskolin," *Chemico-Biological Interactions*, vol. 185, no. 2, pp. 119–127, 2010.

[51] A. le Maire, M. Grimaldi, D. Roecklin et al., "Activation of RXR-PPAR heterodimers by organotin environmental endocrine disruptors," *EMBO Reports*, vol. 10, no. 4, pp. 367–373, 2009.

[52] CDC, "Fourth national report on human exposure to environmental chemicals," 2009, http://www.cdc.gov/exposurereport/.

[53] J. Mathieu-Denoncourt, S. J. Wallace, S. R. de Solla, and V. S. Langlois, "Plasticizer endocrine disruption: Highlighting developmental and reproductive effects in mammals and non-mammalian aquatic species," *General and Comparative Endocrinology*, vol. 216, pp. 74–88, 2015.

[54] N. Kambia, A. Farce, K. Belarbi et al., "Docking study: PPARs interaction with the selected alternative plasticizers to di(2-ethylhexyl) phthalate," *Journal of Enzyme Inhibition and Medicinal Chemistry*, vol. 31, no. 3, pp. 448–455, 2016.

[55] M. K. Sarath Josh, S. Pradeep, K. S. Vijayalekshmi Amma et al., "Phthalates efficiently bind to human peroxisome proliferator activated receptor and retinoid X receptor α, β, γ subtypes: an in silico approach," *Journal of Applied Toxicology*, vol. 34, no. 7, pp. 754–765, 2014.

[56] T. Kaya, S. C. Mohr, D. J. Waxman, and S. Vajda, "Computational screening of phthalate monoesters for binding to PPARγ," *Chemical Research in Toxicology*, vol. 19, no. 8, pp. 999–1009, 2006.

[57] Z. Wang, I. T. Cousins, M. Scheringer, and K. Hungerbuehler, "Hazard assessment of fluorinated alternatives to long-chain perfluoroalkyl acids (PFAAs) and their precursors: Status quo, ongoing challenges and possible solutions," *Environment International*, vol. 75, pp. 172–179, 2015.

[58] J. C. DeWitt, A. Shnyra, M. Z. Badr et al., "Immunotoxicity of perfluorooctanoic acid and perfluorooctane sulfonate and the role of peroxisome proliferator-activated receptor alpha," *Critical Reviews in Toxicology*, vol. 39, no. 1, pp. 76–94, 2009.

[59] A. J. Filgo, E. M. Quist, M. J. Hoenerhoff, A. E. Brix, G. E. Kissling, and S. E. Fenton, "Perfluorooctanoic acid (PFOA)–induced liver lesions in two strains of mice following developmental exposures: PPARα is not required," *Toxicologic Pathology*, vol. 43, no. 4, pp. 558–568, 2015.

[60] A. Mattsson, A. Kärrman, R. Pinto, and B. Brunström, "Metabolic profiling of chicken embryos exposed to perfluorooctanoic acid (PFOA) and agonists to peroxisome proliferator-activated receptors," *PLoS ONE*, vol. 10, no. 12, 2015.

[61] Y. Zhao, Y. S. Tan, S. Z. Haslam, and C. Yang, "Perfluorooctanoic acid effects on steroid hormone and growth factor levels mediate stimulation of peripubertal mammary gland development in C57Bl/6 mice," *Toxicological Sciences*, vol. 115, no. 1, pp. 214–224, 2010.

[62] D. A. Savitz, C. R. Stein, S. M. Bartell et al., "Perfluorooctanoic acid exposure and pregnancy outcome in a highly exposed community," *Epidemiology*, vol. 23, no. 3, pp. 386–392, 2012.

[63] D. A. Savitz, C. R. Stein, B. Elston et al., "Relationship of perfluorooctanoic acid exposure to pregnancy outcome based on birth records in the mid-Ohio valley," *Environmental Health Perspectives*, vol. 120, no. 8, pp. 1201–1207, 2012.

[64] L. A. Darrow, C. R. Stein, and K. Steenland, "Serum perfluorooctanoic acid and perfluorooctane sulfonate concentrations in relation to birth outcomes in the Mid-Ohio Valley, 2005-2010," *Environmental Health Perspectives*, vol. 121, no. 10, pp. 1207–1213, 2013.

[65] J. A. Bjork and K. B. Wallace, "Structure-activity relationships and human relevance for perfluoroalkyl acid-induced transcriptional activation of peroxisome proliferation in liver cell cultures," *Toxicological Sciences*, vol. 111, no. 1, pp. 89–99, 2009.

[66] T. Buhrke, A. Kibellus, and A. Lampen, "In vitro toxicological characterization of perfluorinated carboxylic acids with different carbon chain lengths," *Toxicology Letters*, vol. 218, no. 2, pp. 97–104, 2013.

[67] Z. Shi, H. Zhang, L. Ding, Y. Feng, M. Xu, and J. Dai, "The effect of perfluorododecanoic acid on endocrine status, sex hormones and expression of steroidogenic genes in pubertal female rats," *Reproductive Toxicology*, vol. 27, no. 3-4, pp. 352–359, 2009.

[68] L. Aghajanova and L. C. Giudice, "Effect of bisphenol A on human endometrial stromal fibroblasts in vitro," *Reproductive BioMedicine Online*, vol. 22, no. 3, pp. 249–256, 2011.

[69] W. V. Welshons, K. A. Thayer, B. M. Judy, J. A. Taylor, E. M. Curran, and F. S. vom Saal, "Large effects from small exposures. I. Mechanisms for endocrine-disrupting chemicals with estrogenic activity," *Environmental Health Perspectives*, vol. 111, no. 8, pp. 994–1006, 2003.

[70] F. Acconcia, V. Pallottini, and M. Marino, "Molecular mechanisms of action of BPA," *Dose-Response*, vol. 13, no. 4, 2015.

[71] A. Riu, A. le Maire, M. Grimaldi et al., "Characterization of Novel Ligands of ERα, Erβ, and PPARγ: The Case of Halogenated Bisphenol A and Their Conjugated Metabolites," *Toxicological Sciences*, vol. 122, no. 2, pp. 372–382, 2011.

[72] E. Honkisz and A. K. Wójtowicz, "Modulation of estradiol synthesis and aromatase activity in human choriocarcinoma JEG-3 cells exposed to tetrabromobisphenol A," *Toxicology in Vitro*, vol. 29, no. 1, pp. 44–50, 2015.

[73] E. Honkisz and A. K. Wójtowicz, "The role of PPARγ in TBBPA-mediated endocrine disrupting effects in human choriocarcinoma JEG-3 cells," *Molecular and Cellular Biochemistry*, vol. 409, no. 1-2, pp. 81–91, 2015.

[74] E. Sérée, P.-H. Villard, J.-M. Pascussi et al., "Evidence for a new human CYP1A1 regulation pathway involving PPAR-α and 2 PPRE sites," *Gastroenterology*, vol. 127, no. 5, pp. 1436–1445, 2004.

[75] F. Fallone, P.-H. Villard, L. Decome et al., "PPARα activation potentiates AhR-induced CYP1A1 expression," *Toxicology*, vol. 216, no. 2-3, pp. 122–128, 2005.

[76] A. Ben Slima, Y. Chtourou, M. Barkallah, H. Fetoui, T. Boudawara, and R. Gdoura, "Endocrine disrupting potential and reproductive dysfunction in male mice exposed to deltamethrin," *Human & Experimental Toxicology*, vol. 36, no. 3, pp. 218–226, 2017.

[77] H. Ding, W. Zheng, H. Han et al., "Reproductive toxicity of linuron following gestational exposure in rats and underlying mechanisms," *Toxicology Letters*, vol. 266, pp. 49–55, 2017.

[78] S. L. Meng, L. P. Qiu, G. D. Hu et al., "Responses and recovery pattern of sex steroid hormones in testis of Nile tilapia (*Oreochromis niloticus*) exposed to sublethal concentration of methomyl," *Ecotoxicology*, vol. 25, no. 10, pp. 1805–1811, 2016.

[79] S. Takeuchi, T. Matsuda, S. Kobayashi, T. Takahashi, and H. Kojima, "In vitro screening of 200 pesticides for agonistic activity via mouse peroxisome proliferator-activated receptor (PPAR)α and PPARγ and quantitative analysis of in vivo induction pathway," *Toxicology and Applied Pharmacology*, vol. 217, no. 3, pp. 235–244, 2006.

[80] T. Nakanishi, J.-I. Nishikawa, Y. Hiromori et al., "Trialkyltin compounds bind retinoid X receptor to alter human placental endocrine functions," *Molecular Endocrinology*, vol. 19, no. 10, pp. 2502–2516, 2005.

[81] J. Ernst, J.-C. Jann, R. Biemann, H. M. Koch, and B. Fischer, "Effects of the environmental contaminants DEHP and TCDD on estradiol synthesis and aryl hydrocarbon receptor and peroxisome proliferator-activated receptor signalling in the human granulosa cell line KGN," *Molecular Human Reproduction*, vol. 20, no. 9, pp. 919–928, 2014.

[82] J. L. Lyche, R. Nourizadeh-Lillabadi, C. Karlsson et al., "Natural mixtures of POPs affected body weight gain and induced transcription of genes involved in weight regulation and insulin signaling," *Aquatic Toxicology*, vol. 102, no. 3-4, pp. 197–204, 2011.

[83] J. L. Lyche, R. Nourizadeh-Lillabadi, C. Almaas et al., "Natural mixtures of persistent organic pollutants (POP) increase weight gain, advance puberty, and induce changes in gene expression associated with steroid hormones and obesity in female zebrafish," *Journal of Toxicology and Environmental Health, Part A: Current Issues*, vol. 73, no. 15, pp. 1032–1057, 2010.

[84] Y. Lin, L. Min, Q. Huang et al., "The combined effects of DEHP and PCBs on phospholipase in the livers of mice," *Environmental Toxicology*, vol. 30, no. 2, pp. 197–204, 2015.

14

PPAR-γ Agonists and their Role in Primary Cicatricial Alopecia

Sarawin Harnchoowong and Poonkiat Suchonwanit

Division of Dermatology, Faculty of Medicine, Ramathibodi Hospital, Mahidol University, Bangkok, Thailand

Correspondence should be addressed to Poonkiat Suchonwanit; poonkiat@hotmail.com

Academic Editor: Ling Xu

Peroxisome proliferator-activated receptor γ (PPAR-γ) is a ligand-activated nuclear receptor that regulates the transcription of various genes. PPAR-γ plays roles in lipid homeostasis, sebocyte maturation, and peroxisome biogenesis and has shown anti-inflammatory effects. PPAR-γ is highly expressed in human sebaceous glands. Disruption of PPAR-γ is believed to be one of the mechanisms of primary cicatricial alopecia (PCA) pathogenesis, causing pilosebaceous dysfunction leading to follicular inflammation. In this review article, we discuss the pathogenesis of PCA with a focus on PPAR-γ involvement in pathogenesis of lichen planopilaris (LPP), the most common lymphocytic form of PCA. We also discuss clinical trials utilizing PPAR-agonists in PCA treatment.

1. Introduction

Cicatricial alopecias, or scarring alopecias, are a group of hair loss disorders that are characterized by the permanent destruction of pilosebaceous units. Loss of follicular ostia in the alopecic area and subsequent replacement with fibrous tissue is an important clinical sign [1]. The condition can be classified as primary cicatricial alopecia (PCA) and secondary cicatricial alopecia (SCA). PCA refers to disorders in which the hair follicles are the main targets of destructive inflammatory processes; inflammatory cells destroy the stem cells in the bulge region of hair follicles. In SCA, the hair follicle stem cells are secondarily destroyed by more generalized skin conditions, such as blistering diseases, cancers, trauma, burns, infection, or radiation [1, 2]. PCA is further classified by (predominantly) inflammatory cell type, as shown in Table 1 [3].

Like the loss of follicular ostia in the area of alopecia, clinical signs of PCA include evidence of scalp inflammation, for example, perifollicular erythema and perifollicular scales, hair tufting, pustules, skin atrophy, and hypertrophic scarring (Figure 1) [4]. Histopathologically, inflammatory cell infiltration can be observed, distinguished by subtype. Histopathology, together with immunofluorescent staining, can be used to help make a definitive diagnosis of the specific condition [5]. At later stages of the disease, the inflammatory cells will be replaced with fibrous tissues. The etiology and pathogenesis of PCA remain under discussion [6], and there are several hypothesized mechanisms for different types of PCA. This review article summarizes up-to-date knowledge and hypotheses of PCA, especially in pathogenesis and treatment, focusing on one of the latest ideas: peroxisome proliferator-activated receptor γ (PPAR-γ) involvement in lipid homeostasis within pilosebaceous units. As shown in Figure 2, disruption of this pathway can lead to hair follicle inflammation and permanent destruction [7].

2. Pathogenesis of PCA

One of the most widely discussed hypotheses for PCA pathogenesis is hair follicle stem cell destruction. Hair follicles normally regenerate, beginning with the rapidly growing anagen phase, transforming through the catagen phase and resting at the telogen phase [8]. The main requirement for this regeneration capacity is functional epithelial hair follicle stem cells, and these are located within the bulge area at the lower end of the upper half of the hair follicle [9]. However, epithelial stem cells alone cannot initiate the hair cycle; the interaction between hair follicle epithelium and mesenchyme also plays a role. The bulge region is the location of inflammation in scarring alopecia, in contrast to bulb area involvement in other inflammatory nonscarring alopecias,

TABLE 1: Classification of primary cicatricial alopecia.

Classification of cicatricial alopecia
Lymphocytic
(i) Discoid lesions of lupus erythematosus
(ii) Lichen planopilaris
(a) Classic LPP
(b) Frontal fibrosing alopecia
(c) Graham Little syndrome
(iii) Pseudopelade of Brocq
(iv) Central centrifugal cicatricial alopecia
(v) Alopecia mucinosa
(vi) Keratosis follicularis spinulosa decalvans
Neutrophilic
(i) Folliculitis decalvans
(ii) Dissecting cellulitis
Mixed cell
(i) Acne keloidalis
(ii) Acne necrotica
(iii) Erosive pustular dermatosis

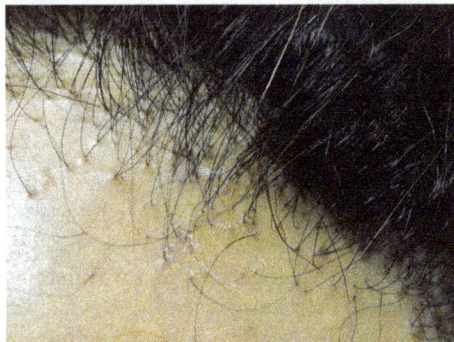

FIGURE 1: Clinical signs of cicatricial alopecia. The scalp shows a loss of follicular ostia, and the residual hairs show perifollicular erythema and scaling.

such as alopecia areata [10, 11]. Therefore, the hypothesis that bulge stem cells are associated with hair follicle destruction has merit. Evidence supporting this hypothesis came from a transgenic keratin-15 mouse model in which bulge stem cell destruction led to the permanent loss of hair follicles [12]. Immunostaining of PCA tissues, such as lichen planopilaris (LPP) and chronic cutaneous lupus erythematosus (CCLE), also shows decreased levels of keratin-15, which is almost exclusively limited to the bulge region [13]. Nevertheless, this hypothesis might not adequately explain the pathogenesis of PCA, because dermal papilla-derived and peribulbar dermal sheath cells transplanted into the skin also show the ability to regenerate hair follicles [14].

Immune privilege is another point of interest for investigators. Scientists hypothesize that immune privilege collapse, leading to immunologic responses, could subsequently cause PCA. Immune privilege sites are defined by their low expression levels of major histocompatibility complex (MHC) class Ia and β-2 microglobulin and increased levels

of immunosuppressive substances such as α-melanocyte-stimulating hormone (α-MSH), transforming growth factor β-1 (TGF β-1), and insulin-like growth factor-1 (IGF-1). Normally, the immune privilege area of hair follicles is located around the hair bulb region; this is the area of exclusive autoantigen-induced autoimmunologic attack, as proposed for the pathogenesis of alopecia areata [15]. However, a recent study suggests that the bulge area also demonstrates immune privilege characteristics of reduced MHC-I and II and β-2 microglobulin levels and upregulation of cluster of differentiation (CD) 200+, α-MSH, TGF-β2, macrophage migratory inhibitory factor, and indoleamine-2,3-dioxygenase [16]. This leads to the idea that any immune attack during the failure of this state of immune privilege in the bulge area would lead to epithelial stem cell destruction and, later, permanent loss of hair follicles. Evidence for an initial causal mechanism leading to immune privilege collapse remains inconclusive. One of the upregulated potent immune-regulatory glycoproteins, CD200 is markedly expressed in the bulge area [16, 17]. CD200 shows anti-inflammatory effects and is suspected to be the hair follicle "no danger" signal [18]. Danger/no danger is the latest proposed model of immunologic response; when presented cells are recognized as dangerous invaders, the immune response will be activated [19]. In a CD200-deficient skin model, hair follicles showed inflammation that caused immune-mediated alopecia, correlating to a mouse model showing that CD200 knockdown mice suffer from peri- and intrafollicular inflammation and terminally scarring alopecia [20]. Other substances found to be involved in the maintenance of immune privilege in the hair follicle are somatostatin and programmed death ligand 1 (PD-L1). Somatostatin is upregulated and strongly expressed in the hair follicle outer root sheath relative to the epidermis [21]. When somatostatin is activated, levels of proinflammatory cytokine-like interferon-γ (IFN-γ) are diminished, leading to the hypothesis that somatostatin has a role in immune privilege preservation. PD-L1 has also been found to have a role in immune privilege maintenance. This substance is highly expressed in dermal papillae and the dermal sheath cup area and epithelium cultured with PD-L1 shows lower levels of IFN-γ [22]. Neuroendocrine substances, such as α-MSH, prolactin, and thyrotropin-releasing hormone (TRH), are also believed to contribute to the maintenance of hair follicle immune privilege [23].

Besides stem cell destruction, epithelial-mesenchymal inhibition is hypothesized to be one of the mechanisms behind PCA pathogenesis. Epithelial-mesenchymal communication is another essential component for hair follicle cycling, and primary inflammation events cause disruption of this communication. This hypothesis holds that inflammation can attack any region of the hair follicles and is not restricted to the bulge region. However, it could not be confirmed that epithelial-mesenchymal communication failure is the primary event of the disease [24].

In CCLE, cytotoxic cell-mediated hair follicle destruction is hypothesized to be one of the pathogeneses of the disease. Early histologic findings showed that CD4 predominates CD8 in lesional skin [25, 26], and levels of cutaneous lymphocyte antigen (CLA) and cytotoxic marker granzyme

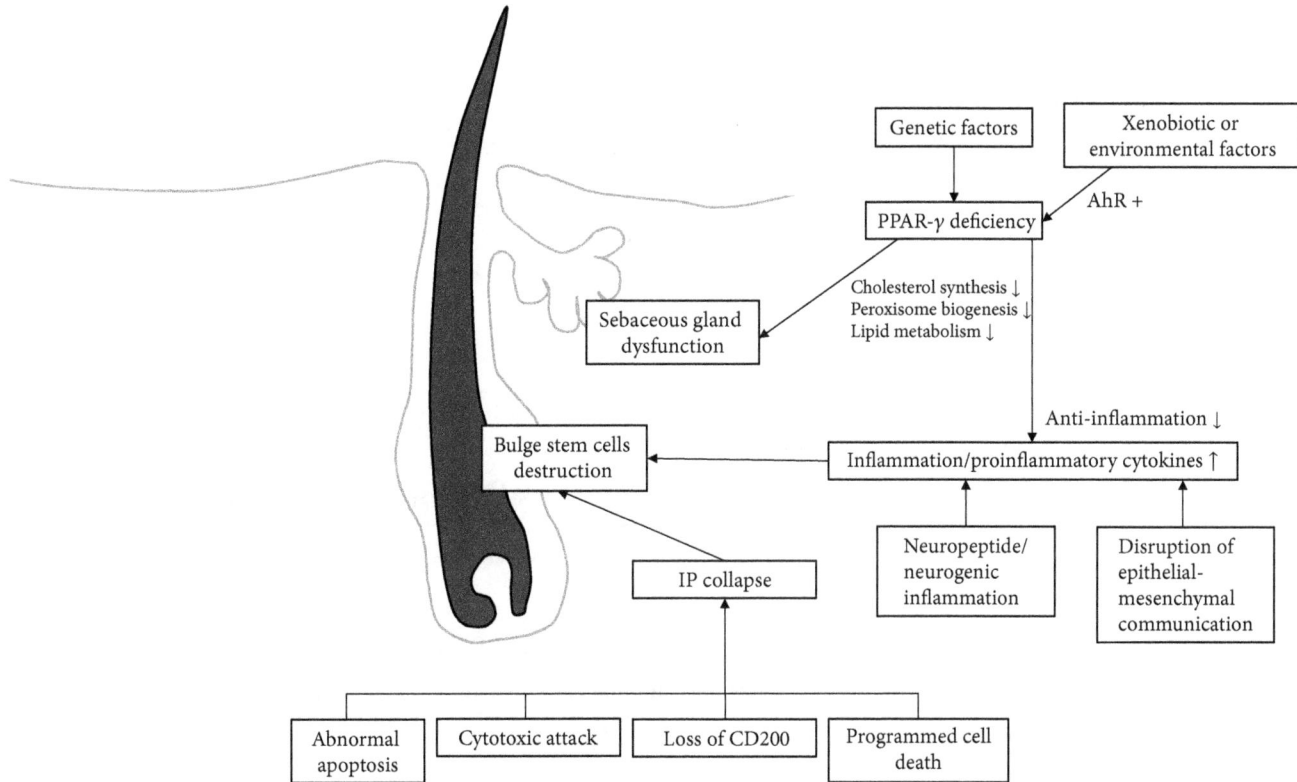

FIGURE 2: Possible pathogenic pathways in primary cicatricial alopecia.

B were higher in CCLE scar tissue [26]. These findings suggest that CD4 might invade the follicular epithelium, induce inflammation and apoptosis, and cause scarring at later stages of the disease. IFN-γ, or type 1 IFN, is believed to be a possible responsible proinflammatory cytokine. When IFN type 1 is activated, it induces production of various inflammatory chemokines, including CXCL9 and CXCL10, recruits chemokines such as CLA, E-selectin, CCR4, and CXCR3 to diseased skin, and causes local inflammation [27]. Apoptosis is one of the pathogenic processes in CCLE. Fas ligand, an essential component of the apoptotic mechanism, is increasingly expressed in CCLE skin compared to controls, and decreased anti-Bcl-2 staining is evidence of significant apoptosis in CCLE [28]. However, it remains unknown what stimulates the IFN response and apoptosis induction. In a recent study, LPP also showed these characteristics of immune privilege collapse together with cytotoxic cell-mediated follicle destruction. Thus, there is a possibility that LPP might also be an autoimmune hair disorder, similar to alopecia areata, but the location of immune attack is at the bulge region [29].

Another proposed hypothesis for PCA pathogenesis is sebaceous gland dysfunction. In an asebia mouse model with defective stearoyl-CoA desaturase-1 (SCD1), mice exhibit scarring alopecia, sebaceous gland atrophy, and abnormal sebum production [30]. Sebaceous gland atrophy and defective sebum production are alleged to be the causes of foreign body reaction, inflammation, and permanent hair follicle destruction. PPAR-γ deficiency has also

been raised as a possible pathogenetic mechanism of PCA, as demonstrated by a PPAR mouse model [31]. PPAR-γ mediates lipid metabolism and inflammation, especially in pilosebaceous units. Hence, defective PPAR-γ could lead to failure of pilosebaceous units and cause permanent hair follicle loss [31]. The following sections of this review will discuss PPAR-γ and PCA association in greater depth.

Other possible causes of PCA have been proposed, but no definitive mechanism explaining how these pathogens cause the disease has been found. For example, LPP was found to be associated with exposure to gold [32]. Other drugs that have been associated with PCA are hepatitis B vaccines causing Graham-Little-Piccardi-Lasseur syndrome [33], anticonvulsants and cyclosporine causing acne keloidalis nuchae (AKN) [34–36], and imatinib causing follicular mucinosis [37]. UV exposure is related to erosive pustular dermatosis (EPD) [38], and folliculitis decalvans (FD), AKN, and EPD can be koebnerized by trauma [39]. A series of cases of LPP and FFA following hair transplant or facelift surgeries have been reported, without describing a specific mechanism [40–42]. Staphylococcus aureus is the main pathogen in FD [43]. Genetic factors also play a role in PCA development, and there are multiple genes associated with PCA [11]. African ancestry is associated with AKN [44]. Stress and neuropeptides also have an impact on alopecia development [45, 46]; however, they will not be discussed here as they are not the primary objective of this review article.

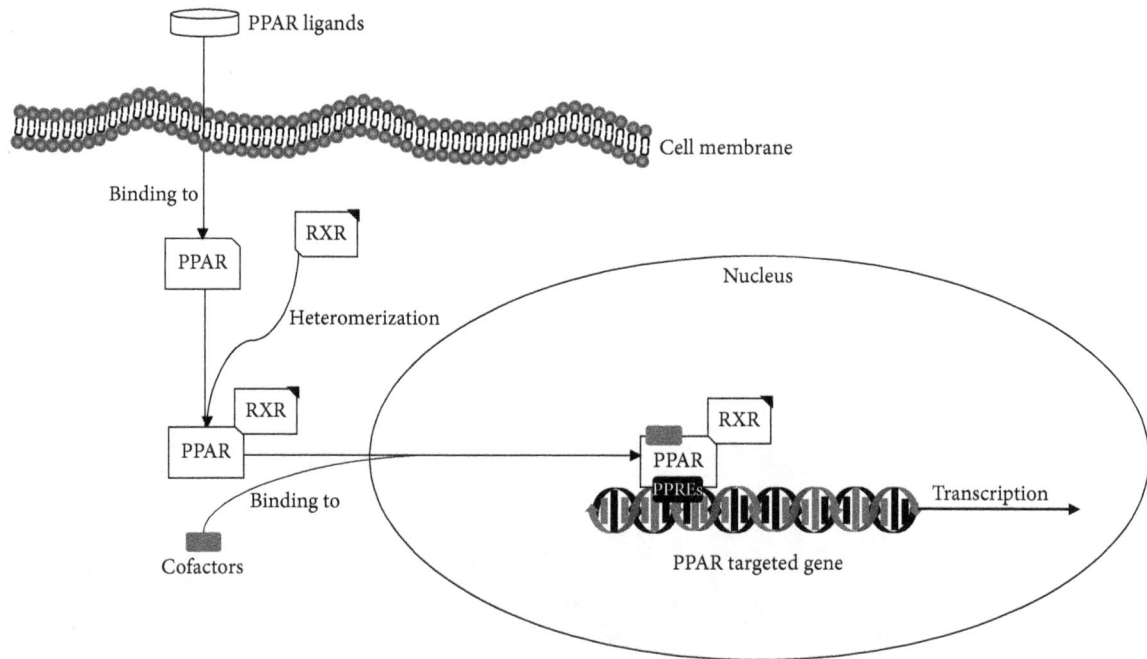

FIGURE 3: Activation of PPAR-RXR complex, leading to PPAR-targeted genes transcription.

3. Molecular Structure and Function of PPARs

PPARs are members of the ligand-activated nuclear receptors superfamily, regulating the transcription of various genes. PPARs are named for their function in peroxisome proliferator substance activation. There are three isoforms, PPAR-α, PPAR-β/δ, and PPAR-γ, each encoded by different genes and distributed differently [47]. PPARs are transferred into the nucleus and heterodimerized with retinoid X receptors (RXR) [48]; then heterodimeric PPAR complexes can bind to specific DNA sequences in the promotor region of target genes containing peroxisome proliferator response elements (PPREs), in the absence of ligands. Several PPAR ligands, both endogenous and exogenous, have been discovered. When specific ligands trigger the PPAR complex, conformational changes occur which lead to transcription of the targeted genes and subsequent translation into specific proteins (Figure 3) [49, 50]. Endogenous ligands for all PPARs include fatty acids and eicosanoid acids. Binding is specific to different types of PPARs; PPAR-α and PPAR-β/δ can bind both saturated and unsaturated fatty acids, but only polyunsaturated fatty acids bind PPAR-γ [51]. In addition, exogenous ligands, such as thiazolidinediones (TZDs) and fibrates, have recently been developed for the treatment of various PPAR-associated diseases [7].

PPARs are expressed in several components of human skin (Table 2) [7]. They are composed of 4 main functional domains: the A/B domain that contains the activation function-1 motif, a target of phosphorylation kinase, the C domain, a DNA binding domain that functions as a binding site for PPREs, the D domain, a hinge domain functioning as the docking site for cofactors, and the E/F domain, a ligand-binding domain that functions as a binding site for

specific ligands, activating PPARs and promoting target gene expression (Figure 4) [56].

PPAR-α is located on chromosome 22q12.2–13.1. Its main function is to regulate fatty acid homeostasis, both mitochondrial and peroxisomal, especially fatty acid catabolism and β-oxidation. Apart from fatty acid regulation, it is also believed to have anti-inflammatory properties; data has shown that PPAR-α inhibits proinflammatory gene expression in vascular smooth muscles, leading to reduced prevalence of atherosclerosis. PPAR-α is significantly expressed in tissues with high fatty acid oxidation, including the liver, heart, and skeletal muscles [57, 58]. Cells and tissues with lower expression include brown adipose tissue, kidneys, adrenal glands, macrophages, smooth muscles, and endothelial cells [59]. PPAR-α is proposed as one of the pathogeneses of various hepatic conditions. The important endogenous ligands for PPAR-α are unsaturated fatty acids, eicosanoids, leukotriene derivatives, and very low-density lipoprotein (VLDL) [7, 60–63]. Important synthetic PPAR-α agonists are known lipid lowering agents, such as the fibrate group [64].

The role of PPAR-β/δ has not been completely elucidated. There is a lack of information about its function and characteristics due to its ubiquitous expression [57, 58]. It is located on chromosome 6p21.1–21.2 and is expressed widely throughout body, highly so in adipose tissue. It has also been found in the liver, cardiac and skeletal muscles, the brain, kidneys, and colon and in vascular and epidermal tissues [59]. PPAR-β/δ is involved with metabolic diseases; it increases lipid oxidation in adipose cells, skeletal muscles, and the heart and improves HDL and insulin resistance status. Other functions include cell proliferation/differentiation induction, weight gain limitation, and inflammatory inhibition, especially in the vascular walls [65]. Its endogenous ligands

TABLE 2: Peroxisome proliferator-activated receptors (PPARs) in human skin.

Skin components	Type of PPAR expression
Epidermis and dermis	
(i) Epidermal keratinocytes	PPAR-α, PPAR-β/δ, and PPAR-γ
(ii) Melanocytes	PPAR-α, PPAR-β/δ, and PPAR-γ
(iii) Fibroblasts	PPAR-γ
(iv) T lymphocytes	PPAR-α, PPAR-β/δ, and PPAR-γ
(v) Langerhan cells	PPAR-α, PPAR-β/δ, and PPAR-γ
(vi) Mast cells	PPAR-β/δ and PPAR-γ
Follicular units	
(i) Hair matrix keratinocytes	PPAR-α, PPAR-β/δ, and PPAR-γ
(ii) Hair shaft cortex	PPAR-α, PPAR-β/δ, and PPAR-γ
(iii) Hair cuticle	PPAR-α, PPAR-β/δ, and PPAR-γ
(iv) Inner root sheath	PPAR-β/δ and PPAR-γ
(v) Outer root sheath	PPAR-α, PPAR-β/δ, and PPAR-γ
(vi) Dermal papilla cells	PPAR-α, PPAR-β/δ, and PPAR-γ
(vii) Connective tissue sheath	PPAR-α, PPAR-β/δ, and PPAR-γ
(viii) Sebocytes	PPAR-α, PPAR-β/δ, and PPAR-γ

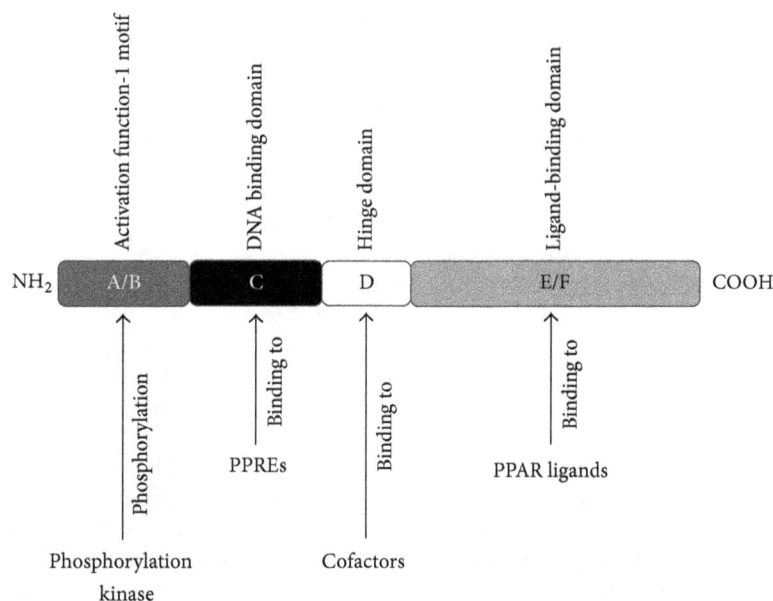

FIGURE 4: Diagram of the functional domain of PPARs.

are unsaturated fatty acids, carbaprostacyclin, and VLDL [7].

PPAR-γ is the most widely discussed PPAR and is our focus in this review article. PPAR-γ is located on chromosome 3p25. It is the most important PPAR; numerous studies relate it with the pathogeneses of different diseases. Its expression is mainly in adipose tissue and sebocytes, but it is also found in the liver, intestinal system, kidneys, retinas, spleen, immune system, skin, sebaceous glands, and thyroid cells and is sparsely expressed in muscles [57–59, 66–70]. PPAR-γ helps to maintain glucose metabolism via insulin sensitization and regulate adipocyte differentiation and lipid storage and acts as an anti-inflammatory agent. Essential fatty acids and their derivatives, for example, eicosanoid

and prostaglandin J2, are common ligands for PPAR-γ [7, 71]. Other recognized PPAR-γ agonists are TZDs [49] and nonsteroidal anti-inflammatory drugs (NSAIDs) [72]. Once activated, PPAR-γ produces 7 mRNA transcripts that are later transcribed into 3 proteins [73]. PPAR-γ1 transcript is found in adipose tissue, liver, pancreatic β-cells, intestines, bone, kidney, adrenal glands, vascular cells, and few in skeletal muscles. PPAR-γ2 is almost exclusively found in adipose tissues under normal circumstances. PPAR-γ 3, 6, and 7 are also found in adipose tissues, and nearly all PPAR mRNAs are found in macrophages [74]. PPAR-γ1 protein is translated from transcripts 1, 3, 5, and 7, PPAR-γ2 protein from transcripts 1 and 2, and PPAR-γ4 protein from transcripts 4 and 6 [73, 75, 76]. PPAR-γ2 protein is involved

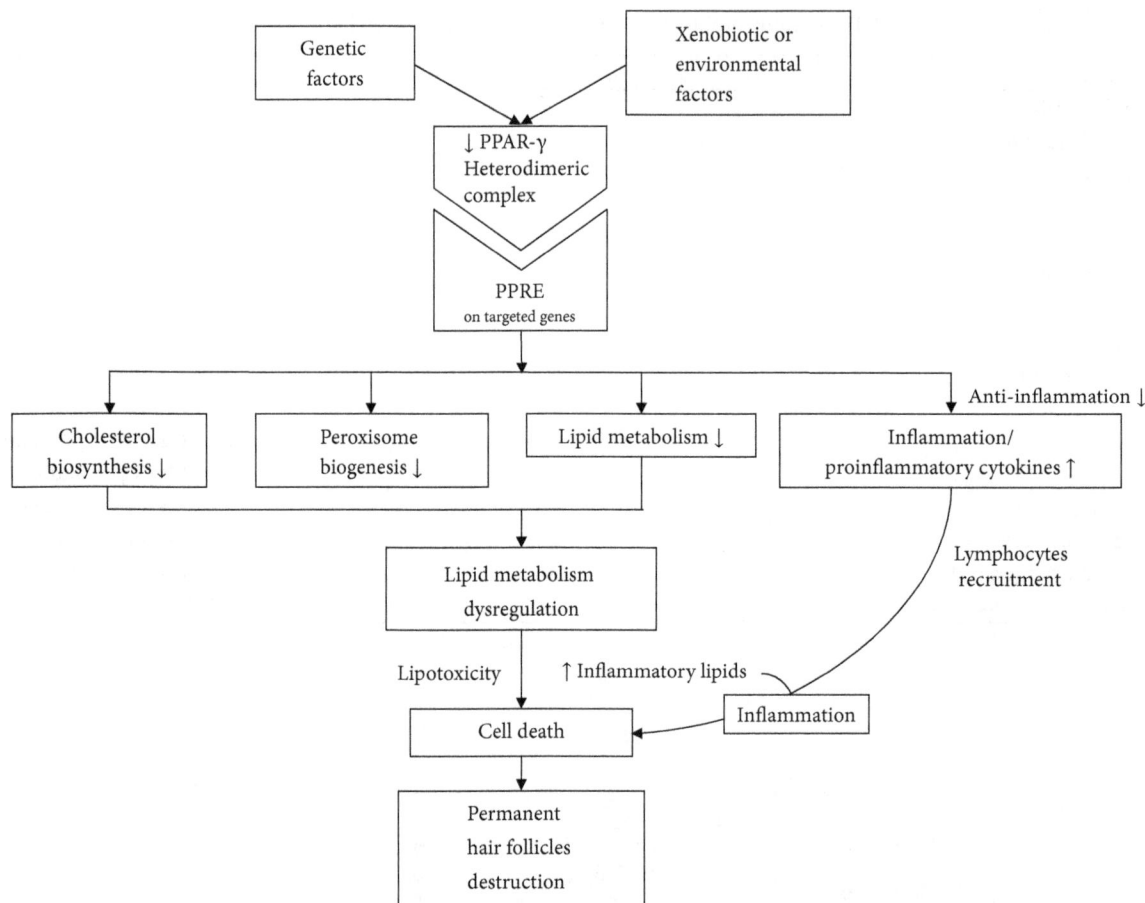

FIGURE 5: The role of PPAR-γ in the pathogenesis of primary cicatricial alopecia.

in adipogenesis with synergistic assistance from PPAR-γ1 [77].

As PPAR-γ is found discretely through multiple systems, defects are thought to be associated with the pathogenesis of various diseases. A prominent association has been found between PPAR-γ expression and multiple cardiovascular diseases, including hypertension, atherosclerosis, heart failure, diabetic cardiomyopathy, angiogenesis, and cardiac fibrosis [78, 79]. It also participates in many metabolic diseases, such as diabetes mellitus, obesity, and weight regulation through its effects on lipid homeostasis and insulin sensitivity [80]. Through its anti-inflammatory properties and immune system involvement, it is also believed to have a role in systemic sclerosis, autoimmune thyroid diseases, astrocyte-associated neurodegenerative diseases, and LPP, the type of scarring alopecia that is the focus of this article; countless other associations remain to be discovered in the future [31, 81–83].

4. The Role of PPAR-γ in PCA Pathogenesis

As mentioned above, PPAR-γ is believed to be one of the possible pathogeneses of PCA. PPAR-γ is linked to lipid homeostasis and inflammatory regulation of various systems including sebaceous glands. Sebaceous glands function in sebum production and are critical for hair follicle cycling

[84, 85]. They are formed together with hair follicles, producing pilosebaceous units which are frequently the target sites of inflammatory reactions that result in sebaceous gland dysfunction (Figure 5) [1]. Several mouse models with dysfunctional sebaceous glands present alopecia phenotypes, mimicking scarring alopecia [11, 30, 31]. However, in humans, sebaceous gland atrophies present differently in each patient with PCA, so it is controversial to call sebaceous gland failure the primary event of the disease [31]. Nevertheless, there is one important factor linking all events together and that is PPAR-γ.

In skin biology, PPAR-γ is expressed in various structures, including epidermal keratinocytes, dendritic cells, T lymphocytes, and hair follicle outer root sheaths and is almost exclusively expressed in fibroblasts, mast cells, hair follicle inner root sheaths, and active sebocytes [7]. PPAR-γ is found abundantly expressed in active or young sebocytes due to its roles in sebocyte and keratinocyte differentiation and epidermal lipid homeostasis [68, 86], while it is sparsely expressed during terminal sebaceous differentiation [7].

PPAR-γ is evidently a primary defect of LPP pathogenesis by comparison of histopathology, gene expression, gene activity, and other profiling methods of the scalp of normal subjects and nonlesional and lesional areas of LPP. First of all, clinical samples from the active edge of early diagnosed LPP, unaffected scalp, and normal hosts show that the active area comprises follicular erythema and scaling, and features easily pulled off anagen hairs, but unaffected areas show features similar to that of normal scalp. Histopathology of unaffected areas shows only mild lymphocytic infiltration with minimal atrophic sebaceous glands, compared to dense lymphocytic infiltration and follicular involvement in active phase, and fibrosis and scarring of follicles at the terminal stage [31].

Gene expression comparison among affected and unaffected areas and normal scalp shows that some genes are downregulated in hair follicle cycling, lipid homeostasis, and peroxisome biogenesis, including PEX3 and PEX16, and some genes involved in the inflammatory cascade and apoptotic pathways are upregulated. Expression of genes involved in fatty acid metabolism and desaturation and cholesterol synthesis is downregulated in both lesional and nonlesional areas, so we could hypothesize that these events take place earlier in the course of the disease. In contrast, CD40, SPG21, and reticulum aminopeptidase-1 (ARTS-1) are the only three factors found to be upregulated in nonlesional scalp areas, being part of cytochrome P450 and xenobiotic NF-kB pathways. Both pathways are believed to be an important part of early pathogenesis. Macrophage activation, T-cell lymphocyte chemotaxis, and apoptosis occur later on [31].

Peroxisomes function in various metabolic activities, including lipid metabolism. They require peroxins (PEXs) for their biogenesis, especially PEX3 and PEX16, which are both quite specific to PPAR-γ. Evidence from keratinocyte culture of all PPAR isoform agonists with PEX3 and PEX16 shows that only PPAR-γ agonists can stimulate PEX3 and PEX16 expression. This correlates with RT-PCR results of affected tissues showing significantly decreased levels of PPAR-γ while other PPAR levels remained unchanged. PEX3 expression was downregulated in both lesional and nonlesional areas of LPP scalp; in contrast PEX16 and PEX22 were downregulated only in affected areas. It might be possible to conclude that PEX3, or peroxisome biogenesis, is one of the earliest events of disease progression. Immunofluorescence staining shows that the disappearance of peroxisomes is an early event because sebaceous glands are still found stained in early lesions [31].

Using analysis of Positions and Patterns of Elements of Regulation, PPREs are involved in all downregulated genes. COX2 expression is found to be upregulated. COX2, an inflammation regulation gene, and PPAR-γ have negative feedback loop as evidenced by COX2 inhibition after application of PPAR-γ agonists to the hair follicle outer root sheath. Supporting these lines of evidence with lipid profile evaluation, levels of cholesterol ester and sapienic acid were decreased. On the contrary, levels of triglycerol and arachidonic acid were found to be increased within lesions [31].

The next point to consider is the trigger factor for PPAR-γ dysfunction. A xenobiotic pathway was found to be upregulated in the assay mentioned above. Aryl hydrocarbon receptor (AhR) is the xenobiotic or environmental trigger of PPAR-γ suppression. Supporting evidence from microarray data shows increased expression of the CYP1A1 gene, which

is associated with AhR. Thus, environmental factors could be a trigger factor of this condition [31].

The last evidence to support the role of PPAR-γ in LPP pathogenesis comes from mouse models, including both PPAR-γ knock out and Gsdma3^{Dfl}/+ mouse models [31, 87]. These presented phenotypes and molecular characteristics consistent with LPP. More recently, another study highlighted the relationship between PPAR-γ and hair follicle cycling by showing the effect of PPAR-γ modulation on proliferation of hair follicle progenitor cells, keratin-15, and keratin-19 [88].

Despite all the evidence supporting the hypothesis of a role for PPAR-γ, several points should be noted. The RNA extraction, gene-profiling, and other microarray sampling in the study mentioned above were performed on whole tissue samples, not from individual hair follicles and sebaceous glands. It could not be definitively concluded that these changes actually occur in our sites of interest, because there could be some interference and overshadowing from other tissues. Further analysis of PPAR-γ protein levels, especially in hair follicle and sebaceous glands, would be more specific and helpful to support the hypothesis that PPAR-γ disruption is the most important and earliest event of LPP pathogenesis. Other small comments must be made on xenobiotic effects and mouse models. In the study mentioned above, confounding effects were not included in significance analysis, so these could potentially affect the results [89]. The major objection to a role for PPAR-γ in LPP pathogenesis comes from a recent study comparing levels of PPAR-γ in lesional and nonlesional biopsies. This study specifically assessed PPAR-γ in bulge epithelium, the site of epithelial hair follicle stem cells. The results showed no difference in PPAR-γ expression in these areas and this raises the question of why globally decreased expression of PPAR-γ would affect only focal areas of the hair follicle and not the entire follicle [29]. Thus, we hesitate to conclude that PPAR-γ plays a major role, but it might be said that PPAR-γ dysfunction precipitates early stage hair follicle changes that lead to inflammatory recruitment or autoimmune attack at bulge stem cells.

5. PPAR-γ Implications in PCA

TZDs, PPAR-γ agonists, have been discovered to be useful in diabetes mellitus [64]. They increase insulin sensitivity leading to a reduction in blood glucose levels. They are also used as anti-inflammatory agents, inhibiting the secretion of inflammatory-related cytokines such as IL-1, IL-6, IFN-γ, CXCL 10 [90], and CXCR 3 [72, 91, 92]. In addition to diabetes mellitus, many TZDs are used to treat ulcerative colitis, rheumatoid arthritis, atherosclerosis, asthma, systemic lupus erythematosus (SLE), renal fibrosis, and psoriasis, and other inflammatory skin diseases [7, 93–98].

Linking PPAR-γ to the pathogenesis of LPP, several pieces of information focusing on TZDs, PPAR-γ agonists, as alternative treatment options for PCA have been reported. Information from the 2011 cicatricial alopecia symposium revealed that pioglitazone, a TZD, could improve LPP symptoms, both clinically and pathologically, in more than half of patients [99]. In addition, 4 clinical trials reported the

TABLE 3: Clinical trials of pioglitazone in the treatment of primary cicatricial alopecia.

Authors, year	Study type	Treatment	Outcome
Mirmirani and Karnik, 2009 [52]	Case report: (i) 1 patient with LPP	(i) Oral pioglitazone hydrochloride 15 mg/day for 14 months	(i) 2 months: clinical improvement (ii) 6 months: marked decrease of inflammation (iii) 1 year: remained symptom-free
Baibergenova and Walsh, 2012 [53]	Case series: (i) 21 patients with LPP (ii) 2 patients with FAPD (iii) 1 patient with FFA	(i) Oral pioglitazone hydrochloride 15 mg/day, increased to 30 mg/day if there is no ADR (ii) Concurrent treatments were variably used as needed	(i) 5 patients: remission (ii) 12 patients: improvement (iii) 3 patients: no improvement (iv) ADR in 4 patients leading to withdrawal: calf pain, lightheadedness, dizziness and hives
Spring et al., 2013 [54]	Case series: (i) 22 patients with LPP	(i) Oral pioglitazone hydrochloride 15 mg/day for 1 year (ii) Adjuvant treatments were variably used as needed	(i) 3 patients: remission and no relapse (ii) 5 patients: improvement with lower disease activity (iii) 4 patients: improvement but symptoms relapsed (iv) 10 patients: negative result
Mesinkovska et al., 2015 [55]	Case series: (i) 18 patients with LPP (ii) 4 patients with FFA	(i) Oral pioglitazone hydrochloride 15 mg/day for median of 10.5 months	(i) 16 patients: marked improvement (ii) 5 patients: stable of disease (iii) 1 patient: progression of disease (iv) ADR: lower extremities edema, weight gain, dizziness, resistant hypertension, mild transaminitis

LPP: lichen planopilaris, FFA: frontal fibrosing alopecia, FAPD: fibrosing alopecia in pattern distribution, and ADR: adverse drug reactions.

efficacy and safety of using pioglitazone in patients with PCA who failed to respond to ordinary treatments. All trials are summarized in Table 3.

The first case report of LPP was published in 2009. A 47-year-old man was diagnosed with LPP and received a series of treatments, including oral prednisolone, oral hydroxychloroquine, oral antibiotic, mycophenolate mofetil, intralesional corticosteroid injection, topical tacrolimus, topical high-potency corticosteroid, and antiseborrheic shampoo. He later received oral pioglitazone at 15 mg/day dose as an alternative regimen. After having treatment for 8 months, he recovered fully and remained symptom-free for 1 year after drug discontinuation [52]. In another clinical trial of 24 patients with LPP, half of the group showed improvement after using oral pioglitazone, while 5 achieved disease remission. Four patients dropped out of study due to adverse reaction and intolerability [53]. In 2013, 22 patients with resistant LPP were given oral pioglitazone at a starting dose of 15 mg/day. Only 3 patients showed a good recovery, while the others were considered to show negative effectiveness. Four patients showed clinical improvement but the symptoms relapsed after pioglitazone discontinuation. Two of these four patients were rechallenged but found to be resistant to pioglitazone [54]. In the latest study in 2015, Mesinkovska et al. retrospectively reported a case series of all-female patients with LPP. Patients receiving oral pioglitazone for at least 1 month and follow-up of up to 3 months were included to this study. The initial dose of pioglitazone started at 15 mg/day and stabilized disease progression in nearly 73% of patients, while 6 patients out of 22 showed hair regrowth. Disease relapsed in two patients (9%) after drug discontinuation. The most common side effect in this study was edema of the lower extremities

(50%) leading to 9 out of 22 patients withdrawing from the study [55].

The results of these trials show the same trend that pioglitazone at least helps to stabilize the disease. There are conflicting results between trials in terms of improvement, ranging from perceived improvement to great improvement or even resolution. However, the findings from these clinical trials suggest the use of PPAR-γ agonists as a treatment option for PCA, especially LPP. TZDs inhibit the inflammatory stages of disease by increasing activation of PPAR-γ resulting in inhibition of interleukins, proinflammatory nuclear transcription factors, and proteolytic enzymes. Further prospective, randomized, double-blind, controlled trials with large numbers of subjects will be necessary to confirm the role of PPAR-γ in PCA pathogenesis and the efficacy and safety of TZDs in PCA treatment.

6. Conclusion

PCA is a diverse group of inflammatory hair diseases involving the destruction of pilosebaceous units and replacement with fibrosis. There are several hypotheses for PCA pathogenesis, including hair follicle stem cell destruction, immune privilege collapse, autoimmune attack, and sebaceous gland dysfunction, among others. It is difficult to prove definitively which event comes first in disease progression and pathogenesis. PPAR-γ, part of the nuclear receptors superfamily, plays a remarkable role in PCA pathogenesis. PPAR-γ is involved in sebocyte differentiation, lipid homeostasis, peroxisome biogenesis, and inflammatory regulation. It is believed that PPAR-γ deficiency, triggered by unknown factors, leads to pilosebaceous dysfunction and failure of peroxisome biogenesis, decreased sebum secretion, and increases in proinflammatory lipid levels. Inflammation occurs and leads to apoptosis of stems cells and hair follicles. However, recent evidence opposing this hypothesis shows no difference in PPAR-γ expression between lesional and nonlesional scalp areas of patients with LPP. We might only conclude that PPAR-γ disruption has a predisposing role in PCA pathogenesis but is not the key factor. From clinical trials, pioglitazone, a PPAR-γ agonist, is effective in stabilizing patients' clinical symptoms. Hence, PPAR-γ agonists might be a good alternative choice of treatment in LPP, the lymphocytic PCA. Development of PPAR-agonists is important to increase specificity and improve efficacy in the near future.

Conflicts of Interest

The authors declare that there are no conflicts of interest regarding the publication of this paper.

References

[1] K. S. Stenn and J. P. Sundberg, "Hair follicle biology, the sebaceous gland, and scarring alopecias," *JAMA Dermatology*, vol. 135, no. 8, pp. 973-974, 1999.

[2] J. T. Headington, "Cicatricial alopecia," *Dermatologic Clinics*, vol. 14, no. 4, pp. 773-782, 1996.

[3] E. A. Olsen, W. F. Bergfeld, G. Cotsarelis et al., "Summary of North American Hair Research Society (NAHRS) - Sponsored workshop on cicatricial alopecia, Duke University Medical Center, February 10 and 11, 2001," *Journal of the American Academy of Dermatology*, vol. 48, no. 1, pp. 103-110, 2003.

[4] M. J. Harries, R. M. Trueb, A. Tosti et al., "How not to get scar(r)ed: Pointers to the correct diagnosis in patients with suspected primary cicatricial alopecia," *British Journal of Dermatology*, vol. 160, no. 3, pp. 482-501, 2009.

[5] S. Trachsler and R. M. Trüeb, "Value of direct immunofluorescence for differential diagnosis of cicatricial alopecia," *Dermatology*, vol. 211, no. 2, pp. 98-102, 2005.

[6] M. J. Harries, R. D. Sinclair, S. MacDonald-Hull, D. A. Whiting, C. E. M. Griffiths, and R. Paus, "Management of primary cicatricial alopecias: Options for treatment," *British Journal of Dermatology*, vol. 159, no. 1, pp. 1-22, 2008.

[7] Y. Ramot, A. Mastrofrancesco, E. Camera, P. Desreumaux, R. Paus, and M. Picardo, "The role of PPARγ-mediated signalling in skin biology and pathology: New targets and opportunities for clinical dermatology," *Experimental Dermatology*, vol. 24, no. 4, pp. 245-251, 2015.

[8] R. Paus and G. Cotsarelis, "The biology of hair follicles," *The New England Journal of Medicine*, vol. 341, no. 7, pp. 491-497, 1999.

[9] M. R. Schneider, R. Schmidt-Ullrich, and R. Paus, "The hair follicle as a dynamic miniorgan," *Current Biology*, vol. 19, no. 3, pp. R132-R142, 2009.

[10] A. Gilhar, R. Paus, and R. S. Kalish, "Lymphocytes, neuropeptides, and genes involved in alopecia areata," *The Journal of Clinical Investigation*, vol. 117, no. 8, pp. 2019-2027, 2007.

[11] M. J. Harries and R. Paus, "The pathogenesis of primary cicatricial alopecias," *The American Journal of Pathology*, vol. 177, no. 5, pp. 2152-2162, 2010.

[12] M. Ito, Y. Liu, Z. Yang et al., "Stem cells in the hair follicle bulge contribute to wound repair but not to homeostasis of the epidermis," *Nature Medicine*, vol. 11, no. 12, pp. 1351-1354, 2005.

[13] M. J. Harries, K. C. Meyer, I. H. Chaudhry, C. E. M. Griffiths, and R. Paus, "Does collapse of immune privilege in the hair-follicle bulge play a role in the pathogenesis of primary cicatricial alopecia?" *Clinical and Experimental Dermatology*, vol. 35, no. 6, pp. 637-644, 2010.

[14] K. J. McElwee, S. Kissling, E. Wenzel, A. Huth, and R. Hoffmann, "Cultured peribulbar dermal sheath cells can induce hair follicle development and contribute to the dermal sheath and dermal papilla," *Journal of Investigative Dermatology*, vol. 121, no. 6, pp. 1267-1275, 2003.

[15] R. Paus, B. J. Nickoloff, and T. Ito, "A 'hairy' privilege," *Trends in Immunology*, vol. 26, no. 1, pp. 32-40, 2005.

[16] K. C. Meyer, J. E. Klatte, H. V. Dinh et al., "Evidence that the bulge region is a site of relative immune privilege in human hair follicles," *British Journal of Dermatology*, vol. 159, no. 5, pp. 1077-1085, 2008.

[17] M. Ohyama, A. Terunuma, C. L. Tock et al., "Characterization and isolation of stem cell-enriched human hair follicle bulge cells," *The Journal of Clinical Investigation*, vol. 116, no. 1, pp. 249-260, 2006.

[18] M. D. Rosenblum, K. B. Yancey, E. B. Olasz, and R. L. Truitt, "CD200, a "no danger" signal for hair follicles," *Journal of Dermatological Science*, vol. 41, no. 3, pp. 165-174, 2006.

[19] P. Matzinger, "The danger model: a renewed sense of self," *Science*, vol. 296, no. 5566, pp. 301-305, 2002.

[20] M. D. Rosenblum, E. B. Olasz, K. B. Yancey et al., "Expression of CD200 on epithelial cells of the murine hair follicle: A role in tissue-specific immune tolerance?" *Journal of Investigative Dermatology*, vol. 123, no. 5, pp. 880-887, 2004.

[21] T. Breitkopf, B. K. K. Lo, G. Leung et al., "Somatostatin expression in human hair follicles and its potential role in immune privilege," *Journal of Investigative Dermatology*, vol. 133, no. 7, pp. 1722-1730, 2013.

[22] X. Wang, A. K. Marr, T. Breitkopf et al., "Hair follicle mesenchyme-associated PD-L1 regulates T-cell activation induced apoptosis: a potential mechanism of immune privilege," *Journal of Investigative Dermatology*, vol. 134, no. 3, pp. 736-745, 2014.

[23] R. Paus, E. A. Langan, S. Vidali, Y. Ramot, and B. Andersen, "Neuroendocrinology of the hair follicle: Principles and clinical perspectives," *Trends in Molecular Medicine*, vol. 20, no. 10, pp. 559-570, 2014.

[24] K. J. McElwee, "Etiology of cicatricial alopecias: A basic science point of view," *Dermatologic Therapy*, vol. 21, no. 4, pp. 212-220, 2008.

[25] J. E. Kloepper, S. Tiede, J. Brinckmann et al., "Immunophenotyping of the human bulge region: The quest to define useful in situ markers for human epithelial hair follicle stem cells and their niche," *Experimental Dermatology*, vol. 17, no. 7, pp. 592-609, 2008.

[26] J. Wenzel, M. Uerlich, E. Wörrenkämper, S. Freutel, T. Bieber, and T. Tüting, "Scarring skin lesions of discoid lupus erythematosus are characterized by high numbers of skin-homing cytotoxic lymphocytes associated with strong expression of the type I interferon-induced protein MxA," *British Journal of Dermatology*, vol. 153, no. 5, pp. 1011-1015, 2005.

[27] J. Wenzel and T. Tüting, "Identification of type I interferon-associated inflammation in the pathogenesis of cutaneous

lupus erythematosus opens up options for novel therapeutic approaches," *Experimental Dermatology*, vol. 16, no. 5, pp. 454–463, 2007.

[28] P. Dupuy, C. Maurette, J. C. Amoric, and O. Chosidow, "Apoptosis in different cutaneous manifestations of lupus erythematosus," *British Journal of Dermatology*, vol. 144, no. 5, pp. 958–966, 2001.

[29] M. J. Harries, K. Meyer, I. Chaudhry et al., "Lichen planopilaris is characterized by immune privilege collapse of the hair follicle's epithelial stem cell niche," *The Journal of Pathology*, vol. 231, no. 2, pp. 236–247, 2013.

[30] Y. Zheng, K. J. Eilertsen, L. Ge et al., "Scd1 is expressed in sebaceous glands and is disrupted in the asebia mouse," *Nature Genetics*, vol. 23, no. 3, pp. 268–270, 1999.

[31] P. Karnik, Z. Tekeste, T. S. McCormick et al., "Hair follicle stem cell-specific PPARγ deletion causes scarring alopecia," *Journal of Investigative Dermatology*, vol. 129, no. 5, pp. 1243–1257, 2009.

[32] N. P. Burrows, J. W. Grant, A. J. Crisp, and S. O. Roberts, "Scarring alopecia following gold therapy," *Acta Dermato-Venereologica*, vol. 74, no. 6, article 486, 1994.

[33] F. Bardazzi, C. Landi, C. Orlandi, I. Neri, and C. Varotti, "Graham little-Piccardi-Lasseur syndrome following HBV vaccination," *Acta Dermato-Venereologica*, vol. 79, no. 1, p. 93, 1999.

[34] R. M. Azurdia, R. M. Graham, K. Weismann, D. M. Guerin, and R. Parslew, "Acne keloidalis in caucasian patients on cyclosporin following organ transplantation," *British Journal of Dermatology*, vol. 143, no. 2, pp. 465–467, 2000.

[35] L. Carnero, J. F. Silvestre, J. Guijarro, M. P. Albares, and R. Botella, "Nuchal acne keloidalis associated with cyclosporin," *British Journal of Dermatology*, vol. 144, no. 2, pp. 429–430, 2001.

[36] M. H. Grunwald, M. Ben-Dor, E. Livni, and S. Halevy, "Acne Keloidalis-like Lesions on the Scalp Associated with Antiepileptic Drugs," *International Journal of Dermatology*, vol. 29, no. 8, pp. 559–561, 1990.

[37] T. Yanagi, D. Sawamura, and H. Shimizu, "Follicular mucinosis associated with imatinib (STI571)," *British Journal of Dermatology*, vol. 151, no. 6, pp. 1276–1278, 2004.

[38] V. Lopez, I. Lopez, V. Ramos, and J. M. Ricart, "Erosive pustular dermatosis of the scalp after photodynamic therapy," *Dermatology Online Journal*, vol. 18, no. 9, article 13, 2012.

[39] C. E. H. Grattan, R. D. Peachey, and A. Boon, "Evidence for a role of local trauma in the pathogenesis of erosive pustular dermatosis of the scalp," *Clinical and Experimental Dermatology*, vol. 13, no. 1, pp. 7–10, 1988.

[40] Y. Z. Chiang, A. Tosti, I. H. Chaudhry et al., "Lichen planopilaris following hair transplantation and face-lift surgery," *British Journal of Dermatology*, vol. 166, no. 3, pp. 666–670, 2012.

[41] M. R. Crisóstomo, M. G. R. Crisóstomo, M. R. Crisóstomo, M. C. C. Crisóstomo, V. J. T. Gondim, and A. N. Benevides, "Hair loss due to lichen planopilaris after hair transplantation: A report of two cases and a literature review," *Anais Brasileiros de Dermatologia*, vol. 86, no. 2, pp. 359–362, 2011.

[42] J. Donovan, "Lichen planopilaris after hair transplantation: Report of 17 cases," *Dermatologic Surgery*, vol. 38, no. 12, pp. 1998–2004, 2012.

[43] J. J. Powell, R. P. R. Dawber, and K. Gatter, "Folliculitis decalvans including tufted folliculitis: Clinical, histological and therapeutic findings," *British Journal of Dermatology*, vol. 140, no. 2, pp. 328–333, 1999.

[44] A. O. George, A. O. Akanji, E. U. Nduka, J. B. Olasode, and O. Odusan, "Clinical, biochemical and morphologic features of acne keloidalis in a black population," *International Journal of Dermatology*, vol. 32, no. 10, pp. 714–716, 1993.

[45] E. M. J. Peters, V. A. Botchkarev, N. V. Botchkareva, D. J. Tobin, and R. Paus, "Hair-cycle-associated remodeling of the peptidergic innervation of murine skin, and hair growth modulation by neuropeptides," *Journal of Investigative Dermatology*, vol. 116, no. 2, pp. 236–245, 2001.

[46] E. M. J. Peters, S. Liotiri, E. Bodó et al., "Probing the effects of stress mediators on the human hair follicle: Substance P holds central position," *The American Journal of Pathology*, vol. 171, no. 6, pp. 1872–1886, 2007.

[47] C. Dreyer, G. Krey, H. Keller, F. Givel, G. Helftenbein, and W. Wahli, "Control of the peroxisomal beta-oxidation pathway by a novel family of nuclear hormone receptors," *Cell*, vol. 68, no. 5, pp. 879–887, 1992.

[48] S. A. Kliewer, K. Umesono, D. J. Noonan, R. A. Heyman, and R. M. Evans, "Convergence of 9-cis retinoic acid and peroxisome proliferator signalling pathways through heterodimer formation of their receptors," *Nature*, vol. 358, no. 6389, pp. 771–774, 1992.

[49] W. S. Cheang, X. Y. Tian, W. T. Wong, and Y. Huang, "The peroxisome proliferator-activated receptors in cardiovascular diseases: Experimental benefits and clinical challenges," *British Journal of Pharmacology*, vol. 172, no. 23, pp. 5512–5522, 2015.

[50] J. Direnzo, M. Söderström, R. Kurokawa et al., "Peroxisome proliferator-activated receptors and retinoic acid receptors differentially control the interactions of retinoid X receptor heterodimers with ligands, coactivators, and corepressors," *Molecular and Cellular Biology*, vol. 17, no. 4, pp. 2166–2176, 1997.

[51] H. E. Xu, M. H. Lambert, V. G. Montana et al., "Molecular recognition of fatty acids by peroxisome proliferator-activated receptors," *Molecular Cell*, vol. 3, no. 3, pp. 397–403, 1999.

[52] P. Mirmirani and P. Karnik, "Lichen planopilaris treated with a peroxisome proliferator-activated receptor γ agonist," *JAMA Dermatology*, vol. 145, no. 12, pp. 1363–1366, 2009.

[53] A. Baibergenova and S. Walsh, "Use of pioglitazone in patients with lichen planopilaris," *Journal of Cutaneous Medicine and Surgery*, vol. 16, no. 2, pp. 97–100, 2012.

[54] P. Spring, Z. Spanou, and P. A. De Viragh, "Lichen planopilaris treated by the peroxisome proliferator activated receptor-γ agonist pioglitazone: Lack of lasting improvement or cure in the majority of patients," *Journal of the American Academy of Dermatology*, vol. 69, no. 5, pp. 830–832, 2013.

[55] N. A. Mesinkovska, A. Tellez, D. Dawes, M. Piliang, and W. Bergfeld, "The use of oral pioglitazone in the treatment of lichen planopilaris," *Journal of the American Academy of Dermatology*, vol. 72, no. 2, pp. 355-356, 2015.

[56] D. J. Mangelsdorf, C. Thummel, M. Beato et al., "The nuclear receptor super-family: the second decade," *Cell*, vol. 83, no. 6, pp. 835–839, 1995.

[57] O. Braissant, F. Foufelle, C. Scotto, M. Dauça, and W. Wahli, "Differential expression of peroxisome proliferator-activated receptors (PPARs): tissue distribution of PPAR-α, -β, and -γ in the adult rat," *Endocrinology*, vol. 137, no. 1, pp. 354–366, 1996.

[58] D. Bishop-Bailey, "Peroxisome proliferator-activated receptors in the cardiovascular system," *British Journal of Pharmacology*, vol. 129, no. 5, pp. 823–834, 2000.

[59] B. Grygiel-Górniak, "Peroxisome proliferator-activated receptors and their ligands: nutritional and clinical implications—a review," *Nutrition Journal*, vol. 13, article 17, 2014.

[60] S. A. Kliewer, S. S. Sundseth, S. A. Jones et al., "Fatty acids and eicosanoids regulate gene expression through direct interactions with peroxisome proliferator-activated receptors α and γ," *Proceedings of the National Acadamy of Sciences of the United States of America*, vol. 94, no. 9, pp. 4318–4323, 1997.

[61] B. M. Forman, J. Chen, and R. M. Evans, "Hypolipidemic drugs, polyunsaturated fatty acids, and eicosanoids are ligands for peroxisome proliferator-activated receptors alpha and delta," *Proceedings of the National Acadamy of Sciences of the United States of America*, vol. 94, no. 9, pp. 4312–4317, 1997.

[62] V. R. Narala, R. K. Adapala, M. V. Suresh, T. G. Brock, M. Peters-Golden, and R. C. Reddy, "Leukotriene B4 is a physiologically relevant endogenous peroxisome proliferator-activated receptor-α agonist," *The Journal of Biological Chemistry*, vol. 285, no. 29, pp. 22067–22074, 2010.

[63] M. A. Ruby, B. Goldenson, G. Orasanu, T. P. Johnston, J. Plutzky, and R. M. Krauss, "VLDL hydrolysis by LPL activates PPAR-α through generation of unbound fatty acids," *Journal of Lipid Research*, vol. 51, no. 8, pp. 2275–2281, 2010.

[64] F. Lalloyer and B. Staels, "Fibrates, glitazones, and peroxisome proliferator-activated receptors," *Arteriosclerosis, Thrombosis, and Vascular Biology*, vol. 30, no. 5, pp. 894–899, 2010.

[65] Y.-X. Wang, C.-H. Lee, S. Tiep et al., "Peroxisome-proliferator-activated receptor δ activates fat metabolism to prevent obesity," *Cell*, vol. 113, no. 2, pp. 159–170, 2003.

[66] E. D. Rosen and B. M. Spiegelman, "PPARγ: a nuclear regulator of metabolism, differentiation, and cell growth," *The Journal of Biological Chemistry*, vol. 276, no. 41, pp. 37731–37734, 2001.

[67] K. S. Gustafson, V. A. LiVolsi, E. E. Furth, T. L. Pasha, M. E. Putt, and Z. W. Baloch, "Peroxisome proliferator-activated receptor γ expression in follicular-patterned thyroid lesions: caveats for the use of immunohistochemical studies," *American Journal of Clinical Pathology*, vol. 120, no. 2, pp. 175–181, 2003.

[68] R. L. Rosenfield, A. Kentsis, D. Deplewski, and N. Ciletti, "Rat preputial sebocyte differentiation involves peroxisome proliferator- activated receptors," *Journal of Investigative Dermatology*, vol. 112, no. 2, pp. 226–232, 1999.

[69] S. Kuenzli and J.-H. Saurat, "Peroxisome proliferator-activated receptors in cutaneous biology," *British Journal of Dermatology*, vol. 149, no. 2, pp. 229–236, 2003.

[70] A. Cabrero, J. C. Laguna, and M. Vázquez, "Peroxisome proliferator-activated receptors and the control of inflammation.," *Curr Drug Targets Inflamm Allergy*, vol. 1, no. 3, pp. 243–248, 2002.

[71] T. Varga, Z. Czimmerer, and L. Nagy, "PPARs are a unique set of fatty acid regulated transcription factors controlling both lipid metabolism and inflammation," *Biochimica et Biophysica Acta*, vol. 1812, no. 8, pp. 1007–1022, 2011.

[72] C. Jiang, A. T. Ting, and B. Seed, "PPAR-γ agonists inhibit production of monocyte inflammatory cytokines," *Nature*, vol. 391, no. 6662, pp. 82–86, 1998.

[73] Y. Chen, A. R. Jimenez, and J. D. Medh, "Identification and regulation of novel PPAR-γ splice variants in human THP-1 macrophages," *Biochimica et Biophysica Acta (BBA)—Gene Structure and Expression*, vol. 1759, no. 1-2, pp. 32–43, 2006.

[74] S. Azhar, "Peroxisome proliferator-activated receptors, metabolic syndrome and cardiovascular disease," *Future Cardiology*, vol. 6, no. 5, pp. 657–691, 2010.

[75] C. Christodoulides and A. Vidal-Puig, "PPARs and adipocyte function," *Molecular and Cellular Endocrinology*, vol. 318, no. 1-2, pp. 61–68, 2010.

[76] G. Medina-Gomez, S. L. Gray, L. Yetukuri et al., "PPAR gamma 2 prevents lipotoxicity by controlling adipose tissue expandability and peripheral lipid metabolism," *PLoS Genetics*, vol. 3, no. 4, p. e64, 2007.

[77] Y. Takenaka, I. Inoue, T. Nakano et al., "A Novel Splicing Variant of Peroxisome Proliferator-Activated Receptor-γ (Pparγ1sv) Cooperatively Regulates Adipocyte Differentiation with Pparγ2," *PLoS ONE*, vol. 8, no. 6, Article ID e65583, 2013.

[78] W. S. Lee and J. Kim, "Peroxisome proliferator-activated receptors and the heart: lessons from the past and future directions," *PPAR Research*, vol. 2015, Article ID 271983, 18 pages, 2015.

[79] H.-J. Liu, H.-H. Liao, Z. Yang, and Q.-Z. Tang, "Peroxisome proliferator-activated receptor-γ is critical to cardiac fibrosis," *PPAR Research*, vol. 2016, Article ID 2198645, 2016.

[80] A. J. Vidal-Puig, R. V. Considine, M. Jimenez-Liñan et al., "Peroxisome proliferator-activated receptor gene expression in human tissues: effects of obesity, weight loss, and regulation by insulin and glucocorticoids," *The Journal of Clinical Investigation*, vol. 99, no. 10, pp. 2416–2422, 1997.

[81] J. Iglesias, L. Morales, and G. E. Barreto, "Metabolic and Inflammatory Adaptation of Reactive Astrocytes: Role of PPARs," *Molecular Neurobiology*, vol. 54, no. 4, pp. 2518–2538, 2017.

[82] A. T. Dantas, M. C. Pereira, M. J. B. de Melo Rego et al., "The role of PPAR gamma in systemic sclerosis," *PPAR Research*, vol. 2015, Article ID 124624, 12 pages, 2015.

[83] S. M. Ferrari, P. Fallahi, R. Vita, A. Antonelli, and S. Benvenga, "Peroxisome proliferator-activated receptor-γ in thyroid autoimmunity," *PPAR Research*, vol. 2015, Article ID 232818, 8 pages, 2015.

[84] M. M. T. Downie and T. Kealey, "Lipogenesis in the human sebaceous gland: Glycogen and glycerophosphate are substrates for the synthesis of sebum lipids," *Journal of Investigative Dermatology*, vol. 111, no. 2, pp. 199–205, 1998.

[85] K. S. Stenn and R. Paus, "Controls of hair follicle cycling," *Physiological Reviews*, vol. 81, no. 1, pp. 449–494, 2001.

[86] M. Schmuth, Y. J. Jiang, S. Dubrac, P. M. Elias, and K. R. Feingold, "Peroxisome proliferator-activated receptors and liver X receptors in epidermal biology," *Journal of Lipid Research*, vol. 49, no. 3, pp. 499–509, 2008.

[87] F. Ruge, A. Glavini, A. M. Gallimore et al., "Delineating immune-mediated mechanisms underlying hair follicle destruction in the mouse mutant defolliculated," *Journal of Investigative Dermatology*, vol. 131, no. 3, pp. 572–579, 2011.

[88] Y. Ramot, A. Mastrofrancesco, E. Herczeg-Lisztes et al., "Advanced inhibition of undesired human hair growth by pparγ modulation?" *Journal of Investigative Dermatology*, vol. 134, no. 4, pp. 1128–1131, 2014.

[89] M. J. Harries and R. Paus, "Scarring alopecia and the PPAR-γ connection," *Journal of Investigative Dermatology*, vol. 129, no. 5, pp. 1066–1070, 2009.

[90] K. L. Schaefer, S. Denevich, C. Ma et al., "Intestinal antiinflammatory effects of thiazolidenedione peroxisome proliferator-activated receptor-γ ligands on T helper type 1 chemokine regulation include nontranscriptional control mechanisms," *Inflammatory Bowel Diseases*, vol. 11, no. 3, pp. 244–252, 2005.

[91] N. Marx, F. Mach, A. Sauty et al., "Peroxisome proliferator-activated receptor-γ activators inhibit IFN-γ- induced expression of the T cell-active CXC chemokines IP-10, Mig, and I-TAC in human endothelial cells," *The Journal of Immunology*, vol. 164, no. 12, pp. 6503–6508, 2000.

[92] Y. Liu, J. Shi, J. Lu et al., "Activation of peroxisome proliferator-activated receptor-γ potentiates pro-inflammatory cytokine production, and adrenal and somatotropic changes of weaned pigs after *Escherichia coli* lipopolysaccharide challenge," *Journal of Innate Immunity*, vol. 15, no. 3, pp. 169–178, 2009.

[93] E. D. A. Lima, M. M. D. de Andrade Lima, C. D. L. Marques, A. L. B. Pinto Duarte, I. D. R. Pita, and M. G. D. R. Pita, "Peroxisome proliferator-activated receptor agonists (PPARs): A promising prospect in the treatment of psoriasis and psoriatic arthritis," *Anais Brasileiros de Dermatologia*, vol. 88, no. 6, pp. 1029–1035, 2013.

[94] H. A. Pershadsingh, "Peroxisome proliferator-activated receptor-γ: Therapeutic target for diseases beyond diabetes: Quo vadis?" *Expert Opinion on Investigational Drugs*, vol. 13, no. 3, pp. 215–228, 2004.

[95] X. Dou, J. Xiao, Z. Jin, and P. Zheng, "Peroxisome proliferator-activated receptor-γ is downregulated in ulcerative colitis and is involved in experimental colitis-associated neoplasia," *Oncology Letters*, vol. 10, no. 3, pp. 1259–1266, 2015.

[96] W. Zhao, C. C. Berthier, E. E. Lewis, W. J. McCune, M. Kretzler, and M. J. Kaplan, "The peroxisome-proliferator activated receptor-γ agonist pioglitazone modulates aberrant T cell responses in systemic lupus erythematosus," *Clinical Immunology*, vol. 149, no. 1, pp. 119–132, 2013.

[97] T. Kawai, T. Masaki, S. Doi et al., "PPAR-γ agonist attenuates renal interstitial fibrosis and inflammation through reduction of TGF-β," *Laboratory Investigation*, vol. 89, no. 1, pp. 47–58, 2009.

[98] L. F. Da Rocha Junior, M. J. B. De Melo Rêgo, M. B. Cavalcanti et al., "Synthesis of a novel thiazolidinedione and evaluation of its modulatory effect on IFN-γ, IL-6, IL-17A, and IL-22 production in PBMCs from rheumatoid arthritis patients," *BioMed Research International*, vol. 2013, Article ID 926060, 2013.

[99] P. Karnik and K. Stenn, "Cicatricial alopecia symposium 2011: Lipids, inflammation and stem cells," *Journal of Investigative Dermatology*, vol. 132, no. 6, pp. 1529–1531, 2012.

15

PPARγ Antagonizes Hypoxia-Induced Activation of Hepatic Stellate Cell through Cross Mediating PI3K/AKT and cGMP/PKG Signaling

Qinghui Zhang[iD],[1] Shihao Xiang,[2] Qingqian Liu,[1] Tao Gu,[1] Yongliang Yao,[1] and Xiaojie Lu[iD][3]

[1]Department of Clinical Laboratory, Kunshan First People's Hospital, Affiliated to Jiangsu University, Kunshan, Jiangsu Province 215300, China
[2]Department of Gastroenterology, Shanghai Tongren Hospital, Shanghai Jiaotong University School of Medicine, Shanghai 200336, China
[3]Department of Liver Surgery, The First Affiliated Hospital of Nanjing Medical University, Nanjing, China

Correspondence should be addressed to Qinghui Zhang; zhangqinghui1983@126.com and Xiaojie Lu; 189@whu.edu.cn

Academic Editor: Antonio Brunetti

Background and Aims. Accumulating evidence reveals that PPARγ plays a unique role in the regulation of hepatic fibrosis and hepatic stellate cells (HSCs) activation. This study was aimed at investigating the role of PPARγ in hypoxia-induced hepatic fibrogenesis and its possible mechanism. *Methods*. Rats used for CCl4-induced hepatic fibrosis model were exposed to hypoxia for 8 hours each day. Rats exposed to hypoxia were treated with or without the PPARγ agonist rosiglitazone. Liver sections were stained with HE and Sirius red staining 8 weeks later. HSCs were exposed to hypoxic environment in the presence or absence of rosiglitazone, and expression of PPARγ and two fibrosis markers, α-SMA and desmin, were measured using western blot and immunofluorescence staining. Next, levels of PPARγ, α-SMA, and desmin as well as PKG and cGMP activity were detected using PI3K/AKT and a cGMP activator or inhibitor. *Results*. Hypoxia promoted the induction and progress of hepatic fibrosis and HSCs activation. Meanwhile, rosiglitazone significantly antagonized the effects induced by hypoxia. Signaling by sGC/cGMP/PKG promoted the inhibitory effect of PPARγ on hypoxia-induced activation of HSCs. Moreover, PI3K/AKT signaling or PDE5 blocked the above response of PPARγ. *Conclusion*. sGC/cGMP/PKG and PI3K/AKT signals act on PPARγ synergistically to attenuate hypoxia-induced HSC activation.

1. Introduction

Fibrosis is a common response to hepatic damage, which is characterized by producing and depositing extracellular matrix (ECM) [1]. Excessive fibrosis characterizes a series of liver diseases, such as chronic hepatitis, alcoholism-induced liver damage, and hepatic autoimmune disorders [2]. During this pathological process, hepatic stellate cells (HSCs) are the main executor of fibrogenesis. HSC activation increases the expression and secretion of collagen and other ECM components. It also stimulates hepatic microenvironment cells, such as macrophages, endothelial cells, and inflammatory cells, resulting in the promotion of fibrogenesis in an autocrine

or paracrine manner [3, 4]. Therefore, understanding the molecular mechanism based on HSC activation is essential for diagnosis and treatment of hepatic fibrosis.

Peroxisome proliferator-activated receptor (PPAR)γ is a fundamental nuclear receptor that regulates lipid metabolism, insulin sensitivity, and fat deposition. It plays an extremely important role in liver physiological metabolism [5]. However, increasing researches have implicated that PPARγ is a key mediator in HSC activation and phenotypic alteration, thus maintaining HSCs in a quiescent phase [6, 7]. Recently, oxidative stress is considered to be involved in HSC activation and hepatic fibrogenesis [8]. A large amount of publications has also reported that HSCs exposed to hypoxia could be activated through HIF1α and its downstream target genes or signaling pathways [9–11]. Based on those evidences, we hypothesized that the effect of PPARγ on HSCs is the mechanisms underlying the role of hypoxia in liver fibrogenesis. In fact, PPARγ has been found to be regulated by hypoxia in several diseases. Wang et al. reported that hypoxia decreased UCP2 via HIF-1-mediated suppression of PPARγ, leading to chemoresistance of non-small cell lung cancer [12]. Jiang et al. found that hypoxia inhibited PKG-PPARγ axis in rat distal pulmonary arterial smooth muscle cells (PASMCs) and distal pulmonary arteries [13]. However, it is not clear whether these cellular events are associated with the pathogenesis of hepatic fibrosis and its key functionary mechanisms. We therefore performed *in vivo* and *in vitro* experiments to test the above hypothesis.

2. Materials and Methods

2.1. Animals and Experimental Protocol. This study was performed on 35 male SD rats with weight of 200–250 g from Shanghai SLAC Laboratory Animal Co. Ltd. (Shanghai, China), housed in regular cages, situated in an animal room at 22 ± 2°C and maintained on a 14-hour light/10-hour dark cycle. The rats were randomly divided into 4 groups as follows: Group I ($n = 5$), serving as controls, were maintained in a standard normoxic chamber (FiO$_2$ 0.21). Group II ($n = 10$) rats were injected with 40% CCl4 (the mixture of CCl4 and olive oil) in a standard normoxic chamber (FiO$_2$ 0.21). Group III ($n = 10$) rats were injected with 40% of CCl4 mixture in normobaric hypoxic chamber (FiO$_2$ 0.07) with hypoxia exposures 8 hours each day. Group IV ($n = 10$) were modeled in the same manner as Group III (40% CCl4 mixture injection plus hypoxia exposures) but treated with PPARγ agonist rosiglitazone (RSG). RSG was added to the liquid diet at a daily intake of 10 mg/kg body wt for feeding.

All rats were sacrificed after 8 weeks, and blood was collected from the abdominal aorta. Serum was separated and stored at −80°C for measurement of hyaluronic acid (HA), laminin (LN), N-terminal peptide of type III procollagen (PIIINP), and collagen type IV (CIV). Then, liver was immediately removed. One part of the liver was used for the extraction of protein for western blotting. The other part of liver was fixed in 4% paraformaldehyde, embedded in paraffin, and cut into sections (5 μm thick) for HE and Sirius red staining. Animal care and procedures were approved by Medical Ethics Committee of Jiangsu University, China.

2.2. Reagents. 8-Br-cGMP, Rp-8-Br-PET-cGMPS, LY294002, rosiglitazone, and zaprinast were purchased from Sigma-Aldrich. 740 Y-P was supplied by R&D systems. LY294002, rosiglitazone, and zaprinast were dissolved in dimethyl sulfoxide (final concentration 0.2%). The other drugs were prepared using distilled water.

2.3. Serum Parameters Examination. Serum levels of HA, LN, PIIINP, and CIV were detected by using ELISA Kits (Elabscience, Wuhan, China) according to the manufacturer's instruction.

2.4. HE and Sirius Red Staining. Tissue slices were fixed in 4% paraformaldehyde, embedded with paraffin, and sectioned using standard techniques. Sections were subjected to HE and Sirius red staining. Each sample was assessed independently and scored by two pathologists for a blind evaluation, according to the modified Scheuer fibrosis score system [14, 15]. The fibrosis stage score was categorized into five stages (0–4): 0: none, 1: zone 3 perisinusoidal fibrosis; 2: zone 3 perisinusoidal fibrosis plus portal fibrosis; 3: perisinusoidal fibrosis and portal fibrosis, plus bridging fibrosis; and 4: cirrhosis.

2.5. Cell Culture. Rat HSC-T6 cell line was a gift from Dr. Ke AiWu (Liver Cancer Institute, Zhongshan Hospital, Fudan University, China). Cells were maintained in Dulbecco's modified Eagle's medium (Hyclone, USA) containing 10% fetal bovine serum (Hyclone, USA), penicillin (100 IU/ml), and streptomycin (100 IU/ml) (Amresco, USA). Cells were cultured at 37°C in a humidified atmosphere of 5% CO2.

2.6. Measurement of Total Cellular cGMP. The supernatant of HSC-T6 cells were collected and stored at −80°C. Total levels of cGMP were measured using a competitive ELISA assay (Cayman Chemical, USA) according to the manufacturer's recommendations.

2.7. Measurement of PKG Activity. The activity of PKG including PKG-I and PKG-II in each sample was measured according to the protocol of the ELISA kit (CycLex, Japan), in which the phosphorylated antibody can identify the phosphorylation of threonine (Thr 68/119) residues on substrate of PKG.

2.8. Immunofluorescence Staining. Immunofluorescence staining assays were performed as we described previously [15]. Cells were incubated overnight with the primary antibody against α-SMA (ab5694) and desmin (ab15200) (1 : 50 dilution; Abcam, USA) at 4°C. The cells were washed three times with PBS (5 min each) and then incubated in the dark for 1 h at room temperature with Alexa Fluor 488 and 550 conjugated goat anti-rat secondary antibody (1 : 200 dilution; ab150157 and ab150083, Abcam, USA). Nuclei of cells were stained with 4′,6-diamidino-2-phenylindole (DAPI) (Sigma-Aldrich, USA). Images were obtained using a Zeiss LSM 510 META Confocal microscope using 20x/0.5 w and 40x/1.2 w objectives.

2.9. Western Blot Analysis. Western blot analysis was performed as described in a previous report from ours [16]. Primary antibodies used in this study are as follows: PPARγ (ab209350) (1 : 1,500), α-SMA (ab5694), desmin (ab15200), AKT (ab8805), Phospho-AKT (ab81283), PI3K p110β (ab151549), PDE5 (ab14672) (1 : 1,000; ABcam, USA), and PI3K p110α (#4249) (1 : 1,200; Cell Signaling Technology, USA). The primary antibody of GAPDH was diluted at 1 : 1,000–1,500 (Santa Cruz, USA). The secondary HRP-conjugated antibodies were diluted at 1 : 2,500. The blots were detected using the ECL system (Beyotime Biotechnology, China). A LI-COR Odyssey scanner (LICOR) was used to analyze the intensity of bands on the blots.

TABLE 1: Grades of fibrosis in rat liver.

Groups	n	Grades				
		0	1	2	3	4
Control	5	5 (100%)	0 (0%)	0 (0%)	0 (0%)	0 (0%)
CCl4 + FiO2 (0.21)	10	0 (0%)	2 (20%)	5 (50%)	2 (20%)	1 (10%)[a]
CCl4 + FiO2 (0.07)	10	0 (0%)	0 (0%)	4 (40%)	4 (40%)	2 (20%)[a,b]
CCl4 + FiO2 (0.07) + RSG (10 mg/kg)	10	0 (0%)	7 (70%)	3 (30%)	0 (0%)	0 (0%)[a,b,c]

[a]$P < 0.01$ as compared with control group. [b]$P < 0.05$ as compared with CCl4 + FiO2 (0.21) group. [c]$P < 0.05$ as compared with CCl4 + FiO2 (0.07) group.

TABLE 2: Serum levels of HA, LN, PIIINP, and C IV (mean ± SD).

Groups	HA (μg/L)	LN (μg/L)	PIIINP (μg/L)	C IV (μg/L)
Control	85.45 ± 13.77	40.46 ± 9.74	21.02 ± 3.81	24.63 ± 6.72
CCl4 + FiO2 (0.21)	190.83 ± 20.23[a]	120.29 ± 22.59[a]	87.73 ± 15.82[a]	81.286 ± 15.28[a]
CCl4 + FiO2 (0.07)	256.29 ± 29.05[a,b]	188.08 ± 28.06[a,b]	142.16 ± 23.34[a,b]	119.36 ± 15.40[a,b]
CCl4 + FiO2 (0.07) + RSG (10 mg/kg)	182.73 ± 26.25[a,d]	103.63 ± 20.82[a,c,d]	72.39 ± 17.48[a,c,d]	62.27 ± 11.12[a,b,d]

[a]$P < 0.01$ as compared with control group. [b]$P < 0.01$ and [c]$P < 0.01$ as compared with CCl4 + FiO2 (0.21) group. [d]$P < 0.01$ as compared with CCl4 + FiO2 (0.07) group.

2.10. Statistical Analysis. All statistical analyses were performed using SPSS 17.0 software. Data are expressed as mean ± SE, and mean values were compared using the Student's t-test and ANOVA. Data were as mean ± SE. Western blot, ELISA, PKG activity, and cGMP analysis were examined using one-way ANOVA. The χ^2 and Fisher's exact test were used to analyze the differences of fibrosis grades in each group. Values of $P < 0.05$ were considered statistically significant.

3. Results

3.1. Low Expression of PPARγ Is Associated with Hypoxia-Induced Hepatic Fibrosis. Consistent with previous studies, we found that hypoxia can promote the progress of hepatic fibrosis (Tables 1 and 2 and Figure 1). Meanwhile, the PPARγ agonist rosiglitazone (RSG) significantly antagonized hypoxia-induced development of hepatic fibrosis. Hypoxia resulted in a trend towards increasing serum markers (HA, LN, PIIINP, and C IV), but also elevated fibrosis histological grade. However, the activation of PPARγ ameliorated this effect (Tables 1 and 2 and Figure 1). To examine the possible correlation of PPARγ with hepatic fibrosis, the correlation between the expression levels of PPARγ and other two markers of fibrosis, α-SMA and desmin, was measured. As shown in Figures 1(b)-1(c), PPARγ was negatively correlated with α-SMA and desmin expression ($r = -0.78613$, $P < 0.001$, and $r = -0.83517$, $P = 0.017$, resp.). These results suggest that PPARγ is associated with hypoxia-induced hepatic fibrosis.

3.2. PPARγ Antagonizes HSCs Activation Caused by Hypoxic Stress. It is well known that HSCs are important effectors inducing hepatic fibrosis. Previously, we demonstrated that hypoxia promoted hepatic fibrogenesis through the regulation of PPARγ *in vitro*. To clarify if HSC is a modulator of this process, HSC was exposed to hypoxic stress with oxygen concentration decreased from 21% to 7% at different time. In comparison to control groups, PPARγ protein level was significantly decreased in a time-dependent manner,

accompanied by an obvious increased expression in two markers of fibrosis, α-SMA and desmin (Figure 2(a)). At the same time, based on our observation, the trend reached plateau after 6 hours of hypoxia exposure. These results demonstrated that the early phase of hypoxic stress might cause HSCs activation.

Then, the expression of α-SMA and desmin were analyzed in HSCs exposed to hypoxia in the presence or absence of the PPARγ agonist, rosiglitazone (RSG, 50 nM), by western blotting and immunofluorescence. As expected, hypoxia exposure to HSCs alone led to significant PPARγ downregulation and α-SMA and desmin rise, whereas cotreatment with hypoxia and RSG reversed these effects (Figure 2(b)), indicating that PPARγ antagonizes HSCs activation caused by hypoxic stress.

3.3. PI3K/AKT Signals Involved in Hypoxia-Induced PPARγ Low Expression. The PI3K/AKT signaling pathway is an essential mechanism by which cells regulate oxidative stress effect and induces HSC activation and proliferation dependent on HIF-1α in response to hypoxia. Here, we analyzed whether PI3K/AKT signaling is associated with PPARγ inhibition of hypoxia-induced HSCs activation. Results showed that hypoxia-induced HSCs activation when AKT phosphorylation was significantly enhanced (Figure 3(c)). Inhibition of PI3K with LY294002 (20 μM) distinctly opposed the above-mentioned activation. Simultaneously, PPARγ expression was also recovered (Figures 3(c) and 3(d)). Similarly, activation of PI3K with 740 Y-P (25 μg/ml) of HSCs exposed to hypoxia in the presence of RSG (50 nM) significantly reduced PPARγ expression, along with increased level of α-SMA and desmin (Figures 3(a) and 3(b)). These results imply that PI3K/AKT signaling blocked the inhibitory effect of PPARγ on hypoxia-induced activation of HSCs.

3.4. The Cross Talk of sGC/cGMP/PKG and PI3K/AKT Signaling Adjusts PPARγ Attenuating Hypoxia-Induced HSC Activation. According to previous studies, sGC/cGMP/PKG

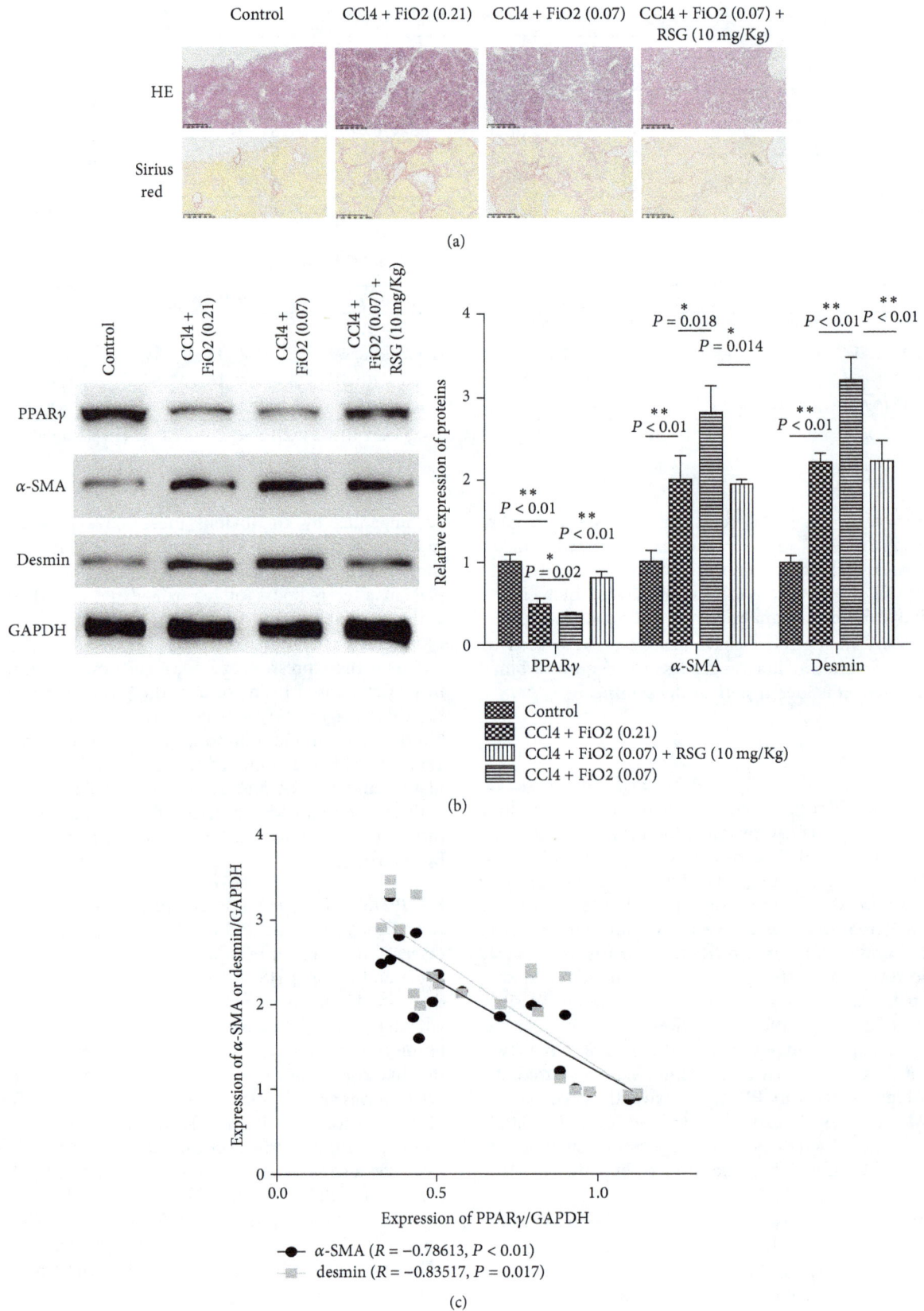

(a)

(b)

(c)

FIGURE 1: Effects of PPARγ on hypoxia-induced hepatic fibrosis. (a) HE and Sirius red staining for liver tissues (magnification, ×200). (b) PPARγ, α-SMA, and desmin expression of liver tissues in experimental groups were detected by western blotting analysis. (c) The correlation between the expression levels of PPARγ and α-SMA or desmin. Bars stand for mean ± SD (same for all figures). For each assay, $n = 3$. *$P < 0.05$, **$P < 0.01$.

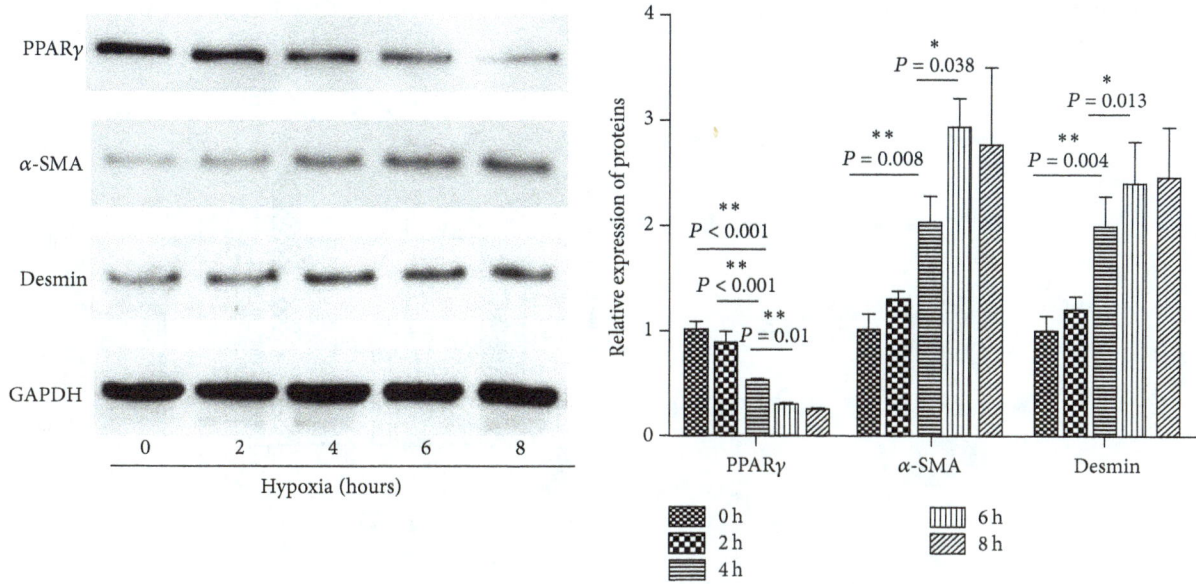

(a)

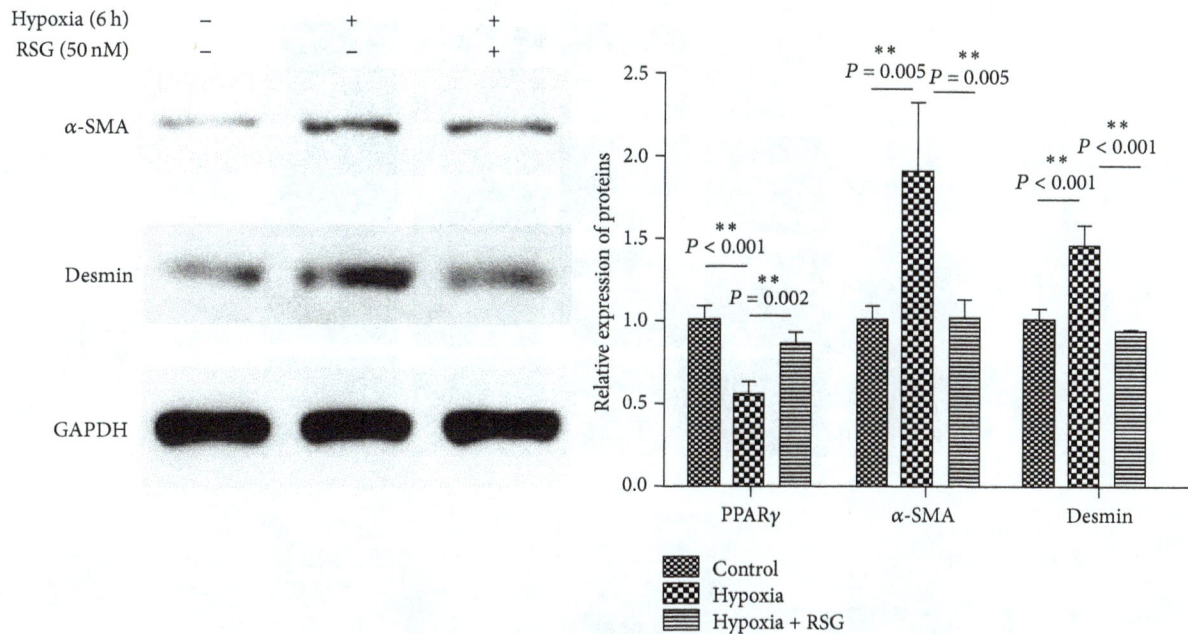

(b)

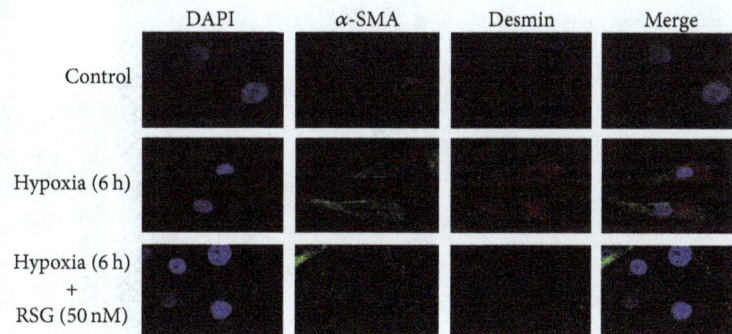

(c)

FIGURE 2: PPARγ inhibits hypoxic-induced HSCs activation. (a) HSCs were exposed to hypoxia for the designated time. Protein expressions of PPARγ, α-SMA, and desmin were tested by western blotting. HSCs were exposed to hypoxia for 6 hours in the presence or absence of PPARγ agonist, rosiglitazone (RSG, 50 nM). (b) PPARγ, α-SMA, and desmin expression of HSCs in experimental groups were analyzed by western blotting. (c) α-SMA and desmin expression in HSCs in experimental groups were detected by immunofluorescence using Confocal microscopy. For each assay, $n = 3$. $^*P < 0.05$, $^{**}P < 0.01$.

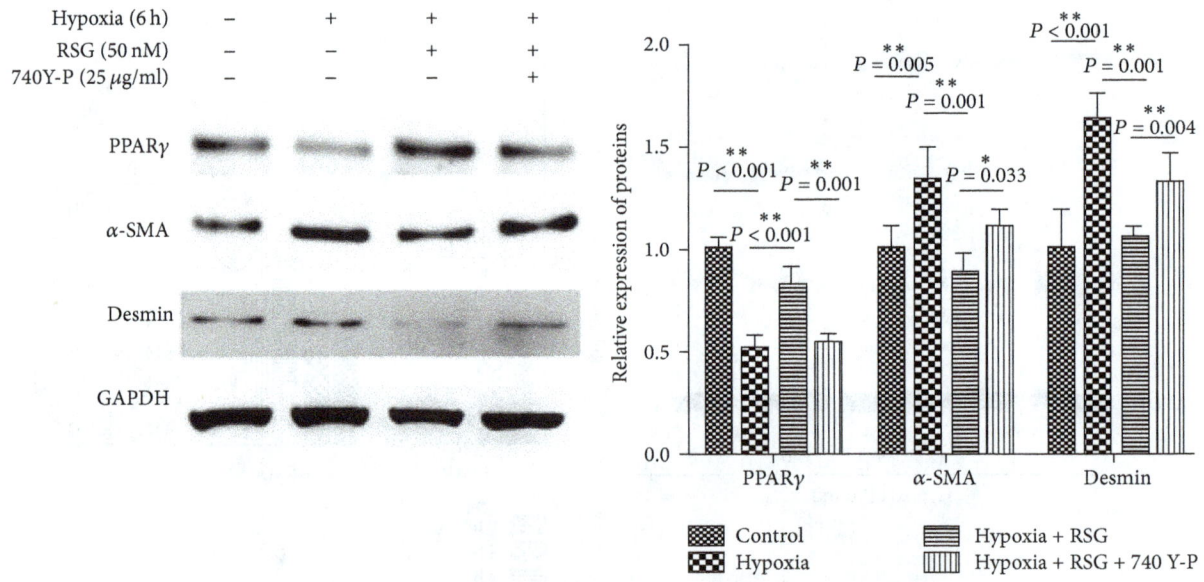

(a)

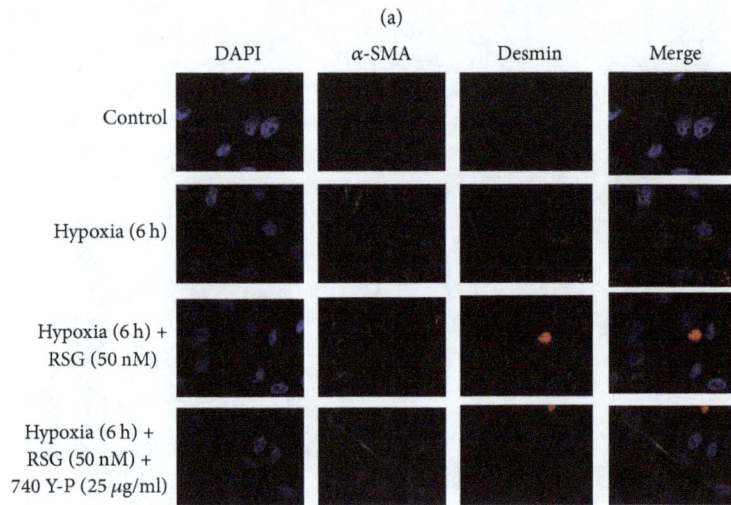

(b)

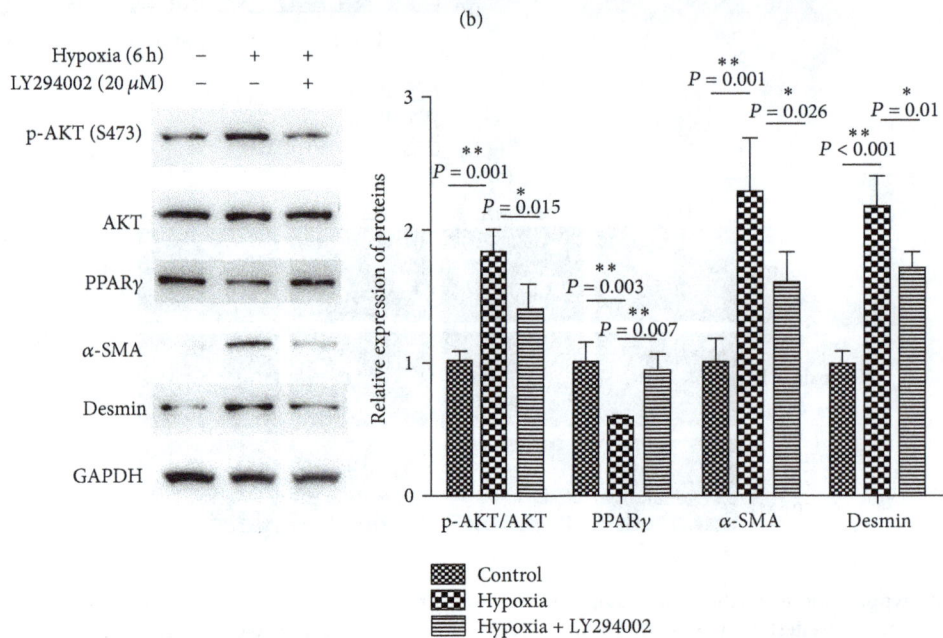

(c)

FIGURE 3: Continued.

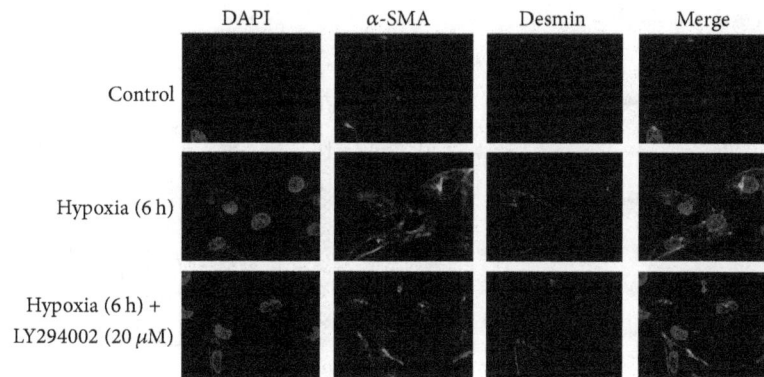

(d)

FIGURE 3: PI3K/AKT signaling blocks the inhibitory effect of PPARγ on hypoxic-induced HSCs activation. Activation of PI3K with 740 Y-P (25 μg/ml) of HSCs exposed to hypoxia in the presence or absence of RSG (50 nM). (a) PPARγ, α-SMA, and desmin expression of HSCs in experimental groups were analyzed by western blotting. (b) α-SMA and desmin expression of HSCs in experimental groups were detected by immunofluorescence using Confocal microscopy. Inhibition of PI3K with LY294002 (20 μM) in HSCs exposed to hypoxia. (c) Phosphorylated AKT, total AKT, PPARγ, α-SMA, and desmin expression of HSCs in experimental groups were measured by western blotting. (d) α-SMA and desmin expression of HSCs in experimental groups were detected by immunofluorescence using Confocal microscopy. For each assay, $n = 3$. $^{*}P < 0.05$, $^{**}P < 0.01$.

contributes to the treatment of cirrhosis. In addition, this signal also modulates various cellular events induced by hypoxic stress. To investigate the potential role of sGC/cGMP/PKG signaling in HSC hypoxia responses modulated by PPAR and PI3K/AKT signaling, HSCs were incubated for 90 min under hypoxia with or without 8-Br-cGMP (1 mM) which was widely used as sGC/cGMP/PKG agonist and in the presence or absence of Rp-8-Br-cGMP (20 μM), a sGC/cGMP/PKG antagonist. We found that cotreated 8-Br-cGMP with hypoxia showed a significant decrease in protein levels of PI3K p110α, PI3K p110β, and phosphorylated AKT in comparison with the hypoxia group. In consequence of this decline, PPARγ expression increased. Moreover, just as we speculated, α-SMA and desmin level also reduced. The effect induced by 8-Br-cGMP was blocked by the inclusion of Rp-8-Br-cGMP (Figure 4(a)). These results indicated that sGC/cGMP/PKG directly inhibited PI3K/AKT signaling and on the other hand increased PPARγ, eventually affecting the hypoxia-induced HSCs activation.

To further confirm the above findings, we used zaprinast, a specific inhibitor of phosphodiesterase type 5 (PDE5), to inhibit cGMP hydrolysis and to observe the subsequent effects on PPARγ and PI3K/AKT signaling on hypoxia-induced HSC activation. Results showed that the hypoxic environment significantly improved the cGMP and PKG activity in HSCs (Figures 4(c)-4(d)). PDE5 inhibition restored cGMP and PKG activity (Figures 4(c)-4(d)), followed by increased PPARγ expression and repressed HSCs activation (decreased expression of α-SMA and desmin) (Figure 4(b)). These data suggested that sGC/cGMP/PKG and PI3K/AKT signals synergistically act on PPARγ, and the latter inhibited hypoxia-induced HSC activation.

4. Discussion

PPARγ, as a transcription factor, controls gene transcription and cell differentiation both in vitro and in vivo and plays a

key role in inhibiting HSC activation and maintaining the morphological and biochemical reversal of activated HSC to quiescent cells [17–19]. Current evidences have shown that hypoxia is a common stimulus to the development of hepatic fibrosis and HSCs activation [20, 21]. In fact, hypoxia is capable of connecting a variety of signals. It not only affects the activation of HSCs but also acts on a variety of other cells, such as sinusoidal cells, hepatocytes, adipocytes, and liver-resident macrophages (Kuppfer cells) [1, 22–24]. Secondly, hypoxia-induced structural changes in hepatic fibrosis aggravate the hypoxic environment, thus, in turn, accelerating its pathologic progression of hepatic fibrosis.

However, little is known regarding the effect of PPARγ on HSC activation and hepatic fibrosis under hypoxia stress. To elucidate the interrelationship and molecular mechanism between HSCs activation and PPARγ in hypoxic environment, we designed experiments both in vitro and in vivo. For this purpose, by exposing CCl4 modeling rats to hypoxic environment, we validated the hypothesis that hypoxic stress promoted hepatic fibrosis. Notably, expression of PPARγ was inhibited by hypoxia. Moreover, expression of two markers of fibrosis, α-SMA and desmin, significantly increased. To further explore the effects of PPARγ in hypoxia, RSG, a PPARγ agonist, was added to hypoxia exposed groups. As expected, hepatic fibrosis induced by hypoxia was ameliorated with increasing PPARγ level. These results were also confirmed by HSC experiments in vivo. Our findings confirmed that PPARγ antagonizes hepatic fibrosis caused by hypoxia stress through inhibiting HSCs activation.

However, the underlying mechanism that PPARγ mediated hypoxia-induced HSC activation must be further explored. Recent studies displayed that AKT signaling and PPARγ have a mutual inhibitory effect [25–27], but this theory is still controversial. Kilter et al. suggested that PPARγ facilitates AKT phosphorylation in cardiomyocytes during hypoxia/reoxygenation [28]. However, another independent

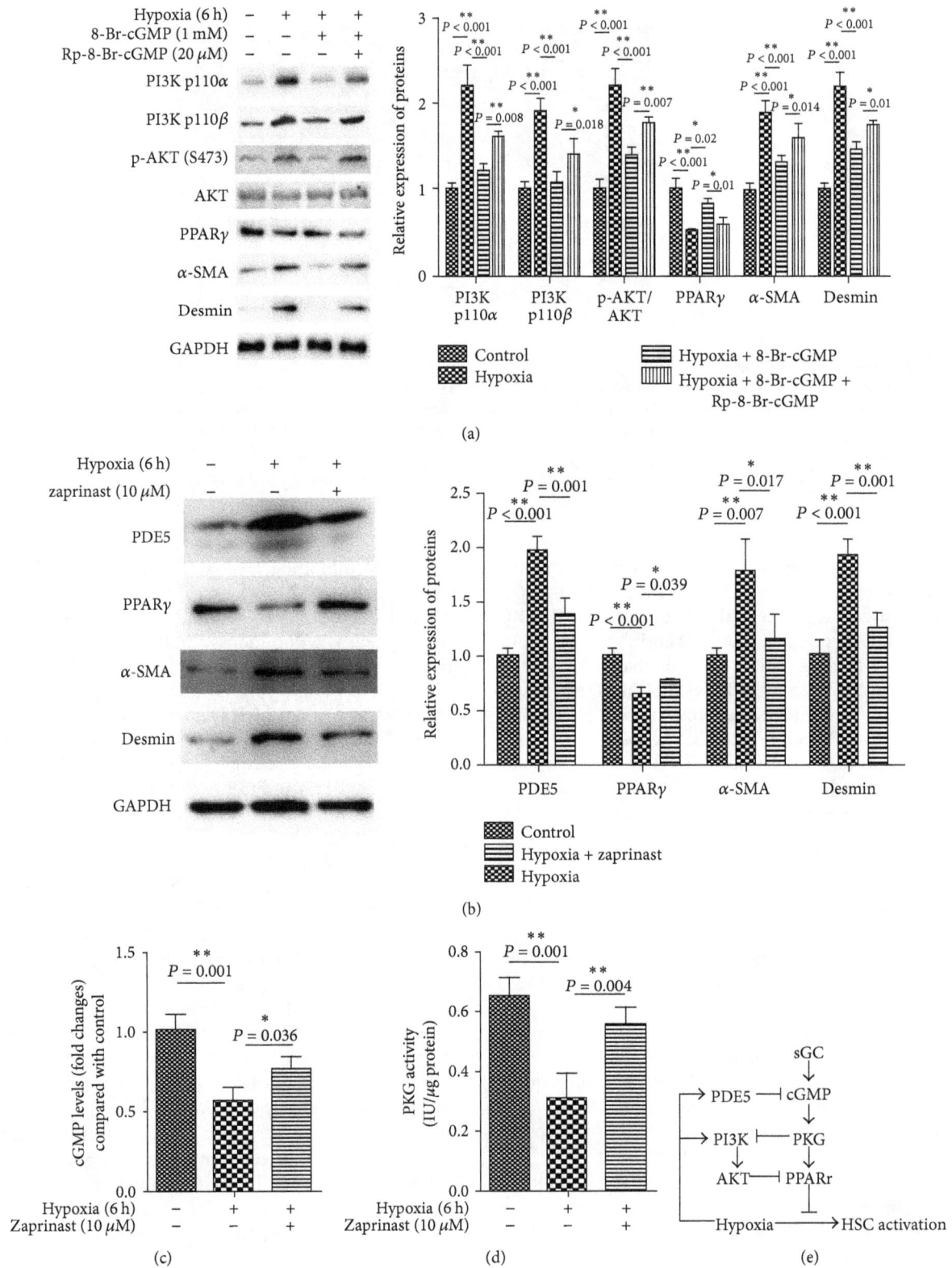

FIGURE 4: sGC/cGMP/PKG and PI3K/AKT signals synergistically act on PPARγ to inhibit hypoxia-induced HSC activation. (a) HSCs were exposed to hypoxia in the presence of cGMP analog, 8-Br-cGMP (1 mM), or agonist, Rp-8-Br-cGMPs (20 μM). PI3K p100 α, p100β, phosphorylated AKT, total AKT, PPARγ, α-SMA, and desmin expression of HSCs in experimental groups were detected by western blotting. HSCs were exposed to hypoxia in the presence of PDE5 agonist, zaprinast (10 μM). (b) PDE5, PPARγ, α-SMA, and desmin expression of HSCs in experimental groups were measured by western blotting. (c)-(d) cGMP and PKG activity were tested, respectively. (e) Possible signal pathway involved in this study. Hypoxia induces HSCs activation. However, PPARγ inhibits this effect, which is triggered by sGC/cGMP/PKG signaling. Hypoxia promotes PI3K/AKT signaling and PDE5, which inhibit cGMP and PPARγ, respectively. Finally, sGC/cGMP/PKG and PI3K/AKT signals synergistically act on PPARγ to inhibit hypoxia-induced HSC activation. For each assay, $n = 3$. $^{*}P < 0.05$, $^{**}P < 0.01$.

study found that PPARγ inhibits endothelial cell migration by inhibiting PI3K/AKT signaling [29]. Our present study showed that PI3K/AKT signaling blocked the inhibitory effect of PPARγ on hypoxia-induced HSCs activation. Next, cGMP analogs and antagonists were used, and results showed that sGC/cGMP/PKG directly inhibited PI3K/AKT signaling and increased PPARγ expression, eventually affecting the hypoxia-induced HSCs activation. In contrast, inhibition of PDE5 and resisting cGMP hydrolysis restore cGMP and PKG activity, followed by increased PPARγ expression and repressed HSCs activation.

Given the synergistic effect of hypoxia and insulin resistance in liver fibrosis, previous study showed that hypoxia leads to a decrease in PPARγ expression, followed by inhibition of IR transcription, resulting in the blockade of IGF-1 and subsequent signals. When TZD restores PPARγ, IR activation occurs directly and indirectly, initiating IGF-1/PI3K signaling [30]. However, we found that the hypoxic environment induced the PI3K signals, leading to the decrease of PPARγ expression, indicating that there is a complex negative feedback mechanism in this process.

Based on these data, we speculated that sGC/cGMP function on PKG activation to activate PPARγ, which attenuates hypoxia-induced HSCs activation and hepatic fibrogenesis. On the other side, hypoxia directly and indirectly inhibits the expression of PPAR, by inducing PI3K/AKT signaling or activating PDE5 to cGMP hydrolysis, which is ultimately beneficial to hypoxia-induced HSCs activation. Our findings may provide new insights into the mechanisms leading to fibrosis in the liver. It would be interesting to establish whether the same signals are operative in tissues in which both hypoxia and PPARγ are present, like in adipose tissue in obesity [31, 32]. New studies are necessary to address the potential of new therapeutic tools able to counteract the pathophysiological processes leading to fibrosis.

Disclosure

Qinghui Zhang and Shihao Xiang are co-first authors.

Conflicts of Interest

The authors have declared that no conflicts of interest exist.

Authors' Contributions

Qinghui Zhang conceived and designed the experiments; Qinghui Zhang and Shihao Xiang performed the experiments; Qingqian Liu and Tao Gu analyzed the data; Yongliang Yao contributed the reagents and materials; Qinghui Zhang wrote the manuscript; Xiaojie Lu supported supplement tests in the revised manuscript and provided a language service for the revised manuscript. Qinghui Zhang and Shihao Xiang are equal contributors.

Acknowledgments

This work was supported by Shanghai Science and Technology Commission Foundation (Grant no. 16411972700).

References

[1] E. Seki and R. F. Schwabe, "Hepatic inflammation and fibrosis: functional links and key pathways," *Hepatology*, vol. 61, no. 3, pp. 1066–1079, 2015.

[2] R. Bataller and D. A. Brenner, "Liver fibrosis," *The Journal of Clinical Investigation*, vol. 115, no. 2, pp. 209–218, 2005.

[3] E. Seki and D. A. Brenner, "Recent advancement of molecular mechanisms of liver fibrosis," *Journal of Hepato-Biliary-Pancreatic Sciences*, vol. 22, no. 7, pp. 512–518, 2015.

[4] R. Weiskirchen and F. Tacke, "Liver fibrosis: from pathogenesis to novel therapies," *Digestive Diseases*, vol. 34, no. 4, pp. 410–422, 2016.

[5] Y. Jia, C. Wu, J. Kim, B. Kim, and S.-J. Lee, "Astaxanthin reduces hepatic lipid accumulations in high-fat-fed C57BL/6J mice via activation of peroxisome proliferator-activated receptor (PPAR) alpha and inhibition of PPAR gamma and Akt," *The Journal of Nutritional Biochemistry*, vol. 28, pp. 9–18, 2016.

[6] D. Zhou, J. Wang, L. N. He et al., "Prolyl oligopeptidase attenuates hepatic stellate cell activation through induction of Smad7 and PPAR-γ," *Experimental and Therapeutic Medicine*, vol. 13, no. 2, pp. 780–786, 2017.

[7] H. Jin, N. Lian, F. Zhang et al., "Activation of PPARγ/P53 signaling is required for curcumin to induce hepatic stellate cell senescence," *Cell Death & Disease*, vol. 7, no. 4, pp. e2189–e2189, 2016.

[8] Z. Liu, W. Dou, Y. Zheng et al., "Curcumin upregulates Nrf2 nuclear translocation and protects rat hepatic stellate cells against oxidative stress," *Molecular Medicine Reports*, vol. 13, no. 2, pp. 1717–1724, 2016.

[9] Y. Wang, Y. Huang, F. Guan et al., "Hypoxia-inducible factor-1alpha and mapk co-regulate activation of hepatic stellate cells upon hypoxia stimulation," *PLoS ONE*, vol. 8, no. 9, Article ID e74051, 2013.

[10] B. L. Copple, S. Bai, L. D. Burgoon, and J.-O. Moon, "Hypoxia-inducible factor-1α regulates the expression of genes in hypoxic hepatic stellate cells important for collagen deposition and angiogenesis," *Liver International*, vol. 31, no. 2, pp. 230–244, 2011.

[11] L. Zhan, C. Huang, X.-M. Meng et al., "Hypoxia-inducible factor-1alpha in hepatic fibrosis: a promising therapeutic target," *Biochimie*, vol. 108, pp. 1–7, 2015.

[12] M. Wang, G. Li, Z. Yang et al., "Uncoupling protein 2 downregulation by hypoxia through repression of peroxisome proliferator-activated receptor γ promotes chemoresistance of non-small cell lung cancer," *Oncotarget*, vol. 8, no. 5, pp. 8083–8094, 2017.

[13] Q. Jiang, W. Lu, K. Yang et al., "Sodium tanshinone IIA sulfonate inhibits hypoxia-induced enhancement of SOCE in pulmonary arterial smooth muscle cells via the PKG-PPAR-γ signaling axis," *American Journal of Physiology-Cell Physiology*, vol. 311, no. 1, pp. C136–C149, 2016.

[14] E. M. Brunt, "Nonalcoholic steatohepatitis: definition and pathology," *Seminars in Liver Disease*, vol. 21, no. 3, pp. 3–16, 2001.

[15] D. E. Kleiner, E. M. Brunt, M. van Natta et al., "Design and validation of a histological scoring system for nonalcoholic fatty liver disease," *Hepatology*, vol. 41, no. 6, pp. 1313–1321, 2005.

[16] Q.-H. Zhang, Y.-L. Yao, X.-Y. Wu et al., "Anti-miR-362-3p inhibits migration and invasion of human gastric cancer cells by its target CD82," *Digestive Diseases and Sciences*, vol. 60, no. 7, pp. 1967–1976, 2015.

[17] W. Guan, F. Cheng, H. Wu et al., "GATA binding protein 3 is correlated with leptin regulation of PPARγ1 in hepatic stellate

cells," *Journal of Cellular and Molecular Medicine*, vol. 21, no. 3, pp. 568–578, 2017.

[18] F. Zhang, D. Kong, Y. Lu, and S. Zheng, "Peroxisome proliferator-activated receptor-γ as a therapeutic target for hepatic fibrosis: from bench to bedside," *Cellular and Molecular Life Sciences*, vol. 70, no. 2, pp. 259–276, 2013.

[19] Y. Ogawa, M. Yoneda, W. Tomeno, K. Imajo, and Y. Shinohara, "Peroxisome proliferator-activated receptor gamma exacerbates concanavalin a-induced liver injury via suppressing the translocation of NF-κB into the nucleus," *PPAR Research*, vol. 2012, Article ID 940384, 5 pages, 2012.

[20] S. C. Iyer, A. Kannan, A. Gopal, N. Devaraj, and D. Halagowder, "Receptor channel TRPC6 orchestrate the activation of human hepatic stellate cell under hypoxia condition," *Experimental Cell Research*, vol. 336, no. 1, pp. 66–75, 2015.

[21] Y. Jin, Y. Bai, H. Ni et al., "Activation of autophagy through calcium-dependent AMPK/mTOR and PKCθ pathway causes activation of rat hepatic stellate cells under hypoxic stress," *FEBS Letters*, vol. 590, no. 5, pp. 672–682, 2016.

[22] S. Mueller, "Does pressure cause liver cirrhosis? the sinusoidal pressure hypothesis," *World Journal of Gastroenterology*, vol. 22, no. 48, pp. 10482–10501, 2016.

[23] E. Ceni, T. Mello, S. Polvani et al., "The orphan nuclear receptor COUP-TFII coordinates hypoxia-independent proangiogenic responses in hepatic stellate cells," *Journal of Hepatology*, vol. 66, no. 4, pp. 754–764, 2017.

[24] L. M. Risør, M. Fenger, N. V. Olsen, and S. Møller, "Hepatic erythropoietin response in cirrhosis," *Scandinavian Journal of Clinical & Laboratory Investigation*, vol. 76, no. 3, pp. 234–239, 2016.

[25] Y. Lecarpentier, V. Claes, A. Vallée, and J. Hébert, "Thermodynamics in cancers: opposing interactions between PPAR gamma and the canonical WNT/beta-catenin pathway," *linical and Translational Medicine*, vol. 6, no. 1, p. 14, 2017.

[26] Z. Ge, P. Zhang, T. Hong et al., "Erythropoietin alleviates hepatic insulin resistance via PPARγ-dependent AKT activation," *Scientific Reports*, vol. 5, Article ID 17878, 2015.

[27] A. M. E. Zuckermann, R. M. La Ragione, D. L. Baines, and R. S. B. Williams, "Valproic acid protects against haemorrhagic shock-induced signalling changes via PPARγ activation in an in vitro model," *British Journal of Pharmacology*, vol. 172, no. 22, pp. 5306–5317, 2015.

[28] H. Kilter, M. Werner, C. Roggia et al., "The PPAR-γ agonist rosiglitazone facilitates Akt rephosphorylation and inhibits apoptosis in cardiomyocytes during hypoxia/reoxygenation," *Diabetes, Obesity and Metabolism*, vol. 11, no. 11, pp. 1060–1067, 2009.

[29] S. Goetze, F. Eilers, A. Bungenstock et al., "PPAR activators inhibit endothelial cell migration by targeting Akt," *Biochemical and Biophysical Research Communications*, vol. 293, no. 5, pp. 1431–1437, 2002.

[30] V. Costa, D. Foti, F. Paonessa et al., "The insulin receptor: A new anticancer target for peroxisome proliferator-activated receptor-γ (PPARγ) and thiazolidinedione- PPARγ agonists," *Endocrine-Related Cancer*, vol. 15, no. 1, pp. 325–335, 2008.

[31] P. Trayhurn, "Hypoxia and adipose tissue function and dysfunction in obesity," *Physiological Reviews*, vol. 93, no. 1, pp. 1–21, 2013.

[32] M. Greco, E. Chiefari, T. Montalcini et al., "Early effects of a hypocaloric, mediterranean diet on laboratory parameters in obese individuals," *Mediators of Inflammation*, vol. 2014, Article ID 750860, 8 pages, 2014.

Peroxisome Proliferator-Activated Receptor γ Induces the Expression of Tissue Factor Pathway Inhibitor-1 (TFPI-1) in Human Macrophages

G. Chinetti-Gbaguidi,[1,2] **C. Copin,**[1] **B. Derudas,**[1] **N. Marx,**[3] **J. Eechkoute,**[1] **and B. Staels**[1]

[1]*Inserm, CHU Lille, Institut Pasteur de Lille, U1011, EGID, Université de Lille, 59000 Lille, France*
[2]*CHU, CNRS, Inserm, IRCAN, Université Côte d'Azur, Nice, France*
[3]*Department of Cardiology, RWTH Aachen University, Aachen, Germany*

Correspondence should be addressed to B. Staels; bart.staels@pasteur-lille.fr

Academic Editor: Nanping Wang

Tissue factor (TF) is the initiator of the blood coagulation cascade after interaction with the activated factor VII (FVIIa). Moreover, the TF/FVIIa complex also activates intracellular signalling pathways leading to the production of inflammatory cytokines. The TF/FVIIa complex is inhibited by the tissue factor pathway inhibitor-1 (TFPI-1). Peroxisome proliferator-activated receptor gamma (PPARγ) is a transcription factor that, together with PPARα and PPARβ/δ, controls macrophage functions. However, whether PPARγ activation modulates the expression of TFPI-1 in human macrophages is not known. Here we report that PPARγ activation increases the expression of TFPI-1 in human macrophages in vitro as well as in vivo in circulating peripheral blood mononuclear cells. The induction of TFPI-1 expression by PPARγ ligands, an effect shared by the activation of PPARα and PPARβ/δ, occurs also in proinflammatory M1 and in anti-inflammatory M2 polarized macrophages. As a functional consequence, treatment with PPARγ ligands significantly reduces the inflammatory response induced by FVIIa, as measured by variations in the IL-8, MMP-2, and MCP-1 expression. These data identify a novel role for PPARγ in the control of TF the pathway.

1. Introduction

Macrophages are heterogeneous cells displaying a spectrum of functional phenotypes ranging from M1 proinflammatory to M2 anti-inflammatory, depending on their microenvironment [1]. Macrophages play crucial roles in the pathogenesis of atherosclerosis. Indeed, within the atherosclerotic plaque, macrophages control the inflammatory response, lipid handling (cholesterol accumulation, trafficking, and efflux) and efferocytosis [2–4]. Moreover, macrophages are also involved in atherosclerotic plaque thrombogenicity by their ability to produce both tissue factor (TF) and its natural inhibitor TFPI-1 [5, 6].

TF is a transmembrane glycoprotein member of the cytokine receptor superfamily acting as the key factor in the initiation of the blood coagulation cascade [7]. TF is expressed by endothelial cells and monocytes/macrophages

after stimulation with oxidized low-density lipoproteins, lipopolysaccharide (LPS), or tumor necrosis factor (TNF)α [8]. Inappropriate expression of TF within the vasculature upon atherosclerotic plaque rupture leads to interaction with circulating FVIIa resulting in the formation of the TF/FVIIa complex that initiates the extrinsic coagulation pathway through a cascade of enzymatic reactions driving the conversion of FX to FXa and the production of thrombin, ultimately leading to thrombosis [9].

Beside its functions in haemostasis, the TF/FVIIa complex also plays a major role in cell migration, metastasis, and angiogenesis, probably through intracellular signalling events [10, 11]. Indeed, the TF/FVIIa complex leads to the generation of proinflammatory cytokines, such as IL-6 and IL-8 [12, 13]. The TF/FVIIa-mediated extrinsic coagulation pathway is inhibited by the tissue factor pathway inhibitor-1 (TFPI-1), a Kunitz-type inhibitor which prevents generation of FXa [8].

TABLE 1: Sequences of primers used.

Gene	Forward	Reverse
TFPI-1	AGA TGG TCC GAA TGG TTT CC	ATC CTC TGT CTG CTG GAG TGA G
IL-8	CCA CCC CAA ATT TAT CAA AGA A	CAG ACA GAG CTC TCT TCC ATC A
MCP-1	TCA TAG CAG CCA CCT TCA TTC C	GGA CAC TTG CTG CTG GTG ATT C
MMP-2	TAT TTG ATG GCA TCG CTC AG	GCC TCG TAT ACC GCA TCA AT
TF	ATG TGA AGC AGA CGT ACT TGG CAC G	ATT GTT GGC TGT CCG AGG TTT GTC
Cyclophilin	GCA TAC GGG TCC TGG CAT CTT GTC C	ATG GTG ATC TTC TTG CTG GTC TTG C

TFPI-1 is mainly synthesized by vascular endothelium and macrophages and is also present in plasma as free form or associated with lipoproteins or platelets [8]. The imbalance between TF and TFPI-1 ratio will thus impact both the TF/FVIIa-mediated coagulation and inflammation.

The peroxisome proliferator-activated receptor gamma (PPARγ), together with PPARα and PPARβ/δ, belongs to a family of transcription factors expressed in macrophages where they control the inflammatory response, cholesterol metabolism, and phagocytosis [14, 15]. PPARs also regulate macrophage thrombogenicity; indeed, PPARα ligands reduce LPS-induced expression of TF [16, 17] whereas the role of PPARγ in the control of TF expression is less clear; in some reports PPARγ is described as having no effect [17] while others showed PPARγ to decrease TF expression [18]. However, no data are available regarding the regulation of TFPI-1 expression by PPARγ in human macrophages.

2. Materials and Methods

2.1. Cell Culture. Monocytes were isolated by density gradient centrifugation from healthy volunteers and differentiated into macrophages by 7 days of culture in RPMI1640 medium (Invitrogen, France) supplemented with gentamicin (40 μg/mL), L-glutamine (2 mM) (Sigma-Aldrich, France), and 10% human serum (Abcys, France) [19]. M2 macrophages were obtained by differentiating monocytes in the presence of human IL-4 (15 ng/mL, Promocell, Germany), while M1 macrophages were obtained by activating differentiated macrophages with LPS (100 ng/mL, 4 h) [20]. Where indicated, synthetic ligands for PPARγ (GW1929, 600 nM or rosiglitazone, 100 nM), for PPARα (GW647, 600 nM), and for PPARβ/δ (GW1516, 100 nM) were added for 24 h to differentiated macrophages. Some experiments were performed on differentiated macrophages which were activated for 24 h with GW1929 (600 nM), washed, and subsequently treated in the absence or in the presence of activated FVII (FVIIa, 10 nM, Cryoprep) for further 24 h.

2.2. RNA Extraction and Analysis. Total cellular RNA was extracted using Trizol (Life Technologies, France). RNA was reverse transcribed and cDNAs were quantified by Q-PCR on a MX3000 apparatus (Stratagene) using specific primers (Table 1). mRNA levels were normalized to those of cyclophilin. The relative expression of each gene was calculated by the ΔΔCt method, where ΔCt is the value obtained by subtracting the Ct (cycle threshold) value of cyclophilin from the Ct value of the target gene. The amount of target relative to the cyclophilin mRNA was expressed as $2^{-(\Delta\Delta Ct)}$.

2.3. In Vivo Study. Forty nondiabetic patients after coronary stent implantation were treated with pioglitazone (30 mg daily for 8 weeks) (Supplemental Table 1 available online at http://dx.doi.org/10.1155/2016/2756781) [21]. RNA was extracted from peripheral blood mononuclear cells (PBMC) using the Paxgene Blood RNA system at both the beginning of the study and at eight-week follow-up.

2.4. Protein Extraction and Western Blot Analysis. After washing in cold PBS, cells were harvested in cold lysis buffer (RIPA). Cell homogenates were collected by centrifugation and protein concentrations determined using the BCA assay (Pierce Interchim). Protein lysate (20 μg) was resolved by 10% SDS-PAGE, transferred to nitrocellulose membranes (Amersham), and then revealed with rabbit monoclonal antibody against TFPI-1 (Abcam) or goat polyclonal antibody against β-actin (Santa Cruz Biotechnology). After incubation with a secondary peroxidase-conjugated antibody (Santa Cruz Biotechnology), immunoreactive bands were revealed by chemiluminescence ECL detection kit (Amersham) and band intensity was quantified using the Quantity One software.

2.5. Measurement of TFPI-1 and MCP-1 Secretion by ELISA. Amounts of TFPI-1 protein were measured in culture media of macrophages treated for 24 h with GW1929 (600 nM) in the absence or in the presence of unfractionated heparin (1 U/mL, Sanofi Aventis, added 1 h before medium collection) [22], using the human TFPI Quantikine ELISA kit (R&D systems). MCP-1 secretion was measured by ELISA (Peprotech, France) according to the manufacturer's instructions.

2.6. Measurement of TFPI-1 Specific Activity. TFPI-1 specific activity was measured using the Actichrome TFPI activity assay (American Diagnostica) following the manufacturer's instructions in culture medium of cells treated or not for 24 h with GW1929 (600 nM).

2.7. Short-Interfering (si)RNA Transfection and Adenoviral Infection. Differentiated RM macrophages were transfected with siRNA specific for human PPARγ and nonsilencing control scrambled siRNA (Ambion), using the transfection reagent DharmaFECT4 (Dharmacon). After 16 h, cells were incubated with GW1929 (600 nM) or vehicle (DMSO) and

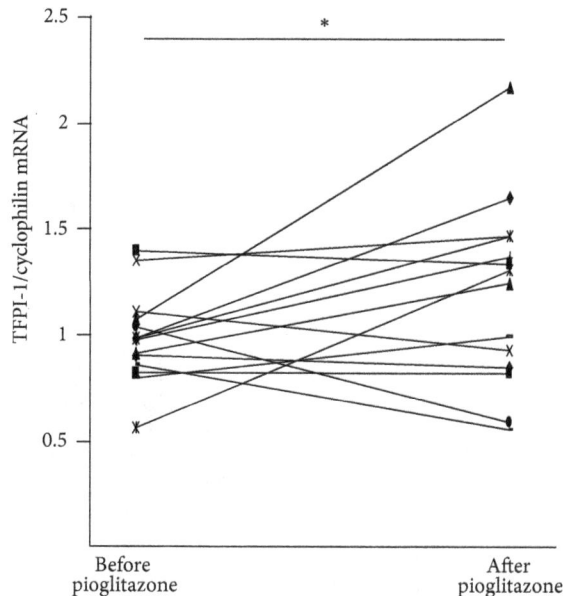

FIGURE 1: PPARγ activation induces TFPI-1 expression in human blood mononuclear cells in vivo. RNA was extracted from PBMC isolated from 14 patients before and after 2 months of pioglitazone treatment (30 mg/day). TFPI-1 mRNA levels were measured by Q-PCR and normalized to cyclophilin mRNA. Statistically significant differences are indicated (t-test; $^{*}p < 0.05$).

harvested 24 h later. For adenoviral infection, macrophages were infected with recombinant adenovirus coding for GFP (Green Fluorescent Protein, Ad-GFP) or for PPARγ (Ad-PPARγ) as described [23, 24]. After 16 h of infection, cells were incubated for further 24 h in the absence or in the presence of rosiglitazone (Rosi, 100 nM).

2.8. ChIP-seq Data Processing and Analysis.
Chromatin immunoprecipitation followed by high-throughput sequencing (ChIP-seq) was performed to monitor H3K9ac levels in M2 macrophages using an antibody against H3K9ac (Millipore (17-658)) [25]. ChIP-seq data were mapped to Hg18 and signals were normalized to the total number of tags before visualization using the Integrated Genome Browser (IGB) [26]. PPARγ ChIP-seq data from human primary adipocytes were obtained from [27] and PPARγ response elements (PPRE) were searched using Dragon PPAR Response Element (PPRE) Spotter v.2.0 (http://www.cbrc.kaust.edu.sa/ppre/).

2.9. Statistical Analysis.
Statistical differences between groups were analyzed by Student's t-test and considered significant when $p < 0.05$.

3. Results

3.1. PPARγ Activation Increases the Expression and Secretion of TFPI-1 in Primary Human Macrophages.
To investigate whether PPARγ activation regulates TFPI-1 expression, peripheral blood mononuclear cells (PBMC), a cell population including circulating monocytes, were isolated from patients before and after pioglitazone administration.

Interestingly, pioglitazone treatment significantly increased the expression of TFPI-1 mRNA in PBMC (Figure 1).

Moreover, activation of human primary differentiated macrophages with the synthetic PPARγ ligands GW1929 and rosiglitazone (Rosi) resulted in the induction of TFPI-1 gene expression in a time and dose-dependent manner (Figures 2(a) and 2(b)). This regulation also occurred at the protein level in macrophages treated for 24 h or 48 h with GW1929 (600 nM) (Figure 2(c)). Induction of TFPI-1 gene expression was also observed upon PPARβ/δ and PPARα activation by GW1516 and GW647 ligands, respectively (Supplemental Figure 1). Moreover, culture media TFPI-1 concentration was increased by PPARγ activation with GW1929 both in the absence as well as in the presence of heparin, a factor known to enhance TFPI-1 release [22] (Figure 2(d)). However, TFPI-1 specific activity was not modified by PPARγ activation in human macrophages (Supplemental Figure 2). Taken together these data indicate that PPARγ activation in human macrophages increases expression and release of TFPI-1 without modifying its activity.

3.2. PPARγ Activation Induces TFPI-1 Gene Expression Both in M1 and M2 Human Macrophages.
Since macrophages can present different functional phenotypes related to the microenvironment [1], the effects of PPARγ activation by GW1929 were studied in nonpolarized macrophages (RM) as well as in M1 proinflammatory and in M2 anti-inflammatory macrophages. The basal expression level of TFPI-1 was significantly higher in M2 macrophages compared to both RM and M1 macrophages (Figure 3). Moreover, PPARγ activation significantly induced TFPI-1 gene and protein expression in all the three different macrophage subtypes (Figure 3).

3.3. PPARγ Ligands Regulate the TFPI-1 Expression in a PPARγ-Dependent Manner.
In support of a direct regulation of TFPI-1 gene expression by PPARγ, we found that active regulatory regions encompassing or localized near the promoter of this gene, identified through enrichment for histone H3 lysine 9 acetylation (H3K9ac) in M2 macrophages, comprise putative PPARγ-response elements (PPRE) and recruit PPARγ in human adipocytes, a cell-type where it is highly expressed (Figure 4(a)). In order to confirm that TFPI-1 regulation induced by GW1929 treatment is due to PPARγ, experiments were performed in macrophages after modulation of PPARγ expression levels. The induction of TFPI-1 gene expression by GW1929 treatment was significantly reduced in the presence of the PPARγ siRNA (Figure 4(b)). Complementary gain of function experiments using an adenovirus coding for PPARγ (Ad-PPARγ) showed that the induction of TFPI-1 gene expression by the PPARγ ligand rosiglitazone was significantly enhanced in Ad-PPARγ-infected macrophages, compared to Ad-GFP infected cells used as control (Figure 4(c)). These results indicate that both GW1929 and rosiglitazone activate TFPI-1 expression in a PPARγ-dependent manner.

3.4. PPARγ Activation Blocks the FVIIa-Induced Inflammatory Response in Human Macrophages.
To determine the

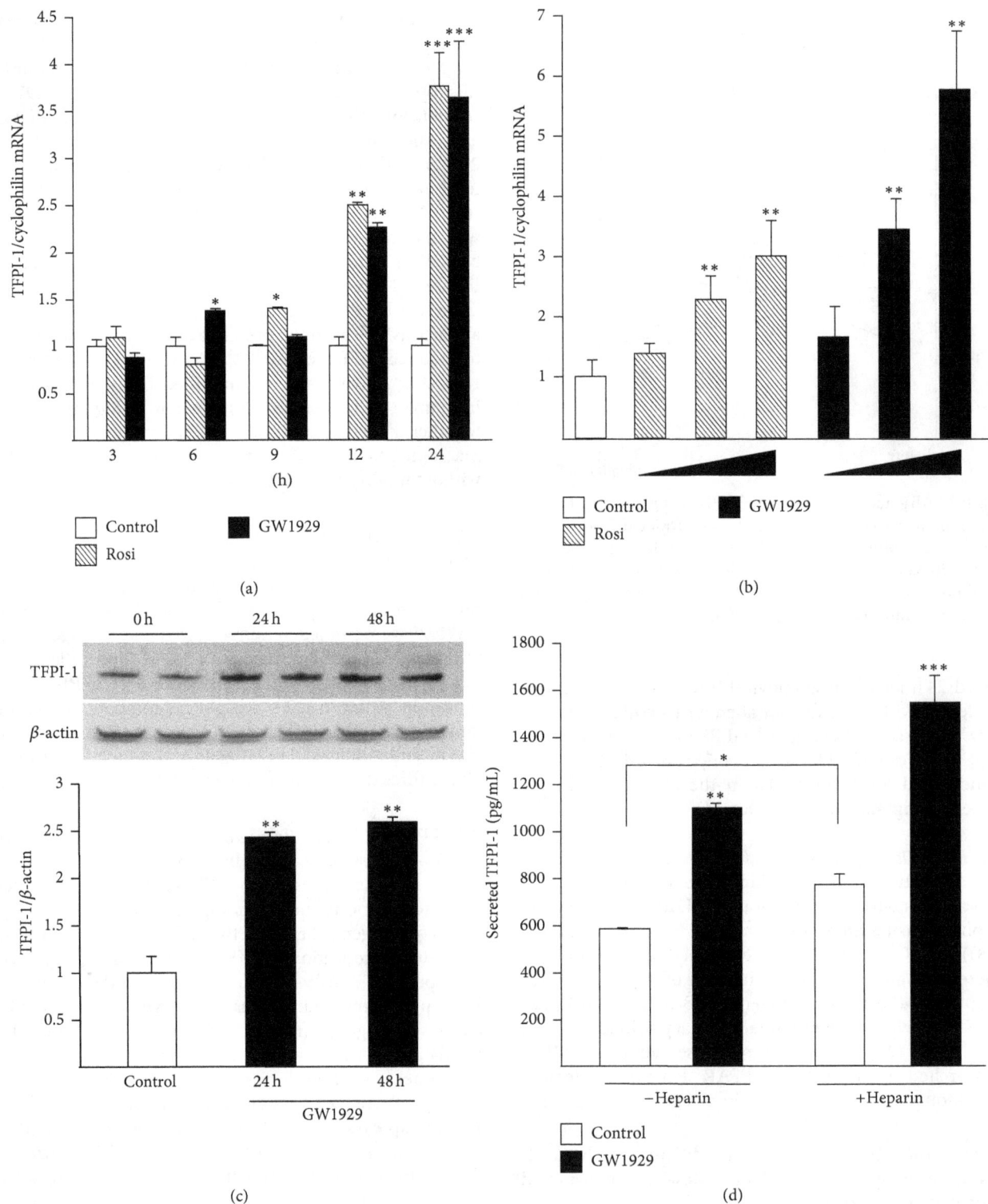

FIGURE 2: Expression of TFPI-1 is enhanced by PPARγ activation in primary human macrophages. Differentiated macrophages were treated in the absence or in the presence of GW1929 (600 nM) and rosiglitazone (Rosi, 100 nM) for 3 h, 6 h, 9 h, 12 h, or 24 h (a) or with increasing concentrations of Rosi (50 nM, 100 nM, and 1 μM) or GW1929 (300 nM, 600 nM, and 3 μM) for 24 h (b). Total RNA was extracted and TFPI-1 mRNA levels were measured by Q-PCR and normalized to those of cyclophilin. (c) Differentiated macrophages were treated with GW1929 (600 nM) for 24 h and 48 h and TFPI-1 protein expression analyzed by western blot. TFPI-1 bands intensity was measured and normalized to those of β-actin. (d) Differentiated macrophages were treated with GW1929 (600 nM) in the absence or in the presence of heparin (1 U/mL), as described above. Culture media were collected and TFPI-1 protein release measured by ELISA. Results are expressed as the mean value ± SD of triplicate determinations, representative of three independent experiments. Statistically significant differences are indicated ($^{*}p < 0.05$, $^{**}p < 0.01$, and $^{***}p < 0.001$).

(a)

(b)

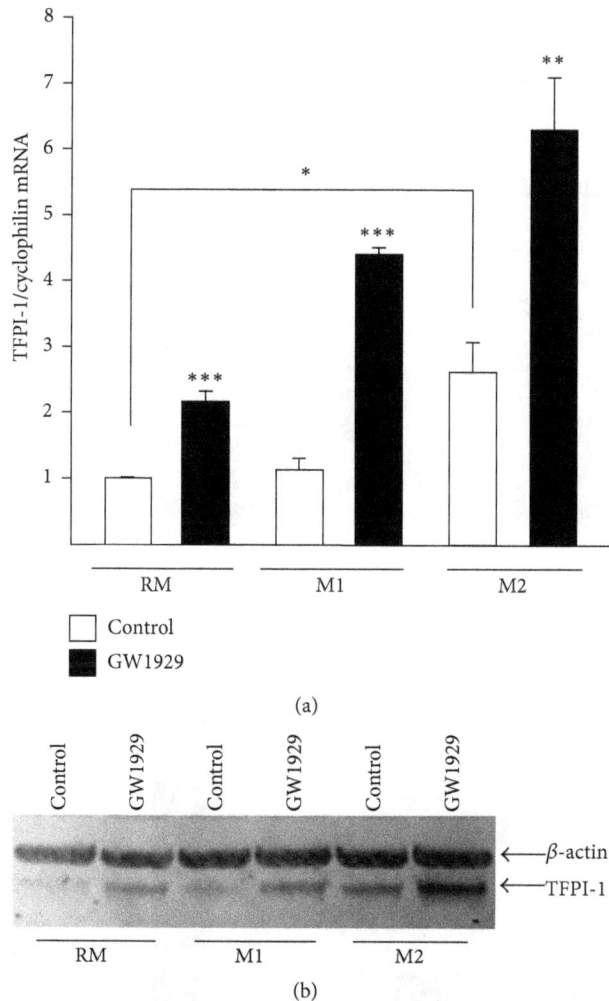

FIGURE 3: PPARγ activation induces the expression of TFPI-1 in human primary macrophages irrespectively of their phenotype. Primary human monocytes were differentiated into resting unpolarized (RM) or M2 macrophages in the absence or in the presence of IL-4 (15 ng/mL) for 7 days, respectively, and then treated for 24 h with GW1929 (600 nM). M1 macrophages were obtained by activation of RM macrophages with LPS (100 ng/mL) for 4 h in the absence or in the presence of GW1929 treatment (24 h, 600 nM). (a) TFPI-1 mRNA levels were measured by Q-PCR, normalized to cyclophilin mRNA, and expressed relative to the levels in untreated cells set as 1. Results are representative of those obtained from 3 independent macrophage preparations. Each bar is the mean value ± SD of triplicate determinations. Statistically significant differences between treatment and control groups are indicated ($^*p < 0.05$; $^{**}p < 0.01$; $^{***}p < 0.001$). (b) TFPI-1 protein expression was analyzed by western blot. β-actin was used as loading control.

potential biological significance of TFPI-1 induction by PPARγ and given that TF/FVIIa complex can enhance an inflammatory response [12, 13], experiments were performed in macrophages treated with GW1929 (600 nM for 24 h), washed, and subsequently stimulated with FVIIa (10 nM). FVIIa induced gene expression of MMP-2, IL-8, and MCP-1, all proinflammatory molecules (Figures 5(a)–5(c)). Interestingly, treatment of macrophages with GW1929 (600 nM) significantly blocked the proinflammatory response mediated

by FVIIa (Figures 5(a)–5(c)). Incubation with GW1929 also decreased FVIIa-induced secretion of MCP-1 (Figure 5(d)). These data suggest that PPARγ activation can counteract the proinflammatory effects mediated by TF/FVIIa complex, the TF being expressed by macrophages [5], likely through the increase of TFPI-1 expression. Indeed, the TF/TFPI-1 ratio was significantly reduced in the presence of the PPARγ agonist (Supplemental Figure 3), thus corroborating that PPARγ activation blocks the FVIIa-induced inflammatory response.

4. Discussion

TF and FVIIa are key components of the coagulation cascade that lead to the formation of a fibrin clot. Within atherosclerotic plaque rupture this provokes thrombus generation, one of the major causes of acute ischemic syndromes such as myocardial infarction [28]. The TF/FVIIa complex has however other potential roles, since it is involved in mediating cell migration and metastasis as well as angiogenesis [29]. Indeed, TF/FVIIa can induce the production of proinflammatory cytokines and factors in keratinocytes and cancer cells [12, 13, 30].

The TF/FVIIa actions are blocked by the natural inhibitor TFPI-1. The presence of TFPI-1 has been reported in human atherosclerotic lesions where it is expressed by macrophages in areas physically close to those expressing TF and FVIIa [6]. This suggests that also in vivo, in human atherosclerotic plaques, TFPI-1 controls the TF-driven coagulation pathways as well as the thrombogenicity and can prevent complications associated with plaque rupture. However, an imbalanced expression of TF and TFPI-1 in atherosclerotic plaques can have consequences in thrombus formation as well as in inflammation.

Whether the transcription factor PPARγ controls the TF-activated pathway as well as the expression of its inhibitor TFPI-1 has been matter of different studies leading to contradictory results. While it has been first reported that PPARγ activation has no effect on LPS-induced TF expression in macrophages [17], other studies have shown an inhibitory effect by a mechanism involving the interference with the AP1 signalling pathway [18]. Moreover, expression of TFPI-1 has been shown to be induced by rosiglitazone in smooth muscle cells but not in THP1 macrophage cell line [18]. Here, we provide evidence that PPARγ activation enhances gene, protein expression and release of TFPI-1 in human primary differentiated macrophages without affecting its specific activity. Interestingly, PPARγ activation by pioglitazone treatment significantly increased the expression of TFPI-1 in PBMC, a heterogeneous cell population including circulating monocytes, thus suggesting that PPARγ activation regulates TFPI-1 expression also in vivo. We have also demonstrated that the induction of TFPI-1 expression upon PPARγ activation occurs in M1 proinflammatory as well as in M2 anti-inflammatory polarized macrophages. Moreover, we found that the basal expression level of TFPI-1 is higher in M2 macrophages compared to both unpolarized and M1 macrophages, suggesting that these M2 macrophages can play a major role in the control of plaque thrombosis and fibrin deposition. These data, generated in monocyte-derived

(a)

(b)

(c)

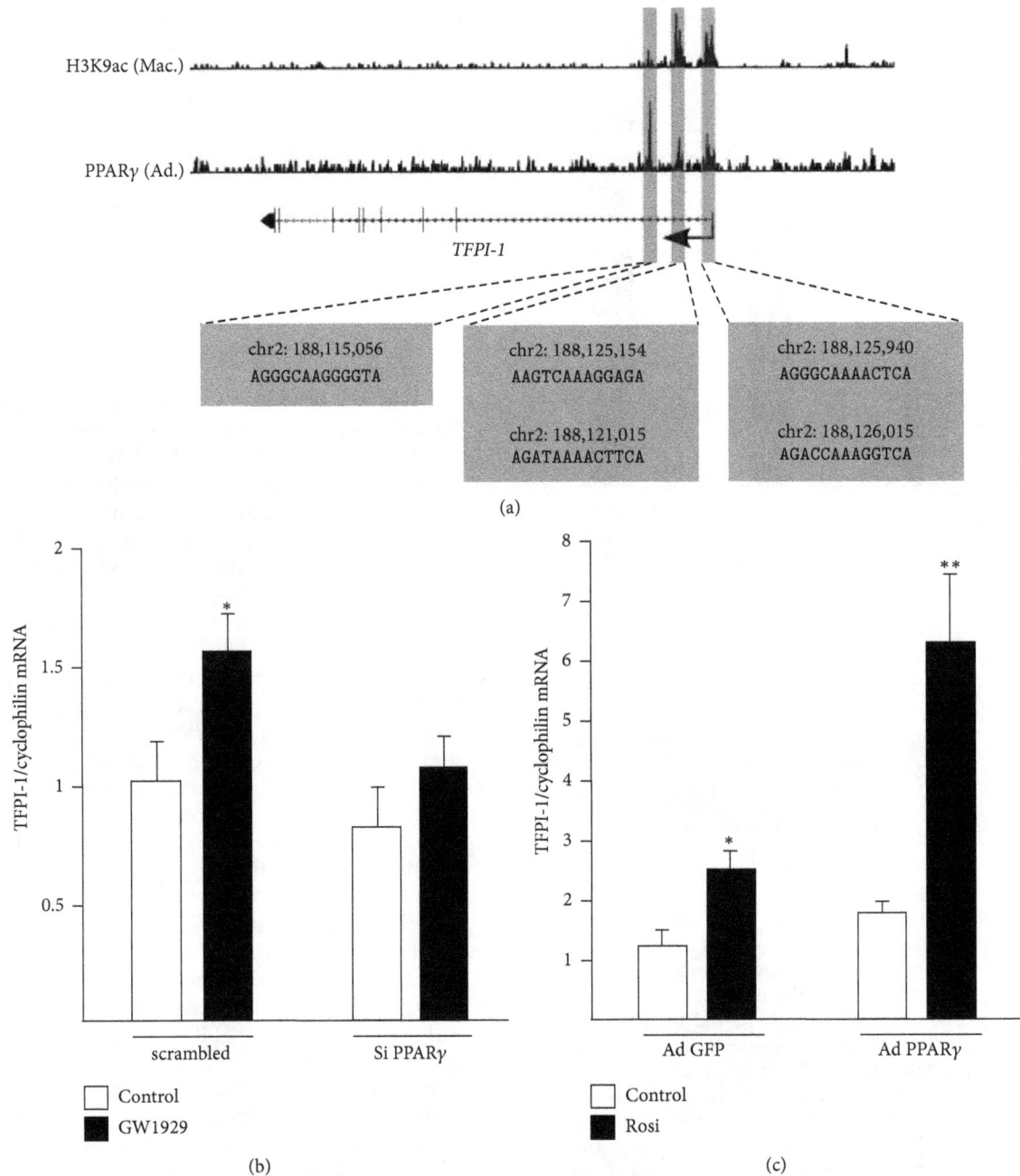

FIGURE 4: PPARγ activation induces the expression of TFPI-1 in a PPARγ-dependent manner. (a) H3K9ac ChIP-seq signals from M2 macrophages (Mac.) as well as PPARγ ChIP-seq signal from human primary adipocytes (Ad.) are shown for the *TFPI-1* gene. Active regulatory regions are highlighted in gray and chromosomal localization (Hg18) and sequences of PPRE identified within these regions are provided at the bottom. (b) Differentiated macrophages were transfected with scrambled or human PPARγ siRNA and subsequently treated with GW1929 (600 nM) or DMSO (Control) during 24 h or were infected with a GFP (Ad-GFP) or a PPARγ (Ad-PPARγ) adenovirus and then treated with rosiglitazone (24 h, 100 nM) (c). Statistically significant differences between treatment and control groups are indicated ($^*p < 0.05$; $^{**}p < 0.01$).

macrophages isolated from healthy volunteers, are in agreement with those obtained in M2 macrophages isolated from atherosclerotic patients, in which the gene expression level of TFPI-1 is also higher in M2 compared to M1 macrophages [31]. The higher expression of TFPI-1 in M2 macrophages could thus contribute to their suggested beneficial role in plaque stabilization [32, 33].

Interestingly, in a rat carotid balloon injury model in vivo, characterized by increased neointima formation and TF overexpression, rosiglitazone injection enhances the expression of TFPI-1 protein in the injured arteries [18]. However, in vitro treatment of human atheroma specimens with rosiglitazone results in a reduced expression of TFPI-1 protein while treatment with pioglitazone led to an increased TFPI-1 expression

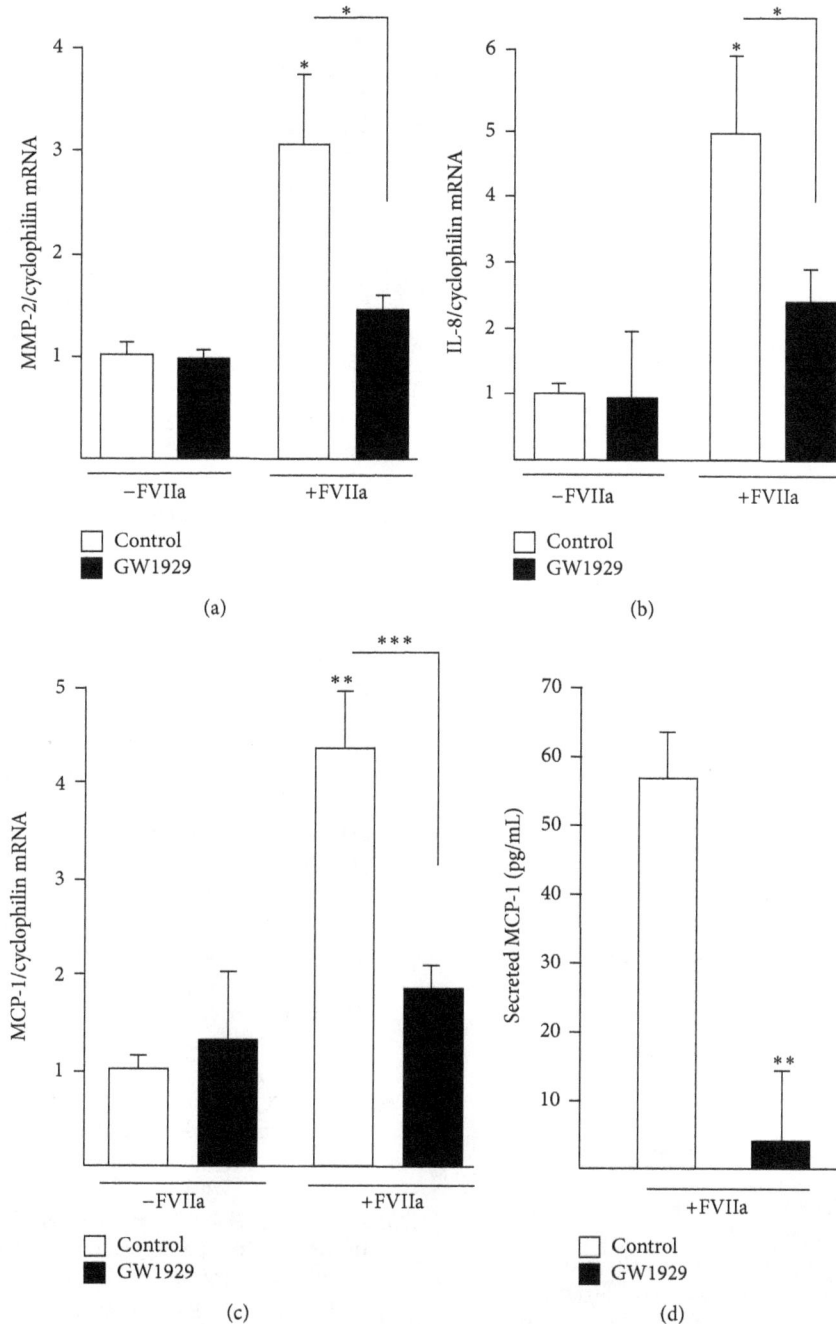

FIGURE 5: PPARγ activation blocks the FVIIa-induced inflammatory response in primary human macrophages. Differentiated macrophages were treated with GW1929 (24 h, 600 nM), washed and then incubated in the absence or in the presence of FVIIa (10 nM) for further 24 h. Total RNA was extracted and MMP-2 (a), IL-8 (b), and MCP-1 (c) mRNA levels were measured by Q-PCR and normalized to those of cyclophilin. Secretion of MCP-1 was measured by ELISA in culture medium (d). Results are expressed as the mean value ± SD of triplicate determinations, representative of three independent experiments. Statistically significant differences are indicated ($^*p < 0.05$, $^{**}p < 0.01$, and $^{***}p < 0.001$).

[34]. These discrepant effects can be explained by the action of PPARγ on other cellular components of the atherosclerotic plaques. Moreover, they have been obtained using high concentrations of the ligands (10 μM for rosiglitazone and 5 μM for pioglitazone, resp.) [34] that cannot guarantee a specificity of action over PPARγ activation [35]. The induction of TFPI-1 expression upon stimulation by rosiglitazone and the

GW1929 compounds in human macrophages are dependent on PPARγ as demonstrated here in PPARγ silencing or overexpression experiments.

Finally, we report that PPARγ preactivation of macrophages significantly reduced the FVIIa-driven inflammatory response, an effect that can be mediated at least partially by the induced TFPI-1 production by PPARγ.

5. Conclusions

In conclusion, we describe a novel function for PPARγ in human macrophages in the control of the TF pathway via the induction of TFPI-1 expression, a regulation that can impact both the thrombogenicity of the atherosclerotic plaques as well as the inflammatory status induced by the TF/FVIIa complex.

Disclosure

B. Staels is a member of the Institut Universitaire de France.

Competing Interests

The authors declare that they have no competing interests.

Acknowledgments

This work was supported by grants from the Fondation de France, the Fondation pour la Recherche Médicale (DPC2011122981), the Agence Nationale de la Recherche (AlMHA project), and the "European Genomic Institute for Diabetes" (EGID, ANR-10-LABX-46).

References

[1] G. Chinetti-Gbaguidi, S. Colin, and B. Staels, "Macrophage subsets in atherosclerosis," *Nature Reviews Cardiology*, vol. 12, no. 1, pp. 10–17, 2015.

[2] P. Libby, "Inflammation in atherosclerosis," *Nature*, vol. 420, no. 6917, pp. 868–874, 2002.

[3] P. Libby, M. Aikawa, and U. Schönbeck, "Cholesterol and atherosclerosis," *Biochimica et Biophysica Acta—Molecular and Cell Biology of Lipids*, vol. 1529, no. 1–3, pp. 299–309, 2000.

[4] I. Tabas, "Macrophage death and defective inflammation resolution in atherosclerosis," *Nature Reviews Immunology*, vol. 10, no. 1, pp. 36–46, 2010.

[5] L. Petit, P. Lesnik, C. Dachet, M. Moreau, and M. J. Chapman, "Tissue factor pathway inhibitor is expressed by human monocyte—derived macrophages: relationship to tissue factor induction by cholesterol and oxidized LDL," *Arteriosclerosis, Thrombosis, and Vascular Biology*, vol. 19, no. 2, pp. 309–315, 1999.

[6] J. Crawley, F. Lupu, A. D. Westmuckett, N. J. Severs, V. V. Kakkar, and C. Lupu, "Expression, localization, and activity of tissue factor pathway inhibitor in normal and atherosclerotic human vessels," *Arteriosclerosis, Thrombosis, and Vascular Biology*, vol. 20, no. 5, pp. 1362–1373, 2000.

[7] K. G. Mann, C. Van't Veer, K. Cawthern, and S. Butenas, "The role of the tissue factor pathway in initiation of coagulation," *Blood Coagulation and Fibrinolysis*, vol. 9, no. 1, pp. S3–S7, 1998.

[8] B. A. Lwaleed and P. S. Bass, "Tissue factor pathway inhibitor: structure, biology and involvement in disease," *Journal of Pathology*, vol. 208, no. 3, pp. 327–339, 2006.

[9] N. Mackman, "Role of tissue factor in hemostasis, thrombosis, and vascular development," *Arteriosclerosis, Thrombosis, and Vascular Biology*, vol. 24, no. 6, pp. 1015–1022, 2004.

[10] B. M. Mueller, R. A. Reisfeld, T. S. Edgington, and W. Ruf, "Expression of tissue factor by melanoma cells promotes efficient hematogenous metastasis," *Proceedings of the National Academy of Sciences of the United States of America*, vol. 89, no. 24, pp. 11832–11836, 1992.

[11] J. L. Yu, L. May, V. Lhotak et al., "Oncogenic events regulate tissue factor expression in colorectal cancer cells: implications for tumor progression and angiogenesis," *Blood*, vol. 105, no. 4, pp. 1734–1741, 2005.

[12] X. Wang, E. Gjernes, and H. Prydz, "Factor VIIa induces tissue factor-dependent up-regulation of interleukin-8 in a human keratinocyte line," *Journal of Biological Chemistry*, vol. 277, no. 26, pp. 23620–23626, 2002.

[13] G. Demetz, I. Seitz, A. Stein et al., "Tissue Factor-Factor VIIa complex induces cytokine expression in coronary artery smooth muscle cells," *Atherosclerosis*, vol. 212, no. 2, pp. 466–471, 2010.

[14] E. Rigamonti, G. Chinetti-Gbaguidi, and B. Staels, "Regulation of macrophage functions by PPAR-α, PPAR-γ, and LXRs in mice and men," *Arteriosclerosis, Thrombosis, and Vascular Biology*, vol. 28, no. 6, pp. 1050–1059, 2008.

[15] G. Chinetti-Gbaguidi, M. Baron, M. A. Bouhlel et al., "Human atherosclerotic plaque alternative macrophages display low cholesterol handling but high phagocytosis because of distinct activities of the PPARγ and LXRα pathways," *Circulation Research*, vol. 108, no. 8, pp. 985–995, 2011.

[16] B. P. Neve, D. Corseaux, G. Chinetti et al., "PPARα agonists inhibit tissue factor expression in human monocytes and macrophages," *Circulation*, vol. 103, no. 2, pp. 207–212, 2001.

[17] N. Marx, N. Mackman, U. Schönbeck et al., "PPARα activators inhibit tissue factor expression and activity in human monocytes," *Circulation*, vol. 103, no. 2, pp. 213–219, 2001.

[18] J.-B. Park, B.-K. Kim, Y.-W. Kwon et al., "Peroxisome proliferator-activated receptor-gamma agonists suppress tissue factor overexpression in rat balloon injury model with paclitaxel infusion," *PLoS ONE*, vol. 6, no. 11, Article ID e28327, 2011.

[19] G. Chinetti, S. Lestavel, V. Bocher et al., "PPAR-α and PPAR-γ activators induce cholesterol removal from human macrophage foam cells through stimulation of the ABCA1 pathway," *Nature Medicine*, vol. 7, no. 1, pp. 53–58, 2001.

[20] G. Bories, S. Colin, J. Vanhoutte et al., "Liver X receptor activation stimulates iron export in human alternative macrophages," *Circulation Research*, vol. 113, no. 11, pp. 1196–1205, 2013.

[21] A. J. Balmforth, P. J. Grant, E. M. Scott et al., "Inter-subject differences in constitutive expression levels of the clock gene in man," *Diabetes and Vascular Disease Research*, vol. 4, no. 1, pp. 39–43, 2007.

[22] C. Lupu, E. Poulsen, S. Roquefeuil, A. D. Westmuckett, V. V. Kakkar, and F. Lupu, "Cellular effects of heparin on the production and release of tissue factor pathway inhibitor in human endothelial cells in culture," *Arteriosclerosis, Thrombosis, and Vascular Biology*, vol. 19, no. 9, pp. 2251–2262, 1999.

[23] E. Rigamonti, C. Fontaine, B. Lefebvre et al., "Induction of CXCR2 receptor by peroxisome proliferator-activated receptor γ in human macrophages," *Arteriosclerosis, Thrombosis, and Vascular Biology*, vol. 28, no. 5, pp. 932–939, 2008.

[24] G. Chinetti-Gbaguidi, C. Copin, B. Derudas et al., "The coronary artery disease-associated gene C6ORF105 is expressed in human macrophages under the transcriptional control of PPARγ," *FEBS Letters*, vol. 589, no. 4, pp. 461–466, 2015.

[25] G. Chinetti-Gbaguidi, M. A. Bouhlel, C. Copin et al., "Peroxisome proliferator-activated receptor-γ activation induces 11β-hydroxysteroid dehydrogenase type 1 activity in human alternative macrophages," *Arteriosclerosis, Thrombosis, and Vascular Biology*, vol. 32, no. 3, pp. 677–685, 2012.

[26] J. W. Nicol, G. A. Helt, S. G. Blanchard Jr., A. Raja, and A. E. Loraine, "The Integrated Genome Browser: free software for distribution and exploration of genome-scale datasets," *Bioinformatics*, vol. 25, no. 20, pp. 2730–2731, 2009.

[27] T. S. Mikkelsen, Z. Xu, X. Zhang et al., "Comparative epigenomic analysis of murine and human adipogenesis," *Cell*, vol. 143, no. 1, pp. 156–169, 2010.

[28] M. J. Davies and A. Thomas, "Thrombosis and acute coronary-artery lesions in sudden cardiac ischemic death," *The New England Journal of Medicine*, vol. 310, no. 18, pp. 1137–1140, 1984.

[29] H. H. Versteeg, M. P. Peppelenbosch, and C. A. Spek, "The pleiotropic effects of tissue factor: a possible role for factor VIIa-induced intracellular signalling?" *Thrombosis and Haemostasis*, vol. 86, no. 6, pp. 1353–1359, 2001.

[30] Z.-C. Jia, Y.-L. Wan, J.-Q. Tang et al., "Tissue factor/activated factor VIIa induces matrix metalloproteinase-7 expression through activation of c-Fos via ERK1/2 and p38 MAPK signaling pathways in human colon cancer cell," *International Journal of Colorectal Disease*, vol. 27, no. 4, pp. 437–445, 2012.

[31] C. Roma-Lavisse, M. Tagzirt, C. Zawadzki et al., "M1 and M2 macrophage proteolytic and angiogenic profile analysis in atherosclerotic patients reveals a distinctive profile in type 2 diabetes," *Diabetes and Vascular Disease Research*, vol. 12, no. 4, pp. 279–289, 2015.

[32] K. Y. Cho, H. Miyoshi, S. Kuroda et al., "The phenotype of infiltrating macrophages influences arteriosclerotic plaque vulnerability in the carotid artery," *Journal of Stroke and Cerebrovascular Diseases*, vol. 22, no. 7, pp. 910–918, 2013.

[33] S. Shaikh, J. Brittenden, R. Lahiri, P. A. J. Brown, F. Thies, and H. M. Wilson, "Macrophage subtypes in symptomatic carotid artery and femoral artery plaques," *European Journal of Vascular and Endovascular Surgery*, vol. 44, no. 5, pp. 491–497, 2012.

[34] J. Golledge, S. Mangan, and P. Clancy, "Effects of peroxisome proliferator-activated receptor ligands in modulating tissue factor and tissue factor pathway inhibitor in acutely symptomatic carotid atheromas," *Stroke*, vol. 38, no. 5, pp. 1501–1508, 2007.

[35] G. Orasanu, O. Ziouzenkova, P. R. Devchand et al., "The peroxisome proliferator-activated receptor-γ agonist pioglitazone represses inflammation in a peroxisome proliferator-activated receptor-α-dependent manner in vitro and in vivo in mice," *Journal of the American College of Cardiology*, vol. 52, no. 10, pp. 869–881, 2008.

Permissions

The contributors of this book come from diverse backgrounds, making this book a truly international effort. This book will bring forth new frontiers with its revolutionizing research information and detailed analysis of the nascent developments around the world.

We would like to thank all the contributing authors for lending their expertise to make the book truly unique. They have played a crucial role in the development of this book. Without their invaluable contributions this book wouldn't have been possible. They have made vital efforts to compile up to date information on the varied aspects of this subject to make this book a valuable addition to the collection of many professionals and students.

This book was conceptualized with the vision of imparting up-to-date information and advanced data in this field. To ensure the same, a matchless editorial board was set up. Every individual on the board went through rigorous rounds of assessment to prove their worth. After which they invested a large part of their time researching and compiling the most relevant data for our readers.

The editorial board has been involved in producing this book since its inception. They have spent rigorous hours researching and exploring the diverse topics which have resulted in the successful publishing of this book. They have passed on their knowledge of decades through this book. To expedite this challenging task, the publisher supported the team at every step. A small team of assistant editors was also appointed to further simplify the editing procedure and attain best results for the readers.

Apart from the editorial board, the designing team has also invested a significant amount of their time in understanding the subject and creating the most relevant covers. They scrutinized every image to scout for the most suitable representation of the subject and create an appropriate cover for the book.

The publishing team has been an ardent support to the editorial, designing and production team. Their endless efforts to recruit the best for this project, has resulted in the accomplishment of this book. They are a veteran in the field of academics and their pool of knowledge is as vast as their experience in printing. Their expertise and guidance has proved useful at every step. Their uncompromising quality standards have made this book an exceptional effort. Their encouragement from time to time has been an inspiration for everyone.

The publisher and the editorial board hope that this book will prove to be a valuable piece of knowledge for researchers, students, practitioners and scholars across the globe.

List of Contributors

Arong Zhou, Baodong Zheng, Shaoxiao Zeng and Shaoling Lin
College of Food Science, Fujian Agriculture and Forestry University, Fuzhou, Fujian 350002, China

Jiamiao Hu
College of Food Science, Fujian Agriculture and Forestry University, Fuzhou, Fujian 350002, China
Warwick Medical School, University of Warwick, Coventry, West Midlands, UK

Peter C. K. Cheung
School of Life Sciences,The Chinese University of Hong Kong, Shatin, New Territories, Hong Kong

Tommaso Mello and Maria Materozzi
Clinical Gastroenterology Unit, Department of Biomedical Clinical and Experimental Sciences "Mario Serio", University of Florence, Viale Pieraccini 6, 50129 Florence, Italy

Andrea Galli
Clinical Gastroenterology Unit, Department of Biomedical Clinical and Experimental Sciences "Mario Serio", University of Florence, Viale Pieraccini 6, 50129 Florence, Italy
Careggi University Hospital, Florence, Italy

Robert I. Glazer
Department of Oncology, Georgetown UniversityMedical Center and the Lombardi Comprehensive Cancer Center, 3970 Reservoir Rd, NW,Washington, DC 20007, USA

Yong-Jik Lee and Yoo-Na Jang
Cardiovascular Center, Korea University, Guro Hospital, 148 Gurodong-ro, Guro-gu, Seoul 08308, Republic of Korea

Yoon-Mi Han, Hyun-Min Kim, Jong-Min Jeong and Hong Seog Seo
Cardiovascular Center, Korea University, Guro Hospital, 148 Gurodong-ro, Guro-gu, Seoul 08308, Republic of Korea
Department of Medical Science, Korea University College of Medicine (BK21 Plus KUMS Graduate Program), Main Building 6F Room 655, 73 Inchon-ro (Anam-dong 5-ga), Seongbuk-gu, Seoul 136-705, Republic of Korea

Min Jeoung Son, Chang Bae Jin and Hyoung Ja Kim
Molecular Recognition Research Center, Materials and Life Science Research Division, Korea Institute of Science and Technology, Hwarangno 14 Gil 5, Seoul 136-791, Republic of Korea

Mini Chandra, Sumitra Miriyala and Manikandan Panchatcharam
Department of Cellular Biology and Anatomy, Louisiana State University Health Sciences Center, Shreveport, USA

Borja Bandera Merchan
Unidad de Gestión Clínica Endocrinología y Nutrición, Instituto de Investigación Biomédica de Málaga (IBIMA),Complejo Hospitalario de Málaga (Virgen de la Victoria), Universidad de Málaga, 29010 Malaga, Spain

Francisco José Tinahones and Manuel Macías-González
Unidad de Gestión Clínica Endocrinología y Nutrición, Instituto de Investigación Biomédica de Málaga (IBIMA), Complejo Hospitalario de Málaga (Virgen de la Victoria), Universidad de Málaga, 29010 Malaga, Spain
CIBER Pathophysiology of Obesity and Nutrition (CB06/03), 28029 Madrid, Spain

Asoka Banno
Department of Medicine, Division of Pulmonary, Allergy and Critical Care Medicine, University of Pittsburgh School of Medicine, Pittsburgh, PA 15213, USA

Sowmya P. Lakshmi, Aravind T. Reddy and Raju C. Reddy
Department of Medicine, Division of Pulmonary, Allergy and Critical Care Medicine, University of Pittsburgh School of Medicine,Pittsburgh, PA 15213, USA
Veterans Affairs Pittsburgh Healthcare System, Pittsburgh, PA 15240, USA

Melody Chiu and Lucien McBeth
Center for Hypertension and Personalized Medicine, Department of Physiology & Pharmacology, University of Toledo College of Medicine, Toledo, OH 43614, USA

Terry D. Hinds
Center for Hypertension and Personalized Medicine, Department of Physiology & Pharmacology, University of Toledo College of Medicine, Toledo, OH 43614, USA
Department of Urology, University of Toledo College of Medicine, Toledo, OH 43614, USA

Puneet Sindhwani
Department of Urology, University of Toledo College of Medicine, Toledo, OH 43614, USA

Yadan Chen, Dasheng Zhu and Xiujuan Fu
Department of Pharmacy, The Second Hospital of Jilin University, Changchun 130041, China

Haiming Ma
Department of Pharmacy, China-Japan Union Hospital of Jilin University, Changchun 130041, China

Guowei Zhao
Department of Pharmacy, Beijing Boai Hospital, China Rehabilitation Research Center, Beijing 100068, China

Lili Wang and Wei Chen
Beijing Institute of Pharmacology and Toxicology, Beijing 100850, China

Wenwen Wang, Kan Chen and Yujing Xia
Department of Gastroenterology, Shanghai Tenth People's Hospital, Tongji University School of Medicine, Shanghai 200072, China

Peiqin Niu
Department of Gastroenterology, Shanghai Tenth People's Hospital, Tongji University School of Medicine, Shanghai 200072, China
Shanghai Tenth People's Hospital Chongming Branch, Tongji University School of Medicine, Shanghai 202157, China

Wenhui Mo
Department of Gastroenterology, Minhang Hospital, Fudan University, Shanghai 201100, China

Fan Wang
Department of Oncology, Shanghai General Hospital, Shanghai Jiaotong University School of Medicine, Shanghai 200080, China

Weiqi Dai
Department of Gastroenterology, Zhongshan Hospital, Fudan University, Shanghai 200032, China
Shanghai Institute of Liver Diseases, Zhongshan Hospital, Fudan University, Shanghai 200032, China

Manoj Govindarajulu, Priyanka D. Pinky, Jenna Bloemer and Nila Ghanei
Department of Drug Discovery and Development, Harrison School of Pharmacy, Auburn University, Auburn, AL, USA

Vishnu Suppiramaniam and Rajesh Amin
Department of Drug Discovery and Development, Harrison School of Pharmacy, Auburn University, Auburn, AL, USA
Center for Neuroscience, Auburn University, Auburn, AL, USA

Chang Jiang, Shuhao Liu and Yuanwu Cao
Department of Orthopaedics, Zhongshan Hospital, Fudan University, Shanghai, China

Hongping Shan
Department of Nephrology, Pudong Medical Center, Fudan University, Shanghai, China

Qiansheng Huang
Key Lab of Urban Environment and Health, Institute of Urban Environment, Chinese Academy of Sciences, Xiamen 361021, China
Center for Excellence in Regional Atmospheric Environment, Institute of Urban Environment, Chinese Academy of Sciences, Xiamen 361021, China

Qionghua Chen
The First Affiliated Hospital of Xiamen University, Xiamen 361003, China

Sarawin Harnchoowong and Poonkiat Suchonwanit
Division of Dermatology, Faculty of Medicine, Ramathibodi Hospital, Mahidol University, Bangkok, Thailand

Qinghui Zhang, Qingqian Liu, Tao Gu and Yongliang Yao
Department of Clinical Laboratory, Kunshan First People's Hospital, Affiliated t o J iangsu University, Kunshan, Jiangsu Province 215300, China

Shihao Xiang
Department of Gastroenterology, Shanghai Tongren Hospital, Shanghai Jiaotong University School of Medicine, Shanghai 200336, China

Xiaojie Lu
Department of Liver Surgery, The First Affiliated Hospital of Nanjing Medical University, Nanjing, China

C. Copin, B. Derudas, J. Eechkoute and B. Staels
Inserm, CHU Lille, Institut Pasteur de Lille, U1011, EGID, Universit´e de Lille, 59000 Lille, France

G. Chinetti-Gbaguidi
Inserm, CHU Lille, Institut Pasteur de Lille, U1011, EGID, Université de Lille, 59000 Lille, France

CHU, CNRS, Inserm, IRCAN, Université Côte d'Azur, Nice, France

N. Marx
Department of Cardiology, RWTH Aachen University, Aachen, Germany

Index

www.ingramcontent.com/pod-product-compliance
Lightning Source LLC
Chambersburg PA
CBHW050453200326
41458CB00014B/5162